SECOND EDITION

Manual for Clinical Trials Nursing

EDITORS
Angela D. Klimaszewski, RN, MSN
Monica Bacon, RN
Heidi E. Deininger, PhD, RN, AOCN®
Bertie A. Ford, RN, MS, AOCN®
Joan G. Westendorp, RN, MSN, OCN®

Oncology Nursing Society
Pittsburgh, Pennsylvania

ONS Publishing Division

Publisher: Leonard Mafrica, MBA, CAE

Director, Commercial Publishing/Technical Publications Editor: Barbara Sigler, RN, MNEd

Production Manager: Lisa M. George, BA

Staff Editor: Amy Nicoletti, BA

Copy Editor: Laura Pinchot, BA

Graphic Designer: Dany Sjoen

Manual for Clinical Trials Nursing (Second Edition)

Library of Congress Control Number: 2008926823

ISBN: 978-1-890504-71-7

Publisher's Note

This book is published by the Oncology Nursing Society (ONS). ONS neither represents nor guarantees that the practices described herein will, if followed, ensure safe and effective patient care. The recommendations contained in this book reflect ONS's judgment regarding the state of general knowledge and practice in the field as of the date of publication. The recommendations may not be appropriate for use in all circumstances. Those who use this book should make their own determinations regarding specific safe and appropriate patient-care practices, taking into account the personnel, equipment, and practices available at the hospital or other facility at which they are located. The editors and publisher cannot be held responsible for any liability incurred as a consequence from the use or application of any of the contents of this book. Figures and tables are used as examples only. They are not meant to be all-inclusive, nor do they represent endorsement of any particular institution by ONS. Mention of specific products and opinions related to those products do not indicate or imply endorsement by ONS. Web sites mentioned are provided for imformation only; the hosts are responsible for their own content and availability.

ONS publications are originally published in English. Publishers wishing to translate ONS publications must contact the ONS Publishing Division about licensing arrangements. ONS publications cannot be translated without obtaining written permission from ONS. (Individual tables and figures that are reprinted or adapted require additional permission from the original source.) Because translations from English may not always be accurate or precise, ONS disclaims any responsibility for inaccuracies in words or meaning that may occur as a result of the translation. Readers relying on precise information should check the original English version.

Printed in the United States of America

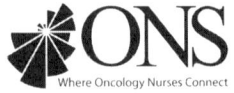

Oncology Nursing Society

Integrity • Innovation • Stewardship • Advocacy • Excellence • Inclusiveness

For Joe, my inspiration and support, and for Michael, my treasure. Always reach for the stars, and do everything with love.

—Angela Klimaszewski

To those patients who have and will participate in clinical trials, to the health professionals who dedicate themselves to clinical trials, with a special thanks to my son, Blair, and my family.

—Bertie Ford

For oncology nurses worldwide—at the bedsides, in the clinics, in the communities and homes; teaching, managing, administrating, researching, and caring—without you, there would be no clinical trials.

—Monica Bacon

To the courageous patients who participated in clinical trials, whom I consider to be heroes. Special thanks to my husband, Wayne, for all of his encouragement and support, and my two wonderful sons, Joseph and Samuel.

—Joan Westendorp

To Peter, Kevin, Madison, Benjamin, and Alexandra—always believe in tomorrow.

— Heidi E. Deininger

Contributors

Editors

Angela D. Klimaszewski, RN, MSN
Nurse Consultant
ADK Communications
Canton, New York
*Chapter 3. Elements of a Protocol; Chapter 14. Informed Consent;
Chapter 19. Psychosocial Considerations*

Monica Bacon, RN
International Intergroup Coordinator
National Cancer Institute of Canada Clinical Trials Group
Queen's University
Kingston, Ontario, Canada
Chapter 56. Canada

Heidi E. Deininger, PhD, RN, AOCN®
President and Founder
ResearchNurse.org
Ann Arbor, Michigan
*Chapter 51. Specialization in Clinical Trials Nursing; Appendix 13.
Internet Resource List*

Bertie A. Ford, RN, MS, AOCN®
Clinical Oncology Specialist
Genentech BioOncology
Westerville, Ohio
Chapter 30. Adherence in Clinical Trials

Joan G. Westendorp, RN, MSN, OCN®
Director, Research/Education
West Michigan Cancer Center
Kalamazoo, Michigan
*Chapter 2. Assurances; Chapter 25. Investigational Agents and Procurement
of Research Study Drugs*

Authors

Susan Anderson, RN, BSN, MFA
Director of the Office of Protocol Review and Monitoring
Yale Cancer Center
New Haven, Connecticut
Chapter 22. Eligibility

Eriko Aotani, RN, MSN, CCRP
Manager, Clinical Trial Coordinating Center
Kitasato University Research Center for Clinical Pharmacology
Tokyo, Japan
Chapter 57. Japan

Carol Anne Bales, RN, MSN, CCRP, AOCN®
CRA Specialist
PPD, Inc.
Wilmington, North Carolina
*Chapter 26. Administration of Protocol Agents; Chapter 50. Interdisciplin-
ary Team Review*

Mechelle Barrick, BSN, RN, OCN®, CCRP
Clinical Research Site Manager
K Force, Inc.
Baltimore, Maryland
*Chapter 10. Educating Staff; Chapter 43. Cancer Trials Support Unit: A
Service of the National Cancer Institute*

Anne E. Belcher, PhD, RN, AOCN®, CNE, FAAN, ANEF
Senior Associate Dean for Academic Affairs
Johns Hopkins University School of Nursing
Baltimore, Maryland
Chapter 18. General Publication and Authorship Policies for Nurses

Deborah T. Berg, RN, BSN
Senior Medical Science Liaison
Genentech
San Francisco, California
Chapter 8. Sponsoring Agencies: Industry

Janelle Bowersox, RN, MSN, OCN®

Program Manager
prIME Oncology
Atlanta, Georgia
Chapter 7. Safety Issues

Michelle A. Brand, RN, OCN®

Gynecology Oncology Nurse Clinician
Marshfield Clinic
Marshfield, Wisconsin
Chapter 27. Symptom Management in Clinical Trials Nursing

Cynthia Brandt, MD, MPH

Associate Professor
Yale University School of Medicine
New Haven, Connecticut
Chapter 44. Clinical Trial Registries

Sheila Breslin, RN, MS

Oncology Research Nurse
Stanford University
Stanford Cancer Center
Stanford, California
Chapter 1. History and Background of Clinical Trials

Mary E. Brimer, RN, MSN, OCN®

Clinical Manager, Cancer Center
Memorial Hermann Hospital
Texas Medical Center
Houston, Texas
Chapter 16. Conflicts of Interest

Sally D. Brown, RN, BSN, MGA, OCN®, CCRP

Coordinator, Research Protocols
Franklin Square Hospital Center
Baltimore, Maryland
Chapter 12. Introduction to Legal and Regulatory Issues

Jane Bryce, RN, MSN, AOCNS®

Research Nurse
Istituto Nazionale dei Tumori Napoli
Naples, Italy
Chapter 58. European Union Directives; Chapter 63. Italy

Fie Budtz, RN

Clinical Trial Nurse
Section of Clinical Research
Department of Oncology
University Hospital of Aarhus
Aarhus, Denmark
Chapter 60. Denmark

Heike Busse, RN

HSK, Dr. Horst Schmidt Klinik
Department of Gynecology and Gynecologic Oncology
Medical Documentation
Wiesbaden, Germany
Chapter 62. Germany

Karen Carty, CCR

Project Manager
CR-UK Clinical Trials Unit
Glasgow, Scotland
Chapter 64. United Kingdom

Marianna Connola, BSN

Research Nurse
Division of Surgical Oncology
Istituto Nazionale dei Tumori Napoli
Naples, Italy
Chapter 63. Italy

Denise Dearing, RN, BSN, OCN®

Home Health Nurse
Four Star Home Health, Inc.
Georgetown, Texas
*Chapter 17. Legislative Issues; Chapter 26. Administration of Protocol
Agents; Chapter 50. Interdisciplinary Team Review*

Kelly J. Dustin, RN, MS, CCRC

Human Subjects Protection Scientist
AMDEX Corporation, in Support of the Office of Research
Protections
Fort Detrick, Maryland
Chapter 46. Standard Operating Procedures

Belinda Egan, RN, PG Cert

Clinical Trials Coordinator
Oncology Service
Christchurch Hospital
Christchurch, New Zealand
Chapter 55. New Zealand

Gabriele Elser, RN

AGO Ovarian Cancer Study Group
Wiesbaden Office
Wiesbaden, Germany
Chapter 58. European Union Directives; Chapter 62. Germany

Rose Ermete, RN, BSN, CCRP, OCN®

Research Nurse Coordinator
St. Mary Mercy Hospital
Livonia, Michigan
Chapter 52. Mentorship

Marzia Falanga, BSN

Research Nurse
Division of Medical Oncology
"S.G. Moscati" Hospital
Avellino, Italy
Chapter 63. Italy

Kelly Filchner, RN, MSN, OCN®, CCRC

Manager, Oncology Integrated Clinical Trials
St. Luke's Hospital and Health Network
Bethlehem, Pennsylvania
Chapter 13. Institutional Review Boards/Protocol Modifications

Marjorie J. Good, RN, BSN, MPH, OCN®

Administrative Director
Wichita Community Clinical Oncology Program
Wichita, Kansas
Chapter 24. Cancer Prevention and Control Study Considerations

Clement K. Gwede, PhD, MPH, RN

Assistant Professor
H. Lee Moffitt Cancer Center, University of South Florida
Tampa, Florida
Chapter 3. Workload Determination and Resource Allocation

Mary Ellen Haisfield-Wolfe, RN, MS, OCN®

Doctoral Candidate
University of Maryland School of Nursing
Baltimore, Maryland
Chapter 36. Off-Treatment Protocol Considerations; Chapter 38. Off-Treatment Documentation

Tasha D. Hall, RN, MS, OCN®, CCRP

Medical Science Liaison
Millennium Pharmaceuticals
Cambridge, Massachusetts
Chapter 37. Long-Term Follow-Up; Chapter 40. Documentation and Forms Submissions

Andrea Harkin, BA, CCR

Head of Trial Co-ordination
CR-UK Clinical Trials Unit
Glasgow, Scotland
Chapter 64. United Kingdom

Patricia Hentschel, RN, MS, ANP, CCRC

Director, Cancer Clinical Trials Office
State University of New York at Stony Brook
Stony Brook, New York
Chapter 15. Compassionate Use of Investigational Drugs

Patricia B. Herman, MSN, RN, AOCN®

Oncology Clinical Nurse Specialist
St. Luke's Hospital and Health Network
Bethlehem, Pennsylvania
Chapter 13. Institutional Review Boards/Protocol Modifications

Carol S. Hill, BSN, RN, OCN®

Clinical Research Nurse
Emory University Winship Cancer Institute
Atlanta, Georgia
Chapter 31. Quality-of-Life Studies; Chapter 32. Pharmacokinetics, Pharmacodynamics, and Pharmacogenomics

Jacquelin Holland, RNC, WHNP-BC

Consultant, Diversity Enhancement Program
The Arthur G. James Cancer Hospital and Richard J. Solove Research Institute at The Ohio State University Medical Center
Columbus, Ohio
Chapter 21. Recruitment and Promotion Strategies for Clinical Trials

June Iesue-Queen, RN, MSN

Clinical Safety Data Manager
Prologue Research International
Columbus, Ohio
Chapter 48. Community-Based Clinical Trials

Catherine Johnson, RN, BSc

Clinical Research Nurse
Calvary Mater Newcastle
Newcastle, New South Wales, Australia
Chapter 54. Australia

David Leos, RN, MBA, OCN®, CCRA

Oncology Clinical Educator
Memorial Hermann Southwest Hospital
Houston, Texas
Chapter 20. Public and Patient Education

Vilma Lopez, RN, MSN, OCN®

Senior Research Nurse
University of Texas M.D. Anderson Cancer Center
Houston, Texas
Chapter 23. Designing a Computerized Tool to Verify Eligibility

Lydia T. Madsen, RN, MSN, OCN®, AOCNS®

Advanced Practice Nurse
University of Texas M.D. Anderson Cancer Center
Houston, Texas
Chapter 6. Statistical Considerations in Protocol Development

Sue Markus, RN, BSN, MS, OCN®, CCRC

Clinical Trials Research Nurse
Johns Hopkins University
Baltimore, Maryland
Chapter 12. Introduction to Legal and Regulatory Issues

Patricia McLaughlin, RN, MSN, AOCN®

Clinical Assistant Professor of Nursing
Drexel University College of Nursing and Health Professions
Philadelphia, Pennsylvania
Chapter 33. Genetic Testing and Storage of Genetic Material; Chapter 34. Pharmacoeconomic Studies

Brigitte Nadeau-Vaissade, BA, Sp.

Formerly International Project Manager
ARCAGY-GINECO Group
Hôpital Hotel-Dieu
Paris, France
Chapter 61. France

Elizabeth Ness, RN, MS

Director, Staff Development
Center for Cancer Research, National Cancer Institute
Bethesda, Maryland
Chapter 53. Professional Continuing Education

Ellen A. Patricia, MS

Assistant Director, HRPP
Quality Improvement Office of Responsible Research Practices
The Ohio State University Medical Center
Columbus, Ohio
Chapter 47. Audit Preparation

Janice Phillips, PhD, RN, FAAN

Nurse Researcher
University of Chicago Medical Center
Chicago, Illinois
Chapter 18. General Publication and Authorship Policies for Nurses

Betty Razvillas, RN, OCN®, CCRC

Research Nurse III
University of Texas Health Science Center at San Antonio
San Antonio, Texas
Chapter 39. The Need for Data Management Tools

Dianne M. Reeves, MSN

Associate Director for Biomedical Data Standards
National Cancer Institute
Center for Biomedical Informatics and Information Technology
Bethesda, Maryland
Chapter 42. Clinical Data Management Systems

Joanne C. Ryan, RN, MS
Director, Medical Oncology
Global Medical Oncology
Pfizer, Inc.
New York, New York
Chapter 41. Electronic Data Capture in Clinical Trials

Yuko Saito, MS, RN, CCRP
Chief Clinical Research Coordinator
Clinical Trial Coordination Office
Shizuoka Cancer Center
Shizuoka, Japan
Chapter 57. Japan

Carolyn R. Schmidt, RN, MSHA, OCN®
Administrative Director, Breast Care Program
St. John Health System
Grosse Pointe Woods, Michigan
Chapter 11. Clinical Research/Interdisciplinary Team

Geri L. Schmotzer, RN, MPH, MSN
Betty Irene Moore Fellow
University of California at San Francisco School of Nursing
San Francisco, California
Chapter 29. Patient and Family Education

Kathleen Scott, BSc(Hons), PhD
Head of Site Management
NHMRC Clinical Trials Centre
The University of Sydney
Camperdown, New South Wales, Australia
Chapter 54. Australia

Belinda Thorwirth, RN
HSK, Dr. Horst Schmidt Klinik
Department of Gynecology and Gynecologic Oncology
Medical Documentation
Wiesbaden, Germany
Chapter 62. Germany

Joyce M. Tokarsky, RN, MSN
Clinical Nurse Specialist
University of Pittsburgh Medical Center Cancer Centers
Pittsburgh, Pennsylvania
Chapter 35. Nursing Companion Studies

Nina M. Trocky, MSN, RN, CCRA
Clinical Instructor and Co-Program Director
Clinical Research Management Specialty
University of Maryland School of Nursing
Baltimore, Maryland
Chapter 44. Clinical Trial Registries

Johanna Ulmer, PhD, SC
Study Coordinator
Medical University Innsbruck
Department of Obstetrics and Gynecology
Innsbruck, Austria
Chapter 59. Austria

Marjorie van der Pas, MS
Product Manager
IMPAC Medical Systems, Inc.
Sunnyvale, California
Chapter 9. Potential Accrual Base

Bénédicte Votan, MSc, Post Graduate
Director of ARCAGY-GINECO Group
Hôpital Hotel-Dieu
Paris, France
Chapter 61. France

Dianna Wellen-Traylor, MSN
Clinical Content Specialist
IMPAC Medical Systems, Inc.
Sunnyvale, California
Chapter 10. Potential Accrual Base

Kelly M. Willenberg, MBA, BSN, RN
Director Research Institute
Spartanburg Regional Healthcare System
Spartanburg, South Carolina
Chapter 5. Budget

Shanita Williams-Brown, PhD, MPH, APRN-BC
Assistant Professor
Morehouse School of Medicine, National Center for Primary Care
Atlanta, Georgia
Chapter 18. General Publication and Authorship Policies for Nurses

Patricia C. Woltz, RN, MS, CCRP
Nurse Consultant
Office of Surveillance and Biometrics
Center for Devices and Radiological Health
U.S. Food and Drug Administration
Rockville, Maryland
Chapter 45. Good Clinical Practice

Siu-Fun Wong, PharmD
Associate Professor of Pharmacy Practice
Western University of Health Sciences
Pomona, California
Chapter 25. Investigational Agents and Procurement of Research Study Drugs; Chapter 49. Drug Accountability

Laura S. Wood, RN, MSN, OCN®
Renal Cancer Research Coordinator
Cleveland Clinic Cancer Center
Cleveland, Ohio
Chapter 28. Adverse Events

Field Reviewers

Pamela H. Carney, RN, OCN®

Research Clinical Specialist
Cancer Information Program
Vanderbilt-Ingram Cancer Center
Nashville, Tennessee

Barbara J. Lane, RN, OCN®, CCRC, CCRP

Clinical Research Coordinator
Florida Hospital Cancer Institute
Tavares, Florida

Patricia McLaughlin, RN, MSN, AOCN®, CCRP

Clinical Assistant Professor of Nursing
Drexel University College of Nursing and Health Professions
Philadelphia, Pennsylvania

Mary Beth Riley, RN, MSN, AOCN®

Clinical Nurse Specialist
Clinical Research Office
Robert H. Lurie Comprehensive Cancer Center of Northwestern
    University
Chicago, Illinois

Colleen M. Ross, RN, OCN®

Oncology Research Nurse
Methodist Hospital Cancer Center
Omaha, Nebraska

Phyllis A. Rudokas, RN, BS, OCN®, CCRP

Oncology Research Nurse
Dayton Clinical Oncology Program Atrium Medical Center
Franklin, Ohio

Camille A. Servodidio, RN, MPH, CRNO, OCN®, CCRP

Nurse/Program Coordinator
Cancer Clinical Research Office
Cancer Program
Hartford Hospital
Hartford, Connecticut

Contents

Preface

The last decade brought with it important advances in the realm of clinical trials, including closer adherence to the requirements set forth in the Declaration of Helsinki, the emergence of the nurse navigator role, an increasing number of clinical trial registries worldwide, and the creation of "metadata" for intergroup and international trials. The medical community is rallying for more disclosure or "transparency" regarding ethics and informed consent, and an increasing number of journals require that all published trials describe informed consent and ethics committee approval (International Committee of Medical Journal Editors, 2007).

The role of clinical trial nurses (CTNs) is rapidly evolving as well. A survey sponsored by the Oncology Nursing Society (Ehrenberger & Lillington, 2004) revealed the multiplicity of titles, job description duties, and educational and professional requirements. CTNs in Italy recently replicated this survey. This is the tip of the iceberg worldwide, where CTN responsibilities are being delegated to non-nursing staff. We believe that national, and ultimately worldwide, consensus on training to obtain CTN certification will add much needed clarity to this rapidly changing role. As we move forward, it is more than the CTN role, but the *position* of the CTN within the global, interdependent clinical research enterprise that must be standardized. That is, the official rank, status, and standing of the CTN. This edition will not only raise but will answer critical questions about the *role* of the CTN. This is intentional. It is our hope that by the third edition, the *position* of the CTN will be solidified globally.

Changes to the second edition of the *Manual for Clinical Trials Nursing* are intended to add clarity and perspective to the broad scope of clinical trials in our world today. For example, the chapters addressing the Internet and World Wide Web resources have been deleted, as this information is now common knowledge. References to Web sites are included in the text or Appendix 13 as required. Chapters on budget, compassionate use of protocol drugs, computerized tool design to verify eligibility, electronic data capture, clinical trial registries, mentorship, and specialization in clinical trial research nursing are new. Also, the appendices are expanded to include key documents in the ethical treatment of human research participants, such as the Nuremberg Code, the Declaration of Helsinki, the National Research Act, and portions of the *Code of Federal Regulations* and the International Committee on Harmonisation's Good Clinical Practice mandate. Finally, a list of abbreviations will help even the savviest CTNs navigate the manual with ease.

The contributions from international colleagues in the first edition are recognized as invaluable. The oncology research world is shrinking, and we are all aware of the many benefits of collaborative clinical trials. As globalization of clinical trials progresses, it behooves us all to become familiar with the processes of our overseas cancer research partners.

Therefore, our international section has more than doubled in size in the second edition. We welcome chapters from Australia, New Zealand, Austria, Canada, Denmark, France, Germany, Italy, Japan, and the United Kingdom, and hail our colleagues who wrote in a language foreign to them. The authors generally followed the order of the Table of Contents, adapting it to their own individual (and national) styles. A new chapter discussing the European Union directives adds insight to the framework within which our European colleagues work.

It is our sincere belief that only increased harmonization at the operations and nursing care levels of cancer research will enable successful international collaboration. Note: Colleagues from nations that are not represented are invited to contact the ONS Publishing Division for future contribution possibilities.

It is both interesting and important to note the number of contributors who asked to have this manual produced in a continually updated online version. The editors hope that as technologies continue to advance, and researchers and CTNs continue to collaborate worldwide, the next edition will be able to fulfill this request.

Angela D. Klimaszewski, RN, MSN, Lead Editor
Monica A. Bacon, RN, Coeditor
Heidi E. Deininger, PhD, RN, AOCN®, Coeditor
Bertie A. Ford, RN, MS, AOCN®, Coeditor
Joan G. Westendorp, RN, MSN, OCN®, Coeditor

References

Ehrenberger, H.E., & Lillington, L. (2004). Development of a measure to delineate the clinical trials nursing role [Online exclusive]. *Oncology Nursing Forum, 31*, E64-E68.

International Committee of Medical Journal Editors. (2007, October). *Uniform requirements for manuscripts submitted to biomedical journals: Writing and editing for biomedical publication.* Retrieved January 18, 2008, from http://www.icmje.org/index.html#top

Acknowledgments

··

The editors would like to acknowledge the following individuals, without whose support this manual would not have been accomplished: the international authors, who embraced the daunting task of writing in a foreign language; Carrie Goudreau, for typing and technical assistance with the International Section; and Barbara Sigler, RN, MNEd, director of Commercial Publishing, Oncology Nursing Society, for support and guidance.

Abbreviations

ABN—Australasian Biospecimens Network (Australia/New Zealand)

ACC—Accident Compensation Corporation

ACoS—American College of Surgeons

ACRP—Association of Clinical Research Professionals

ACS—American Cancer Society

ACTIS—AIDS Clinical Trials Information Service

ACTR—Australian Clinical Trials Registry

ADA—Americans with Disabilities Act

AdEERS—adverse events expedited reporting system

ADR—adverse drug reaction

AEGIS—AIDS Educational Global Information System

AFSSAPS—Agence Française de Sécurité Sanitaire des Produits de Santé (Competent Authority)

AGC—absolute granulocyte count

AGITG—Australian Gastro-Intestinal Trials Group

AGO-OVAR—*Arbeitsgemeinschaft gynäkologische Onkologie – Studiengruppe Ovarialkarzinom* (Germany)

AHEC—Australian Health Ethics Committee

AHRDMA—Australian Health Research Data Manager's Association

AHRQ—Agency for Healthcare Research and Quality

AIFA—*Agenzia Italiana del Farmaco* (Italian National Medicines Agency)

AIIO—Associazione Italiana Infermieri Oncologia (Italian Oncology Nursing Association)

AIOM—*Associazione Italiana di Oncologia Medica* (Italian Association of Medical Oncology)

ALARA—as low as reasonably achievable

AMG (a)—*Arzneimittelgesetzt* (German Drug Law)

AMG (b)—Audit and Monitoring Group

AMG (c)—Austrian medicinal products legislation (Austria)

AMS—account management system

ANC—absolute neutrophil count

ANPRM—advanced notice of proposed rulemaking

ANZBCTG—Australia and New Zealand Breast Cancer Trials Group

ANZGOG—Australia and New Zealand Gynaecological Oncology Group

APN—advanced practice nurse

ARSAC—Administration of Radioactive Substances Advisory Board

ASCO—American Society of Clinical Oncology

ASHP—American Society of Health-System Pharmacists

AUC—area under concentration-time curve

BCBS—Blue Cross Blue Shield Insurance

BfArM—*Bundesinstitut für Arzneimittel und Medizinprodukte* (competent authority for pharmaceuticals and medicine products in Germany)

BLA—biologic license application

BMGF—Austrian Ministry of Health and Women Bundesministerium für Gesundheit und Frauen (competent authority in Austria)

BODMA—British Oncology Data Managers Association

BRM—biologic response modifier

BSA—body surface area

BSC—biological safety cabinet

CAEPR—complete adverse events and potential risks

CALGB—Cancer and Leukemia Group B

CANO—Canadian Association of Nurses in Oncology

CANR—Canadian Association of Nurses in Research

CBC—complete blood count

CCCG—Coalition of Cancer Cooperative Groups

CCOP—Community Cooperative Oncology Program

CCS—Canadian Cancer Society

CDC—Centers for Disease Control and Prevention

CDE—common data elements

CDER—Center for Drug Evaluation and Research

CDMS—clinical data management systems

CEM—continuing education credits in medicine

CFR—*Code of Federal Regulations*

CHA—Canadian Health Act

CHCP—community hospital cancer program

CI—chief investigator

CICRS—CTSU Independent Clinical Research Site

CIRB—central institutional review board

CMS—Centers for Medicare and Medicaid Services

CNSA—Cancer Nurses Association of Australia

CNS—clinical nurse specialist

CoC—Commission on Cancer

COMP—community-based cancer program

CON—certified oncology nurse

CONJ—*Canadian Oncology Nursing Journal*

COREC—Central Office for Research Ethics Committees

COSA—Clinical Oncological Society of Australia

COSHH—Control of Substances Hazardous to Health

COTS—commercial off-the-shelf

CPA—cooperative project assurance

CPI—Centre Performance Index

CPMP/ICH/135/95—note for guidance on Good Clinical Practice

CPRP—cooperative protocol research program

CRA/DM—clinical research associate/data manager

CRA—clinical research associate

CRADA—cooperative research and development agreement

CRC—clinical research coordinator

CRD—Cancer Research Database

CRF—case report form

CRG—Cancer Research Group (Australia)

CRO (a)—clinical research organization (also known as sponsor)

CRO (b)—contract research organization (Australia)

CRPG—Clinical Research Professionals Group

CRSC—Clinical Research Support Centre

CR-UK—Cancer Research United Kingdom

CSGS—Clinical Studies Group

CSO—Chief Scientists Office

CSPOR—Comprehensive Support Program for Oncology Research (Japan)

CTAAC—Clinical Trials Advisory and Awards Committee

CTA—clinical trials agreement (United States)

CTA—Clinical Trials Authorization

CTCAE—Common Terminology Criteria for Adverse Events

CTCAEv3—Common Terminology Criteria for Adverse Events, version 3.0

CTC—Clinical Trials Committee

CT—clinical trial

CTCv2—Common Toxicity Criteria, version 2.0

CTD—Clinical Trial Directive (European Union)

CTEP—Cancer Therapy Evaluation Program

CTES—cancer clinical trials education series

CTG—Clinical Trials Group

CTIMP—Clinical Trial Involving an Investigational Medicinal Product

CTMS—clinical trial monitoring service

CTN—Clinical Trial Notification Scheme (Australia)

CTN—clinical trial nurse

CTNZ—Cancer Trials New Zealand

CTO—clinical trials office

CTRN—clinical trial research nurse (Canada)

CTSU—Cancer Trials Support Unit

CTU—clinical trials unit

CTX—Clinical Trial Exemption Scheme (Australia)

DAR—drug accountability record

DCI—data collection instruments

DCTD—Division of Cancer Treatment and Diagnosis

DDE—direct data entry

DF/PCC—Dana-Farber/Partners CancerCare

DHB—District Health Board (New Zealand)

DHHS—U.S. Department of Health and Human Services

DKG—*Deutsche Krebsgesellschaft* (German Cancer Society)

DLT—dose-limiting toxicity

DMC—data monitoring committee

DM—data manager

DMSB—data monitoring and safety board

DoD—Department of Defense

DOH—Department of Health

DOT—Department of Transportation

DRO—Department of Research Organization (Austria)

DSMC—data safety monitoring committee

ECCO (a)—European Convention of Clinical Oncology

ECCO (b)—European Cancer Conference (Federation of European Cancer Societies)

EC—ethics committee

ECG—electrocardiogram

ECHO—economic, clinical and humanistic outcomes

ECOG—Eastern Cooperative Oncology Group

e-CRF—electronic case report form

ECTC—Expanded Common Toxicity Criteria

EDC—electronic data capture

EEOC—Equal Employment Opportunity Commission

ELSI—Ethical, Legal, and Social Implications research program

EMEA—European Medicines Agency

EMR—electronic medical record

EONS—European Oncology Nursing Society

EORTC—European Organization for the Research and Treatment of Cancer

ESO—European School of Oncology

EudaCT—European Clinical Trials Database

EU—European Union

EWG—expert working group

FAA—Federal Aviation Administration

FACT Act—Fair Access to Clinical Trials Act

FAQ—frequently asked questions

FCA—False Claims Act

FDA—U.S. Food and Drug Administration

FHWA—Federal Highway Administration

FRA—Federal Railroad Administration

FSK—*Faglig Sammenslutning af Kræftsygeplejersker* (Denmark)

FWA—federalwide assurance

GBG—German Breast Group

GCP—good clinical practice

GCRP—Good Clinical Research Practice (New Zealand)

GFR—glomerular filtration rate

GIRC—*Gruppo Italiano Infermieri di Ricerca Clinica* (Italian Clinical Research Nurse Working Group)

GMP—good manufacturing practice

GP—general practitioner

GSK—GlaxoSmithKline

GTAC—Gene Therapy Advisory Committee

H&P—history and physical

HBM—Health Belief Model

HBV—Hepatitis B virus

HCV—Hepatitis C virus

HIPAA—Health Insurance Portability and Accountability Act

HMB—Hospital Management Board (Austria)

HMIP—Her Majesty's Inspectorate of Pollution (United Kingdom)

HON—Health on the Net code

HPB—Health Protection Branch

HREC—Human Research Ethics Committee (Australia)

HSC—Health and Safety Commission

HSE—Health and Safety Executive

IATA—International Air Transport Association

IBC—Institutional Biosafety Committee

IB—investigator's brochure

ICAO—International Civil Aviation Organization

ICH—International Conference on Harmonisation of Technical Requirements for Registration of Pharmaceuticals for Human Use

IC—informed consent

ICMJE—International Committee of Medical Journal Editors

ICORG—All Ireland Co-operative Oncology Research Group

ICR (a)—intelligent character recognition

ICR (b)—Institute of Clinical Research

ICT—information and communication technology

ICTRP—International Clinical Trials Registry Platform

IDB—investigator's drug brochure

IDE—investigational device exemption

IDMSC—Independent Data Monitoring and Safety Committee (Germany)

IEC—independent ethics committee

IFPMA—International Federation of Pharmaceutical Manufacturers and Associations

IND—investigational new drug

IOM—Institute of Medicine

IRB—institutional review board

ISD—Information Services Division

ISNCC—International Society of Nurses in Cancer Care

ISO—International Organization for Standardization

ISPOR—International Society for Pharmacoeconomics and Outcome Research

ISS—*Instituto Superiore di Sanita'* (National Health Institute, Italy)

IST—Investigator Sponsored Trial (Germany)

IT—information technology

IVRS—interactive voice response system

JALSG—Japan Adult Leukemia Study Group

Japic CTI—Japan Pharmaceutical Information Center Clinical Trials Information

JASMO—Japan SMO association

JCOG—Japan Clinical Oncology Group

JGOG—Japanese Gynecologic Oncology Group

JNA—Japanese Nursing Association

JPMA—Japanese Pharmaceutical Manufacturers Association

JSCN—Japanese Society of Cancer Nursing

JSCO—Japan Society of Clinical Oncology

JSCPT—Japanese Society of Clinical Pharmacology and Therapeutics

KKS—*Koordinierungszentrum klinische Studien* (Germany)

KOK—*Konferenz Onkologischer Kranken und Kinderkrankenpflege* (Germany)

LAR—legally authorized representative

LREC—local research ethics committee

MASCC—Multinational Association of Supportive Care in Cancer

MCA—Medicines Control Agency

MDA—Medical Devices Agency

MDT—multidisciplinary teams

MEC—Multiregional Ethics Committees (New Zealand)

MEXT—Ministry of Education, Culture, Sports, Science of Technology (Japan)

MHLW—Ministry of Health, Labour and Welfare (Japan)

MHRA—Medicines and Healthcare Products Regulatory Agency

MI—myocardial infarction

MPA—multiple project assurance

MPG—*Medizinproduktegesetzt* (German medical products law)

MRC—Medical Research Council

mRCT—metaRegister of Controlled Trials

MS—member states of European Union

MTD—maximum tolerated dose

MURB—Medical University Research Boards (Austria)

NAI—no action indicated

NAPBC—National Action Plan on Breast Cancer

NCCN—National Comprehensive Cancer Network

NCCTG—North Central Cancer Treatment Group

NCD—national coverage determination

NCIC—National Cancer Institute of Canada

NCI—National Cancer Institute

NCRI—National Cancer Research Institute

NCRN—National Cancer Research Network

NCR—no carbon required

NDA—new drug application

NExT—NCI Experimental Therapeutics

NHGRI—National Human Genome Research Institute

NHMRC—National Health and Medical Research Council (Australia)

NHS—National Health Service

NHS—National Health System (United Kingdom)

NIA—noninstitutional investigator agreement

NIH—National Institutes of Health

NI—Northern Ireland

NLM—National Library of Medicine

NOGGO—*Nordostdeutsche Gesellschaft für Gynäkologie und Onkologie* (Germany)

non-PHI—non-protected health information

NPO—non-profit organization (Japan)

NPRM—notice of proposed rulemaking

NRR—National Research Registry (United Kingdom)

NSW—New South Wales

NTRAC—National Translational Cancer Research Network

NZACRES—New Zealand Association of Clinical Researchers

NZ—New Zealand

OAI—official action indicated

OCR—optical character recognition

OHRP—Office for Human Research Protections

OMA—Office of Management Assessment

OMR—optical marking recognition

ONS (a)—Office of National Statistics

ONS (b)—Oncology Nursing Society

ONS (c)—UK Oncology Nursing Society

OPRR—Office for Protection from Research Risk

ORI—Office of Research Integrity

OSHA—Occupational Safety and Health Administration

OsSC—National Monitoring Centre for Clinical Trials (*Osservatorio Nazionale della Sperimentazione Clinica*) (Italy)

PC—physician coordinator

PCP—primary care physician

PDA—personal digital assistant

PEI—Paul-Ehrlich-Institute (competent authority for medicine products in Germany)

PHI—protected health information

PhRMA—Pharmaceutical Researchers and Manufacturers of America

PI—principal investigator

PIV—peripheral IV

PK—pharmacokinetics

PKS—pharmacokinetic sampling

PLA—product license application

PLT—platelet count

PMB—Pharmaceutical Management Branch

PMDA—Pharmaceuticals and Medical Devices Agency

POG—Pediatric Oncology Group

PRO—patient-reported outcomes

PR—proposed rule

QA—quality assurance

QI—quality improvement

QOL—quality of life

R&D—research and development

RAID—rapid access to intervention and development

RAPS—Regulatory Affairs Professionals Society

RA—regulatory authority (Austria)

RA—research associate

RBC—red blood cell count

RCN—Royal College of Nursing (United Kingdom)

RDC—remote data capture

RDE—remote data entry

REB—Research Ethics Board (Canada)

RECIST—Response Evaluation Criteria in Solid Tumors

REC—Regional Ethics Committee (New Zealand, European Union)

REC—Research Ethics Committee

RFP—request for proposals

RSS—regulatory support system

RTOG—Radiation Therapy Oncology Group

SAE—serious adverse event

SAS*—Statistical Analysis System (Canada)

SCLD—State Cancer Legislated Database

SCOTT—Standing Committee on Therapeutic Trials (NZ)

SCRN—Scottish Cancer Research Network

SC—study coordinator

SCT—Society for Clinical Trials

SDV—source document verification

SGCTG—Scottish Gynaecological Cancer Trials Group

SGNO—Society of Gynecologic Nurse Oncologists

SIG—special interest group

SoCRA—Society of Clinical Research Associates

SOP—standard operating procedure

SPA—single project assurance

SSA—site-specific assessment

SSOP—summary of standard operating procedures

SST—serum separator tube

SUSAR—suspected unexpected serious adverse reaction

SWOG—Southwest Oncology Group

TCCA—The Cancer Council Australia

TGA—Therapeutic Goods Administration (Australia)

TPD—Therapeutic Products Directorate

TRC—Treatment Referral Center

TRICC—Translational Research in Clinical Trials Committee

TROG—Trans Tasman Radiation Oncology Group (New Zealand)

TSC—Trial Steering Committee

TTM—Transtheoretical Model

UK—United Kingdom

UMIN-CTR—University Hospital Medical Information Network Clinical Trials Registry (Japan)

UP—universal precautions

VAI—voluntary action indicated

VA—Veterans Affairs

VPN—virtual private network

WBC—white blood cell

WCTN—Wales Cancer Trials Network

WHO—World Health Organization

WJTOG—West Japan Thoracic Oncology Group

WMA—World Medical Association

SECTION I.

History and Background

CHAPTER 1
History and Background of Clinical Trials

CHAPTER 1
History and Background of Clinical Trials

Sheila Breslin, RN, MS

History

Experimental research studies on human subjects can be traced to ancient times. Early clinical trials often were comparative studies that largely focused on the prevention of communicable diseases and on nutritional disorders, which were prevalent up until the latter half of the 20th century (Lilienfeld, 1982). In an effort to promote public health in the United States, a one-room laboratory was created in 1887 within the Marine Hospital Service (predecessor to the U.S. Public Health Service). Called the Hygienic Laboratory, the facility was established to provide funding for research on the prevention, detection, and treatment of disease. The Ransdell Act of 1930 legislated public funding of medical research and changed the name of the Hygienic Laboratory to the National Institute of Health (Harden, n.d.). The name was later changed to the National Institutes of Health (NIH) to reflect the addition of new institutes.

The first documented clinical trial in the United States using a matched control group, random assignment, and single-blinding was reported in 1931 by J. Burns Amberson and colleagues. The trial evaluated the use of sanocrysin, a gold compound, in the treatment of patients with pulmonary tuberculosis treated at the W.H. Maybury Sanatorium in Northville, MI. Twenty-four patients were matched and then randomized to either group I (sanocrysin-treated) or group II (control). Subjects were not aware of the differences in the treatment regimens between the groups (Lilienfeld, 1982).

In 1937, President Franklin D. Roosevelt signed the National Cancer Institute Act, which established the National Cancer Institute (NCI) as a division of NIH. The act mandated funding to support cancer research and training (Jenkins & Lake, 1988; White-Hershey & Nevidjon, 1990). The following year saw passage of the Food and Drug Act, implemented to ensure that a drug demonstrated safety in humans before it could be marketed to the public (Swann, 1998).

NCI began to fund cooperative oncology groups in an effort to expand enrollment in clinical trials in the mid-1950s. Cooperative oncology groups are composed of groups of physicians at various institutions who collaboratively design and implement clinical trials. Today, the Clinical Trials Cooperative Group Program comprises 12 groups (NCI, 2005a) (see Figure 1-1). The Cancer Therapy Evaluation Program, a branch of NCI's Division of Cancer Treatment, oversees the cooperative oncology groups (Cheson, 1991).

The National Cancer Act of 1971 resulted in a large increase in NCI funding. NCI was charged with the responsibility of conducting basic scientific research in oncology and applying the results to clinical practice. The National Cancer Act also promoted the development of oncology training programs, facilities, and public-education services (Jenkins & Hubbard, 1991; Jenkins & Lake, 1988).

By 1973, most oncology clinical trials were conducted at NCI-designated comprehensive cancer centers that received core grants from NCI to fund operations. Community oncologists, however, still were treating patients with

---

Figure 1-1. Clinical Trials Cooperative Groups*

- American College of Radiology Imaging Network (ACRIN)
- American College of Surgeons Oncology Group (ACOSOG)
- Cancer and Leukemia Group B (CALGB)
- Children's Oncology Group (COG)
- Eastern Cooperative Oncology Group (ECOG)
- European Organisation for Research and Treatment of Cancer (EORTC)
- Gynecologic Oncology Group (GOG)
- National Cancer Institute of Canada, Clinical Trials Group (NCIC CTG)
- National Surgical Adjuvant Breast and Bowel Project (NSABP)
- North Central Cancer Treatment Group (NCCTG)
- Radiation Therapy Oncology Group (RTOG)
- Southwest Oncology Group (SWOG)

*The above list is current as of the time of writing. For a list that is current at the time of reading, visit www.cancer.gov/cancertopics/factsheet/NCI/clinical-trials-cooperative-group.

cancer who might be eligible for enrollment in a clinical trial. In response, NCI developed outreach programs in an attempt to make clinical trials available to larger numbers of patients with cancer and to improve accrual of patients into these trials. These programs provided funding for community physicians to participate in NCI-sponsored clinical trials (Cheson, 1991; Jenkins & Hubbard, 1991).

The Cooperative Group Outreach Program, established in 1976 by NCI's Division of Cancer Treatment, allows community physicians to affiliate with a cooperative group to offer their patients access to cooperative group trials. The Community Clinical Oncology Program, instituted in 1983, differs from the Cooperative Group Outreach Program in its funding source, research focus, accrual requirements, and affiliation policies. NCI's Division of Cancer Prevention and Control (DCPC) funds the Cooperative Group Outreach Program. Community physicians affiliate with cancer centers and cooperative groups to form a research base. In addition to cancer treatment, DCPC-sponsored clinical trials focus on prevention and early detection of cancer. The High-Priority Clinical Trials Program, established in 1988, targets phase III cooperative group trials as high priority, thus increasing accrual (Cheson, 1991).

Growth of Regulation

Fraudulent claims of safety and efficacy, as well as abuses in drug and device manufacturing, were rampant in the United States in the late 1800s, leading to untold numbers of serious injuries and deaths. As a result of these abuses, the 1906 Food and Drug Act was signed into law, establishing the first federal regulatory standards to ensure food and drug purity and truth in labeling. The Bureau of Chemistry, whose name was changed in 1930 to the Food and Drug Administration (FDA), implemented these laws. In 1938, a new, more stringent law was enacted that mandated drug safety testing and, for the first time, FDA approval prior to marketing. This legislation also brought the marketing of medical devices under the FDA's regulatory purview. The Kefauver-Harris Amendment to the Food and Drug Act was passed in 1962 after the discovery that thalidomide could cause fetal abnormalities. The amendment required preclinical testing of drugs, as well as proof of efficacy and safety before use in humans. It also required that research subjects provide informed consent before participating in clinical trials (Swann, 1998).

Research on vulnerable populations, such as slaves, prison inmates, the mentally handicapped, the poor, children, and minority groups, was conducted in the United States from the mid-1800s to the mid-1900s without participants' informed consent (Allen, 1994; Merkatz & Junod, 1994). However, it was not until the exposure of medical atrocities performed on prisoners during World War II that a code of ethics for human experimentation was developed. The resulting Nuremberg Code of 1947 serves as the foundation for the ethical principles governing clinical research today (McCarthy, 1994; Merkatz & Junod) (see Appendix 1).

In 1964, the World Medical Association developed a set of international ethical guidelines for physicians involved in biomedical research. These guidelines, the Declaration of Helsinki (see Appendix 2), mandated preclinical studies prior to the implementation of human clinical trials, scientific justification for experimentation in humans, and a written protocol document with review by an independent committee. In addition, the declaration posited that research be conducted only by qualified medical personnel and offered guidelines for the provision of informed consent from human subjects (World Medical Organization, 1996).

After the passage of the National Research Act in 1974 (see Appendix 3), the National Commission for the Protection of Human Subjects of Biomedical and Behavioral Research was created to develop written policies for the protection of human subjects. Published in 1979, the resulting Belmont Report (see Appendix 4) led to the establishment of institutional review boards (IRBs), outlined protocol design criteria, and required that written informed consent be obtained from all research subjects (Jenkins & Hubbard, 1991). These policies were codified in 1981 in the *Code of Federal Regulations* (see Appendix 5) (Sparks, 2002).

One of the most important of these regulations, known as "the Common Rule" (Basic HHS Policy for Protection of Human Research Subjects, 2001), outlines specific measures that investigators and institutions must follow to protect subjects who participate in federally funded research. The Common Rule includes criteria for the provision of informed consent, guidelines for the conduct of IRBs, and requirements for the protection of vulnerable populations, as well as other subject protections such as the mandate for data and safety monitoring boards, regulations regarding investigator conflict of interest, and training of clinical research personnel (NCI, 2005a).

In 1996, members of the International Conference on Harmonisation (ICH) of Technical Requirements for Registration of Pharmaceuticals for Human Use finalized a set of good clinical practice (GCP) standards for the conduct of clinical trials. Officially known as the *ICH Harmonised Tripartite Guideline for Good Clinical Practice* (see Appendix 6), its 13 principles have been adopted by the United States, the European Union, Japan, Australia, Canada, and a number of other countries, as well as the World Health Organization. In addition to establishing consistent principles for the protection of human subjects, the goal of the ICH GCP guidelines is to streamline regulatory approvals of new drugs by developing consistent recommendations for the design, implementation, reporting, and interpretation of clinical trials worldwide (Dixon, 1999; Lin, 1998). (See Chapter 46 for additional information.)

Passed by Congress in 1996 and implemented by the U.S. Department of Health and Human Services (DHHS) in 2003, the Health Insurance Portability and Accountability Act (HIPAA) has influenced the conduct of clinical trials, mandating specific privacy protections for trial participants. For a detailed examination of the impact of HIPAA on clinical trials, the reader is referred to NIH Publication Number 04-5495 (DHHS, 2004).

Federalwide Assurance (FWA) for the Protection of Human Subjects (see Appendices 7 and 8) was passed in 2005 with the intent of enforcing that all research involving human subjects is subject to federal regulations and must be guided by ethical principles. The ethical principles specifically cited include the *Belmont Report: Ethical Principles and Guidelines for the Protection of Human Subjects of Research of the National Commission for the Protection of Human Subjects of Biomedical and Behavioral Research,* in addition to other appropriate ethical standards recognized by federal departments and agencies that have adopted the federal policy for the protection of human subjects (i.e., the Common Rule).

The Office for Human Research Protections (OHRP) oversees the safety of participants in federally funded clinical trials. FWA is the only type of assurance of compliance currently accepted and approved by OHRP for institutions engaged in nonexempt human subjects research conducted or supported by DHHS. For an in-depth discussion of assurances and FWA, see Chapter 2.

Treatment of Minorities and Women

Despite the increasing incidence of and mortality from cancer in the African American community, this group has been underrepresented in clinical trials (Powe, 1995; Thomas, Pinto, Roach, & Vaughn, 1994). The reason for the lack of participation by minorities in general, and African Americans in particular, largely had been attributed to fears of exploitation generated by the Tuskegee syphilis experiment conducted by the U.S. Public Health Service from the 1930s to the 1970s. This study allowed African American men with syphilis to go untreated, even after curative treatment was available, in order to study the natural progression of the disease. In addition, no attempt was made to educate these men about preventing the spread of syphilis, which placed the general population at risk for infection (Allen, 1994; McCarthy, 1994; Thomas et al.).

Lack of access to state-of-the-art health care, cultural or ethnic factors, economic status, language or literacy barriers, and long-standing fear, apprehension, and skepticism have been identified as obstacles to minority participation in clinical trials (Millon-Underwood, Sanders, & Davis, 1993; NCI, 2005a; Powe, 1995; Thomas et al., 1994). However, because 40% of Community Clinical Oncology Program annual referrals are from minority populations, NCI provides funding to institutions that serve a high percentage of minority groups through its Minority-Based Community Clinical Oncology Program, begun in 1990 (NCI, 2005a; Thomas et al.). A study demonstrating equal minority access to NCI-sponsored cancer treatment trials from 1991 to 1994 (Tejeda et al., 1996) and the work of

Hutchins, Unger, Crowley, Coltman, and Albain (1999) suggested a reversal in the trend of low minority participation. In the African American and Hispanic communities, participation in clinical trials in patients younger than age 30 has, in fact, become proportional to incidence, although inequities still exist among older age groups (NCI, 2004; Sateren et al., 2002). Additionally, the Minority-Based Community Clinical Oncology Program accrues 10% of all ethnic minorities participating in NCI-approved clinical trials (NCI, 2005a).

In 1977, women were excluded from participation in clinical trials because of concerns about the potential teratogenic effects of untested drugs on a developing fetus. This exclusion, which was mandated by the FDA partially as a result of severe birth defects caused by the drug thalidomide, applied to phase I clinical trials involving the use of untested drugs in pregnant women or women of childbearing potential. However, in practice, the exclusion was extended to all women in all phases of clinical trials (McCarthy, 1994).

These policies severely limited our knowledge about gender- and race-related differences in drug safety and efficacy (Allen, 1994; McCarthy, 1994; Merkatz & Junod, 1994; Millon-Underwood et al., 1993). The AIDS epidemic highlighted the potentially discriminatory nature of these exclusionary practices (Kelly & Cordell, 1996; McCarthy). Between 1992 and 1993, 15% of all new AIDS cases reported were in women, and almost 75% of these women were either African American or Hispanic (Allen).

In 1986, NIH drafted its first policy promoting the inclusion of women in clinical trials (La Rosa, 1994). Women of childbearing potential may participate in phase I clinical trials as long as they are not pregnant. They must be advised of the potential for fetal damage if they become pregnant and must agree to use effective contraception while participating in the study (Merkatz & Junod, 1994). In 1990, NCI created the Office of Research on Women's Health to promote research on women's health issues and the participation of women in clinical trials (Pinn, 1994). The NIH Revitalization Act, passed by Congress in 1993, mandated the inclusion of women and minorities in all NIH-sponsored clinical trials (Pinn). Women now account for 60% of participants enrolled in NCI-sponsored treatment trials (NCI, 2004).

Treatment of Children and Older Adults

Historically, participation of children in cancer clinical trials has far exceeded adult participation. This is, in part, because childhood cancers are rare, and most children with cancer are treated at major academic institutions with access to clinical trials (NCI, 2004; Sateren et al., 2002). However, because children represent a vulnerable population, special protections have been implemented to safeguard their treatment. In 1983, laws to protect children in clinical trials were added to the *Code of Federal Regulations* (Burns, 2003; Hirtz & Fitzsimmons, 2002; Sparks, 2002).

Concerns have been raised that drugs used to treat adults were being used without adequate testing in children (Hutchins et al., 1999; Sateren et al., 2002). Consequently, NIH issued a policy mandating the inclusion of children in clinical trials unless scientifically or ethically contraindicated. In 2002, the Best Pharmaceuticals for Children Act was passed, amending the Food, Drug, and Cosmetic Act to improve drug safety and efficacy testing prior to use in children (Burns, 2003). Until recently, parental consent alone was sufficient for children younger than the age of 18 to participate in clinical trials. Federal regulations now require, except under certain circumstances, that children age 7 and older also sign a consent form—tailored to their developmental level—to participate in the process (Burns; NCI, 2005b) (see Chapter 14).

Underrepresentation of the older adult population has been another concern in clinical trials. In 1989, the FDA published recommended guidelines for inclusion of older adults in clinical trials. However, they continue to be proportionally underrepresented in clinical trials, despite the fact that cancer incidence and mortality rates are highest in this population. Suggested reasons for underrepresentation include concerns about toxicities, the presence of comorbid conditions, perceived lack of benefit, advanced stage of disease at diagnosis, lack of awareness, quality-of-life concerns, and a variety of socioeconomic barriers (Hutchins et al., 1999; Lewis et al., 2003; Talarico, Chen, & Pazdur, 2004).

Lack of participation by older adults in clinical trials may not only limit the generalizability of results to older patients but actually may result in less aggressive approaches to treatment because of misconceptions about tolerability, thereby compromising survival outcomes (Hutchins et al., 1999; Talarico et al., 2004). It is estimated that by 2030, the incidence of some cancers may double in this age group (Yancik, 1997). Increased representation of older adults in clinical trials, therefore, is critically important. Today, cooperative group trials, such as treatment (e.g., chemotherapy) and quality-of-life trials, are designed specifically to include older adults. Table 1-1 summarizes the significant events in the history of clinical trials development.

Types and Phases of Trials

The goals of cancer clinical trials are to develop new approaches to prevent, detect, and treat the disease and to improve the quality of life and care of people with cancer or those at high risk for developing it (NCI, 2005a). The major types of clinical trials include prevention, screening and early detection, diagnostic, genetics, treatment, and quality-of-life and supportive care trials (NCI, 2005a).

Treatment (therapeutic) clinical trials are studies that evaluate the efficacy of a particular intervention in preventing or eradicating a disease or improving patient care or treatment. Clinical trials involving new drugs or devices in humans are preceded by preclinical studies in animals. The

FDA must approve the use of a new drug in a clinical trial by review and approval of an investigational new drug (IND) application (Jenkins & Hubbard, 1991; White-Hershey & Nevidjon, 1990). Only about 5% of IND applications for new oncology drugs eventually receive FDA approval (NCI, 2007).

Treatment clinical trials consistently are assigned a phase (e.g., phase I) and are moved through the other phases of the drug development process. This process involves conducting the trial, collecting and analyzing data, and evaluating the data to determine whether the drug should move forward to the next phase. Then, the process is repeated. Thus, it may take many years for a drug to move through phases I, II, III, and IV of a clinical trial.

The *therapeutic index* of most conventional chemotherapy drugs is very narrow. That is, an effective dose is almost at the dose where side effects occur (NCI, 2007). These drugs move through the standard process (phases I–IV) of drug development. Molecularly targeted therapeutic drugs have a wide therapeutic index; the desired effect may be reached without significant side effects. Thus, the NCI instituted *phase 0* clinical trials in 2006 specifically to study the biologically effective dose of molecularly targeted drugs (NCI, 2007).

Phase 0 clinical trials study the pharmacodynamic and pharmacokinetic properties of a drug. They are part of the NCI Experimental Therapeutics (NExT) Program, which combines the expertise of drug development of NCI's Division of Cancer Treatment and Diagnosis with the in-house research and access to NIH at NCI's Center for Cancer Research. In the NExT Program, researchers hope to significantly shorten the standard drug development process. An FDA guidance issued in January 2006 specifies that phase 0 clinical trials are to be conducted under an "exploratory new drug" application (NCI, 2007). For additional information about phase 0 clinical trials, go to www.cancer.gov/newscenter/pressreleases/PhaseZeroNExTQandA.

Phase I studies of anticancer agents, or other modes of therapy in combination, are designed to evaluate the maximum tolerated dose (the dose above which a dose-limiting toxicity is observed), dosing schedule, and toxicity profile of a new treatment. They are offered to a small number of patients (< 30) with a variety of tumor types who have exhausted all other treatment options. These participants then are divided into cohorts of three to six patients, and each cohort is treated with an increased dose of the drug (NCI, 2005a). Phase I trials involve, in the case of a new drug, pharmacokinetic studies and the dose-escalation cohorts to determine the maximum tolerated dose (Jenkins & Hubbard, 1991; Melink & Whitacre, 1991).

Phase II trials are offered to less than 100 patients with a given tumor type. The goal is to evaluate efficacy in subsets of patients with the same tumor. Objective tumor response is the usual end point. Patients usually are treated at the recommended dose determined in phase I

Table 1-1. History of Clinical Trials	
Year	**Event**
1747	Lind conducts the first documented comparative study on patients with scurvy.
1800s	Drugs and vaccines to treat smallpox, diphtheria, and cholera are developed and tested.
1887	The National Institutes of Health (NIH) is founded.
1900s	Research on prevention and treatment of infectious diseases begins.
1906	The Food and Drug Act is signed into law, regulating drug purity, safety, and labeling.
1937	The National Cancer Institute Act establishes the National Cancer Institute (NCI).
1938	The Food, Drug, and Cosmetic Act, replacing the 1906 Food and Drug Act, requires that drugs be tested for safety prior to marketing.
1947	The Nuremberg Code establishes a basic code of ethics for experimentation on human subjects.
1962	The Kefauver-Harris Amendment to the Food, Drug, and Cosmetic Act mandates preclinical testing and the provision of informed consent.
1964	The Declaration of Helsinki establishes specific guidelines for physicians conducting human research.
1966	U.S. Surgeon General policy mandates independent review of all research on human subjects, proposing the establishment of institutional review boards.
1971	The National Cancer Act mandates NCI to conduct and apply basic cancer research.
1974	The National Research Act establishes the National Commission for the Protection of Human Subjects of Biomedical and Behavioral Research.
1976	NCI initiates the Cooperative Group Outreach Program.
1979	The Belmont Report outlines ethical principles and guidelines for protection of human subjects.
1981	Laws governing the protection of human subjects in research funded by the U.S. Department of Health and Human Services (DHHS) are added to the *Code of Federal Regulations.*
1983	NCI funds Community Cancer Outreach Programs.
1986	NIH establishes policies for the inclusion of women in clinical trials.
1988	NCI establishes the High-Priority Clinical Trials Program.
1989	FDA publishes guidelines for the inclusion of older adult patients in clinical trials.
1990	The Office of Research on Women's Health is created.
1991	Sixteen federal agencies adopt the federal policy for the protection of human subjects, known as the "Common Rule."
1993	The NIH Revitalization Act mandates the inclusion of women and minorities in NIH-sponsored clinical trials.
1996	The International Conference on Harmonisation establishes good clinical practice guidelines for human subjects research. Congress passes the Health Insurance Portability and Accountability Act (HIPAA).
1997	The Food and Drug Modernization Act mandates establishment of a public resource for information on clinical trials.
1998	NIH Policy and Guidelines on the Inclusion of Children as Participants in Research Involving Human Subjects mandates that children must be included in all NIH-sponsored research except under certain circumstances.
2000	The World Health Organization establishes international guidelines for ethics committees involved in the review of biomedical research.
2002	The Best Pharmaceuticals Act for Children amends the Federal Food, Drug, and Cosmetic Act to improve drug safety and efficacy testing for children.
2003	The DHHS implements HIPAA.
2004	The International Committee of Medical Journal Editors issues a statement mandating public registration of clinical trials, including a description of informed consent and ethics committee approval as prerequisites for manuscript publication.
2005	Federalwide Assurance for the Protection of Human Subjects is required for all studies funded or conducted by the DHHS that involve human subjects.
2006	NCI initiates phase 0 clinical trials to study the pharmacokinetics and pharmacodynamics of molecularly targeted drugs.

studies, and additional safety and toxicity data are evaluated (Jenkins & Hubbard, 1991; Melink & Whitacre, 1991; NCI, 2005a).

In *phase III* trials, a treatment that has demonstrated efficacy in phase II studies is compared to standard treatment in a randomized, prospective fashion. If a standard treatment for a disease does not exist, a placebo control group may be used. The primary end points in phase III clinical trials include response rates, survival, and quality of life. Phase III trials must be conducted with large numbers of patients (hundreds to thousands) to have sufficient statistical power to assess treatment group differences. Thus, they often are conducted in multiple institutions simultaneously and may be single- or double-blinded (Jenkins & Hubbard, 1991; Melink & Whitacre, 1991; NCI, 2005a).

Phase IV clinical trials are postmarketing studies designed to evaluate long-term safety and efficacy, new formulations, or additional indications after a treatment is approved for standard use (Hubbard, 1982; NCI, 2005a). Table 1-2 summarizes the phases of clinical trials.

Summary

The evolution of clinical trials has resulted in dramatic improvements in the prevention and treatment of many diseases, including cancer. Advances in medicine, improved surgical techniques, the development of new drugs and devices, the application of statistical techniques to research studies, recognition of the need for regulation, and the development of ethical codes all have influenced the way clinical trials are now conducted both in the United States and internationally.

References

Allen, M. (1994). The dilemma for women of color in clinical trials. *Journal of the American Medical Women's Association, 49,* 105–109.

Basic HHS Policy for Protection of Human Research Subjects, 45 C.F.R. § 46 (2001).

Burns, J.P. (2003). Research in children. *Critical Care Medicine, 31,* S-31–S136.

Cheson, B.D. (1991). Cancer clinical trials: Clinical trials programs. *Seminars in Oncology Nursing, 7,* 235–242.

Dixon, J.R., Jr. (1999). The International Conference on Harmonization good clinical practice guideline. *Quality Assurance, 6,* 65–74.

Harden, V.A. (n.d.). *A short history of the National Institutes of Health.* Retrieved March 17, 2007, from http://history.nih.gov/exhibits/history/index.html

Hirtz, D.G., & Fitzsimmons, L.G. (2002). Regulatory and ethical issues in the conduct of clinical research involving children. *Current Opinion in Pediatrics, 14,* 669–675.

Hubbard, S.M. (1982). Cancer treatment research: The role of the nurse in clinical trials of cancer therapy. *Nursing Clinics of North America, 17,* 763–783.

Hutchins, L.F., Unger, J.M., Crowley, J.J., Coltman, C.A., & Albain, K.S. (1999). Underrepresentation of patients 65 years of age or older in cancer-treatment trials. *New England Journal of Medicine, 341,* 2061–2067.

Jenkins, J., & Hubbard, S. (1991). History of clinical trials. *Seminars in Oncology Nursing, 7,* 228–234.

Jenkins, J.F., & Lake, P.C. (1988). Celebration of an era of public service at the National Institutes of Health and the National Cancer Institute. *Cancer Nursing, 11,* 58–64.

Kelly, P.J., & Cordell, J.R. (1996). Recruitment of women into research studies: A nursing perspective. *Clinical Nurse Specialist, 10,* 25–28.

La Rosa, J.H. (1994). Office of research on women's health: National Institutes of Health and the women's health agenda. *Annals of the New York Academy of Sciences, 736,* 196–204.

Lewis, J.H., Kilgore, M.L., Goldman, D.P., Trimble, E.L., Kaplan, R., Montello, M.J., et al. (2003). Participation of patients 65 years of age or older in cancer clinical trials. *Journal of Clinical Oncology, 21,* 1383–1389.

Lilienfeld, A.M. (1982). Ceteris paribus: The evolution of the clinical trial. *Bulletin of the History of Medicine, 56,* 1–18.

Lin, M.H. (1998). Ethical considerations in clinical trials: An international perspective. *Drug Information Journal, 32,* 1293S–1297S.

Table 1-2. Phases of Cancer Clinical Trials		
Phase and Number of Participants	**Primary Goals**	**Characteristics**
Phase 0 10–12 people	• Study pharmacodynamic and pharmacokinetic properties of a drug. • Identify drugs that do not produce desired effect, and avoid moving them into phase I trials. • Determine a dosing regimen for testing in standard clinical trials.	• Limited number of doses • Lower doses administered • Less risk to participant • Useful for molecularly targeted drugs with wide therapeutic indexes • Also useful for drugs that require development of biomarkers for future studies
Phase I 20–25 people	• Establish maximum tolerated dose and dosing schedule. • Evaluate toxicity. • Determine pharmacokinetics.	• Relapsed/refractory disease • Small number of patients • Dose-escalating cohorts • Variety of tumor types • Pharmacokinetic studies
Phase II < 100 people	• Determine antitumor activity in specific tumor types. • Evaluate toxicity.	• Groups of patients with same tumors • Measurable disease to assess response rates
Phase III 100–thousands	• Establish efficacy by assessing survival and time to progression. • Compare with current standard.	• Randomization between experimental treatment and standard treatment and/or control group • Large numbers of patients
Phase IV Hundreds to thousands	• Expand "off-label" use. • Further assess toxicity data and long term safety. • Assess long-term effectiveness.	• Postmarketing trials and commercially available drugs

McCarthy, C.R. (1994). Historical background of clinical trials involving women and minorities. *Academic Medicine, 69,* 695–698.

Melink, J., & Whitacre, M.Y. (1991). Planning and implementing clinical trials. *Seminars in Oncology Nursing, 7,* 243–251.

Merkatz, R.B., & Junod, S.W. (1994). Historical background of changes in FDA policy on the study and evaluation of drugs in women. *Academic Medicine, 69,* 703–707.

Millon-Underwood, S., Sanders, E., & Davis, M. (1993). Determinants of participation in state-of-the-art cancer prevention, early detection/ screening, and treatment trials among African-Americans. *Cancer Nursing, 16,* 25–33.

National Cancer Institute. (2004, September). *NCI-supported cancer clinical trials: Facts and figures.* Retrieved October 15, 2005, from http://www. nci.nih.gov/clinicaltrials/facts-and-figures

National Cancer Institute. (2005a). *Cancer clinical trials: The in-depth program* [NIH Publication No. 05-5051]. Bethesda, MD: Author.

National Cancer Institute. (2005b, May). *Children's assent to clinical trial participation.* Retrieved October 15, 2005, from http://www.cancer. gov/clinicaltrials/understanding/childrensassent0101/

National Cancer Institute. (2007). *New approaches to cancer drug development and clinical trials: Questions and answers.* Retrieved June 12, 2007, from http://www.cancer.gov/newscenter/pressreleases/ PhaseZeroNExTQandA/print?page=&keyword=

Pinn, V.W. (1994). The role of the NIH's Office of Research on Women's Health. *Academic Medicine, 69,* 698–702.

Powe, B.D. (1995). Cancer fatalism among elderly Caucasians and African-Americans. *Oncology Nursing Forum, 22,* 1355–1359.

Sateren, W.B., Trimble, E.L., Abrams, J., Brawley, O., Breen, N., Ford, L., et al. (2002). How sociodemographics, presence of oncology specialists, and hospital cancer programs affect accrual to cancer treatment trials. *Journal of Clinical Oncology, 20,* 2109–2117.

Sparks, J. (2002). *Timeline of laws related to the protection of human subjects.* Retrieved July 31, 2005, from http://history.nih.gov/01Docs/ historical/2020b.htm

Swann, J.P. (1998). The Food and Drug Administration. In G.T. Kurian (Ed.), *Historical guide to the U.S. government* (pp. 248–254). New York: Oxford University Press.

Talarico, L., Chen, G., & Pazdur, R. (2004). Enrollment of elderly patients in clinical trials for cancer drug registration: A 7-year experience by the U.S. Food and Drug Administration. *Journal of Clinical Oncology, 22,* 4626–4631.

Tejeda, H.A., Green, S.B., Trimble, E.L., Ford, L., High, J.L., Ungerleider, R.S., et al. (1996). Representation of African-Americans, Hispanics, and Whites in National Cancer Institute cancer treatment trials. *Journal of the National Cancer Institute, 88,* 812–816.

Thomas, C.R., Pinto, H.A., Roach, M., & Vaughn, C.B. (1994). Participation in clinical trials: Is it state-of-the-art treatment for African-Americans and other people of color? *JAMA, 86,* 177–182.

U.S. Department of Health and Human Services. (2004). *Clinical research and the HIPAA privacy rule* [NIH Publication No. 04-5495]. Bethesda, MD: Author.

White-Hershey, D., & Nevidjon, B. (1990). Fundamentals for oncology nurse/data managers—preparing for a new role. *Oncology Nursing Forum, 17,* 371–377.

World Medical Organization. (1996). Declaration of Helsinki. *British Medical Journal, 313,* 1448–1449.

Yancik, R. (1997). Cancer burden in the aged: An epidemiologic and demographic overview. *Cancer, 80,* 1273–1283.

SECTION II.

....

Protocol Development

CHAPTER 2
Assurances

Joan Westendorp, RN, MSN, OCN®

Introduction

The protection of human subjects is extremely important to organizations involved in clinical research and the entire research enterprise. Every institution engaged in human subjects research has a responsibility to protect the participants. Federal regulations and policies are in place to protect participants' safety and privacy. Organizations conducting clinical research may handle human research protection differently. All institutions should have policies in place for human research protection; however, some may have a department that develops and conducts quality improvement activities to improve human research protection programs, establishes a human research protections program, coordinates conferences focusing on issues in human subjects protection, or responds to requests for clarification and guidance regarding ethical issues within the institution. Whether the institution is small or large and has many items in place for human subjects protection, every institution must be aware of and adhere to these regulations and policies.

Office for Human Research Protections

The Office for Human Research Protections (OHRP), formerly known as the Office for Protection from Research Risks (OPRR), is an administrative unit within the U.S. Department of Health and Human Services (DHHS). OHRP is physically located in Bethesda, MD, and is organizationally located in the Office of Public Health and Science, under the direction of the Assistant Secretary for Health (ASH). The ASH serves as the primary adviser to the Secretary of the DHHS on matters involving the nation's public health and oversees the DHHS's Public Health Service.

OHRP supports, strengthens, and provides leadership to the United States' system for protecting participants in research conducted or supported by DHHS. To accomplish this, OHRP provides clarification and guidance to research institutions, develops educational programs and materials, and promotes innovative approaches to enhancing human subject protections. It helps to ensure that such research is carried out in accordance with the highest ethical standards and in an environment where all who are involved in the conduct or oversight of human subjects research understand their primary responsibility for protecting the rights, welfare, and well-being of subjects. OHRP is able to ensure the highest ethical standards by developing and enforcing laws and regulations that govern the protection of human subjects. The four goals of the OHRP are depicted in Figure 2-1.

Figure 2-1. Goals of the Office for Human Research Protections

1. Establish criteria for—and approve assurances of—compliance for the protection of human subjects with institutions engaged in Department of Health and Human Services (DHHS)-conducted or DHHS-supported human subjects research.
2. Provide clarification and guidance on involving humans in research.
3. Develop and implement educational programs and resource materials.
4. Promote the development of approaches to enhance human subject protections.

Note. Based on information from Office for Human Research Protections, 2005.

Historical Development of the Office for Human Research Protections

From 1966 until 1974, DHHS operated according to the Policies for the Protection of Human Subjects issued by what is now the OHRP. On May 30, 1974, these policies were upgraded to regulations for the protection of human subjects. The Public Health Service Act (Title IV, Part G, Section 491[a]) regulated the policies for the protection of human subjects. This regulation was codified at Title 45, Part 46 of the *Code of Federal Regulations.* It is, therefore, called 45 CFR 46 (see Appendix 5).

On July 12, 1974, the National Research Act (Public Law 93-348) was signed into law as part of 45 CFR 46. This led to the creation of the National Commission for the Protection of Human Subjects of Biomedical and Behavioral Research. This act challenged the newly formed commission to regulate any entity with a grant or contract involving the conduct of biomedical or behavioral research involving human subjects, and it also required such agencies to establish an institutional review board (IRB) and comply with ethical issues in research (OPRR, 1992, 1993, 1998).

The area of ethical issues in research had not been addressed before; therefore, the first item on the agenda for the commission was to identify the basic ethical principles that should underlie the conduct of biomedical and behavioral research involving human subjects. In addition, the commission was to recommend steps for improving 45 CFR 46 and for ensuring that such research complies with the ethical principles of the act.

In 1979, the commission issued its "Ethical Principles and Guidelines for Protection of Human Subjects of Research," also known as the Belmont Report (see Appendix 4). The Belmont Report identified three basic principles of ethics that are particularly relevant to the protection of human participants in biomedical and behavioral research: respect for persons, beneficence, and justice (see Table 2-1).

Table 2-1. Definitions of the Principles of Ethics	
Principle of Ethics	**Definition**
Respect for persons	Recognition of personal dignity and autonomy of individuals and special protection of those with diminished autonomy
Beneficence	Obligation to protect individuals from harm by maximizing unanticipated benefits and minimizing possible risk of harm
Justice	Fairness in the distribution of research benefits and burdens

Roles of the Office for Human Research Protections

Compliance

The OHRP's Division of Compliance Oversight evaluates all written substantive allegations or indications of noncompliance with DHHS regulations. The relevant institution is notified of the allegation and is asked to investigate the basis for the complaint. The institution then must provide a written report of its investigation, along with relevant IRB and research records, to OHRP. OHRP subsequently determines what, if any, regulatory action needs to be taken.

Education

The OHRP's Division of Education and Development provides guidance to individuals and institutions involved in conducting DHHS-supported human subject research. Assistance is provided to IRB members and staff, as well as to scientists and research administrators, on the complex ethical and regulatory issues relating to human subject protections in medical and behavioral research. The division conducts national and regional educational workshops and conferences, participates in professional, academic, and association conferences, and develops and distributes resource materials in an effort to improve protections for research participants. OHRP also helps institutions to assess and improve their human research protection programs through quality improvement consultations.

Policy and Assurances

The OHRP's Division of Policy and Assurances prepares policies and guidance documents, and interpretations thereof, on human subject protections and disseminates this information to the research community. In addition, every institution engaged in human subject research conducted or supported by DHHS must obtain an assurance of compliance approved by OHRP. However, federal rules and regulations still apply to all other work with human subjects (e.g., pharmaceutical industry research).

Assurance Document

Any institution engaged in federally conducted or supported human subject research must commit itself in writing to the protection of those subjects. This written commitment is called an assurance of compliance. For human subject research conducted or supported by DHHS, an institution's assurance must be approved before the funds can be awarded and research can begin. An institution is engaged in human subject research whenever (a) the institution's employees or agents intervene or interact with human subjects for research purposes, (b) the institution's employees or agents obtain individually identifiable private information about human subjects for research purposes, or (c) the institution receives a direct DHHS award to conduct human subject research, even if all activities involving human subjects are carried out by a subcontractor or collaborator (DHHS, 2005b). The awarded institution bears the ultimate responsibility for protecting subjects involved in research conducted under the award. Seeking or obtaining informed consent from a research participant also is considered engagement in research (DHHS, 2005a).

Assurance of Compliance

In 2005, OHRP revised its assurance program and replaced the previous assurance types (see Table 2-2) with federalwide assurance (FWA). FWA is the only type of assurance accepted for review and approval by OHRP as of January 1, 2006 (see Appendix 7). Each legally distinct entity that is engaged in federally supported human subjects research must file its own separate assurance.

Table 2-2. Previous Assurance Types	
Assurance Types	**Description**
Multiple project assurance (MPA)	Covers multiple research projects. Department of Health and Human Services (DHHS)-conducted or DHHS-funded research at institutions with an MPA-type assurance may be reviewed by the approved institutional review board (IRB) at the MPA site without the further involvement of the Office for Human Research Protections (OHRP).
Cooperative project assurance (CPA)	Used with OHRP-recognized Cooperative Protocol Research Program activities. These protocols, conducted or sponsored by DHHS, are approved and monitored by DHHS Protocol Review Committees that are recognized by OHPR as satisfactorily addressing the quality of human subject protection. Participation in other federally supported research involving human subjects requires a separate assurance of compliance.
Single project assurance (SPA)	Limited to an individual research activity. A SPA institution usually relies on its own IRB. A modification to a standard SPA may be used when an institution utilizes the IRB of a neighboring co-participating institution that either has an MPA from OHRP, an OHRP-approved SPA, or another applicable assurance for a given project. The modified SPA requires signatures by the IRB chair and officials of both institutions. Use of this type of assurance requires careful prior review of the underlying circumstances and approval by OHRP before preparation and submission to OHRP.
Interinstitutional agreement	May be considered for an affiliated performance site where employees of an institution with an MPA routinely conduct their DHHS research at a neighboring affiliated institution. This mechanism avoids the need for a SPA for each separate project performed at such sites by employees of the MPA institution.
Noninstitutional investigator assurance	Used when a performance site involves no institution. If research investigators or physicians accrue patients into DHHS-funded or DHHS-conducted research in their private offices, they are nevertheless responsible for the protection of human research subjects under their control (Office for Protection from Research Risks, 1983). Therefore, they are required to assure DHHS of their compliance with the terms of 45 CFR 46 and the Belmont Report. If investigators are covered under a CPA but accrue subjects in their private offices, they must obtain a noninstitutional investigator assurance in cooperation with the local institution used for IRB review.
Note. Based on information from Office for the Protection from Research Risks, 1998.	

Obtaining FWA is a two-step process for institutions. The first step is that the institution filing an assurance must designate one or more institutional review boards (IRBs) that have registered with and provided a membership roster to the DHHS to be responsible for oversight of the research conducted under the assurance. Institutions can register the necessary IRB with DHHS and OHRP by going to the OHRP's IRB registration and assurance Web site (www.hhs. gov/ohrp/assurances/index.html) and completing the IRB registration form. Within three to five days, the applicant can check the OHRP's IRB registration listings to verify that the application has been processed.

The second step is the completion of the FWA application. The form can be found on the OHRP Web site at www. hhs.gov/ohrp/assurances/assurances_index.html. Before completing the application, the institution must designate individuals who will serve as the human protections administrator (HPA) and the signatory official. The HPA is the primary contact person for human subjects protection issues and exercises operational responsibility for the institution's program for protecting human research participants. The HPA should have comprehensive knowledge of all aspects of the institution's system of these protections and should be familiar with the institution's commitments under the FWA. The HPA plays a key role in ensuring that the institution fulfills its responsibilities under the FWA. The signatory official must be a senior institutional official who has the authority to commit the entire institution, as well as all of the institutional components listed, to a legally binding agreement. This individual also must have the authority to ensure compliance of the institution and all of its components with the terms of assurance. Generally, this is someone at the level of president or chief executive officer, unless another official has been specifically delegated this authority. The IRB chair or IRB members are not appropriate personnel to serve as the signatory official.

Once an FWA application is completed and submitted, the receipt of the form can be tracked on the OHRP Web site at http://ohrp.cit.nih.gov/search/logqry.asp. The information regarding when it was received, in addition to which assurance coordinator is reviewing it and how to contact that person, is available on this site. When the FWA is approved, the submitter, the human protections administrator, and the signatory official will receive an automatically generated e-mail informing them of FWA approval.

In an FWA, an institution commits to DHHS that it will comply with the requirements set forth in 45 CFR 46 (see Appendix 5), as well as the terms of assurance (see Figure 2-2). The FWA is effective for three years and must be renewed at the end of that period in order to remain effective.

Figure 2-2. Key Components of the Federalwide Assurance (FWA)

- The identifying information for the institution filing the FWA, the human protections administrator (or a reliable point of contact) at the institution, and the institutional official signing the FWA
- A list of the institution's legal components where human subjects research will be conducted (Legal components are generally defined as parts of the institution that may be viewed as separate organizations but remain part of the legal entity or institution.)
- A statement of ethical principles to be followed in protecting human subjects of research
- An applicability statement indicating that the institution commits to comply with the terms of the FWA for institutions within the United States for all federally conducted or supported human subject research covered by the FWA
- The designation of one or more institutional review boards that will review the research covered by the FWA (These boards must be registered with the Office for Human Research Protections before the FWA can be approved.)
- The signature of an official authorized to represent the institution

Note. Based on information from Office for Human Research Protections, 2005.

If the FWA information on record with OHRP needs to be altered, those alterations should be submitted within 90 days of the change. Updates of the FWA using the electronic submission system do not automatically renew the FWA for another three years. The FWA must be fully completed and updated and submitted in hard copy to renew the FWA for another three years, whereas limited updates (i.e., if the FWA is partially updated) submitted in hard copy will not alter the FWA expiration date (DHHS, 2005a).

Once an institution has an approved FWA, all employees and agents of the institution are covered whenever they are involved in the conduct of research defined by the FWA. Employees and agents, including students, are individuals performing institutionally designated activities and acting on behalf of the institution or exercising institutional authority or responsibility. An institution holding an OHRP-approved FWA may extend the applicability of its FWA to cover two types of collaborating individual investigators: collaborating independent investigators and collaborating institutional investigators.

A collaborating independent investigator is (a) not otherwise an employee or agent of the assured institution, (b) conducting collaborative research activities outside the facilities of the assured institution, and (c) not acting as an employee of any institution with respect to his or her involvement in the research being conducted by the assured institution.

A collaborating institutional investigator is (a) not otherwise an employee or agent of the assured institution, (b) conducting collaborative research activities outside the facilities of the assured institution, or (c) acting as an employee or agent of an institution that does not hold an OHRP-approved FWA with respect to his

or her involvement in the research being conducted by the assured institution and does not routinely conduct human subject research (DHHS, 2005a). The extension of an assured institution's FWA to cover a collaborating individual investigator should be documented using an individual investigator agreement (see Appendix 9). This agreement can be found at www.hhs.gov/ohrp/humansubjects/assurance/guidanceonalternativetofwa.htm.

Summary

Research involving human subjects is essential to finding the best treatments and cures for diseases. DHHS and OHRP mandate and monitor federal regulations and policies to protect the safety and privacy of research participants. Assurance of compliance is a vital part of the research process. OHRP is available to answer questions concerning the protection of human participants as well as compliance with policies and applicable OHRP regulations. More information is available at OHRP's Web site, www.hhs.gov/ohrp/about.

Clinical trial nurses (CTNs) should be concerned about the safety and privacy of research participants, but what does assurance of compliance have to do with CTNs, as this is an institutional issue and not part of a CTN's day-to-day operations? CTNs are well aware of the type of research being conducted, whether pharmaceutical or DHHS funded; therefore, the CTNs need to be aware of the necessary compliance with regulations in order to be mediators for human subjects. At some smaller institutions, the responsibility of one of the CTNs is to be the human protections administrator of the assurance of compliance. If this is the situation, the CTN must have an in-depth knowledge of the institution's compliance program. It is essential for all CTNs to have knowledge of the OHRP and FWA to assist them in the overall picture of what is involved with the protection of human subjects, beyond informed consent.

References

Office for Human Research Protections. (2005). *About the Office for Human Research Protections.* Retrieved October 30, 2005, from http://www.hhs.gov/ohrp/about/

Office for Protection from Research Risks. (1983). *Code of federal regulations* (Title 45, Vol. 1, Part 46). Washington, DC: U.S. Government Printing Office.

Office for Protection from Research Risks. (1992). *Sample human subjects assurance.* Washington, DC: U.S. Government Printing Office.

Office for Protection from Research Risks. (1993). *Cooperative project assurance information packet.* Washington, DC: U.S. Government Printing Office.

Office for Protection from Research Risks. (1998). *Answers to questions concerning protection of human subjects when involved in clinical trials research.* Washington, DC: U.S. Government Printing Office.

U.S. Department of Health and Human Services. (2005a). *Questions and answers.* Retrieved October 22, 2005, from http://answers.hhs.gov/

U.S. Department of Health and Human Services. (2005b). *Step-by-step instructions for filing a federalwide assurance for institutions within the United States.* Retrieved October 10, 2005, from http://www.hhs.gov/ohrp/humansubjects/assurance/filasuri.htm

CHAPTER 3
Elements of a Protocol

Angela D. Klimaszewski, RN, MSN

Introduction

During the past two decades, emerging technologies have unleashed almost unbelievable discoveries in medicine. For example, animals have been cloned, the human genome has been mapped, and, in 2006, the U.S. Food and Drug Administration (FDA) approved the first vaccine to prevent cancer, Gardasil® (Merck & Co., Inc.) (FDA, 2006). The speed with which we are moving into a new age of discovery has resulted in the formulation of numerous highly sophisticated clinical trials. For clinical trial nurses (CTNs), this translates into scientific studies with more complex and comprehensive protocol documents. Understanding the essential elements of the protocol document is more critical than ever before. This chapter will identify and discuss those elements and how they relate to the daily practice of CTNs.

The Protocol

A protocol is a formal document that delineates specific actions to be taken to protect participants while answering one or more research questions and maintaining the scientific integrity of the clinical trial (McCabe, 2005). It is viewed as the "written agreement between the investigator, the subject, and the scientific community" (Friedman, Furberg, & DeMets, 1985, p. 7). To ensure consistency and enable communication among those working on the clinical trial, the same protocol is used at every participating site (National Cancer Institute [NCI], 2005). Execution of the same protocol also allows for the data from multiple sites to "be combined and compared" (NCI, p. 23).

Every protocol has common or essential elements (see Figure 3-1). Protocol templates contain these essential elements and are used within a particular class of studies. For example, NCI's Cancer Therapy Evaluation Program (CTEP) has links from its "Guidelines and Tools for Protocol Development" Web site (http://ctep.cancer.gov/guidelines) to the following items (NCI CTEP, 2006).

- Phase I and II templates (single and multiple drug)

- Phase III template (single and multiple drug)
- Organ dysfunction templates
- Protocol submission worksheet, version 4.3
- CTEP amendment requests
- Treatment assignment instructions and guidelines

Similarly, NCI's Division of Cancer Prevention (n.d.) offers chemoprevention protocol template instructions in the "Consortia" section of its Web site. To view these, go to http://prevention.cancer.gov/clinicaltrials/management/pio/instructions and select "DCP Consortia Protocol Template" to bring up the instructions.

These templates and applications enable investigators to easily insert research specifics into a protocol template. Template instructions are detailed and provide telephone, e-mail, and fax contact information to reach the CTEP help desk. NCI's *Investigator Handbook: Manual for Participants in Clinical Trials of Investigational Agents Sponsored by DCTD,*

Figure 3-1. Protocol Elements Required by the U.S. Food and Drug Administration

- General information
- Background information (with relevant references from the scientific literature)
- Trial objectives and purpose
- Trial design
- Participant selection and withdrawal
- Participant treatment
- Efficacy assessment
- Safety assessment
- Statistics
- Direct access to source data and documents
- Quality control and quality assurance
- Ethics
- Data handling and recordkeeping
- Financing and insurance
- Publication policy
- Supplements

Note. From *The Federal Register* [Electronic version], by the U.S. Food and Drug Administration, 1997. Retrieved June 1, 2006, from http://www.fda.gov/cder/guidance/iche6.htm

---

NCI encourages the use of a protocol template to facilitate rapid review when the protocol is submitted (NCI CTEP, 2002).

NCI (2005) identified six types of clinical trials, including prevention trials, screening trials, diagnostic trials, treatment trials (including adjuvant or neoadjuvant trials), quality-of-life or supportive care trials, and genetics trials. Every trial has a unique protocol with detailed essential elements. Each of the FDA essential protocol elements will now be described briefly.

Essential Elements

The *general information* section of the protocol contains the information found on the face sheet and the following one to two pages. It presents the title of the protocol with an identifying number (and cooperative group letters, if applicable) and the date. The identification number, the corresponding cooperative group letters, and the date should be clearly documented on all protocol amendments. The name, title (if applicable), address, and phone numbers of key individuals and departments are presented, including the investigator conducting the trial, the physician responsible for all of the trial site–related medical decisions, and, if applicable, the sponsor, nurse contact, and monitor. Names and addresses of clinical laboratories or other technical departments or institutions also are noted in this section (FDA, 1997a).

The *background* section of the protocol includes sufficient background information so that the rationale of the study is clear (NCI CTEP, 2002). This section includes the name and a description of the investigational product(s), findings from nonclinical studies and unpublished data that might have clinical significance, and a summary of both known and potential risks and benefits to human subjects. A description and justification of the treatment(s)—radiation, surgery, or drug therapy, the route of administration, dosage, dosage regimen, and treatment periods—are presented in the background section, as well.

A statement that the trial will be conducted in compliance with the protocol, good clinical practice guidelines (FDA, 1997a), and all regulatory requirements also should be included. A brief description of the population to be studied and references to relevant literature are both presented in the background section (FDA, 1997b; NCI CTEP, 2002). The reader is referred to Chapter 45 for additional information.

The *trial objectives and purpose* section has a detailed description of the primary and complementary objectives, including hypotheses to be tested and the purpose of the trial. CTEP (NCI CTEP, 2002) includes the statistical section here, whereas the FDA advises that statistics be written later in the protocol document. See Chapter 6 for a more complete look at trial objectives.

The *trial design* section determines the scientific integrity of the study and the credibility of the data (FDA, 1997b). Trial design includes primary and secondary end points to be measured, a description of the type of trial to be conducted, and a schema of the trial design, procedures, and stages. In this section, the steps taken to avoid bias, such as randomization and blinding, are explained. If investigational agents are to be used, a description of the trial treatments, dosage and dosage regimen, dosage form, packaging, and labeling of the investigational product(s) must be included (FDA, 1997b).

Details include an explanation of the expected length of time that participants will be on study. Participant time required for follow-up and a description of the discontinuation criteria are delineated, as well. This section explains the accountability for storage of the investigational products, the method of maintaining randomization codes, and the procedure for breaking codes if the trial is to be blinded (FDA, 1997a, 1997b; NCI CTEP, 2002).

Also included in the trial design section of the protocol is a specific list of any data that are to be recorded on case report forms and any data that are to be considered as source data (FDA, 1997b). See Chapters 6 and 37 for additional information on statistical considerations and long-term follow-up, respectively.

The next section, *selection and withdrawal of subjects,* identifies inclusion, exclusion, off-study, and withdrawal criteria. Participant withdrawal criteria must include specific procedures regarding when and how to withdraw participants, type and timing of data to be collected and follow-up for withdrawn participants, and whether and how participants are to be replaced (FDA, 1997a, 1997b; Melink & Whitacre, 1991; NCI CTEP, 2002). See Chapter 22 for a more in-depth discussion.

Treatment of subjects provides a detailed description of the products used in the trial, including treatment and follow-up periods for the participant. This includes names of all investigational agents, as well as doses and dosing schedules (FDA, 1997b). The following topics are found in this section of a protocol (FDA, 1997a; NCI CTEP, 2002).

- Storage requirements (see Chapter 49)
- Stability
- Route of administration
- Toxicities and dose modification criteria for each study drug (see Chapter 28)
- Medications permitted for patients to use and those not permitted
- Procedures to monitor patient compliance (see Chapter 30)

For surgery and radiation therapy, this section presents detailed explanations of devices or procedures.

The procedure for entering a participant on study, including a description of the randomization process, patient characteristics, and stratification factors, is provided in the treatment of subjects section.

Assessment of efficacy describes the criteria for scoring responses for both measurable and evaluable disease. In this section, if disease-specific criteria are required, the required method of tumor measurement, such as scans, must be indicated. Additionally, the timing (schedule) for assessing, recording, and analyzing efficacy parameters must be clearly identified (FDA, 1997a, 1997b; NCI CTEP, 2002). Time measures for responses, including time to event comments, time to progression, and survival, also will be delineated in the assessment of efficacy. See Chapter 6 for additional information.

The *assessment of safety* section specifies the safety parameters along with the methods and timing for assessing, recording, and analyzing them (FDA, 1997b). The plan of dose change for adverse events must be clearly stated for *each* study agent. The current version of the NCI Common Terminology Criteria for Adverse Events (CTCAE) should be used to evaluate toxicities unless otherwise specified. Procedures for reporting and recording adverse events are explained in this section, as well as post-treatment follow-up for participants who experience adverse events (FDA, 1997a; NCI CTEP, 2002). Chapter 28 presents a more thorough review of the topic of adverse events.

The *statistical considerations* section of a protocol presents a description of the statistical methods used as well as the schedule for any interim analysis. Specific statistical elements of a protocol are detailed in Figure 3-2. In multi-center trials, the number of enrolled subjects projected for each trial site may be specified. See Chapter 6 for a comprehensive presentation of clinical trial statistics.

The section titled *source documents* identifies the document type, file location, and schema of filing for each of the following: on-study information including participant

---

Figure 3-2. Statistical Elements of a Protocol

- Method of randomization and stratification
- Total sample size justified for adequate testing of primary and secondary hypotheses
- Error levels (alpha and beta) in phase III studies
- Differences to be detected for comparative studies
- Size of the confidence interval to be constructed around the estimated outcome
- Estimated accrual rate and/or study duration, with supporting documentation
- Stopping guidelines, including statistical and administrative procedures for monitoring the progress of the trial to implement early termination for positive results, or for results sufficiently negative to preclude the eventual achievement of statistically significant positive results
- Expected outcome parameters as appropriate (response rate, time to progression, survival times)
- Primary end point for interim and final analysis
- Clear specification of primary and secondary hypotheses
- Maximum number of patients
- Plan for analysis

Note. From "The Drafting of a Protocol" (pp. 24–25), by the National Cancer Institute Cancer Therapy Evaluation Program, 2002, in *The Investigator's Handbook: A Manual for Participants in Clinical Trials of Investigational Agents Sponsored by DCTD, NCI.* Retrieved July 12, 2007, from http://ctep.cancer.gov/handbook/hndbk_toc.html

---

eligibility data and participant history, flow sheets, specialty forms for pathology, radiation, or surgery, and an off-study summary sheet that includes a final assessment by the treating physician. Also included in this section is a statement that specifies agreement by the investigators to permit trial-related monitoring, audits, institutional review board review, and regulatory inspections that include direct access to data and source documents (FDA, 1997a, 1997b; NCI CTEP, 2002). The reader is referred to Sections IX and X of this manual for additional information.

The *quality control and quality assurance* measures provide a description of the prospective monitoring system built into the study. The system is designed to assess completeness and accuracy of everything from the qualifications of the investigator-physician to specific dates to submit forms (FDA, 1997a; NCI CTEP, 2002).

The *ethics* section addresses the ethical considerations and regulatory issues associated with the trial (FDA, 1997a). This section includes a protocol-specific informed consent document that contains the elements required by federal regulation (see Chapter 14). Because of the importance of the informed consent process, an additional separate section may be included to solely address informed consent. The ethics section also may include compliance issues, patients lost to follow-up, early discontinuation of the trial, medical emergencies, confidentiality of data, and who at the institution will address any ethical concerns raised about the study.

The *data handling and recordkeeping* content presents an explanation of electronic data transmission and the accompanying security measures employed to ensure confidentiality. See Section IX of this manual for a more in-depth discussion.

Financing and insurance issues, if not addressed in a separate document, are presented next. The study sponsor and any external funding for the study should be identified here. Plans by the sponsor or investigator to pay stipends to patients or institutions on a "per patient" basis should be clearly delineated (FDA, 1997b).

A statement regarding the *publication policy* for the abstracts, papers, reports, and other publications that result from the study should be included in the protocol. This is particularly important in multicenter trials, where many investigators, coinvestigators, CTNs, statisticians, pharmacists, and data managers are involved. See Chapter 18 for more detailed information on publication and author guidelines.

The last section contains any *supplements,* including the informed consent form, documents addressing multicenter logistics issues, and any appendices.

Future Directions

Sheible (2006) stated that "the clinical network model has begun a transformation to a more centralized approach with e-Clinical processes" because of "market changes;

demands for better access to more cutting-edge therapies at lower costs; shrinking research and development budgets; increasing regulatory requirements leading to larger, longer trials; and the impact of an aging population" (p. 709). Noting that the virtual revolution is upon us, Sheible cited as proof the efficiency gains of e-clinical tools, such as virtual training via webcast, secure Web sites for document delivery, and e-data capturing systems that "allow for centralized monitoring and more rapid data access and review" (p. 712). Ultimately, we have just scratched the surface of where research networks can go.

Advances in information and communication technology (ICT) may make it possible in the future for clinical trial design to be based on the interoperability of each single task in the clinical trial process (Fazi et al., 2006). The development of an ICT system that standardizes data exchange between stages of a clinical trial and manages and automates the entire process at multiple sites may be on the horizon. Such a system would "enable organizational interoperability by defining a virtual community of organizations playing roles such as clinical trial coordinator, participant center, etc." (Fazi et al., p. 4). The future of clinical trials design may begin by standardizing tasks internationally and then evolve into universal software that allows for unlimited resources to support patients and advance medicine.

Summary

Creating clearly organized protocol documents can be a monumental task. Using a multidisciplinary approach to creating a protocol helps to ensure that an expert in each area addresses all sections. The protocol document will be used daily by members of many disciplines, including but not limited to investigators, CTNs, pharmacists, data managers, and staff nurses. CTNs generally are afforded the opportunity to contribute to the study design and conduct through analysis, scientific presentation, and publication. The greater the involvement of the CTN in the design of a clinical trial protocol, the greater the likelihood that he or she will know the subtleties and nuances of it. CTNs working with today's complex and comprehensive studies ensure superior patient treatment and high-quality clinical trials through their knowledge of the protocol document.

References

Fazi, P., Ali, L.C., Luzi, D., Ricci, F.L., Serbanati, L.D., & Vignetti, M. (2006, January 1). A proposed clinical trial model: Analyzing the CT process. *Applied Clinical Trials.* Retrieved June 28, 2006, from http://www.actmagazine.com/appliedclinicaltrials/content/printContentPopup.jsp?id=283029

Friedman, L.M., Furberg, C.D., & DeMets, D.L. (1985). Introduction to clinical trials. In L.M. Friedman, C.D. Furberg, & D.L. DeMets (Eds.), *Fundamentals of clinical trials* (2nd ed., pp. 1–10). St. Louis, MO: Mosby.

McCabe, M. (2005). Principles of clinical research and development. In C.H. Yarbro, M.H. Frogge, & M. Goodman (Eds.), *Cancer nursing: Principles and practice* (6th ed., pp. 201–211). Sudbury, MA: Jones and Bartlett.

Melink, T.J., & Whitacre, M.Y. (1991). Planning and implementing clinical trials. *Seminars in Oncology Nursing, 7,* 243–251.

National Cancer Institute. (2005). *Cancer clinical trials: The in-depth program* [NIH Publication No. 05-5051]. Bethesda, MD: Author.

National Cancer Institute Cancer Therapy Evaluation Program. (2002). *The investigator's handbook: A manual for participants in clinical trials of investigational agents sponsored by DCTD, NCI.* Retrieved July 5, 2006, from http://ctep.cancer.gov/forms/Hndbk.pdf

National Cancer Institute Cancer Therapy Evaluation Program. (2006). *Guidelines and tools for protocol development.* Retrieved June 1, 2006, from http://ctep.cancer.gov/guidelines

National Cancer Institute Division of Cancer Prevention. (n.d.). *Instructions, templates and forms.* Retrieved October 17, 2007, from http://prevention.cancer.gov/clinicaltrials/management/pio/instructions

Scheible, L.S. (2006). The clinical network: A different approach. *Community Oncology, 3,* 709–712.

U.S. Food and Drug Administration. (1997a). *Federal register, Vol. 62, No. 90* [Electronic version]. Retrieved June 1, 2006, from http://www.fda.gov/cder/guidance/iche6.htm

U.S. Food and Drug Administration. (1997b). *Good clinical practice: Consolidated guideline.* Rockville, MD: U.S. Government Printing Office.

U.S. Food and Drug Administration. (2006, June 8). *FDA licenses new vaccine for prevention of cervical cancer and other diseases in females caused by human papillomavirus* [FDA news release P06-77]. Retrieved June 10, 2006, from http://www.fda.gov/bbs/topics/NEWS/2006/NEW01385.html

CHAPTER 4
Workload Determination and Resource Allocation

Clement K. Gwede, PhD, MPH, RN

Introduction

As the clinical research profession continues to grow, little published and validated information is available to guide research administrators on key issues, such as
- Assignment of studies to clinical research coordinators (CRCs)
- Appropriate coordinator-to-study ratios
- Appropriate patient-to-coordinator ratios
- Determining the cost of doing clinical trial "work," and
- Determining the most efficient staff mix to maximize clinical trial productivity and cost-effectiveness.

These fundamental questions remain unanswered despite recent interest in the topic. Many in the field continue to ponder very basic workload questions:
- How many clinical trial protocols can each coordinator handle?
- How many patients can each coordinator handle?
- How many coordinators does it take?
- How busy is coordinator A versus coordinators B or C?
- At what point should a coordinator be provided with ancillary resources?

The universal answer to these questions is, "It depends." Recognizing that both clinical trial workload measurement and resource allocation are monumental, volatile issues, this chapter seeks only to highlight and summarize selected aspects of these topics and to suggest solutions for managing workload and resources in an ever-changing landscape. Perhaps the synthesis provided here will inform the novice as well as the expert clinical research professional and administrator.

Factors Affecting Workload Determination and Resource Allocation

Factors that affect workload determination and resource allocation include but are not limited to

- The research personnel and organization of clinical research services in a research center (Gwede, Johnson, & Daniels, 2001; Gwede, Johnson, & Trotti, 2000a, 2000b)
- The type (sponsor or clinical phase [i.e., I, II, III, IV]) and acuity or complexity of protocols involved (Fowler & Thomas, 2003; Gwede et al., 2000a, 2000b; Roche et al., 2002)
- The actual time it takes to do the work (Fowell & Wilson, 2002; Fowler & Thomas, 2003; Roche et al., 2002)
- Associated costs (Chirikos, 2003; Emanuel, Schnipper, Kamin, Levinson, & Lichter, 2003; Johnson, 2003).

Thus, determining the workload and resources needed for clinical trial management can be a challenging task. The CRC provides cohesiveness that holds together the clinical trial process. As the total number of cancer cases is expected to double by 2050 if current incidence rates remain stable (Edwards et al., 2002), and given projections that by 2030 one in five Americans will be 65 years or older (Yancik, 1997; Yancik & Ries, 2004), increased representation of older adults in clinical trials is an important consideration for CRCs. More importantly, having adequate resources to coordinate their care in trials is paramount.

Over the past decade, many models for managing clinical trials have been developed, including a variety of administrative and organizational structures (Gwede et al., 2001), as well as an evolving and increasingly delineated role of CRCs (Ehrenberger & Lillington, 2004). Specifically, numerous distinct clinical trial tasks have been identified, and the expansive scope of the work of CRCs is now better understood (Devine, Nagel, Benson, & Krailo, 2005; Fowler & Thomas, 2003; Gwede et al., 2000a, 2000b; Roche et al., 2002).

The work of CRCs involves wide-ranging responsibilities, including regulatory processing, contracts management, patient accrual and monitoring, collection and

The author would like to acknowledge Carol L. Verderese, RN, MS, and Suzanne Fioravanti, RN, BSN, OCN®, for their contribution that remains unchanged from the first edition.

processing of research specimens, dispensing of study drugs, data collection and management, auditing, and billing, as detailed later. As a result, new CRC roles/positions, such as regulatory specialist, clinical trial nurse, data manager, specimen processing specialist, and clinical trial pharmacist, have emerged and are evolving in research centers. A critical mix of multidisciplinary personnel now exists to cover the different facets and many responsibilities of CRCs. Yet, despite these developments, many CRCs remain burdened by the vast scope of work required of them, as they sometimes feel as though they have to "do it all."

With regard to quantitative, objective workload measurement and determination, no precise reliable, valid, and universally accepted tools are available, and numerous challenges remain largely unresolved (Gwede et al., 2000a, 2000b, 2001; Roche et al., 2002). Table 4-1 summarizes selected studies aimed at addressing clinical trial workload measurement tools.

Workload determination and resource allocation are cornerstone issues in defining a profession. They are directly related to productivity, quality, and satisfaction—all important values for patients, CRCs, employers and managers, and study sponsors who have a financial stake in successful clinical trial management.

Key Lessons Learned About Workload Measurement

Many lessons about clinical trial workload determination have been documented elsewhere (Fowler & Thomas, 2003; Gwede et al., 2000a, 2000b; Neuer, 2002). Three lessons that are most relevant as background for resource planning and allocation are summarized here.
1. The workload of CRCs continues to increase.
2. Measuring the actual work (task times) rather than number of patients or protocols managed by a CRC seems to be the better approach.
3. One size does not fit all—customized approaches that take the local realities into consideration are needed.

First, the workload of CRCs, as determined by crude measures such as the number of clinical trials or the number of patients actively managed by a single CRC, is increasing annually (Fowler & Thomas, 2003; Gwede et al., 2000a, 2000b; Neuer, 2002). Reasons for this include increasing costs of conducting clinical research, a growing trend in health care to do more work with fewer resources, and the growing recognition that more patient participation in clinical trials improves quality of care—hence, many healthcare organizations seek to increase the number of patients participating in clinical trials (West, Wright, Tuffnell, Jankowicz, & West, 2005).

However, given the increasing responsibilities of CRCs and the decreasing time allotted to complete them, mounting professional and social pressure creates a burden on CRCs. One recent study demonstrated that some CRCs experience employment-related distress and burnout

(Gwede, Johnson, Roberts, & Cantor, 2005). Such distress may lead to coordinator turnover and loss of experienced personnel (Fowler & Thomas, 2003; Gwede et al., 2000a, 2000b; Neuer, 2002). Studies have found that the majority of CRCs have been in their current positions for less than three to five years (Gwede et al., 2000a, 2000b; Neuer). One analysis of CRCs (N = 500) found that 56% have been in their current positions for less than three years in 2002, compared to 40% in 1999 (Neuer). Although this change may reflect increased growth in the profession as well as staff turnover (Fowler & Thomas; Gwede et al., 2000a, 2000b; Neuer), it also demonstrates that the overall experience level of CRCs is declining. Consequently, the retention and training of clinical research staff is a paramount effort at investigative sites, and accurate determinations of workload with subsequent assignment of resources remain important priorities for the clinical research administrator.

Regarding the question "How much workload can one CRC handle?", the answer is that the measurement of CRC workload does not entail measuring merely the number of patients or protocols managed (Devine et al., 2005; Fowler & Thomas, 2003; Gwede et al., 2000a, 2000b; Roche et al., 2002). Rather, it is best to identify specific work tasks and determine how much time it takes to complete them. Once the tasks and times have been delineated (Devine et al.; Fowler & Thomas; Gwede et al., 2000a, 2000b; Roche et al.), the relevant costs and resources can be estimated and assigned. Two studies have addressed this issue directly (Fowler & Thomas; Roche et al.), but the findings are preliminary (see Tables 4-1 and 4-2) and have not been evaluated rigorously in the various clinical research settings.

The third lesson is that one size does not fit all. That is, it is not clear to what extent a system developed in one research center may be applicable (or adaptable) for use in other settings where research operations (i.e., organization, structure, and culture) and resources differ significantly. For example, can a protocol acuity system developed for a cardiology practice work as well in an oncology setting? What minimal adaptations are required to refine and validate the system across disciplines (e.g., adult oncology, pediatric oncology)?

Until the profession matures and uniform standards in role delineation, employment practices, and professional training are widely adopted, a need for customized approaches remains. Other qualitative solutions to match the structure and culture of each organization are needed. Administrators are faced with the challenge of how to create a sensible local solution that takes into account the many variables and realities of each center.

For example, staff mix and role delineation, type and phase of clinical trial protocols (i.e., industry sponsored, cooperative group, or locally authored trials), organization of the clinical research operations, and the institutional culture and mindset about clinical research participation on the part of investigators and treating physicians vary widely among centers across the United States. These factors are

Table 4-1. Selected Workload Studies in Clinical Trial Management

Author/Year	Purpose/Key Findings	Author Conclusions/Utility in Workload Management
Gwede et al., 2000a, 2000b	To report the number of patients enrolled by a typical clinical research coordinator (CRC) in a cooperative group and to identify factors associated with this measure of workload. Self-reported workload (number of patients) varied widely by CRC and type of study. Focusing on the "work" tasks is perhaps a better measure of workload than number of patients. No definitive workload formula was provided or recommended.	In the absence of reliable, valid, and universally accepted clinical trial workload measures, administrators must take a broader approach and focus on the time required to do tasks rather than the number of patients.
Gwede et al., 2001	To document the structure and organization of clinical research services and evaluate the impact on the workload of CRCs. Organization of clinical research services may account for efficiencies and productivity. Three primary data management models (centralized, decentralized, and mixed) were identified, and workload (number of patients) varied by data management model.	Within each of the three primary data management models, the challenges and determinants of workload vary. The data management model provides an all-important context and environmental milieu in which workload and resource utilization dynamics occur.
Roche et al., 2002	To measure time required to complete specific protocol tasks and identify factors associated with task times. Early-phase trials had longer task times than phase III trials, and industry-sponsored trials had longer task times than local or cooperative group studies. Task times were identified, but no definitive workload formula was provided or recommended.	The study showed the importance of consideration of sponsor type and study phase in estimating costs, workload, and resource allocation. A close examination of the time required for individual tasks may influence daily decisions about workload distribution among CRCs. Further research is needed to improve accuracy of time estimates.
Fowler & Thomas, 2003	To quantify protocol acuity and task times (workload threshold) based on actual coordinator time and activities in order to guide prospective staffing and budgetary decisions. Task times and acuity score were identified.	Each research center has to determine the acuity load for each coordinator or protocol. The preliminary tool presented here may be refined or adapted for other centers to generate a numbers-driven workload measurement system.
Devine et al., 2005	To determine what percentage of time CRCs spend on different work tasks. Results indicated that focusing on trial tasks rather than on enrollment numbers is the best approach. No definitive workload formula was provided or recommended.	For daily management, CRCs may be assigned based on appreciation of the tasks and percent effort required. This study informs role delineation to reduce scope of work.

important influences on both productivity and workload-related distress for CRCs (Fowler & Thomas, 2003; Gwede et al., 2000a, 2000b, 2001, 2005; Roche et al., 2002).

When a coordinator senses that his or her workload is increasing, few objective tools are available to help to quantify this situation and provide justification for additional resources. The workload is measured based on crude tools that do not capture the true intensity and scope of work. However, the literature has increased (from virtually none) since the 1990s—and research administrators are becoming cognizant of the discrepancy between the work and the workload measures. Although current efforts at identifying an objective clinical research workload measure are preliminary at best, there is incremental progress and promise (Fowler & Thomas, 2003; Gwede et al., 2000a, 2000b, 2001, 2005; Roche et al., 2002). Much like other professions, such as nursing, where workload and acuity measures and resource allocation systems continue to evolve and attract scrutiny (Jones, Cusack, & Chisholm, 2004; Rozich & Resar, 2002; Van Slyck, 1995; Walts & Kapadia, 1996), workload systems for clinical research will see much contention and

refinement. Even if a purely quantitative universal measure is not imminent, a practical, functional workload measurement approach that facilitates daily staffing decisions is conceivable based on the growing body of work.

Time- and Task-Based Workload Measurement Systems

How much time does it take to complete specific protocol tasks? Only a few studies have sought a direct answer to this question (Fowler & Thomas, 2003; Gwede et al., 2000a, 2000b, 2001, 2005; Roche et al., 2002). The conclusion from these studies is that a quantitative system for measuring workload is feasible, but the data are not ready for general use without careful adaptation. That is, the validity and general applicability of data in the various research settings has not been established. Hence, a specific "magic" number or formula is not provided in this chapter. Instead, readers can make their own assessment of the published data and adapt it to their own clinical setting (Fowler & Thomas; Gwede et al., 2000a, 2000b, 2001,

2005; Roche et al.). Table 4-2 summarizes key elements of published time- and task-based outcomes primarily to identify two quantitative workload measures: acuity score and task times (Fowler & Thomas; Roche et al.).

Table 4-2. Empirically Developed Task-Based Workload Measures

Author/ Year	Measure/ Tool	Possible Final Outcome Product	Possible Utility in Workload Management
Fowler & Thomas, 2003	a) Protocol acuity score b) Protocol task time estimates	Protocol acuity score Hours per task/patient/ protocol/coordinator	Prospective uses: • Budgeting • Comparison of individual studies or coordinator • Staff assignments Authors concluded: • Is a preliminary measure; may be adapted for different research centers.
Roche et al., 2002	Protocol task time estimates	Hours per task/patient/ protocol/coordinator	Prospective uses: • Budgeting • Comparison of individual studies or coordinator • Staff assignments • Staff role delineation Authors concluded: • Is a preliminary measure; task times are underestimates; needs further development to better and more accurately capture the true scope of work. Not yet ready for dissemination or wide application.

An important methodologic contribution is that these studies (Fowler & Thomas, 2003; Gwede et al., 2000a, 2000b, 2001, 2005; Roche et al., 2002) surveyed CRCs to identify actual work tasks and estimate the time it takes to do specific protocol tasks. Figure 4-1 summarizes the core work tasks identified in this literature.

Within these general or core work categories exist numerous time-intensive subtasks to be completed, which constitute an important part of the *actual* workload of CRCs. Although crude measures such as number of patients

or number of protocols managed by a CRC are important and commonly recognized outcomes, they are not entirely accurate or direct measures of workload—the actual work should be measured. Nevertheless, these tools are, in essence, good *measures of productivity*, and as such should be considered in the context of the time and resources needed to produce those outcomes. Validated and reliable estimates of the time and resources required to perform the broad protocol-directed tasks, and the many distinct subtasks, still are needed.

The implications of reliable protocol task time estimates are clear. As a new protocol is developed locally or received from an external sponsor, it is possible to outline the tasks involved in the specific protocol, estimate the time and costs, and budget for the appropriate level of resources (see Chapter 5). In principle, prospective cost estimating and resource planning is ideal, but practical challenges in funding, hiring, training, and retention of experienced research personnel still remain. When trained CRCs are not available for hiring, the workload will continue to increase. Limited personnel still are expected to manage the work and to meet compliance and quality standards. Moreover, patient accrual and budget projections may not be accurate, and an overestimation or underestimation of either or both elements will result in undesirable workload and resource imbalances. Thus, qualitative approaches for day-to-day management of workload burden will remain a meaningful alternative as we await a robust quantitative workload measure.

A Prospective Approach for Workload Determination and Resource Planning

Given the existing challenges, day-to-day resource allocation and management in a busy clinical research environment can be a monumental task to those inexperienced in the endeavor. As funding constraints have increased, more precise estimates of costs, as well as methods, to monitor productivity and effectiveness are needed (Bjornson-Benson et al., 1993; Coleman, 1995; Fowler & Thomas, 2003; Gwede et al., 2000a, 2000b, 2001; Roche et al., 2002).

Figure 4-1. Core Work Tasks of Clinical Research Coordinators

• Initial and continuing institutional review board regulatory processing
• Contracting, budgeting, and billing
• Patient eligibility screening, work-up, and enrollment
• Patient monitoring during active treatment and follow-up
• Study drug dispensing and accountability
• Research (lab) specimen processing
• Data collection/management and case report completion
• Administrative and other coordination activities
• Audit preparation and clarification of data

Note. Based on information from Fowler & Thomas, 2003; Gwede et al., 2000a, 2000b, 2001, 2005; Roche et al., 2002.

Several key variables must be considered when determining resource allocation. Variables such as the *phase of the trial* (i.e., I, II, III, or IV), the *type and stage of disease* being treated, and *anticipated complications* all must be evaluated before beginning the process of determining and allocating resources. Other less obvious factors, such as quality-of-life issues, life expectancy, ethical values, and online data entry versus data collection via case report forms, also must be considered.

Depending on the institution planning to conduct the trial, resource allocation can be calculated as presented in the next section. The information presented is intended to evoke ideas, lend suggestions, and provide a possible template for determining resource allocation in various clinical research settings. The key to this effort is recognizing the positive impact that protocol-directed resource planning and allocation has in an institution's capacity when an appropriate workload and resource analysis is completed before protocol implementation.

Protocol-Directed Resource Planning

To begin, formulate questions addressing the "who, what, when, and why" of performing the resource analysis and allocation. A thorough analysis of specific protocol tasks and appropriate knowledge of the institutional resources to be used are required before accurate protocol task-based costs are determined. Outlining the steps and procedures a patient would go through to complete the protocol is a natural way to break down the protocol into smaller tasks (see Figure 4-2).

The distinct subtasks then create a timeline of the life of the protocol, thereby identifying individual quantifiable events and frequency and duration of occurrence and providing a picture of the scope of work. This timeline can be divided into manageable segments of time, such as days, cycles, or admissions. Within a defined time frame, resources can be broken down by the department (or person) who will provide a specific service. This process culminates in a protocol budget and resource plan that will guide implementation of the project (Johnson, 2003). A protocol-based timeline or plan of work can be used to enhance the multidisciplinary approach to implementing a new clinical trial. Figure 4-3 lists questions to ask when designing a timeline.

Figure 4-2. A Basic Algorithm for Determining Resource Allocation

Written draft (or final) of clinical trial protocol
↓
Protocol reviewed by key investigator and research nurse
↓
Protocol reviewed by budget personnel
↓
Protocol resources analyzed
↓
Budget proposes cost estimates and resource allocation for institution.
↓
Principal investigator assesses projection.
↓
Modification of protocol, if needed
↓
Resource projections distributed to affected departments
↓
Multidisciplinary team meetings to review impact on departments
↓
Protocol implementation
↓
Protocol billing and collections
↓
Revenue recovery to departments performing the work

Figure 4-3. Questions to Ask When Designing a Timeline

- Does the protocol contain a table of assessments listing activities to be performed?
- Is there information to help understand how a patient goes through the entire protocol?
- Will the information be used as part of a recruitment tool that can be shown to referring physicians or prospective patients so that they can readily understand what the protocol will entail?
- Can this information be used to prospectively plan for resources to be put in place for a patient to successfully complete the protocol?
- Will a cost estimate be generated? If so, how will it be used?
- Will the cost estimate be used to create a budget for the protocol?
- Will the cost estimate be used as part of the analysis in determining whether the protocol is approved to be implemented?
- Will this information provide a sense of protocol intensity or extent of time required to implement?
- What additional information is needed (e.g., case report forms) to make an assessment of workload and to complete cost estimates?
- Is the additional information forthcoming? Can the protocol be approved for implementation without this additional information?
- Is the method used to derive costs appropriate, adequate, and balanced for all involved?

Graphics Used for Resource Planning and Allocation

Computer-generated graphics, formulas, or algorithms may be used to plot resource information. A flow chart or grid is an example of a graphic (see Figure 4-4). To facilitate implementation, financial billing, and collection, the activities are divided into sections of who provided the service, thus allowing the service provider to see at a glance what services are expected from each department and guide a plan for cost recovery when collections are received.

Another example of a visual resource allocation graphic is the protocol planning map (see Figure 4-5). The planning map is an excellent tool to help departments to visualize when their services are required. The protocol map can be several pages in length and depicts all of the costs that will be incurred, as well as costs related to unplanned events. The map's timeline starts at the beginning of the protocol and proceeds through long-term follow-up and the patient's discharge from the protocol (as applicable). The principal

Figure 4-4. Sample Flow Chart of Resources Needed for One Subject to Go Through a Protocol

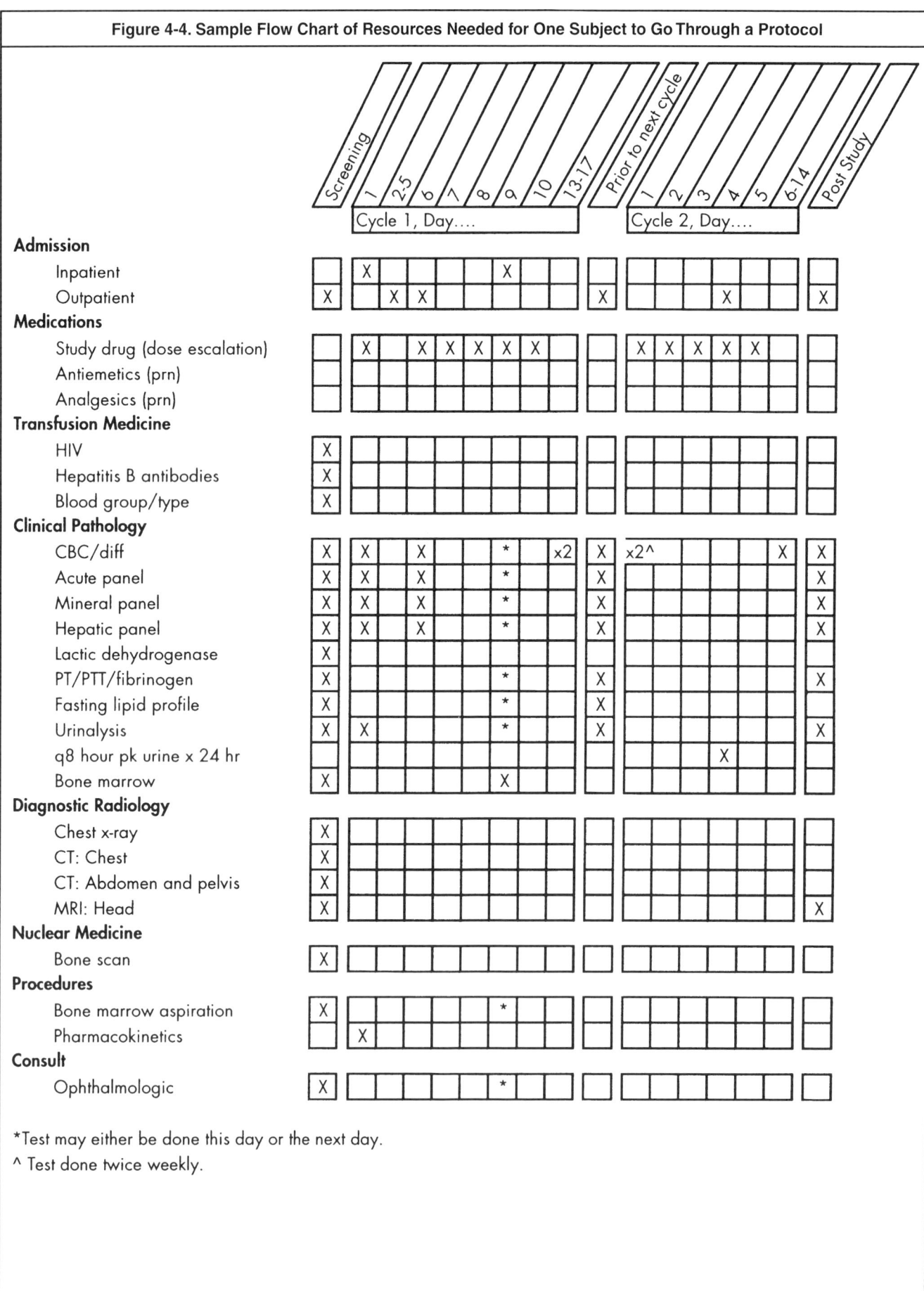

	Screening	Cycle 1, Day 1	Cycle 1, Day 2-5	Cycle 1, Day 6	Cycle 1, Day 7	Cycle 1, Day 8	Cycle 1, Day 9	Cycle 1, Day 10	Cycle 1, Day 13-17	Prior to next cycle	Cycle 2, Day 1	Cycle 2, Day 2	Cycle 2, Day 3	Cycle 2, Day 4	Cycle 2, Day 5	Cycle 2, Day 6-14	Post Study
Admission																	
Inpatient		X				X											
Outpatient	X		X	X						X				X			X
Medications																	
Study drug (dose escalation)		X		X	X	X	X	X			X	X	X	X	X		
Antiemetics (prn)																	
Analgesics (prn)																	
Transfusion Medicine																	
HIV	X																
Hepatitis B antibodies	X																
Blood group/type	X																
Clinical Pathology																	
CBC/diff	X	X		X		*		x2		X	x2^					X	X
Acute panel	X	X		X		*				X							X
Mineral panel	X	X		X		*				X							X
Hepatic panel	X	X		X		*				X							X
Lactic dehydrogenase	X																
PT/PTT/fibrinogen	X					*				X							X
Fasting lipid profile	X					*				X							
Urinalysis	X	X				*				X							X
q8 hour pk urine x 24 hr														X			
Bone marrow	X					X											
Diagnostic Radiology																	
Chest x-ray	X																
CT: Chest	X																
CT: Abdomen and pelvis	X																
MRI: Head	X																X
Nuclear Medicine																	
Bone scan	X																
Procedures																	
Bone marrow aspiration	X					*											
Pharmacokinetics		X															
Consult																	
Ophthalmologic	X					*											

*Test may either be done this day or the next day.

^ Test done twice weekly.

Figure 4-5. Sample Protocol Planning Map

Protocol Planning Map (Date)

(For example, questions one would ask to complete map)

Name of Protocol: Treatment of cancer

Principal Investigator (PI): Dr. Smith   Branch: Medical Oncology

Max N: 50 patients (entire study)   N (projected): 40   N (for first year): 15

Sign off by PI: Electronic sign-off

Clinical Research Coordinator: Ma Jones, RN, Phone #/Beeper #: 104-104-7

Date	Screening	Cycle 1	Post–Cycle 1 Follow-Up Visit
Site	**Oncology Clinic**	**Inpatient Unit**	**Oncology Clinic**
Assessment and interventions	Eligibility requirements Life expectancy Karnofsky performance status Past medical history and treatment	Care requirements for staff Frequent vital signs or monitoring Special bed or equipment needs	Care requirements for staff Frequent vital signs or monitoring
Medications	List patient's medications. Will patient use his own supply or hospital's? Who is supplying treatment for protocol? Hospital pharmacy, drug company, grant-sponsored?	Chemotherapy Immunotherapy treatment of side effects (e.g., nausea and vomiting, diarrhea, headache, fatigue, neutropenia) Radiation therapy Wound care Mouth care	Chemotherapy Immunotherapy treatment of side effects (e.g., nausea and vomiting, diarrhea, headache, fatigue, neutropenia) Radiation therapy
Labs	Eligibility labs Tumor markers HIV Hepatitis profile 24-hour urine Pregnancy tests Type and cross Protocol research labs required	Pharmacokinetics: peripheral or venous access device Daily labs: phlebotomy or RN draw Urine specimen collection Transportation of specimens	Pharmacokinetics: peripheral or venous access device Daily labs: phlebotomy or RN draw Urine specimen collection Transportation of specimens
Diagnostic tests	Chest x-ray Electrocardiogram Multigated acquisition scan Computed tomography scans Magnetic resonance imaging Ultrasound Radiation simulation for treatment	Treatment of side effects Chest x-ray after line placement Restaging scans Follow-up scans	Treatment of side effects Restaging scans Follow-up scans
Consults	Surgery for line placement Biopsies needed for study or diagnosis Dental work before bone marrow transplant Vision or hearing tests Pain team consult Anesthesiology Radiation therapy Pathology labs Apheresis/department of transfusion medicine Neurology Anticipated intensive care unit admission	Blood product transfusions Pharmacy Nurse practitioner On-call physician Outpatient cancer center for follow-up	Long-term follow-up issues Pain control Surgery for future biopsies
Teaching	Informed consent and education about the protocol Treatment schema Admission procedure	Management of side effects Colony-stimulating factor injections Blood product transfusions Inpatient and outpatient procedures	Follow-up issues Management of long-term side effects
Miscellaneous	Bed space issues Sedation of patients Transportation issues Family support Social work issues Third-party reimbursement issues	Dietary issues Staffing issues 1:1 patient care Frequent pharmacokinetics Emotional support Advance directives	Fear of recurrence, emotional support issues Transportation Insurance coverage issues

investigator and the research administrator or CRC are responsible for confirming that the map is an accurate reflection of the proposed protocol and associated work.

After the timeline is established for one patient to receive the full treatment of the protocol and estimates have been made for the number of patients that will go through each phase of the protocol, the next step is to develop a master timeline. A master timeline plots each participant's usage of critical, limiting *threshold* resources, such as specialized care areas, over time. How patients are accrued onto a protocol often will determine if certain resources will be overtaxed (see Figure 4-6).

Threshold resources guide the determination of what resources must be added to successfully implement the protocol as planned. It is important not to undercut this process by imposing unrealistic estimates. For example, some investigators may want to implement the protocol for academic gain and will waive investigator fees in order to meet a sponsor's arbitrary or predetermined funding level. Although such a practice may achieve important goodwill with sponsors, it may lead to poor project performance when resources are inadequate. The potential negative implications are far-reaching.

Of course, unexpected events do occur. Patients may develop complications related to their disease or to the interventions. It may be helpful to create and compare several timelines regarding a critical resource, with one indicating the worst-case scenario and the other demonstrating a timeline that goes according to the planned protocol.

Once a listing of resources has been determined, the next step is to establish who will provide each service and whether the service provider has the resources to accommodate the request. For planning purposes, rewriting the list of resources and grouping them by service provider can be helpful. The service provider then can be notified of the requested resources, and provisions can be made to have the necessary resources available when the patient arrives. This communication process is a key factor in smooth and accurate implementation of the protocol.

After a resource allocation proposal is designed, a cost estimate can be generated per task, per protocol interval, per patient, and for the entire protocol. Both direct and indirect costs must be included in the protocol budget. Direct costs will be identified as activity and resource allocation lists are generated and prepared. Indirect costs may include fees for the initiation of the trial, administrative costs, data management, institutional review board submissions, publicity and advertisements, pharmacy charges, and long-term follow-up (see Chapter 5). Many institutions have a preset percentage of total costs for indirect costs. These fees may be charged to the study sponsor above the cost of the direct patient services.

The complexity of this process requires the use of a computer—clinical trials software—to set up, track, and manage the process. Consequently, a host of homegrown and commercially developed software programs are emerging to address this need.

Figure 4-6. Sample Master Timeline for a Protocol																										

Effect of Limited Resources on Rate of Patient Accrual Onto a Protocol
Example: One research magnetic resonance imaging (MRI) test space per week

Week

Patient	1	2	3	4	5	6	7	8	9	10	11	12	13	14	15	16	17	18	19	20	21	22	23	24	25	26
A	x								x																	
B		x								x																
C			x								x															
D				x								x														
E					x								x													
F						x								x												
G							x								x											
H								x								x										
I																	x								x	
J																		x								x

Notes/Assumptions: Each patient needs baseline research MRI immediately prior to initiation of protocol therapy and a post-treatment MRI nine weeks later. In this example, the research team has only one opening for a research MRI per week. Patients I and J must wait until weeks 17 and 18 to begin the protocol.

Summary

The future of clinical trial workload, funding, and staffing cannot be predicted; thus, workload measurement and resource allocation continue to be key concerns. It is increasingly clear that utilization of protocol task–based and activity time–based cost estimation can be a positive, proactive way to estimate and obtain appropriate levels of funding for clinical trials. The healthcare industry is in an era of rapid computerization of patient-care–related information, clinical trial data, and financial information at different phases of implementation. Thus, the integration of computer resources and technology in prospective task-based workload and resource planning and allocation is key to managing clinical trials in the future. We remain cautiously optimistic that a uniform workload determination formula or algorithm eventually will emerge from current and future experiences.

References

Bjornson-Benson, W.M., Stibolt, T.B., Manske, K.A., Zavela, K.J., Youtsey, D.J., & Buist, A.S. (1993). Monitoring recruitment effectiveness and cost in a clinical trial. *Controlled Clinical Trials, 14*(Suppl. 2), 52–67.

Chirikos, T.N. (2003). Three questions about costs and cancer clinical trials. *Cancer Control, 10,* 71–78.

Coleman, T. (1995). Health system reform and clinical research. *Oncology, 9*(2), 118, 121, 126.

Devine, S., Nagel, K., Benson, L., & Krailo, M. (2005, April). CRA discipline time and effort study: Children's Oncology Group. *Applied Clinical Trials,* (Suppl.), pp. 12–16.

Edwards, B.K., Howe, H.L., Ries, L.A., Thun, M.J., Rosenberg, H.M., Yancik, R., et al. (2002). Annual report to the nation on the status of cancer, 1973–1999, featuring implications of age and aging on U.S. cancer burden. *Cancer, 94,* 2766–2792.

Ehrenberger, H.E., & Lillington, L. (2004). Development of a measure to delineate the clinical trials nursing role [Online exclusive]. *Oncology Nursing Forum, 31,* E64–E68.

Emanuel, E.J., Schnipper, L.E., Kamin, D.Y., Levinson, J., & Lichter, A.S. (2003). The costs of conducting clinical research. *Journal of Clinical Oncology, 21,* 4145–4150.

Fowell, J.P., & Wilson, J.T. (2002, Summer). The six phases of a research site budget. *Monitor,* pp. 31–34.

Fowler, D.R., & Thomas, C.J. (2003). Protocol acuity scoring as a rational approach to clinical research management. *Research Practitioner, 4,* 64–71.

Gwede, C.K., Johnson, D., & Daniels, S. (2001). Organization of clinical research services at investigative sites: Implications for workload measurement. *Drug Information Journal, 35,* 695–705.

Gwede, C.K., Johnson, D.J., Roberts, C., & Cantor, A.B. (2005). Burnout in clinical research coordinators in the United States. *Oncology Nursing Forum, 32,* 1123–1130.

Gwede, C.K., Johnson, D., & Trotti, A. (2000a, January). Measuring the workload of clinical research coordinators, part I: Tools to study workload issues. *Applied Clinical Trials,* pp. 40–44.

Gwede, C.K., Johnson, D., & Trotti, A. (2000b, February). Measuring the workload of clinical research coordinators, part II: Workload implications for sites. *Applied Clinical Trials,* pp. 42–47.

Johnson, G.P. (2003, May). Budget tool helps investigative sites calculate the cost of a coordinator's time for a typical outpatient study visit: Part I. *SoCRA SOURCE,* pp. 33–37.

Jones, A., Cusack, G., & Chisholm, L. (2004). Patient intensity in an ambulatory oncology research center: A step forward for the field of ambulatory care—part II. *Nursing Economics, 22,* 120–123, 107.

Neuer, A. (2002). The rising tide of CRC workload and turnover. *CenterWatch, 9,* 1–7.

Roche, K., Paul, N., Smuck, B., Whitehead, M., Zee, B., Pater, J., et al. (2002). Factors affecting workload of cancer clinical trials: Results of a multicenter study of the National Cancer Institute of Canada Clinical Trials Group. *Journal of Clinical Oncology, 20,* 545–556.

Rozich, J.D., & Resar, R.K. (2002). Using a unit assessment tool to optimize patient flow and staffing in a community hospital. *Joint Commission Journal on Quality Improvement, 28,* 31–41.

Van Slyck, A. (1995). Not all acuity systems are the same. *Nursing Management, 26*(7), 11.

Walts, L.M., & Kapadia, A.S. (1996). Patient classification system: An optimization approach. *Health Care Management Review, 21*(4), 75–82.

West, J., Wright, J., Tuffnell, D., Jankowicz, D., & West, R. (2005). Do clinical trials improve quality of care? A comparison of clinical processes and outcomes in patients in a clinical trial and similar patients outside a trial where both groups are managed according to a strict protocol. *Quality and Safety in Health Care, 14,* 175–178.

Yancik, R. (1997). Epidemiology of cancer in the elderly. Current status and projections for the future. *Rays, 22*(Suppl. 1), 3–9.

Yancik, R., & Ries, L.A. (2004). Cancer in older persons: An international issue in an aging world. *Seminars in Oncology, 31,* 128–136.

CHAPTER 5
Budget

Kelly Willenberg, MBA, BSN, RN

Introduction

The key to a carefully prescribed clinical trial management plan starts with the development of a proper budget. This is a daunting task for even the most experienced research administrator. A clinical trial may be considered a success or failure in the minds of the research team depending on whether it makes or loses money. What are the guidelines to prepare a budget correctly? What are the key ingredients of a successful budget? According to Wright et al. (2005), "The study budget represents the total amount of money required to conduct a trial and is usually negotiated on a per patient basis" (p. 422). The financial impact of conducting a clinical trial in oncology can be thwarted by poor negotiation for proper reimbursement. This chapter will provide the proper tools needed to budget a clinical trial successfully. As Good (2002) noted, "Sweat the small stuff. Attorneys do it; so do CPAs. Don't just record major expenditures . . . but track every phone call and the time your staff spends on it" (p. 163). The research team's success depends on the completeness of the plan at the beginning of the budget process—not after the study is open to accrual, when it is too late.

Administrative Components

First and foremost, the clear starting point for proper budgeting is reading and understanding the protocol. "A detailed budget is an itemized list accounting for every expense required to complete the project" (Higdon & Topp, 2004, p. 924). The administrator must review what the sponsor provides, knowing his or her facility's costs and being secure in that knowledge. If something is unclear or confusing in the protocol regarding what has to be done, the administrator obtains clarification from the sponsor. In investigator-initiated studies, confusing items should be clarified with the principal investigator (PI) *prior* to opening the study for patient accrual. Knowing what is required before opening the trial shows that the administrator's review was thorough.

A careful review of both the study calendar, which graphically depicts the timing of study events, and the clearly defined parameters of what the sponsor considers to be covered under the reimbursement agreement and budget is vital to development of a successful budget. Provide sufficient justification for all components of the study, including materials and labor costs (Koren, 2005).

Delineating the standard of care from what is considered to be part of the research for the protocol is extremely important. A billing grid should be used to build the patient care budget (see Figure 5-1). All research nurses and study coordinators or people responsible for billing need to be trained on how to complete the billing grid, understanding that it displays how they will post charges for the study. The billing grid also is a guide for ordering supplies for each patient visit. The key to successful budget building is verifying up front what constitutes the standard of care versus care that is provided for research purposes only. This can include a rating system to estimate a budget per patient (see Figure 5-1) (Spear, 2005).

The administrator must schedule a meeting with the research team and calculate the complexity of the study to determine the amount of time that will be necessary to complete every aspect of the study. "Financial managers should collaborate with researchers and physicians in implementing and interpreting a standard costing format for clinical trials" (West, Balas, & West, 2000, p. 11). One always must consider future cost and, therefore, price increases for services for the duration of the study. The administrative fees should include an analysis of protocol data to build a budget and negotiate a contract that will define the institutional overhead. The administrative components include all nonrefundable fees (see Figure 5-2). Document travel expenses, investigator fees, and computer-related expenditures. In addition, keep track of time spent on study-related tasks—including time spent on the telephone. This can end up being substantial (Good, 2002). It is vital to track everything; the data may be useful at a later time.

Figure 5-1. Billing Grid

Department of Finance
Research Billing and Compliance

Study Title	0
Study Sponsor	0
Sponsor Protocol #	0
Principal Investigator	
Research Nurse	, nurse

Department		0
Department Administrator		
Study Coordinator/Contact		, nurse

# of Patients Projected	0
Project Duration (Months)	0
Beginning Date	1/0/1900
Ending Date	1/0/1900

Per Patient Cost Analysis Worksheet Conventional Care / SOC (standard of care) label as 0 zero, Research Related, document the charge amount.

HELP

If you have any questions determining conventional care, click here (hyperlink to LMRP/LCD site)

	CDM code	CPT4 Codes	Baseline	Week 1	Week 2	Week 3	Week 4	Week 5	Week 6	Week 7	Week 8	Week 9	Week 10	Week 11	Week 12	Week 13	Week 14	Week 15	Week 16	Week 17	Month 9	Month 12	Month 15	Month 18	Month 21	Month 24	TOTAL charge	Number billed to D & H
					Treatment																		Follow-Up						
Procedures* (itemize)																													
Example Chest X-ray	34301028	71020	$56.00	$56.00	$56.00	$0	0	$0	$56.00	$0	$0	$0	$0	$0	$0	$0	$0	$0	$0	$0	$0	0	$0	$0	$0	$0	$0	3
Totals			$0	$0	$0	$0	$0	$0	$0	$0	$0	$0	$0	$0	$0	$0	$0	$0	$0	$0	$0	$0	$0	$0	$0	$0	$0	0
Professional (itemize)																													
Example Chest X-ray professional	34301028	99204	$43.00	$43.00	$43.00	$0	0	$0	$43.00	$0	$0	$0	$0	$0	$0	$0	$0	$0	$0	$0	$0	0	$0	$0	$0	$0	0	3
professional for these																													
Totals			$0	$0	$0	$0	$0	$0	$0	$0	$0	$0	$0	$0	$0	$0	$0	$0	$0	$0	$0	$0	$0	$0	$0	$0	$0	0
Other directs (itemize)																													
Example Iv tubing	11461118	99070	$35	$0	$35	$0	$35	$0	$35	$0	$0	$0	$0	$0	$0	$0	$0	$35	$0	$0	$0	$35						$210	
Pharmacy Dispensing Fee																											$35	
Monitoring Fee																											$0	
Totals			$0	$0	$0	$0	$0	$0	$0	$0	$0	$0	$0	$0	$0	$0	$0	$0	$0	$0	$0	$0	$0	$0	$0	$0	$0	
Totals for patient expense	63410		$0	$0	$0	$0	$0	$0	$0	$0	$0	$0	$0	$0	$0	$0	$0	$0	$0	$0	$0	$0	$0	$0	$0	$0	$0	0

Signature of Principal Investigator _____   Date _____

"The above listed principal investigator has reviewed the Medicare Coverage Analysis and agrees with the findings documented as conventional care and research related on the Clinical Research Budget Grid attached."

*Conventional Care/SOC (Standard of Care) - Billed to the Patient's Insurance or * Research Related-please document the charge amount (see examples above in the gray rows)

If there are questions regarding CDM/CPT codes or charges, please contact the Clinical Research Financial Compliance Office at E-mail address researchratesrus@vanderbilt.edu

*If any SOC procedures are denied by a patient's insurance, please contact the clinical trial financial analyst as soon as possible.

Note. Figure courtesy of Vanderbilt University Medical Center. Used with permission.

Figure 5-2. Nonrefundable/One-Time Fees		
One-Time Per Study Nonrefundable Fees (insert as applicable)		
Description	5-Digit Account #	Totals
IRB Preparation	61400	$5,000
Consent Form Development	61400	$50
IRB Submission and Review	61400	$400
IRB Amendments Processing	61400	$100
SAE Processing	61400	$250
IRB Annual Review	61400	$500
Total for Account 61400		$6,300
Pharmacy Protocol Management Fee	61910	$100
Archival Fee	61910	$0
Advertising Fee	61910	$250
Clinical Trial Operational Fee	61910	$400
Storage Fee	61910	$1,000
Shipping and Postage Fees	61910	$200
Auditing Fee	61910	$200
Monitoring Fee	61910	
Total for Account 61910		$2,150
Duplication & Xerox	60000	$785
Publication Costs	60010	$125
Printing	60020	$150
Postage	60030	$175
Office Supplies	60040	$700
Lab Supplies	60150	$1,500
Federal Express	60225	$45
Drug Floor Stock	60530	$1,000
Telephone	61300	$225
Misc. Expense	61900	$500
Meeting Expense	62100	$50
Subject Participation	63400	$400

Electing not to open a study because the budget does not meet the site's budget feasibility is perfectly acceptable. John P. Rowell (2005), RN, MSN, of the Louisiana State University (LSU) Health Sciences Center, noted that LSU handles about 100 studies a year but also may turn away that many protocols because the protocol does not meet the institution's budget feasibility. He stated, "One of the advantages of being a big site is [that] we turn some down before we get to the budget phase" (Rowell, 2005, p. 91).

Rowell (2005) further noted that it is not unusual for the budget he has generated to be twice the amount the sponsor originally said it would pay. "But I won't come down below our costs. We won't lose money doing research—we can't afford to" (p. 91). A break-even point and the bottom line should be analyzed. The administrator needs to feel empowered to make a recommendation that a study will lose money. Many academic centers have review committees that have the authority to decide whether the institution will take a financial "hit" to do the study. The key to achieving success is being aware up front of what the study entails financially and planning how to accomplish it without a loss.

Online tools are available to assist in creating a budget. The Cancer Therapy Evaluation Program (CTEP) of the National Cancer Institute (NCI) offers Microsoft Excel® templates online for a cost estimate worksheet (http://ctep.cancer.gov/forms/costest1004.xls) and a cooperative group common budget outline (http://ctep.cancer.gov/guidelines/coop_grp_budget.xls). Additionally, the NCI site titled "States That Require Health Plans to Cover Patient Care Costs in Clinical Trials" provides links to individual state Web sites that allow visitors to retrieve laws, agreements, and key provisions. This Web site can be accessed at www.cancer.gov/clinicaltrials/learning/laws-about-clinical-trial-costs.

Estimating Accrual

Estimating accrual is complicated and must be done for the entire study. "Physicians new to drug and device investigations usually overestimate the ease of obtaining subjects, underestimate the time of complying with regulatory affairs, under-budget for the unexpected, and overestimate their own efficiency" (Iber, Riley, & Murray, 1987, p. 53).

Be realistic when estimating accrual. Check cancer registry data to note how many patients normally are seen. Do not overestimate the total number of patients to be accrued. Know the average number of cycles or days that each patient will be on study, and have a clear understanding of the timeline for finishing the study. The number-one thing to remember is to never agree to the sponsor's initial offer, regardless of how incredible the dollar amount sounds. All sponsors or clinical research organizations have a business plan, and making money is their goal. They will underestimate to the administrator what it will cost the facility to complete the study. The offer may sound good, but unless the budget is prepared carefully, the administrator will have no idea how accurate it truly is.

Nonrefundable Fees

Nonrefundable fees are the only way to collect start-up costs. Examples of these costs include the institutional review board (IRB) fees, IRB preparation and consent form composition, RN coordinator time, budget preparation, contract negotiations, prestudy visits with the sponsor (which can be combined with the initiation visit to save time), and meetings to set up the protocol or review the budget (see Figure 5-2). Nonrefundable fees also can include the pharmacy fees. This prevents the pharmacy fee from being connected to the price per patient, which can result in a loss of the protocol management fees if patient accrual is low. Regardless of the number of patients accrued, the pharmacy incurs fees, such as preparing an itemized budget, developing order entry sets, maintaining drug inventory records and binders established for the study, and carefully reviewing the protocol. The pharmacy expends time and effort prior to any patient ever being registered to the study and should be compensated regardless of whether there is accrual to the study.

IRB fees also are considered nonrefundable and may be predetermined by the research arm and non-negotiable. These fees vary and can be associated with the number of adverse events or amendments submitted. Listing these as "pass-through," or invoiceable, costs can help in preparing an invoice for the sponsor.

Billing Compliance for Medicare and Third-Party Payers

The administrator must assess whether the study is qualified under Medicare guidelines to know how the facility may bill and what must be budgeted in a clinical trial. To be eligible for Medicare reimbursement, the clinical trial must be qualified under National Coverage Determination (NCD). NCD covers all items and services otherwise generally available to Medicare beneficiaries that are provided in either the experimental or control arms of a clinical trial that are considered routine costs that would be medically necessary and would be rendered absent a clinical trial (Centers for Medicare and Medicaid Services [CMS], 2000). Medicare does not cover services, drugs, devices, and tests provided solely for research purposes or related to treatment complications caused by participation in the trial. For more information, see "Clinical Trials Covered Under the Medicare Anti-Cancer Drugs National Coverage Decision" on the NCI Web site at www.cancer.gov/clinicaltrials/developments/NCD179N.

It is imperative to know what the facility is allowed to bill to Medicare and proper coding for clinical trials with Medicare. Routine costs for which Medicare generally does not reimburse include purely experimental medical care, even if there is no other source of payment. If a service or item is provided or reimbursed by another payer, including industry-sponsored trials, federally sponsored clinical trials, and/or private insurance, Medicare cannot be billed. This would be viewed as "double dipping."

Effective September 19, 2000, clinical trials that automatically qualify under Medicare include (CMS, 2000)
- Trials funded by the National Institutes of Health (NIH), the Centers for Disease Control and Prevention (CDC),

the Agency for Healthcare Research and Quality (AHRQ), CMS, the Department of Defense (DoD), and the Department of Veterans Affairs (VA)
- Trials supported by centers or cooperative groups that are funded by the NIH, CDC, AHRQ, CMS, DoD, and VA
- Trials conducted under an investigational new drug (IND) application reviewed by the U.S. Food and Drug Administration (FDA)
- Drug trials that are exempt from having an IND application under 21 CFR 312.2(b)(1) will be deemed automatically qualified until the qualifying criteria are developed and the certification process is in place. At that time, the PIs of these trials must certify that the trials meet the qualifying criteria to maintain Medicare coverage of routine costs. This certification process will only affect the future status of the trial and will not be used to retroactively change the earlier deemed status (CMS, 2000).

Medicare will cover the routine costs of trials that have either been deemed to be automatically qualified or have certified that they meet the qualifying criteria, unless CMS's chief clinical officer subsequently finds that a clinical trial does not meet the criteria or jeopardizes the safety or welfare of Medicare beneficiaries (CMS, 2000).

Device Trials

Device trials need to be assessed up front so that the administrator has the FDA exemption letter stating the category assigned and the investigational device exemption (IDE) number. This information must be submitted to the IRB. The administrator needs to know the category of the device to know whether it is billable under Medicare guidelines. Many different categories of devices exist. It is very important to understand the category of the device being used in the specific clinical trial, as the various categories are supplied and potentially billed differently. A requirement for device studies is the IDE number. This number is required on the bill for Medicare to consider payment.

Category A (Experimental) Devices—Innovative Medical Devices

Devices in category A do not have a functional equivalent that has already been proved to be safe and effective and therefore are considered experimental (CMS, 2000). The initial questions of safety and effectiveness have not been resolved, and the FDA is unsure whether the device can be safe and effective. Billing may include only the standard-of-care costs in clinical trials involving IDE category A devices effective for routine services performed for the trial. *The category A device itself is not covered.* This authorization became effective as of January 1, 2005. It is very important that the "QV" procedure code modifier be applied. The QV modifier indicates that the "item or service is provided as routine care in a qualified clinical trial" (Ingenix, 2005, p. 21).

Category B Devices—Investigational Devices

A category B classification means that incremental risk is being investigated and that the fundamental issues of safety and effectiveness have already been resolved (CMS, 2000). These devices are so similar to other devices on the market that regulators believe they are at least as safe and effective as the ones on the market. Payment for these devices is payable by Medicare. The device must be reasonable and necessary for the treatment or diagnosis of a medical condition or disease (CMS). Devices that are statutorily excluded from coverage are not covered simply because they are part of a clinical trial. *The payment for a category B investigational device is limited to the amount equal to or less than what Medicare would have paid for a comparable approved device.* Payment under Medicare for a category B device will be based on information provided in the IDE submission. The billing for this device must include a QV modifier and the IDE.

Patient Care Costs

To determine the budget necessary to cover the cost of the study, the administrator must price each test and procedure that is *not* considered standard of care (see Figure 5-3). Knowing the procedures being done and *where* they will be done is important. Are they cardiology, radiology, laboratory, or respiratory events? Are special readings to be taken, specific contrast used, or the x-rays copied? All of these items are budgeted in a detailed way. Laboratory shipment fees can be significant if labs must be shipped overseas or even across the country. Tissue and pathology costs and professional fees/physician fees are part of the overall budget; do not forget to include them. Consider not only pathology but also radiology for examples of fees to be charged. A separate fee is assessed for the test and the interpretation.

Common items missed in budget preparation are pharmacy costs, a lengthy consent form process for the coordinator, follow-up visits not included in the original schedule of events, supplies to give IV medications, drawing labs that are sent to a central lab, and screen failure payments. A sample worksheet is presented in Figure 5-4. Other fees include advertising costs, shipping costs, storage of charts, and RN coordinator time.

Laboratory Fees

Laboratory fees need to be accounted for when determining a clinical trial budget. Iber et al. (1987) stated that in all studies, 5%–15% of tests that are performed can be expected to be abnormal, unsatisfactory, or simply confusing to interpret and must be repeated; they recommend budgeting $50 per subject to cover repeat test fees. Laboratory fees also may change during the course of a study. Market adjustments can put the budget into disarray. Know the high-end and low-end amounts required to cover these costs.

If the protocol requires two tests but to obtain results the institution requires an additional test to be done, the additional test must be billed to the sponsor. These may be institutional facility fees or requirements and should be considered in budget preparation. Know these scenarios, and do not forget the consequences of not budgeting properly.

The itemized budget list includes not only the research-related patient care procedures but also the ancillary services that will be utilized in the facility. Will the patients be admitted to the general clinical research center? Will they be in the clinic or treatment room? Will they be admitted as inpatients? These issues must be considered during budget preparation.

Pharmacy Costs

Pharmacy costs can be included in the nonrefundable fees and are published and confirmed in writing to ensure that the pharmacy receives payment regardless of accrual to the study. The fees that usually comprise a per-patient amount are fees for dispensing based on number of visits or cycles. Do not forget supplies in this fee, such as fluid or a pump to administer the provided drug or a special type of tubing. Investigational drug pharmacies charge protocol management fees, which should be considered nonrefundable, and dispensing fees, which are patient-specific.

Pharmacokinetic Sampling

Pharmacokinetic sampling (PKS) is a necessary item in early-phase studies. The administrator must plan and know the number of hours at which samples will need to be drawn. If special supplies are needed to perform PKS, such as a special centrifuge, a freezer that the facility might not have, IV supplies, special syringes, dry ice, tubes, or even a microwave, do not fail to include them in the budget. Always consider the staffing necessary for PKS that must be drawn in the off hours when the clinic is not open. Consider on-call coverage of physicians or research staff as well.

Figure 5-3. Calculating Nonstandard Procedure Costs				
Review items necessary but not standard of care. Find current procedural terminology code that correlates and institutional cost for each item. Budget appropriate number according to study requirements and do not bill to third-party payer or Medicare. See the following table for an example of how to formulate budget costs.				
Procedure	**Current Procedural Terminology Code**	**Cost**	**Research Frequency**	**Total Cost to Budget Per Subject**
Chest x-ray, two views	71020	$185.00	4	$185 × 4 = $740

Figure 5-4. Budget and Schedule of Events (B.A.S.E.)

Study Title:	0		
Study Sponsor:	0	# of Patients Projected:	0
Sponsor Protocol #	0	Project Duration (# of Months):	0
Principal Investigator:	,	Beginning Date:	1/0/1900
Research Nurse:	, nurse	Ending Date:	1/0/1900
Department:	0		
Department Administrator:	,		
Study Contact/Coordinator:	, nurse		

HELP

Fringe Faculty Rate	22.50%
Fringe Staff Rate	23.20%
Adjusted Cost Rate	0.00%
Indirect Cost Rate	29.00%

The fringe rates shown to the left are 2006/07 projected rates. If you prefer another rate, please refer to the website below and enter manually.

http://www.vanderbilt.edu/ocga/fringebenefit/fringebenefit.ht

	Principal Investigator	Research Nurse	Study Coordinator	Other	Total Project Salaries & Fringes
Number of Hours per Month	0	0	0	0	
Annual % Effort	0.0%	0.0%	0.0%	0.0%	
Base Salary	$0	$0	$0	$0	
Annual Projected Salary	$0	$0	$0	$0	$0
Annual Projected Fringe	$0	$0	$0	$0	$0
Annual Projected Sal & Fringe	$0	$0	$0	$0	$0
Project Duration Total	$0	$0	$0	$0	$0
Percent of Total Budget	#DIV/0!	#DIV/0!	#DIV/0!	#DIV/0!	#DIV/0!

Patient Care Expenses		
Lab Supplies - 60150	0	#DIV/0!
Subject Participation - 63400	0	#DIV/0!
Inpatient/Outpatient Expense - 63410	0	#DIV/0!
	0	
Administrative Expense		
Duplication & Xerox - 60000	0	#DIV/0!
Publication Costs - 60010	0	#DIV/0!
Printing - 60020	0	#DIV/0!
Postage - 60030	0	#DIV/0!
Office Supplies - 60040	0	#DIV/0!
Federal Express - 60225	0	#DIV/0!
Drug Floor Stock - 60530	0	#DIV/0!
Telephone - 61300	0	#DIV/0!
Meeting Expense - 62100	0	#DIV/0!
	0	#DIV/0!
TOTAL OPERATING EXPENSES	0	#DIV/0!
Salaries, Fringes, Expenses	0	#DIV/0!
Adjusted Cost VU	0	#DIV/0!
NON-REFUNDABLE FEES		
Fees - 61400	0	
Total Non-Refundable Fee (includes 29% Indirect Rate)	0	
DIRECT COSTS	0	#DIV/0!
INDIRECT COST VU	0	#DIV/0!
TOTAL DIRECT AND INDIRECT COSTS	0	#DIV/0!
Total Fee per Patient	0	#DIV/0!

Consider using the general clinical research center or an infusion center for these blood draws if the facility has these departments. This is a cost to the budget, and the pharmaceutical sponsor should cover the costs of the staffing to draw samples. Thus, it is important to know who will draw off-time labs and who will be responsible for spinning down, separating, and storing them.

If PKS must be done, include in the budget the time needed to package and ship them. If special items are needed, for example, storage boxes, tubes, Styrofoam containers, popcorn pellets for shipping, or the actual payment for shipping, secure these items up front from the sponsor. If items such as these are not accounted for in the initial budget, the facility ends up eating the costs later. These can be rather expensive, especially if the study requires only a small number of samples.

Staff Effort and Budgeting

Principal Investigator

Always budget a minimum number of hours for the PI's effort based on his or her time needed to complete the study requirements. Overseeing the daily operations of a clinical trial can be significant, especially if the institution is acting as the coordinating center for a large study. The PI will sometimes be responsible for reviewing eligibility for all patients. Consider whether the PI helped to develop the study with the sponsor. Some institutions have a minimum percent effort that must be included in each study budget. The PI's true effort in the study completion is what should be budgeted. Do not forget the RN coordinator's time in relation to the PI, and budget for it, as well. Consider the RN's time spent with monitors when the study has begun to accrue patients. This may require a large block of time weekly or monthly with high accruing studies.

The other area where the PI may be required to put in large amounts of time, especially for phase I studies, is conference calls. These sometimes may require an hour or two per week in between cohorts for safety analysis or discussions with the sponsor. "The same process and template are used for each review in order to identify procedures that exceed standard care and the percent effort by the PI" (Wujcik & Willenberg, 1999, p. 5).

A PI's time can be budgeted by different methods. One way is to calculate a percentage of the PI's overall annual salary. Take the number of hours necessary to do the study multiplied by the annual salary, and then divide by 2080 (the number of hours in a year of full-time work). The second way to calculate PI time is based on a timeline per visit. This also provides a budget amount. Some pharmaceutical sponsors will send a template to the administrator to calculate salary. Either way is acceptable as long as the administrator feels that the PI's actual time is reflected.

On government grants, justification and certification of time and effort are equally important. "Some agencies, most notably the federal government, provide detailed templates

for how to prepare the budget. Others do not. In general, all budgets should included estimates for (a) personnel, including consultations if needed; (b) the purchase of rental equipment; (c) local and long distance travel; (d) supplies; and (e) other miscellaneous expenditures" (Ingersoll & Eberhard, 1999, p. 132).

Investigator meetings are a high-dollar time necessity, and not all sponsors cover the travel costs and time to complete these. Consider all of this when building a budget if the sponsor is not covering the time needed to attend.

Study Coordinator

The effort of the study coordinator or research nursing staff should be budgeted by hours (see Figure 5-5) or time points necessary for the staff to be with the patient (see Table 5-1). Review prestudy activities for protocol feasibility and budget preparation. Baseline eligibility for each patient should be *carefully* considered. Phase I studies might require up to two days for review of the patient's eligibility criteria. How long does it take to obtain informed consent from a potential participant? Allow ample time to do a thorough job with each patient. Consider what it takes to create a calendar, patient information packet, or checklist(s) for each patient. Remember to include the time it takes to discuss with each study participant activities such as quality-of-life surveys and questions or phone calls they might require, and budget for the coordinator's time to see the patient as well.

Screen failures (i.e., patients who are screened for eligibility but are deemed ineligible) take time, as well. Learn to rely on the past experience of the team and patient population to sufficiently budget for these, considering how many patients will need to be screened to enroll one. Always remember to include enrollment log completion. Some studies will require that numerous logs be completed. Inquire whether they must be completed within a certain time frame and faxed to the sponsor. The study coordinator should be compensated for this time. This will help to cover the institution's expenses. A minimum number of hours should be budgeted. Allow for at least three to four hours to screen each patient and at least one to two hours per cycle or time point in the study for the study coordinator. This total can be shown as a percentage of their total annual hours in a budget.

The staff will require time to complete treatment activities. Consider the coordinator with the physician, as well as the coordinator alone. Remember to include the lab-only visits if the coordinator will perform the lab tests. Keep

---

Figure 5-5. Calculating Staff Effort

Nurse/Coordinator
Annual salary budget entry = $XX/per hour x 2,080 hours/year

Data Manager/Clinical Research Associate
Annual salary budget entry = $XX/per hour x 2,080 hours/year

Table 5-1. Rating System to Estimate Budget Per Patient					
Acuity Level	Study Phase	Activity	Hours Per Week	Full-Time Employee % Per Week	Cost Per Subject
					$ complete based on annual salary
All levels	All phases	Prescreening	1	2.50%	
4	1	Screening	12	30.00%	
3	2	Screening	12	30.00%	
2	3	Screening	10	25.00%	
1	4	Screening	10	25.00%	
4	1	On treatment	8	20.00%	
3	2	On treatment	6	15.00%	
2	3	On treatment	4	10.00%	
1	4	On treatment	2	5.00%	
4	1	Withdraw/termination	5	12.50%	
3	2	Withdraw/termination	3	7.50%	
2	3	Withdraw/termination	2	5.00%	
1	4	Withdraw/termination	1	2.50%	
All levels	All phases	Auditing/reporting	5	12.50%	

4 = Highest intensity/complex
3 = Moderately intensity/complex
2 = Less intensity/complex
1 = Least intense/not complex

in mind that reporting adverse events and serious adverse events will take time, which is based on the type of drug involved. Take into account the time involved in scheduling lab tests, biopsies, and cardiology or radiology procedures. Record the time it takes to assemble scans or films and to order supplies or equipment for the study. The coordinator's time must be covered in order to do all of these tasks. Work with the coordinator continually to ensure that his or her effort being expended to complete the study is covered.

Screening for accrual can be a time-consuming process. If the study coordinator says that 10 patients will need to be screened in order to accrue one patient, budget for that time. Screen failures should always be a part of the budget, and any sponsor that will not cover screening costs should be considered as not really understanding the clinical trial process. Some sponsors will allow for a limited number of screenings, but, after learning the ratio of the number

screened to the number accrued, they balk on the screening fee. A 20% screen failure is considered to be fair, and most sponsors abide by this figure in their contracts and legal agreements. Do not agree to be paid for five screen failures if you plan to accrue 100 patients. Hold firm on the amount of time required for chart screenings and logs, too. These can take an enormous amount of time, and the institution should be paid to complete this work. Assessment of work can be crucial, and a manager should evaluate at time points (see Figure 5-6).

Data Management/Clinical Research Associate

Every study requires someone to enter data either into a case report form (CRF) or into a Web-based data collection system. Administrators will find that their staff will require a minimum number of hours for complex studies. Base this on the activities of doing eligibility reviews, screening, per-

Figure 5-6. Workload Summary for Study Coordinators		
Workload Summary for Study Coordinators	**Number**	**Comments**
Therapeutic study accrual this month		
Correlative accrual this month		
Open protocols this team manages		
Patients on study		
Patients in follow-up		
Queries received		
Queries pending		
Queries completed		
Outside safety reports processed		
Patients with data > 1 month		

forming routine visits, conducting patient teaching, and so on. NCI's standard is that one full-time employee can manage 25 patients on study and 50 in follow-up. It is not clear whether this standard applies only to data management or includes the nursing and regulatory activities required.

Thus, tracking all activities in monthly reports, which document the amount of work done within a certain time frame, can create benchmarks for standards. Always consider the time needed for monitors to prepare for patients, the time spent with a patient for each visit, the number of hours it takes to complete adverse event reports for each patient, and the review and preparation of outside safety reports that come in from sponsors prior to submitting to the IRB.

Take into account whether the data manager or research associate must travel for training or go to investigator meetings. This can be a substantial amount of time if they have to be away from the workplace for a lengthy period. Many sponsors cover some expenses of personnel to travel, but not all. If the institution must contract the work out of a department, or if personnel must travel on a weekend, include additional money in the budget to cover these institutional expenses.

The data management piece may comprise the most amount of time put into any study that is performed at an institution. Knowing up front whether a study will be done in paper or electronic format is crucial to successful budgeting for the study. Ask to see the CRFs before putting the budget together. If a data log is to be maintained, include the time necessary to do so. If a database has to be maintained, including a file server, storage, and archiving, the administrator must not hesitate to project the true time that is needed to maintain these items. Determine the follow-up schedule, and if the sponsor asks for more

follow-ups than are in the CRFs, verify it and include this time in the budget. The data manager's or clinical research associate's needs might be underreimbursed if the administrator does not review all of the items necessary to complete the CRFs.

Hidden Costs

Every budget includes expenses that cannot be predicted. These can result in a budget shortfall and possibly poor budget management by the study administrator. Incorporating an adjusted cost or administrative rate into the budget will help to account for unexpected market adjustments in salaries or increases in hospital ancillary costs, such as lab or x-ray costs.

Other items that are not tangible costs but that will add to the bottom line are staff training, source document design, obtaining a second or revised consent, phone calls, query resolution, enrollment log completion, advertising and Web fees, and screening of patient charts. Figure 5-4 displays all of the budget items together, showing where to include personnel costs and patient care costs in one budget for a sponsor. Costs can be calculated by reviewing itemized bills and planning for contingencies, such as price increases, as well.

Clinical Trial Budget Checklist

The following checklist may be used to prepare a clinical trial budget.
- Compensation and personnel costs (e.g., salaries, fringe benefits, professional fees)
- Supplies and document storage (e.g., office supplies, tubes for blood draws, shipping materials such as special boxes or cartons)

- Travel (e.g., investigator meetings not covered by the sponsor)
- Budgeting services, including invoicing of sponsors
- Equipment (e.g., dry ice, document storage, beepers)
- Other (e.g., phone, fax, shipping, subject payments, records retention)
- Research pharmacy
- Administrative costs (e.g., IRB fee, clinical trials office fee)
- University fringe and administrative costs (industry sponsors must pay anywhere from 20%–35%)
- Start-up fees (including all screening costs)
- Nonreimbursable start-up fees
- Query resolution fees
- Close-out costs (e.g., long-term storage fees, queries)
- Decision of what is standard of care and what is being done for research purposes only
- Advertising fees

Summary

Clinical trial budgeting is an art. A person who does it day in and day out becomes very savvy at it. The one item to keep in mind is that once actual expenses are tracked, bad budget decisions will be apparent. The administrator should look at the institution's history with certain types of trials and consider this information when preparing a budget. By accurately tracking expenditures, an adminstrator can minimize the chances of problems developing.

References

Centers for Medicare and Medicaid Services. (2000, September). *September 2000 final national coverage decision.* Retrieved July 10, 2006, from http://www.cms.hhs.gov/ClinicalTrialPolicies/Downloads/finalnationalcoverage.pdf

Good, P.I. (2002). *A manager's guide to the design and conduct of clinical trials.* New York: Wiley-Liss.

Higdon, J., & Topp, R. (2004). How to develop a budget for a research proposal. *Western Journal of Nursing Research, 26,* 922–929.

Iber, F.L., Riley, W.A., & Murray, P.J. (1987). *Conducting clinical trials.* New York: Plenum Medical Book Company.

Ingenix. (2005). *HCPCS level II expert 2006.* Salt Lake City, UT: Author.

Ingersoll, G.L., & Eberhard, D. (1999). Grants management skills keep funded projects on target. *Nursing Economics, 17,* 131–141.

Koren, G. (2005). How to increase your funding chances: Common pitfalls in medical grant applications. *Canadian Journal of Clinical Pharmacology, 12,* e182–e185.

Rowell, J.P. (2005). Fair budgets lead to better research. *Clinical Trials Administrator, 3,* 91–93.

Spear, L. (2005). [Effort calculator]. Durham, NC: Duke Comprehensive Cancer Center.

West, D.A., Balas, E.A., & West, T.D. (2000). Financial managers' costing expertise is needed in clinical trials. *Journal of Health Care Finance, 27,* 11–20.

Wright, J.R., Roche, K., Smuck, B., Cormier, J., Cecchetto, S., Akow, M., et al. (2005). Estimating per patient funding for cancer clinical trials: An Ontario based survey. *Contemporary Clinical Trials, 26,* 421–429.

Wujcik, D., & Willenberg, K. (1999). Vanderbilt workload assessment tool validated by nursing committee. *Quarterly Newsletter for the Eastern Cooperative Oncology Group, 4,* 5.

Additional Resource

Kulakowski, E.C., & Chronister, L.U. (Eds.). (2006). *Research administration and management.* Sudbury, MA: Jones and Bartlett. Available at http://nursing.jbpub.com/catalog/076373277X/table_of_contents.htm

CHAPTER 6
Statistical Considerations in Protocol Development

Lydia T. Madsen, RN, MSN, OCN®, AOCNS®

Introduction

The development of a clinical research protocol involves multiple interactions between the statistician and clinicians, regulatory agencies, and, if applicable, industry sponsors. Additional collaborators may be involved in the design and conduct of a protocol, with the clinical trial nurse (CTN) serving as an essential member of the research team. Once the objectives and design of the study protocol have been agreed on, the statistician also is a key team member, with the statistician's initial goal being to develop the appropriate statistical considerations for the study. A greater understanding of the statistician's role and the statistical tools used in clinical research will facilitate an effective interaction between the statistician and the CTN involved in the conduct of the study.

The purpose of this chapter is to give the CTN a general overview of the basic statistical terms commonly used in protocol development. Topics also will address the factors that help to determine the number of subjects to be entered on each treatment or dose specified in the study design of a clinical trial and an overview of the general guidelines for analyses and interim study monitoring.

Clinical research trials are a critical component to the advancement of medical science. The conduct of a clinical trial involves a serious commitment on the part of its subjects. In clinical cancer studies, participants frequently consent to receive treatment with new therapies that have the potential to be toxic or not as effective as standard treatments. However, those new therapies may have the potential to offer greater effectiveness or a lesser side effect profile than standard treatment. Subjects in a trial also may consent to have additional tests performed and samples of blood and other tissue taken solely for research purposes. In addition, the number of subjects eligible for trials may be limited because of the rate of occurrence of the specific tumor type, the stage of disease, or the specific trial objectives.

The conduct of a clinical trial may be expensive to the sponsoring agencies. It may be labor intensive and time consuming at the clinical sites and at the data management and statistical center, as well. For these reasons, determining the appropriate number of subjects needed for a study is important. By calculating the number of subjects needed to answer the proposed protocol research question, the goals of protecting subject safety, conserving resources, and completing the study in a timely manner can be met. The results of a clinical protocol then can be statistically determined, and those results, either positive or negative, can be disseminated to the scientific community.

A clinical trial must be large enough so that the results are statistically valid and can be generalized to the target population as a whole. If the study is too small, an important life-saving advance in therapy could be missed (a statistical type II error), or a toxic or lethal regimen could be accepted for use in a large population (a statistical type I error) (Polit & Beck, 2004). A study that is too small may provide incomplete or incorrect information, potentially resulting in a waste of not only time and effort but also of limited subject and financial resources.

The statistician works with the clinical investigators, the review committees, and agencies to design a study that is large enough to test the study questions but is not oversized. This chapter outlines the *statistical considerations* section of a protocol and provides some detail about how to interpret the statistical language found in this section. For those who either wish to familiarize themselves with the method in which a proposed study sample size is calculated or have an additional interest in this aspect of clinical research, suggested reading materials are provided at the conclusion of the chapter.

The author would like to acknowledge Janet W. Andersen, ScD, and Traci Leong, MS, for their contribution that remains unchanged from the first edition.

Primary and Secondary Objectives

Statistical analysis of data helps to ensure that the information gathered in a study is organized, interpreted, and scientifically presented in an accurate and informative way (Gravetter & Wallnau, 2006). The sponsor, the study chair, or a site-specific research team will determine the study objectives as an initial step to the development of a clinical protocol. The primary objective is a short statement of the purpose of the study. The primary objective should answer the following questions.

- Is this to be a comparative or descriptive study?
- What is/are the end point(s) of primary interest?
- What is the subject population?
- What is/are the treatment(s)?

Some studies have more than one objective. The sample size is based on the stated objectives and must be large enough, with suitable adjustments, to account for the number of intended statistical tests. Secondary objectives are either of lesser importance or are exploratory and hypothesis-generating in nature.

Oncology Trial End Points

The end points of a study are the clinical and biologic parameters that will be measured to evaluate the study's primary and secondary objectives (Gastineau, 2006). The statistical section (or another related section of the protocol document) should define the end points so that they are reproducible and, where relevant, consistent with other studies in the same disease and population.

Reproducible means that different evaluators given the same data will code the end point the same way both within a site and across all the sites that might participate in a study. The purpose of publishing reproducible, detailed statistical results is to provide researchers with a set of standardized tests that are recognized and understood within the scientific community (Gravetter & Wallnau, 2006). This helps to prevent, for example, having the response rate for one site or clinician be much higher than others because of a difference in evaluation rather than a true difference in the clinical result.

Consistency with other studies is important so that the results of a study or treatment can be evaluated within the context of the history of treatment of the given disease and subject population (Gravetter & Wallnau, 2006). These statistical results, therefore, are termed *inferential statistics* and are mathematical calculations based on the laws of probability. This category of statistics is calculated for use within the scientific community to study samples and subsequently make generalizations about the population that is represented by the test or study population.

Study End Points

Common end points of oncology trials include toxic effects and the tumor assessment end points of objective response rate (ORR), progression-free survival (PFS), time to progression, durable complete response, disease-free survival (DFS), and overall survival.

In the 1970s, ORR was the end point used by the U.S. Food and Drug Administration (FDA) for approval of drugs used in oncology. The ORR end point relied solely on physical and radiologic exams to assess tumor status. However, in the 1980s, the FDA began including DFS, overall survival, improvement in quality of life (QOL), and relief of tumor-related symptoms as end points that were given consideration during the approval process (FDA, 2005).

The most recent guidance document from the FDA, however, again focuses on ORR and PFS as the most favorable end points for drug approval at the time of submission. These two assessment end points are based on the evolving radiologic imaging techniques that provide medical imaging evaluation. The tests used to view and measure tumor size over the course of the clinical trial are computed tomography, magnetic resonance imaging, and positron-emission tomography (Gastineau, 2006).

Toxicity

Toxicities are the adverse effects to organ systems and/or to the participant's subjective status produced by therapy (Oken et al., 1982). Early effects include reductions in blood counts or elevated liver function tests and chronic conditions such as pulmonary fibrosis. Examples of late effects are secondary cancers or myelodysplastic syndromes.

Toxicity is "graded" from 0 to 5, with 0 = none, 1 = mild, 2 = moderate, 3 = severe, 4 = life-threatening, and 5 = lethal. The large cancer cooperative groups and the World Health Organization (WHO) each developed similar (but not identical) grading schemes. The Eastern Cooperative Oncology Group (ECOG) toxicity criteria were published in 1982 and served as a guideline for toxicity grading for many single-institution studies (Oken et al., 1982).

In 1988, the National Cancer Institute (NCI) organized a unification of the many grading schemes into standards used to grade, assign attribution to, and report side effects experienced by subjects on clinical trials. The NCI Cancer Therapy Evaluation Program Common Terminology Criteria for Adverse Events (CTCAE) (version 3.0), formerly known as the Common Toxicity Criteria (version 2.0), or WHO criteria should be used in every oncology clinical trial so that reports of both the frequency and severity of adverse events can be compared between studies. The most current version of the NCI CTCAE may be accessed online at http://ctep.cancer.gov/reporting/ctc.html. Although the ECOG toxicity criteria still are in use and can be accessed at www.ecog.org/general/ctc.pdf, the NCI CTCAE is more detailed and has largely replaced the ECOG toxicity criteria for toxicity grading.

Response

ORR is the measurable and observable effect of the therapy on the tumor over a predefined period of time

(Gastineau, 2006). The ECOG Response Criteria (Oken et al., 1982) are used in many studies to define response, although many groups and trials use other definitions tailored to the specific combination of chemotherapy, surgery, radiotherapy, and other modalities included in the treatment strategies. Leukemia studies have specific response criteria based on the status of the bone marrow, platelets, white blood cells, and hematocrit level. Solid tumor response generally is coded as complete response, partial response, progressive disease, or stable disease (see Figure 6-1).

Figure 6-1. Response Criteria

Evaluation of target lesions
- Complete response (CR): Disappearance of all target lesions
- Partial response (PR): At least a 30% decrease in the sum of the longest diameter (LD) of target lesions, taking as reference the baseline sum LD
- Progressive disease (PD): At least a 20% increase in the sum of the LD of target lesions, taking as reference the smallest sum LD recorded since the treatment started or the appearance of one or more new lesions
- Stable disease (SD): Neither sufficient shrinkage to qualify for PR nor sufficient increase to qualify for PD, taking as reference the smallest sum LD since the treatment started

Evaluation of non-target lesions
- CR: Disappearance of all non-target lesions and normalization of tumor marker level
- Incomplete response/SD: Persistence of one or more non-target lesion(s) and/or maintenance of tumor marker level above the normal limits
- PD: Appearance of one or more new lesions and/or unequivocal progression of existing non-target lesions*

*Although a clear progression of "non-target" lesions only is exceptional, in such circumstances, the opinion of the treating physician should prevail and the progression status should be confirmed later by the review panel (or study chair).

Note. From *Response Evaluation Criteria in Solid Tumors (RECIST) Quick Reference,* by Cancer Therapy and Evaluation Program, National Cancer Institute, n.d. Retrieved July 20, 2007, from http://ctep.cancer.gov/forms/quickrcst.doc

---

Time to Recurrence

In adjuvant studies, in which subjects enter after successful treatment so they are disease-free at entry, the end point is time to reappearance (recurrence) of the treated disease. This must be defined carefully in the study so it is clear whether new disease outside the treated area, such as the finding of a contralateral tumor or metastatic disease in a woman treated locally for breast cancer, is considered as a study end point, even if the participant goes off treatment or off study at the finding.

Relapse

Relapse is the reappearance of disease after complete response or the worsening of disease after partial response (FDA, 2005).

Duration of Response

The duration of response is the time from documentation of a complete response or partial response to relapse (FDA, 2005).

Time to Treatment Failure

The time from entry into the study to the first indication of progression, relapse, or death from any cause is referred to as time to treatment failure.

Disease-Free Survival

DFS is the time from entry into the study to recurrence in an adjuvant study or the time from complete response to relapse in a treatment study.

Overall Survival

Overall survival time is the time from the start of therapy until death.

Other End Points

Other end points of interest in oncology studies include measures of drug pharmacology and pharmacokinetics, immunologic and biologic parameters, adherence and compliance, pain control, and the control of toxicity, such as emesis or bone marrow suppression.

QOL assessment is an additional oncology trial end point that is of continued, increasing interest. Although the measures of QOL are subjective, the value of this end point cannot be overemphasized. With the increasing number of potential treatments available to subjects that could prolong life, QOL data as a trial end point will provide information that subjects may use for various treatment considerations.

Design Summary

The statistical section should summarize the study design that was developed to answer the primary objectives. The section should address (FDA, 1998)
- The number of treatment arms
- Whether subjects are assigned treatment by randomization (i.e., by random choice usually directed by a computer-generated coin toss), by direct assignment, or by other means, such as physician or subject choice
- Whether randomization is stratified so that each subgroup of participants, defined by entry characteristics, is balanced between treatment arms
- The phase of the study.

The mathematical calculations needed to determine the sample size must reflect each of these criteria, so it is important for the statistician to clearly state them.

Power and Sample Size

Ultimately, the purpose of the statistical section is to *state and justify the sample size.* Based upon the study's primary objectives, end points, and design, the statistician decides upon the basic type of statistical test that will be used to analyze the data. Often, several different statistical tests will be used. For randomized studies, examples include the chi-square test, Fisher's exact test, and logistic regression for comparisons of categorical data; a log-rank test or Cox regression for comparisons of censored survival data; and a t-test or analysis of variance for comparisons of normally distributed data. Confidence intervals or one-sample tests generally are used for comparing the observed data with a hypothesized or historical control value in single-arm evaluations (FDA, 1998). Nonparametric analogs exist for most of these tests, as well (see Figure 6-2 for a brief glossary of statistical terms).

To calculate the sample size for a randomized phase III study, the statistician identifies the test that will be used to compare the primary outcomes between the treatment arms on the study. The statistician then determines with the study team the values for the α-level (alpha level) for the study, the desired power, and the null and alternative hypotheses of interest.

The study team bases estimates for the probable outcomes on long-term clinical use of standard regimens and on extensive phase II and possibly phase III use of experimental modalities and combinations. Generally, the null hypothesis is that the treatments are comparable, and the alternative hypothesis is that the new treatment is better than the standard (a one-sided alternative) by a stated amount, or that one is different from the other by a stated amount. The magnitude of the alternative hypothesis should be a therapeutic effect that is both clinically relevant and yet realistic. The difference between the null and alternative hypotheses has a direct effect on the sample size—the larger the difference, the smaller the sample size.

Although hypothesizing a huge difference to guarantee a small sample size may be tempting, if that difference is much larger than that which is clinically interesting (or even clinically possible), the resulting small study is likely to fail to detect a smaller but truly important treatment advance. The statistical section therefore must clearly state the α-level, the power, and the null and alternative hypotheses. The statistician uses formulas, published tables, and computer packages to calculate the sample size needed in each arm of the study to detect the specified difference between the null and alternative hypotheses, given the stated values for α and power.

The procedure for calculating the sample size for a single-arm study or for each arm of a randomized, noncomparative phase II study follows the outline for a randomized study in that the statistician elicits the null and alternative hypotheses and the desired α-level and power for the study from the team. In single-arm evaluations, the null hypothesis comes from historical data about prior treatment and outcomes or from a clinical decision about what would constitute an unacceptable outcome. The null hypothesis generally is the therapy under investigation and is either ineffective or too toxic (i.e., the "bad" outcome). The alternative hypothesis is set by a medical decision about what would be a clinically meaningful result. It should be a therapeutic effect that is both clinically relevant and yet realistic.

Efficient procedures are now available for both phase II and III studies that allow the team to stop accrual or follow-up because of clear, early evidence of the results. A simple example would be that if 5 episodes of toxicity in a sample size of 30 on a phase II study would be unacceptable, then the study should stop if 5 are seen in the first 10 entries. Similarly, if a study is designed to detect a 20% difference in survival between arms and an early analysis indicates a 60% difference, perhaps the study should be terminated and the results published. Numerous procedures exist to allow the development of such adaptive designs. Consideration of adaptive designs is valuable because when trials are stopped early, clinical information of significance

---

Figure 6-2. Definitions of Statistical Terms

The **null hypothesis,** or H_0, is the outcome that the trial designers are trying to disprove or to "reject." The H_0 in most randomized studies is that a new therapy is not better than the standard treatment arm or that two experimental treatments have the same efficacy. H_0 in most single-arm studies is that the therapy under consideration has an unacceptable rate of the end point of interest (e.g., a specified unacceptably low rate of response, a stated unacceptably high rate of toxicity).

The **alternative hypothesis,** or H_A, is the outcome that the trial designers hope will occur: that the new therapy is better than the standard in a comparative study or that an investigative therapy has a better response rate (or lower toxicity) than the stated null unacceptable rate. Results of most statistical tests follow a known statistical distribution, such as the normal distribution or "bell-shaped curve" centered at zero. Other common distributions are the t, the χ^2 (chi-square), and the F. Values of the tests near zero are uninteresting because they are very likely, whereas large (positive or negative) values in the "tail" of the distribution are unlikely. The χ-value is the probability that the value of a statistical test of data could be that far from zero by chance. A χ-value of 0.003 means that there is a 0.3% chance that the results of a test were a random event rather than the result of interesting things happening in the data.

The **type I error** or α-level (alpha level) of a study is the probability that the overall results of the study will indicate that the null hypothesis is false or rejected when in fact it is true. The common α-level is 0.05, but other levels are employed when more- or less-stringent criteria are acceptable.

The **type II error** or β-level (beta level) of a study is the probability that the overall results of the study will fail to reject the null hypothesis when the alternative is in fact true. The power of the study, or chance of detecting a true effect, is $1 - \beta$. Commonly, studies are designed to have 80%–90% power (β of 0.10 or 0.20).

The **significance level** is the maximum p-value of a test that will be taken to indicate statistical significance. When many tests are run on the same data, the significance level for any one test may need to be smaller than 0.05 to keep the overall α-level of the study at 0.05.

Note. Based on information from Gravetter & Wallnau, 2006.

may be lost, and questions related to secondary outcomes may go unanswered. In-depth reading materials regarding adaptive trial designs are included in the list of suggested reading materials at the end of this chapter, and readers interested in more detail are referred to these sources and to the large body of literature available on multistage and sequential designs.

Phase I studies are handled differently than phase II and III studies in that the purpose is to identify the maximum tolerated dose (MTD) for use in other studies. Small cohorts of subjects are entered at a dose of drug, and, depending on the toxicity observed and the escalation/de-escalation scheme, either the study is terminated at that dose, more subjects are entered at that dose or a lower dose, or accrual is commenced at a higher dose.

To develop the design, the team decides upon definitions of dose-limiting toxicity (DLT) and the true rate of DLT that would be unacceptable. The statistician uses exact binomial probabilities to develop an algorithm of subject numbers and dose levels. This algorithm has a high probability of allowing dose escalation if the true rate of DLT at that dose is low, yet also has a low chance of approving for further use a dose with an unacceptably high level of DLT. Some phase I studies randomize rather than sequentially assign subjects to doses, but the intent is always to ensure subject comparability, not to contrast the outcomes statistically.

Analysis Plan

The analysis plan details the intended analyses of the primary and secondary end points and often is not included in a protocol document. However, it may be quite lengthy in an industry-sponsored study that will be part of an FDA filing. The analysis plan covers the particular statistical tests that will be used, with specific attention to issues such as handling stratification and missing data. The plan sets forth the rules that will be applied for the inclusion and exclusion of cases, in addition to special coding and transformations of the data.

The number and type of comparisons to be made need to be specified for a study that has more than one primary end point or for a phase III study with more than two treatment arms. Often, the type I error is divided by the number of comparisons. For example, a three-arm study with two comparisons (arm A versus arm B, and arm A versus arm C) might use 0.025 type I error for each comparison. Many statistical issues that arise during data analysis, such as postrandomization dropout or noncompliance to protocol therapy, cannot be foreseen at the time of the design. However, every attempt should be made to anticipate data problems that could compromise the analysis.

Monitoring

Safety is a vital end point in clinical trials (Hindin, 2006). How safety is monitored and interpreted differs by the phase and the objectives of each trial. Although clinical outcomes are not ignored in phase I studies, they are more important in phase II studies and are the focus in phase III trials. Data from clinical trials are evaluated by internal and external reviewers on an ongoing basis to detect unexpected or unacceptable toxicity and to consider whether it is clear early in accrual that a treatment is ineffective and that subjects should not continue on that arm (FDA, 1998). It should be noted that at interim analysis, treatment might be stopped if the significance of the treatment benefit cannot be detected in the projected sampling population.

Also important to consider is whether the study demonstrates early convincing evidence that one or more treatments are an important advance in therapy. If so, the study should be stopped and the results made public. The monitoring section of the statistical considerations not only outlines the monitoring plan but, where not stated in the sample size section, also provides the stopping rules that guide the reviewers.

In phase I studies, usually small numbers of subjects (three to six) are treated at each dose level. Monitoring the safety of subjects, occasionally on a subject-by-subject basis, is essential, as the escalation/de-escalation scheme to determine the MTD depends on the toxicities observed in subjects at a particular dose level.

In phase II studies, monitoring for both response rate and toxicity often occurs. Phase II studies can have two-stage designs in which a small number of subjects are entered and accrual is continued to the planned total only if a minimum number of responses are seen. The statistical section must state the number of responses needed for the accrual to continue to the second stage. Even if no rules are stated, a study can be paused or closed at any time because of unacceptable or unexpected toxicity.

Outcomes of phase III studies often are monitored through group sequential methods. As an alternative to analyzing the data after the study has accrued all of the necessary subjects and had full follow-up, interim analyses may take place at prespecified fractions of the total planned study time, the total planned study accrual, or the number of events needed to obtain the power specified in the sample size section. The group sequential methods specify boundary values for statistical tests (which correspond to χ-values) in a way that preserves the overall α-level of the study.

The type I error (often 0.05) is spread throughout the number of interim analyses, or "looks," with the last look evaluated at a significance level close to but less than 0.05. If, at any analysis, the statistical test for the primary end point exceeds the boundary established in the statistical design, then statistical significance can be declared, and the trial can be terminated. Procedures also exist that allow termination because of a clear lack of a difference. Although these methods allow a study to close early if it shows convincing early evidence that the study objectives have been met, the sample size has to be a bit larger (about 5%) to allow reuse of the data.

A data monitoring and safety board (DMSB) reviews the interim analysis and other administrative reports. DMSBs play an important role in reviewing interim data from a trial that may have implications for subject safety, the early termination of accrual, or greater treatment efficacy. The committee is composed of a variety of experts from different fields and may include clinicians, ethicists, subject advocates, and biostatisticians. The group meets periodically to consider a study's treatment-specific toxicity and outcomes in a strictly confidential, closed meeting. It is common to hold a planned yearly review of a study, even if the accrual has not yet reached a predetermined interim analysis review point. If no monitoring of phase III outcome data by a DSMB is planned, or if a prolonged delay in data review occurs, a justification must be given to the institutional review board.

Descriptive Statistics

Descriptive statistics are another category of statistics that provide essential information to an interdisciplinary group conducting research. Whereas inferential statistics are used by the scientific community to study samples and subsequently make generalizations about the population that is represented by the test or study population, *descriptive statistics* "describe" the data and are necessary to first organize, summarize, and present the study information in a consistent manner (Gravetter & Wallnau, 2006). When the study results are reviewed and presented for publication, the descriptive statistics are always presented in the introductory information to help to frame the results of the study and define the study population. Thus, the descriptive statistics section provides information that allows members of the scientific community to determine whether the published results are applicable to their subject population.

Descriptive statistics are relevant at each interim analysis and may be hypothesis-generating for future studies. From the CTN's perspective, they are an important component of the research role that the CTN should be familiar enough with to discuss at study reviews. These commonly reported statistics include frequency, mean, median, mode, range, minimum, maximum, sum, and variance and are reported for each variable for which data points are collected during the course of the study.

Commonly used descriptive statistics terms include

- *Mean*—The measure of central tendency that is most commonly used when defining a characteristic of the study population. Adding all the scores for the variable and dividing that number by the number of scores will provide the mean.
- *Median*—The number value that is calculated by locating where exactly half of the data set scores have a value less than or equal to. The median is the 50th percentile. This number is used instead of the mean when the average does not provide a good representation of the study population.
- *Mode*—The data score that occurs with the greatest frequency in a distribution of scores
- *Range*—The measure or value representing the variability within the data sample. The number is calculated by subtracting the lowest value (the minimum) from the highest value (the maximum) in the data score distribution.
- *Minimum*—The lowest value represented in a data score distribution
- *Maximum*—The highest value represented in a data score distribution
- *Sum*—The total number reached when adding all the values (data) within a score distribution
- *Variance*—The "spread" or variability that is represented between data values in a data set. Variance is a mathematical calculation that is represented by the standard deviation when it is squared.

Summary

Interaction among the entire research team is important in establishing the design, hypotheses, and end points that will drive the sample size and power considerations for a clinical trial. The entire research team must have clearly defined plans for interim monitoring and the eventual analysis of the study, as all parts affect each other. This has been a brief, non-numeric overview of the considerations important in the development of a statistical plan for a study. Readers interested in the details and mathematics of sample size calculation, or statistics in general, might consider taking a college-level class in statistics, enrolling in a continuing education offering within their institution on a specific statistical software program, such as SPSS, StatView, or Statistica, or conducting further detailed review of the references listed at the end of this chapter.

Issues evolving in clinical trials that bear watching in the next decade include flexible protocol design, proposed regulations to require electronic submission of study data, streamlining of clinical trial data collection, radiology-based end points, and merging of clinical trial phases. Evaluation and consideration of current statistical methods will be necessary as protocol design and data collection continue to evolve.

The FDA (2006) has been working on an initiative to streamline clinical trials. A "Critical Path Opportunities" paper was published in 2006 that listed proposed future issues for consideration. These issues include data analysis using multiple end points, adaptive trial and enrichment designs, noninferiority trial designs, and handling missing data. Additional key aspects of the FDA's initiative include harnessing bioinformatics by improving designs of late-stage clinical testing and establishing standards for novel forms of drug delivery (FDA, 2006). Such issues will directly affect the continuing evolution of the CTN role, and CTNs will benefit by being familiar with the FDA Web sites as they are updated.

References

Gastineau, T. (2006, May 2). FDA guidance document focuses on cancer trial endpoints. *Applied Clinical Trials.* Retrieved August 4, 2006, from http://www.actmagazine.com/appliedclinicaltrials/content/printContentPopup.jsp?id=324334

Gravetter, F.J., & Wallnau, L.B. (2006). *Statistics for the behavioral sciences* (7th ed.). Belmont, CA: Wadsworth/Thomson Learning.

Hindin, T.J. (2006, June 1). The metamorphosis of trials. *Applied Clinical Trials.* Retrieved August 4, 2006, http://www.actmagazine.com/appliedclinicaltrials/content/printContentPopup.jsp?id=334563

Oken, M.M., Creech, R.H., Tormey, D.C., Horton, J., Davis, T.E., McFadden, E.T., et al. (1982). Toxicity and response criteria of the Eastern Cooperative Oncology Group. *American Journal of Clinical Oncology, 5,* 649–655.

Polit, D.F., & Beck, C.T. (2004). *Nursing research: Principles and methods* (7th ed.). Philadelphia: Lippincott Williams & Wilkins.

U.S. Food and Drug Administration. (1998, September). *Guidance for industry—E9 statistical principles for clinical trials.* Retrieved March 27, 2007, from http://www.fda.gov/cder/guidance/ICH_E9-fnl.pdf

U.S. Food and Drug Administration. (2005, April). *Guidance for Industry—Clinical trial endpoints for the approval of cancer drugs and biologics.* Retrieved March 27, 2007, from http://www.fda.gov/cder/guidance/index.htm

U.S. Food and Drug Administration. (2006). *Critical path opportunities initiated during 2006.* Retrieved March 28, 2007, from http://www.fda.gov/oc/initiatives/criticalpath/opportunities06.html

Additional Resources

Bailar, J.C., & Mosteller, F. (1992). *Medical uses of statistics* (2nd ed.). Boston: Massachusetts Medical Society.

Buyse, M.E., Staquet, M.J., & Sylvester, R.J. (Eds.). (1984). *Cancer clinical trials: Methods and practice.* New York: Oxford University Press.

Donner, A. (1984). Approaches to sample size estimation in the design of clinical trials—A review. *Statistics in Medicine, 3,* 199–214.

Friedman, L.M., Furberg, C.D., & DeMets, D.L. (1998). *Fundamentals of clinical trials* (3rd ed.). New York: Springer.

Gravetter, F.J., & Wallnau, L.B. (2006). *Statistics for the behavioral sciences* (7th ed.). Belmont, CA: Wadsworth/Thomson Learning.

Pocock, S. (1983). *Clinical trials: A practical approach.* New York: Wiley.

Wechsler, J. (2006, May 1). FDA outlines critical path opportunities. *Applied Clinical Trials.* Retrieved August 4, 2006, from http://www.actmagazine.com/appliedclinicaltrials/content/printContentPopup.jsp?id=324324

Wierman, C. (2006, May 2). Oncology clinical development: Retooling for MTTs. *Applied Clinical Trials.* Retrieved August 4, 2006, from http://www.actmagazine.com/appliedclinicaltrials/content/printContentPopup.jsp?id=324332

SECTION III.

Preparation and Assessment

CHAPTER 7
Safety Issues

Janelle Bowersox, RN, MSN, OCN®

Introduction

Safety and protection are integral components of research at all levels of the clinical trial process. Biosafety approval may be required from the Institutional Biosafety Committee (IBC) if a protocol contains handling of an infectious agent, a biologic toxin, or recombinant DNA molecules. Clinical trial nurses (CTNs) share the responsibility of maintaining a safe study environment with the principal investigator (PI) and interdisciplinary team members. CTNs' responsibilities include maintaining current knowledge and skills to safely prepare, handle, and dispose of experimental agents, cytotoxic agents, and biologic agents. If a clinical trial involves radiation therapy, knowledge of safety principles and practices related to each radioactive isotope is essential. Adequate knowledge ensures the personal safety of the nurse, the research participant, family, visitors, and other staff members. This chapter will address safety issues and concerns related to the implementation of clinical trials involving several cancer treatment modalities.

Protection From Blood-Borne Pathogens

In 1991, the Occupational Safety and Health Administration (OSHA) published 29 CFR 1910.1030 in the *Code of Federal Regulations* to protect healthcare workers from the risks associated with HIV, the hepatitis B virus, and the hepatitis C virus. This standard requires employers to implement and annually update a written exposure control plan. Included in these measures are the following: personal protective clothing and equipment, training, sharps containers, and vaccinations against hepatitis B. In response to continued concerns for needlestick injuries, Congress passed the Needlestick Safety and Prevention Act, effective April 18, 2001. This act provided a revision to 29 CFR 1910.1030 and requires employers to utilize technology to reduce exposures to blood-borne pathogens, keep a sharps injury log, and solicit input from healthcare workers who are at risk, and it also requires a mandatory hepatitis B declination to be signed by anyone with a risk of occupational exposure who declines vaccination (OSHA, 1991).

Universal precautions, as defined by the Centers for Disease Control and Prevention (CDC), are intended to address healthcare providers' occupational exposure to blood-borne pathogens. The CDC is a federal agency within the U.S. Department of Health and Human Services (DHHS) whose mission is to "promote health and quality of life by preventing and controlling disease, injury, and disability" (CDC, 2006). Universal precautions provide guidelines for healthcare workers when the potential exists for exposure and possible transmission of HIV, the hepatitis B virus, and other blood-borne pathogens when providing health care. The CDC (1987) defined potentially infective materials as blood or the following human body fluids: urine, semen, vaginal secretions, amniotic fluid, peritoneal fluid, pericardial fluid, pleural fluid, sputum, saliva in dental procedures, cerebrospinal fluid, synovial fluid, any body fluid that is visibly contaminated with blood, and all body fluids in situations where differentiating between body fluids is difficult or impossible. When used judiciously, universal precautions guidelines (CDC, 2003) will prevent the spread of disease from healthcare worker to patient and from patient to healthcare worker (see Figure 7-1). The CDC precautions also include recommendations for disinfecting, sterilizing, cleaning, decontaminating blood spills, and disposing of soiled laundry and infective waste.

The OSHA standard outlines the minimum requirements for preventing accidental exposure to blood-borne pathogens in the workplace. Employers formulate individual exposure-control plans based on these requirements. CTNs must be familiar and compliant with the OSHA standards, as well as with specific institutional policies and procedures that direct clinical components of their practice. Clinical trials frequently require collection of blood or other body fluids from study participants. Individual protocols should clearly specify the procedure to be used in the collection, labeling, and safe transport of study specimens.

Figure 7-1. Universal Precautions

- Protective barriers should be used to prevent exposure of skin or mucous membranes to the blood or body fluids of any patient. Proper gloving is necessary for contact with blood or body fluids; mucous membranes, or non-intact skin of patients, for handling linens or materials that are soiled with blood or body fluids, and for performing venipuncture and other vascular-access device procedures. Masks, protective eyewear, face-shields, and gowns should be worn during procedures that may generate droplets or splashes of blood.
- Skin surfaces should be washed immediately if contamination with blood or body fluids occurs. Hand washing should be employed after the handling of viable materials, after removal of gloves, and before leaving the work area.
- Eating, drinking, smoking, handling contact lenses, and applying cosmetics are not permitted in the work areas. Food should be stored outside the work area in cabinets or refrigerators designed for that purpose only.
- Precaution should be taken to prevent injuries caused by needles, scalpels, and other sharp instruments and devices during and after procedures. All sharps and contaminated instruments should be placed in appropriate puncture-resistant containers for disposal or transport to reprocessing areas.
- Protective ventilation devices should be available for use in areas where the potential for resuscitation is predictable.
- Only mechanical pipetting devices are permitted for transferring of blood and or other body fluids.
- Healthcare workers with open lesions should refrain from direct patient care and direct handling of patient-care equipment until the condition resolves.
- Because of the risk of perinatal transmission, pregnant healthcare workers should be particularly aware of and compliant with precautions to minimize the risk of HIV, hepatitis B virus, and hepatitis C virus transmission.
- All pregnant healthcare workers should have HIV screening included with their prenatal testing.

Note. Based on information from CDC, 1987 [Updated 2006]. Available at http://www.cdc.gov/mmwr/preview/mmwrhtml/rr5514a1.htm.

Chemotherapeutic Agents: Safe Handling

In 1986, OSHA issued a set of safety guidelines (not mandates) to protect and assist personnel who deal with cytotoxic agents. These guidelines offer recommendations for the safe preparation, administration, disposal, spill management, medical surveillance, and storage of cytotoxic agents. They also provide recommendations for training and information dissemination (OSHA, 1986). In addition, the Oncology Nursing Society's (ONS's) *Chemotherapy and Biotherapy Guidelines and Recommendations for Practice* (Polovich, White, & Kelleher, 2005) offer a framework for educating oncology nurses in safe practices for handling chemotherapy to protect themselves and their patients. The American Society of Health-System Pharmacists (ASHP) also produced written guidelines that are congruent with those of OSHA and ONS (Carmignani & Raymond, 1997).

The potential routes of occupational exposure to cytotoxic agents include inhalation of drug aerosols, dust, or droplets; absorption through direct contact with the skin;

injection by inadvertent injury from a needlestick or other contaminated sharp; and ingestion of contaminated food (Polovich et al., 2005). Recommended protective measures include using surgical latex gloves and disposable, lint-free, low-permeability gowns for all cytotoxic drug activities, including preparation, administration, patient care, and spills clean-up. People with known or suspected latex sensitivity or allergy should use gloves made from an alternative material, such as nitrile (Polovich et al.). Face protection (e.g., plastic shields, goggles, respirator masks) should be worn when cleaning chemotherapy spills and when preparing and administering drugs as indicated.

Biological safety cabinets (BSCs) are recommended for the preparation of all antineoplastic drugs to reduce the risk of inhalation exposure (Carmignani & Raymond, 1997; Polovich et al., 2005). The benefits of BSCs are well documented in the literature. The reader is referred to the ONS *Chemotherapy and Biotherapy Guidelines and Recommendations for Practice* (Polovich et al.) for further discussion of BSCs. In addition, all food products and cosmetics should be kept away from the drug preparation and administration area to prevent accidental exposure and contamination.

According to current guidelines, precautionary measures are required when handling excreta and body fluids of patients for at least 48 hours following treatment with antineoplastic agents. This timeline should be adjusted based on the pharmacokinetic activity of individual drugs (Polovich et al., 2005). Guidelines include using appropriate personal protective equipment, providing tight-fitting lids for urinals, and emptying waste products and all contaminated material in a hazardous waste container. CTNs must refer to individual institution-specific guidelines for proper disposal of hazardous waste.

Some phase I and II drug and radiolabeled antibody clinical trials may require the collection of blood, urine, and tissue for pharmacokinetic or radiographic analysis at specific time points. CTNs are responsible for using appropriate self-protective measures during procurement and handling, as well as for ensuring safe transport of specimens to their destination.

Radiation Therapy: Safety Principles and Practices

Many clinical trials involve the use of radiation therapy, either alone or in combination with other treatment modalities. Radiation therapy is the use of ionizing radiation in the treatment of malignant disease. Radiation has two main modes of delivery: external-beam radiotherapy (teletherapy) and brachytherapy (internal or implant therapy). External-beam radiotherapy is the more common of the delivery modes. It is delivered within a very controlled environment to ensure safety of patients and personnel. The ionizing rays are generated and delivered by a linear accelerator that aims the beam at a very specific predetermined field. As the beam passes through the patient's body, changes to cells within the treatment field are initiated that ultimately lead to the cells' destruction. Patients do not retain any radioactivity in their bodies and should be reassured that they are in no danger of causing radioactive harm to themselves or to others around them.

Personnel responsible for the daily treatment of patients receiving radiation are required to wear film badges to monitor accidental exposure. The film-monitoring devices are processed for radiation exposure, and the results are reported monthly. The National Council on Radiation Protection and Measurements recommends that occupational exposure limits be *as low as reasonably achievable,* designated by the acronym ALARA (Dow, Bucholtz, Iwamoto, Fieler, & Hilderley, 1997).

Patients receiving external-beam radiation therapy are not a source of radioactivity and do not require special precautions for the handling of body fluids. However, patients who are receiving cytotoxic agents concomitantly with radiation therapy are subject to the safety precautions for the respective agent(s). Clinicians should reference the OSHA guidelines for safe handling of individual cytotoxic agents.

Brachytherapy commonly is referred to as implant or internal radiation. This form of radiation can be delivered through mechanical placement of radioactive sources (i.e., sealed sources). It also can be delivered through metabolized or absorbed sources that can be administered orally, intravenously, intrapleurally, or intraperitoneally (i.e., unsealed sources). The characteristics of the isotope being used will determine what safety practices need to be followed. It is essential to know the half-life, the type of radioactive emission being produced, and the amount and energy of the isotope being used.

The reader is referred to the ONS *Manual for Radiation Oncology Nursing Practice and Education* (Bruner, Haas, & Gosselin-Acomb, 2005) for further information on radiation safety practices and measures.

Biotherapy: Safety Issues

Biotherapy has emerged as one of the four major cancer treatment modalities over the past several decades. Hyde (2000) described biologic response modifiers (BRMs) as natural or synthesized substances capable of enhancing, regulating, or restoring function to the immune system. Biologic agents act by (a) modulating an individual's immune response to the tumor, (b) acting directly against the tumor, or (c) altering other biologic activities that have an effect on the tumor (Reiger, 2001). Biotherapy is categorized into major BRM classifications (see Figure 7-2).

Many clinical trials involve the use of BRMs. CTNs are responsible for maintaining the knowledge required to administer agents safely and effectively. As with antineoplastic agents, universal precautions should be adhered

to for the handling and disposal of all biologic agents and contaminated materials. Readers are referred to the current edition of the ONS *Chemotherapy and Biotherapy Guidelines and Recommendations for Practice* (Polovich et al., 2005).

Figure 7-2. Classifications of Biotherapy Agents

- Interferons
- Interleukins
- Hematopoietic growth factors
- Monoclonal antibodies
- Retinoids
- Gene therapy

Antiangiogenic agents target the vasculature of tumors to halt their growth and are ideal for use with other cancer therapies (Polovich et al., 2005). Antiangiogenic agents include medications such as bevacizumab (anti–vascular endothelial growth factor), thalidomide, shark cartilage, and levamisole. Many of the new agents are combined with conventional treatment and used in clinical trial protocols. CTNs are responsible for reviewing the protocol and knowing the side effects and interventions to apply.

Summary

The safety of patients, nurses, and members of the interdisciplinary team cannot be overemphasized. Universal precautions, introduced in 1987, protect both healthcare providers and patients from accidental exposure to cytotoxic and biologic agents. Furthermore, knowledge of radiation safety measures is necessary before CTNs can provide complete care to patients receiving radiation therapy. Guidelines developed by ONS during the past five years can provide CTNs with the information needed to ensure a safe environment for healthcare providers and patients.

References

Bruner, D.W., Haas, M., & Gosselin-Acomb, T.K. (Eds.). (2005). *Manual for radiation oncology nursing practice and education* (3rd ed.). Pittsburgh, PA: Oncology Nursing Society.

Carmignani, S.S., & Raymond, G.G. (1997). Safe handling of cytotoxic drugs in the physician's office: A procedure manual model. *Oncology Nursing Forum, 24,* 41–48.

Centers for Disease Control and Prevention. (1987, August 21). Recommendations for prevention of HIV transmission in health-care settings. *Morbidity and Mortality Weekly Report, 36*(Suppl. 2), 1.

Centers for Disease Control and Prevention. (2003, July). *Exposure to blood: What healthcare personnel need to know.* Atlanta, GA: Author.

Centers for Disease Control and Prevention. (2006, July 16). *About CDC: Vision, mission, core values, and pledge.* Retrieved July 31, 2007, from http://www.cdc.gov/about/organization/mission.htm

Dow, K.H., Bucholtz, D., Iwamoto, R., Fieler, V., & Hilderley, L.J. (1997). *Nursing care in radiation oncology* (2nd ed.). Philadelphia: Saunders.

Hyde, R.M. (Ed.). (2000). *Immunology* (4th ed.). Philadelphia: Lippincott Williams & Wilkins.

Occupational Safety and Health Administration. (1986). *Work practice guidelines for personnel dealing with cytotoxic (antineoplastic) drugs*

[Publication No. 8-1.1]. Washington, DC: U.S. Government Printing Office.

Occupational Safety and Health Administration. (1991). *Bloodborne pathogens (Code of Federal Regulations, Title 29, 1910.1030)*. Retrieved April 30, 2006, from http://www.osha.gov/pls/oshaweb/owadisp.show_document?p_table=STANDARDS&p_id=10051

Polovich, M., White, J.M., & Kelleher, L.O. (Eds.). (2005). *Chemotherapy and biotherapy guidelines and recommendations for practice* (2nd ed.). Pittsburgh, PA: Oncology Nursing Society.

Rieger, P.T. (2001). Biotherapy. In P.T. Rieger (Ed.), *Biotherapy: A comprehensive overview* (pp. 3–37). Sudbury, MA: Jones and Bartlett.

CHAPTER 8
Sponsoring Agencies: Industry

Deborah T. Berg, RN, BSN

Introduction

Historically, the National Cancer Institute (NCI) Division of Cancer Treatment and Diagnosis (DCTD) was the major sponsor of new anticancer drug development, as its goal is to facilitate bringing novel anticancer drugs to the public as quickly and as safely as possible. NCI, which funds cooperative groups and cancer centers, as well as other investigators, has collaborations with approximately 10,000 investigators from 200 institutions (NCI Cancer Therapy Evaluation Program [CTEP], 2002).

Pharmaceutical and biotech companies are now more involved in anticancer drug development. This is because of the growth of the specialty of medical oncology and successful improvements in the treatment of several cancers (NCI CTEP, 2002). Most of the anticancer drugs currently developed at NCI are by pharmaceutical and biotech companies (NCI CTEP, 2002). Pharmaceutical and biotech companies are active in new drug development in four different ways (see Figure 8-1). Together with NCI, DCTD evaluates agents in a wide variety of tumor types and disease settings.

Agent Codevelopment With the Cancer Therapy Evaluation Program

The codevelopment of an agent with CTEP may begin with the drug being developed at either CTEP or at a pharmaceutical or biotech company. If CTEP discovers a new agent, an industry sponsor is sought early because NCI does not market new agents. Pharmaceutical and biotech companies may seek CTEP codevelopment at any point in the process (e.g., antitumor screening, preclinical toxicology, clinical trials). If the investigational agent is proprietary to the pharmaceutical or biotech company, NCI negotiates and executes one of two types of contracts: either a cooperative research and development agreement (CRADA) or a clinical trials agreement (CTA). The Federal Technology Transfer Act of 1986 created CRADA agreements, which provide

> **Figure 8-1. Pharmaceutical Company Involvement in New Drug Development**
>
> - Codevelopment of an agent with the National Cancer Institute Cancer Therapy Evaluation Program
> - Collaboration with a cooperative group
> - Industry-designed protocol with a selected research base of one or more institutions
> - Institutional protocol with industry support

a means for the government to collaborate with industry. CTA agreements are an initiative of NCI (2000). After either agreement is initiated, CTEP will submit an investigational new drug (IND) application, a legal mechanism under which investigational drug research is conducted in the United States, to the U.S. Food and Drug Administration (FDA). CTEP then seeks investigators through a request for proposals (RFP), a competitive peer review process in which the merits of the scientific question, which dictates support and funding, are decided.

The investigational agent can be used only within the scope of the protocol, though it may involve the study of a combination of other agents including investigational or commercial anticancer agents. Expenses, protocol development, and data are shared in this partnership. Data are made available to the sponsoring pharmaceutical or biotech company, NCI, and the FDA. The pharmaceutical or biotech company may use the clinical trial results for future trial development or in its FDA drug-approval application. This is either a new drug application (NDA) for cytotoxic or cytostatic agents or a biologic license application (BLA) for biologic agents.

Beyond competitive RFP applications, CTEP uses the Treatment Referral Center (TRC) to inform investigators about anticancer therapeutic protocols available at cancer centers or by cooperative groups. A pharmaceutical or biotech company may work with the TRC to develop the protocol provided to the participating cancer centers. These collaborations can enhance the development process, thus providing new agents to patients with cancer more quickly (NCI CTEP, 2002, 2005).

Collaboration With Cooperative Groups

NCI fosters collaboration between pharmaceutical companies and cooperative groups as long as the proposed clinical trial is consistent with the goals of the cooperative group and is scientifically reasonable (Cheson, 1991). Collaboration with a cooperative group provides peer review, centralized data management, statistical consultation, quality assurance, and access to a large number of potentially eligible patients, including minority populations.

NCI created the Cancer Trials Support Unit (CTSU) to facilitate access to phase III clinical trials that primarily are generated by cooperative groups to study treatment options for breast, gastrointestinal, and genitourinary cancers, as well as acute leukemia. If a pharmaceutical or biotech company is working on a phase III trial through a cooperative group, that same trial will be available to other cooperative groups and non-group investigators via the CTSU, thereby enhancing the number of patients possibly eligible for participation in the study. The reader is referred to Chapter 43 for additional information about the CTSU.

The pharmaceutical or biotech company holds the initial IND application for the investigational agent, but the sponsoring organization also must submit an IND to the FDA for the particular trial, as it is responsible for meeting the FDA's IND regulations. As with clinical trials codeveloped within CTEP, the pharmaceutical or biotech company and the cooperative group collaborate in the planning and writing of the protocol document. The protocol document must be reviewed and approved by CTEP's protocol review committee prior to activation. This mandatory review process results in a perception that the cooperative group clinical trial process is slow and bureaucratic.

Once the protocol is activated, the pharmaceutical or biotech company cannot directly contact the cooperative group to discuss any protocol matters (e.g., obtain protocol information, conduct data audits, discuss protocol amendments) without the prior approval of CTEP's Regulatory Affairs Branch (NCI, 2000).

CTEP provides support, funding, and investigational drug per its standard procedures. The cooperative group may accept additional funding from the pharmaceutical or biotech company for the specific clinical trial only if the funds are to support additional costs, such as extra laboratory tests or data collection, as a result of work requested by the pharmaceutical or biotech company (NCI CTEP, 2002).

Ethical review and the collection of regulatory documents are done according to the cooperative group's standard procedures (see Figure 8-2). Investigators may elect to use a central institutional review board (IRB) established by the NCI to try to streamline the review process of cooperative group/national multicenter cancer treatment trials.

Figure 8-2. Standard Regulatory Documents
• Form 596—Protection of human subject assurance/certification/declaration • Form 1572—Statement of investigator • Curriculum vitae of principal investigator and each subinvestigator • Laboratory certification certificates* • Laboratory normal values (hematology, chemistry, and pathology)* • Institutional review board–approved protocol and consent form documents • Institutional review board clinical trial approval letter
*This information must be provided from every laboratory performing laboratory work for a patient involved in the clinical trial.

Other local IRBs also can decide to accept the review of the central IRB, thereby forgoing the need for a local review.

Data collection, including the submission of case report forms (CRFs), is done according to the cooperative group standard operating procedures. The items to be collected, the necessary reporting time points, and the statistical plan are agreed upon during protocol development. The data obtained during the clinical trial are the property of the cooperative group. However, they are made available to the pharmaceutical or biotech company as agreed upon prior to protocol activation (NCI CTEP, 2002). The cooperative group can present and publish the data according to its standard operating procedures. Release of the raw data to the pharmaceutical or biotech company allows the company to perform statistical analyses on the data. In turn, the analyzed data results may be used by the company for future trials or in an NDA or BLA.

Another way for industry to collaborate with cooperative groups is via a collaborator agreement. A collaborator agreement is used for research that involves a cooperative group not directly supported by CTEP. The Regulatory Affairs Branch of CTEP may review the agreement prior to execution to evaluate any possible conflicts of interest (NCI, 2000).

Single- or Multi-Institutional Collaboration With a Pharmaceutical or Biotech Company Clinical Trial

From an institutional perspective, the most labor-intensive clinical trials are done in collaboration with a pharmaceutical or biotech company. This is a result of the numerous procedures, forms, data points, and quick timelines that are required. These are based on the pharmaceutical or biotech company's operating procedures and goals; for example, a study that may be used to obtain FDA approval will require more data (i.e., more work) than a study that will not be used to gain or extend an existing FDA approval.

Unless a prior working relationship exists with a specific pharmaceutical or biotech company, the institution's principal investigator and the study coordinator will meet with a representative of the company for a prestudy site visit. During this visit, the parties discuss the protocol concept, thereby ascertaining the institute's interest in the study, ability to execute the study based on the number of patients, and potential accrual estimates and patterns. The visit includes pharmaceutical or biotech company representatives touring the hospital, paying particular attention to the patient care areas, pharmacy, and laboratories.

The pharmaceutical or biotech company, with little (if any) input from the institutional principal investigators, frequently drafts the actual clinical trial design and protocol document. The pharmaceutical or biotech company will hold the IND for the trial and must comply with all FDA requirements. However, the standard steps for obtaining protocol approval from the institutions must be followed.

The protocol document must be submitted to each participating institution's scientific review committee and IRB and to a central IRB if one is being utilized for the specific trial (Jenkins & Hubbard, 1991). These groups may take issue with items in the protocol that must be submitted to the pharmaceutical or biotech company prior to activation at the institution. Activation of the protocol can be delayed if there is a disagreement about the locally recommended changes to the protocol.

If the company and the local institution cannot come to an agreement regarding the local suggestions, that particular institution will not be able to participate in the trial. Because the protocol document has already been submitted to and approved by the FDA, all changes to the protocol document must be completed as a formal protocol amendment. All documents listed in Figure 8-2 must be submitted to the pharmaceutical or biotech company before protocol activation. In addition, the company and the institution must sign a contract that outlines the roles of parties, adverse event reporting procedures, good clinical practice guidelines, and a budget.

To explain the protocol document and CRFs to the principal investigator and study coordinator, the pharmaceutical or biotech company may hold a single investigators' meeting for all participants, or it may conduct site initiation meetings at each hospital. The process of data collection (paper or electronic submission), including the actual CRFs used, required data items, and submission time points, is done according to the company's rules and regulations. In this case, the data are the property of the pharmaceutical or biotech company and not the participating institutions.

A clinical research monitor, who is an employee of either the pharmaceutical or biotech company or a professional clinical research organization hired by the company, visits the participating institutions approximately every four to eight weeks. During these visits, the monitor audits a predesignated number of protocol patients by cross-checking information documented on the CRFs with the data points found in the patients' medical records (also known as source documents) following the *Code of Federal Regulations* (CFR), good clinical practice guidelines, and Health Insurance Portability and Accountability Act guidelines (NCI CTEP, 2005a).

The study coordinator is expected to provide the monitor with a workspace, completed CRFs, and patients' medical records. The coordinator also must allot time to work with the monitor if there are questions or if clarifications are needed. The principal investigator should be readily accessible to answer questions or provide clarification for the monitor. During the first visit by any monitor, the study coordinator must orient the monitor regarding the location of key areas (e.g., medical records department) and the set-up of the medical record. The monitor will visit the institution regularly until all CRFs have been audited and submitted to the pharmaceutical or biotech company.

During the trial or even after all CRFs have been submitted, the study coordinator may receive written requests for data clarifications, or queries, because of issues noted during data entry, interim data review, or statistical analysis. These queries must be answered promptly and returned to the pharmaceutical or biotech company with supporting CRF pages or source documentation.

The FDA defines in the CFR procedures and requirements governing the use of investigational new drugs and the monitoring of adverse events (21 CFR 312) (NCI CTEP, 2005b). During the course of the study, including during the treatment and protocol-designated follow-up period, the pharmaceutical or biotech company must receive copies of all reports of serious adverse events and IRB continuing review approvals in accordance with CFR and NCI CTEP (2005b) reporting requirements. The reader is referred to Chapter 28: Adverse Events for a detailed discussion of reporting procedures for adverse events.

Once all of the subjects have ended the protocol-designated follow-up period, the IRB will receive written notification of study completion. At this point, the pharmaceutical or biotech company officially closes the trial at that site. Any unused CRFs and study drugs are returned to the company. The institute is required to keep copies of all CRFs and subject records for a minimum of two years after the pharmaceutical company obtains FDA approval of its NDA or BLA (or it closes the IND) for the same indication as that investigated in the clinical trial (NCI CTEP, 2002).

Institutional Protocol With Pharmaceutical or Biotech Company Support

Investigators may seek the support of a pharmaceutical or biotech company for clinical trials of their own design. Such support may range from supplying the IND for the trial to providing financial support. Although these trials are of interest to the pharmaceutical company, the sponsor's primary resources are focused on other areas. In this partnership, the investigator or the study coordinator provides *limited* regulatory documentation to the pharmaceutical company. Usually, only the 1572 form, the IRB approval letter, the protocol, and the FDA IND documents are required.

Adverse event reporting is done according to CFR and NCI CTEP (2005b) guidelines based on the phase of the trial and with assurances that the pharmaceutical or biotech company is notified of each occurrence. Summary reports are submitted to the company as agreed upon in the clinical trial contract. The protocol document is designed by the principal investigator and reviewed by the pharmaceutical company, which may or may not respond with recommendations. Data point requirements, CRFs, data entry, and statistical analysis are completed at the investigator's institution. The pharmaceutical or biotech company is notified of the final clinical trial results upon completion of the statistical analysis. In the case of presentations or publications, this process must occur at least 30 days prior to submission to allow the company to review the data.

Summary

Industry-sponsored clinical trials are an important part of the clinical trial process. The clinical trial research base may be with NCI, a cooperative group, or one or more institutions. The requirements of an individual investigator and research staff vary depending on the method of participation in the particular clinical trial. Because a clinical trial nurse is well-versed in clinical trial procedures, he or she is able to take a leadership role in implementing the trial as written and in contributing to the timely completion of the study. The clinical trial nurse's primary responsibilities involve patient education, patient recruitment, administration of protocol treatment, protocol compliance, data collection, coordination of required testing, and documentation of test results. This is particularly labor intensive in today's healthcare environment. Strict attention to detail and the completion of successful clinical trials validate outcomes that might translate into changes in health care for patients with cancer.

References

Cheson, B.D. (1991). Clinical trials program. *Seminars in Oncology Nursing, 7*, 235–242.

Jenkins, J., & Hubbard, S. (1991). History of clinical trials. *Seminars in Oncology Nursing, 7*, 228–234.

National Cancer Institute. (2000). *Industry relationship guidelines.* Retrieved July 10, 2006, from http://ctep.cancer.gov/industry/industry.html

National Cancer Institute Cancer Therapy Evaluation Program. (2002). *The investigator's handbook: A manual for participants in clinical trials of investigational agents sponsored by DCTD, NCI.* Retrieved August 29, 2006, from http://ctep.cancer.gov/handbook/index.html

National Cancer Institute Cancer Therapy Evaluation Program. (2005a). *Cancer Therapy Evaluation Program.* Retrieved July 10, 2006, from http://ctep.cancer.gov/index.html

National Cancer Institute Cancer Therapy Evaluation Program. (2005b). *CTEP, NCI guidelines: Adverse event reporting requirements.* Retrieved January 7, 2008, from http://ctep.cancer.gov/reporting/newadverse_2006.pdf

CHAPTER 9
Potential Accrual Base

Dianna Wellen-Traylor, MSN, and Marjorie van der Pas, MS

Introduction

Patients are the essence of a clinical trial. However, only approximately 3%–4% of eligible patients with cancer are enrolled in studies. Currently, much interest surrounds this minimal enrollment (Gross & Krumholz, 2005). The clinical trial nurse (CTN), economic and cultural factors, external marketing, the support of the referral community, and internal staff interest contribute to the potential accrual base, which affects recruitment strategies (McCabe, Varricchio, & Padberg, 1994).

Clinical Trial Enrollment Strategies

CTNs can leverage a variety of promotional and communication techniques to increase clinical trial awareness and enrollment in their communities. Internally, an initial assessment can be done at the cancer center to evaluate and expand employee recognition of currently active trials.

CTNs can utilize the management professionals in the center's marketing department to influence trial promotion. Cancer awareness months are becoming widely recognized by communities at large (see Table 9-1). Local radio and television stations often feature topical media spots during these months, and this opportunity should not be overlooked. Highlighting open clinical trials for breast cancer in October and lung cancer in November is an effective way to focus attention on the advanced treatment opportunities available at local cancer centers.

Lance Armstrong, a cyclist who survived stage IV testicular cancer and won seven Tours de France, recently cycled into cities and towns encouraging patients with cancer to enroll in clinical trials. He has said that such

medical studies saved his life. Armstrong's name is nationally recognized, and CTNs can work with pharmaceutical representatives in their region to take advantage of such familiarity in order to publicize the availability of trials in the area (see www.livestrong.org for more information).

Minority and Underserved Populations

The recruitment of patients from minority and underserved populations to participate in research trials continues to increase. The Geriatric Oncology Consortium (GOC, n.d.) (www.thegoc.org), formed in 2001, is a network of healthcare professionals focused on increasing the pace of discovery in geriatric oncology. The GOC provides the organizational infrastructure for large, multisite intervention trials in the community setting. Practitioners participate in clinical research in their own practices, thus providing patient access to these treatments in their own community.

The specific concerns of culturally diverse populations also must be identified and addressed to provide a sensitive and reasonable approach to accrual. Ethnicity, language, religion, insurance concerns, and comprehension and reading level are just some of the concerns with which a consultant should be involved. These issues, however, are beyond the scope of this chapter.

Internal Processes

Increasing community awareness about the availability of studies at a cancer center may create local interest and familiarity with the overall concept of clinical trials. Community marketing strategies are successful even if they

Authors' note: An electronic medical record (EMR) is now extensively used throughout the healthcare system to document the clinical aspects of patient care. This chapter is written with the assumption that the clinical trial staff is using an EMR; however, this content can also be leveraged for paper-based systems.

The author would like to acknowledge Beverly Meadows, RN, MS, OCN®, for her contribution that remains unchanged from the first edition.

Table 9-1. American Cancer Society Cancer Awareness Calendar of Events	
Month	**Cancer Awareness Event**
January	Great American Health Check Healthy Weight Week National Cervical Cancer Awareness Month
February	Screening and Early Detection Awareness Month
March	National Colorectal Cancer Awareness Month National Nutrition Awareness Month
April	National Cancer Control Month National Minority Cancer Awareness Week National Volunteer Week
May	American Cancer Society Relay for Life® Signature Weekend Melanoma Monday (first Monday in May—American Academy of Dermatology) National Physical Fitness and Sports Month National Woman's Health Week Skin Cancer Detection and Prevention Month Women's Health/Cancer Awareness (Mother's Day) World No Tobacco Day
June	Men's Health/Cancer Awareness (Father's Day) National Cancer Survivors Day (first Sunday in June) National Men's Health Week
July	UV Safety Month
August	Great American Eat Right Challenge
September	Childhood Cancer Month Gynecologic Cancer Awareness Month Leukemia and Lymphoma Awareness Month National Ovarian Cancer Month Prostate Cancer Awareness Month Prostate Cancer Awareness Week Take a Loved One for a Checkup Day
October	National Breast Cancer Awareness Month National Mammography Day
November	Coaches vs. Cancer Classic® Weekend Great American Smokeout Lung Cancer Awareness Month National Family Caregivers Month National Healthy Skin Month Pancreatic Cancer Awareness Month
December	National Aplastic Anemia and MDS Awareness Week

Note. Based on information from Huntsman Cancer Institute, 2007; National Cancer Institute, 2007.

do nothing more than increase the knowledge base in a community. However, it will be years before a clinical trial team can sit back, relax, and wait for patients to knock at their door. Today, searching a clinical database for patients with recurrent disease and aggressively pursuing scheduled patients before their first cycle of a potentially disqualifying treatment will continue to be realistic sources for accrual.

The time-consuming activities related to evaluating eligibility still fall to the oncologist. One strategy is to utilize the electronic medical record (EMR) to filter, sort, and create a list of potentially eligible patients to help the oncologist to identify a subset of patients with a higher chance of matching the enrollment criteria. The EMR output can be based upon enrollment parameters such as diagnosis, comorbidities, tumor-node-metastasis stage, disease status, and laboratory values indicating vital organ functionality. The goal is to encourage busy clinicians to consider enrollment for a short list of patients that are 80% qualified, requiring only surgical margin and pathology report review to validate eligibility (Goldwein, van der Pas, Tis, Nickens, & Comis, 2007).

Trial manager activities that make the dissemination of information easier will facilitate enrollment and minimize miscommunication. The cancer center's intranet is a convenient way to store trial schema in an unalterable file format (i.e., portable document format [PDF]). This provides a secure guidelines document for clinicians to reference on any available workstation.

Accrual Responsibilities

Patients are becoming more and more Internet savvy, and many use legitimate Web sites as a source of trial information. Wick and Zanni (2003) noted that the National Cancer Institute's (NCI's) Cancer Information Service helps potential participants to identify appropriate trials. The National Institutes of Health provides a search engine at www.clinicaltrials.gov that is designed to link patients with possible trials located throughout the United States. If a clinical trial is not available at a specific site, it usually is the responsibility of the physician to contact participating centers.

Using Tumor Registry Data to Ensure Enrollment Success

To successfully meet the accrual goals of a trial, it is best to start with the knowledge that an appropriate number of potentially eligible patients can be approached about the trial. Cancer registry data is an underused yet valuable resource for the nurse who plans to activate new trials or recruitment campaigns. Before a contract is signed and human subject applications are prepared, the CTN should contact the cancer registry and request a report on the incidence of the cancer to be studied.

Andersen, Schroeder, Gaul, Moinpour, and Urban (2005), at the Fred Hutchinson Cancer Research Center in Seattle, WA, used their cancer registry to identify newly diagnosed patients with ovarian cancer and their physicians. With the physicians' consent, these patients were contacted about a quality-of-life trial. Pakilit et al. (2001) found that cancer registries were an excellent source for identifying a large sample of breast cancer survivors. Seventy percent of eligible women responded to a mailed invitation and indicated interest in completing questionnaires for a study examining the late reproductive effects of breast cancer treatments.

The University of Wisconsin Clinical Cancer Center began a recruitment campaign for a cancer control trial by reaching out to physicians. Newcomb, Love, Phillips, and Buckmaster (1990) used nine years' worth of cancer registry data to identify more than 3,000 women who were potentially eligible for their study. The patients' physicians were asked to review a roster of their patients and sign letters with study information if they wanted their patients to be contacted. Thirty-eight percent of women who received letters enrolled in the study, and the trial accrual goal was met 18 months after this method of recruitment was initiated.

Accrual Planning and Economic Considerations

According to the Oncology Roundtable (Advisory Board, 2007b), assessing the economic impact of trials is one of the hurdles that community cancer centers face when developing a clinical research program. Central Baptist Hospital in Lexington, KY, uses an assessment template to estimate the research contribution to the hospital's bottom line (Advisory Board, 2007b). A financial summary is created for every protocol as it is undergoing initial review. As the trial nears closure, the research department reviews expected and actual volumes and costs. The analysis helps to catalogue costs of research activities in order to improve the planning process.

Consolidation of research activities decreases research program costs at academic medical centers and at community hospital centers. Dana-Farber/Partners CancerCare (DF/PCC) was formed in the mid-1990s when three medical centers in the Boston area joined together for research activities. A consolidated business office calculated trial costs for the three centers and served as the single contract office. Revenues from research contracts for DF/PCC have increased 10-fold since the business office was established (Advisory Board, 2007a).

Community health systems also can evaluate opportunities for research consolidation, such as establishing one institutional review board for trials used at all hospitals and clinics in a community system or hiring study coordinators whose role will be to travel to physician offices to enroll eligible patients and provide research coordination between the hospital and the private practices.

Billing Considerations

In September 2000, the Center for Medicare and Medicaid Services issued a National Coverage Determination (NCD) that allows Medicare reimbursement for clinical trial services. Medicare will cover medically necessary conventional care, administration of investigational items or services, and the management of complications related to the investigation. In addition, 18 states have passed legislation requiring health plans to cover routine medical care for clinical trial participants. Although this is good news for clinical trial reimbursement, it creates a complex billing process. In fact, the Office of the Inspector General can impose steep penalties for erroneous billing.

Billing staff will need education from research staff to understand how to bill for trial procedures. The University of Alabama Health System in Birmingham, AL, has established a notification system between the billing and research departments (Advisory Board, 2003). The principle investigator is responsible for completing and faxing a clinical trial billing notice to the billing office whenever a trial receives institutional review board approval. As each trial patient is treated, the research coordinator must fax a notice of services to the billing office that indicates if all charges are to be billed to a trial budget or how to split the charges between the trial sponsor and the patient's insurance.

Trial-specific encounter forms have been successfully used by several hospitals and also can prompt staff to provide the required Medicare diagnosis code and modifiers when patients with Medicare coverage are participating in trials. In addition to trial encounter forms, some hospitals appoint a clinical trial billing compliance officer. In addition to serving as a point of contact between the billing and research departments, the officer can conduct random billing audits. As part of the audit process, the officer can issue corrections for any billing errors and review the audit results with the research department to plan any needed billing process changes.

Summary

Community-based marketing may increase the general awareness of trial availability; however, it is the effort required of the trials team that generally leads to enrollment. Offering studies that correspond to a region's statistical cancer incidence will improve the chances for increased accrual. Community consortiums can help to defray operational costs, thus lowering the cost per person when consent is obtained. Information systems, such as EMRs or cancer registry systems, can be used to suggest potential matches of patients to trials or to generate reports to aid accrual efforts.

References

Advisory Board. (2003, July 23). *Oncology roundtable practice brief: Clinical research billing.* Retrieved April 6, 2007, from http://www.advisory.com

Advisory Board. (2007a, January 2). *The oncology leadership agenda: Integrated clinical trials management.* Retrieved April 6, 2007, from http://www.advisory.com

Advisory Board. (2007b, January 22). *Oncology revenue strategy: Clinical research business units.* Retrieved April 6, 2007, from http://www.advisory.com

Andersen, M.R., Schroeder, T., Gaul, M., Moinpour, C., & Urban, N. (2005). Using a population-based cancer registry for recruitment of newly diagnosed patients with ovarian cancer *American Journal of Clinical Oncology, 28,* 17–20.

Geriatric Oncology Consortium. (n.d.). *Membership features.* Retrieved November 19, 2005, from http://www.thegoc.org/features_benefits.html

Goldwein, J.W., van der Pas, M.A., Tis, L., Nickens, R., & Comis, R. (2007). Clinical trial eligibility determination using an oncology electronic medical record system interfaced to a caBIG-certified trial database [Abstract]. *Journal of Clinical Oncology, 2007 ASCO Annual Meeting Proceedings, 25*(Suppl. 18), Abstract 6626.

Gross, C.P., & Krumholz, H.M. (2005). Impact of managed care on cancer trial enrollment. *Journal of Clinical Oncology, 23,* 3811–3818.

Huntsman Cancer Institute. (2007, June 28). *Cancer awareness calendar.* Retrieved August 2, 2007, from http://www.huntsmancancer.org/cancerInformation/awareness.jsp

McCabe, M.S., Varricchio, C.G., & Padberg, R.M. (1994). Efforts to recruit the economically disadvantaged to national clinical trials. *Seminars in Oncology Nursing, 10,* 123–129.

National Cancer Institute. (2007). *Cancer related health observances calendar 2007.* Retrieved August 14, 2007, from http://cis.nci.nih.gov/resources/observance.html

Newcomb, P.A., Love, R.R., Phillips, J.L., & Buckmaster, B.J. (1990). Using a population-based cancer registry for recruitment in a pilot cancer control study. *Preventive Medicine, 19,* 61–65.

Pakilit, A.T., Kahn, B.A., Petersen, L., Abraham, L.S., Greendale, G.A., & Ganz, P.A. (2001). Making effective use of tumor registries for cancer survivorship research. *Cancer, 92,* 1305–1314.

Wick, J., & Zanni, G. (2003, December). Cancer clinical trials and the elderly: Searching for certainty. *Pharmacy Times.* Retrieved November 3, 2005, from http://www.pharmacytimes.com/article.cfm?ID=823

CHAPTER 10
Educating Staff

Mechelle Barrick, BSN, RN, OCN®, CCRP

Introduction

Conducting an effective clinical trial is a multidisciplinary effort. If the trial is to be completed successfully, the training of collaborating staff must be a high priority. As DiGiulio et al. (1996) noted, an effective staff education program assists the investigator in achieving the fundamental goal of the trial: to determine whether the treatment is effective and safe. A well-trained staff will ensure that all patients receive the treatment as delineated in the protocol and that any side effects, especially serious ones, are quickly identified and managed. Education programs help to provide the consistency necessary to obtain valid, accurate results. The clinical trial nurse (CTN) is a resource and guide for staff nurses, and open communication that fosters education will help to maintain the integrity of the clinical trial.

Planning the Program

Cassidy and Macfarlane (1991), Wheeler (1991), and DiGiulio et al. (1996) emphasized that the first step in designing and conducting an effective education program requires that the CTN have a thorough knowledge of the protocol. Understanding the protocol will help to identify the needed resources and assist in analyzing the trial's impact on the responsibility of the healthcare team. Figure 10-1 is an example of the staff representation in a gene therapy study for mesothelioma.

The CTN must identify (a) the targeted population of the trial, (b) the disciplines and departments that will participate in or be affected by the trial, (c) the guidelines for the responsibilities of each staff member, (d) the drug delivery method that will be used, (e) any new skills that are required, and (f) the equipment necessary to perform the trial.

Identifying who will train the staff and what resources will be available to train them is the next step in develop-

> **Figure 10-1. Members of the Healthcare Team in a Gene Therapy Study for Mesothelioma**
>
> - Physicians
> - Nurses
> - Human applications laboratory personnel
> - Pharmacists
> - Laboratory personnel
> - Nursing support personnel
> - Radiology staff
> - Dermatology staff
> - Psychosocial support staff, including pastoral care staff
> - Outpatient services/visiting nurse
> - Outpatient infusion companies
> - Business office/financial department

ing the education program. Meili (1991) explained that the nurse, in the role of educator, is responsible for staff education. Depending on the size of the institution, the educator for clinical trials should be a nurse, and this educator may be one or a combination of the following: clinical nurse specialist, CTN, nurse manager, or staff nurse. Wheeler (1991) identified clinical nurse specialists and nurse practitioners as in-house resources to assist with training. In-house training programs should be used to help to develop or improve skills and to obtain any certification (e.g., chemotherapy) required for the trial. The study sponsor can assist with presenting education programs for staff, as well.

Once the trainer is identified, an assessment of the staff's level of knowledge of clinical trials and of the skills required for the trial may be undertaken. To better identify the training needs of the staff, the trainer should conduct a meeting with the supervisors to discuss individual and group skill requirements and preferred method(s) of learning.

The CTN then introduces the trial to the staff. Ideally, the principal investigator will present the study and explain

The author would like to acknowledge Adri Recio, RN, for her contribution that remains unchanged from the first edition.

the scientific rationale. The CTN explains the specific meaning that participating in a clinical trial has to the patient. For example, in a clinical trial, participation can be offered as treatment for the disease or as palliative treatment. In the event that the principal investigator is not available, the CTN should have the expertise to present the study in its entirety to the staff.

Tools Used in Staff Training

According to DiGiulio et al. (1996), developing effective tools for training is essential (see Figure 10-2). The most valuable instrument in a clinical trial is the actual

---

Figure 10-2. Educational Tools

- Protocol
- Fact sheets
- Abridgments
- Summaries
- Schema
- Calendars
- Instruction sheets
- Videos
- Booklets
- Flyers
- List of open studies
- Laminated pocket cards with study eligibility criteria
- E-mails to staff regarding open studies, eligibility criteria, and closures
- Intranet/Internet

---

protocol itself. This document is the detailed written plan of a clinical experiment and provides step-by-step guidelines for the safe conduct of the trial. A copy of the protocol should be kept in every department and unit involved in the trial, as well as on the institution's intranet. Every copy must be kept current with new protocol recommendations, and staff must be informed of updates, as well.

Although everyone involved in a trial should be familiar with the protocol, using it as a single reference has drawbacks. Often, not enough time is available to read the document, and sometimes it may not provide adequate information on the administration of the drug. Therefore, DiGiulio et al. (1996) recommended that other instructional materials be used as complements to the protocol. Several effective tools can be developed to enhance the educational process, including fact sheets to use as quick reference guides, abridgments (commonly used by the National Cancer Institute) to summarize essential information and identify the staff's responsibilities, and summaries (used by the European Oncology Research and Treatment Consortium) to identify the daily requirements of the protocol and provide practical solutions that will not interfere with the trial's outcome. In addition, calendars and schema (see Figure 10-3) can list standard instructions for the daily requirements of the study. All of these methods help to provide accurate,

concise, and easy-to-read information about the protocol for quick reference.

Wheeler (1991) strongly recommended the use of protocol abridgments because they can be used as a quick referral source and to communicate changes to the protocol. Figure 10-4 is an example of a protocol abridgment that has been adapted from an NCI example. Spilker (1991) recommended the use of written instructional material "to standardize the conduct of the clinical trial and to help prevent problems in communication between the people involved" (p. 272).

Once the protocol opens to enrollment, continued communication with the multidisciplinary team is essential. The CTN should be present to assist and support the team. Frequent updates on new findings and trends should be shared, especially with the personnel providing direct care. Any deficiencies noted in implementation of the study should be identified and corrected, and any areas of concern should be addressed.

Training the Nursing Staff

As the protocol is ready to be activated, special attention and training should be given to the nursing staff. Whether the setting is the hospital, outpatient clinic, or, with the advent of managed care, the home, the staff nurse is integral to clinical research (Melink & Whitacre, 1991). Wheeler (1991) identified nurses as the key to a successful clinical trial because they have the skills necessary to best affect the trial. Figure 10-5 lists what should be included in a training program for the nursing staff.

Based on the many roles of staff nurses and CTNs providing care for patients in a clinical trial, the training and education of these team members is particularly important. The same steps and tools used to train other team members should be used. Attention should be paid to training as many staff nurses as possible. If the patient is hospitalized, in-service programs should be held for all shifts, and a member of the research team should be available to answer any questions that may arise.

Melink and Whitacre (1991) viewed the staff nurse as the one staff member who provides continuity of care and support to the patient enrolled in a clinical trial, as well as information on the treatment, side effects, and response. As the primary caregiver, the staff nurse has a broad base of responsibility (McEvoy, Cannon, & MacDermott, 1991; Melink & Whitacre; Wheeler, 1991). The staff nurse is responsible for educating the patient and the family and for ascertaining their full understanding of the trial, the treatment, its risks and side effects, any special requirements, and follow-up. The staff nurse administers the treatment while providing safety and comfort. Assessing for side effects, recognizing symptoms before the patient is aware of them, and identifying toxicities not experienced in the preclinical studies are valuable nursing skills. The staff nurse manages symptoms within

Figure 10-3. Calendar for Gene Therapy for Mesothelioma																					
Day	PRE	1	2	3	4	5	6	7	8	9	10	11	12	13	14	15	16	17	18	19	20
Date																					
H&P	x	x	x			x		x		x			x		x		x			x	
Weight	x	x	x			x		x		x			x		x		x			x	
CBC/DIFF	x	x		x		x		x		x			x		x		x			x	
Renal/LFTS	x	x		x		x		x		x			x		x		x			x	
UA	x																				
PFTS	x																				
EKG	x			x		x		x													
CXR	x	x	x			x	x			x			x		x		x			x	
CT scan	x																				
Ancillary Test																					
5 green-top tubes[a]			x			x														x	
1 red-top tube[b]			x			x				x			x							x	
Pleural fluid		x	x			x															
AFU Cx swabs[c]			x	x		x							x							x	
GCV Peak & Trough																					
Treatment																					
CT	x																				
Virus instillation		x																			
VTC			x																		
Ganciclovir				x																	
Discharge																					x

Draw bloods at 6 am.
[a] Call immunology lab ext. _____ for pick up.
[b] Coagulate for 30 min., centrifuge for 10 min., separate, and freeze.
[c] Refrigerate.

the parameters allowed in the protocols. Additionally, the staff nurse documents the treatment, side effects, and interventions to facilitate communication and data extraction and also coordinates any tests required by the study, makes the appropriate referrals as necessary, and acts as a patient advocate (see Figure 10-6).

Smith and Buscemi (2005) stressed the role of the clinical nurse in maintaining the integrity of clinical trials. However, they found that the majority of new staff nurses were unsure of their role in the implementation of clinical trials. Rather than wait until specific protocols are initiated, clinical trial education should begin with the initial unit orientation program. As current literature acknowledges the need for staff education, limited resources and educational tools are available to assist in staff preparation. Smith and Buscemi developed a clinical trial module to utilize as part of a staff orientation program, ensuring the appropriate preparation of new oncology nurses.

Summary

The success of a clinical trial relies on the identification of members of the multidisciplinary team involved in

---

Figure 10-4. Example of Protocol Abridgment

Title: Phase I Trial of AdRSVtk Virus with Ganciclovir in Patients With Unresectable Malignant Mesothelioma

Principal Investigator:

Patient Population: Patients with histologically proven malignant mesothelioma of pleural origin that cannot be surgically resected. Patients are excluded if they have brain metastases or have received prior chemotherapy, radiotherapy, immunotherapy, or gene therapy or have undergone successful pleurodesis.

Therapy: A phase I study to evaluate the toxicity and to identify the maximum tolerated dose of AdRSVtk when given with ganciclovir.

Treatment Schema: All patients will have a chest tube (CT) placed on day of admission. On day 2, a one-time dose of AdRSVtk will be instilled over five minutes via the chest tube at bedside. All patients will undergo a videothoracoscopy (VTC) biopsy on day 5. Ganciclovir (GCV) 5 mg/m^2 IV twice a day for 14 days will start on day 6. Dose escalation may occur 30 days after the last patient has received the virus. When the maximum tolerated dose is reached, two more patients are treated at the prior dose.

	CT		AdRSVtk		Videothoracoscopy	Ganciclovir
Day	1	2	3	4	5	6–19

Dose Escalation: All dose escalations require that three patients tolerate the previous dose, 30 days have elapsed since the gene instillation, and no more than grade 3 toxicities have occurred.
1. 10^9 particles
2. 10^{10} particles
3. 10^{11} particles
4. 10^{12} particles

Major Side Effects: This is a phase I study, and toxicities to human beings are unknown. However, expected side effects may include fever, hypotension, anaphylaxis, myelotoxicity, localized skin rash and pruritus, elevated transaminases, pain to site of CT and VTC, as well as complications of CT placement and surgery.

Guidelines for Virus Administration
1. AdRSVtk virus will be thawed and diluted in 100 cc normal saline and provided by the Institute of Human Gene Therapy at the University of XXX to the bedside by 8 am on day 2.
2. The principal investigator will instill the virus via the CT.
3. Normal saline at KVO (keep vein open) will be infused via peripheral line.
4. Patient will be attached to a cardiac monitor for 24 hours.
5. Vital signs and O_2 sats will be taken prior to instillation, every 15 minutes x 4, every 30 minutes x 2, every hour x 2, every four hours x 6, then every shift throughout hospitalization.
6. Patients will be monitored closely for toxicities during the full 19-day hospitalization.

Guidelines for GCV Administration
1. GCV will be reconstituted by the pharmacy in 10 ml of sterile water for injection to provide a solution of 50 mg/ml. The appropriate dose (5 mg/m^2) then will be diluted in 100 ml normal saline.
2. Once reconstituted, GCV is stable for 12 hours and should be kept at room temperature.
3. GCV is administered IV over one hour twice daily. Because of its potential for phlebitis, a central line access (subclavian or peripherally inserted central catheter) should be placed before the start of treatment. Nursing guidelines for central lines must be followed.
4. The nurse administering GCV must follow nursing guidelines for administration of IV fluids.
5. Patients will be monitored for neutropenia and thrombocytopenia, headache, confusion, abnormal liver function, increased serum creatinine, retinal detachment, nausea and vomiting, and phlebitis.

Guidelines for Monitoring
1. Complete blood count, differential, liver function tests, renal panel three times a week
2. Electrocardiogram three times a week
3. Chest x-ray post CT placement, post CT removal, three times a week

Ancillary Studies
1. Two red-top tubes three times a week. Let coagulate for 30 minutes, centrifuge for 10 minutes, separate serum, freeze, and batch.
2. Five green-top tubes on days 2, 5, and 19. Page immunology laboratory staff for pick up.
3. Chest fluid: 5–10 cc from CT on days 1, 2, and 5.
4. Adenoviral forming unit assays (AFU), culture swabs of nose, stool, and urine on days 1, 2, 3, 4, 8, 12, and 16. Refrigerate and batch.

Figure 10-5. Training Program for a Clinical Trial

- Presentation of protocol, scientific rationale, and objectives
- Description of dose and administration of treatment
- Review of the expected and unexpected toxicities
- Monitoring and management of side effects
- Instruction on use of specialized equipment necessary for the conduct of the study (e.g., IV pumps, tubing)
- Review of tests required by study
- Review of instructions on processing ancillary tests (e.g., pharmacokinetics)
- Review of questionnaires to be completed by the subjects
- Review of names and telephone numbers of the clinical trial staff
- Review of the handouts (e.g., articles on agent, protocol abridgment or summaries, calendar of events)
- Review of order forms that will be used for the protocol
- Review of any forms that will require completion by the staff
- Special labeling of charts (e.g., special color, "investigational drug required")
- Highlights of study requirements
- Materials from study sponsor

Figure 10-6. Responsibilities of the Staff Nurse

- Education of patient and family
- Administration of treatment
- Assessment of side effects
- Management of symptoms
- Identification of new toxicities
- Documentation of treatment and side effects
- Notification and communication with clinical trial nurse
- Communication with research team
- Referrals
- Patient advocacy

---

the conduct of the trial as well as on the skills and training required by the team members to perform the individual tasks. Education of the nursing staff, who provides direct care to patients in a clinical trial, will foster accurate treatment, identification and management of toxicities, and continuity of patient care. The CTN needs to be on the forefront of staff education on clinical trials, especially as related to drugs, side effects, and administration. In addition to the protocol document, tools can be designed for quick reference to help team members to better understand the protocol and each member's role in the study. The CTN can coordinate and assist in these efforts, preparing the staff to embark on a trial conducted safely and effectively.

References

Cassidy, J., & Macfarlane, D.K. (1991). The role of the nurse in clinical cancer research. *Cancer Nursing, 14*, 124–131.

DiGiulio, P., Arrigo, C., Gall, J., Mohn, C., Nieweg, R., & Strohbucker, B. (1996). Expanding the role of the nurse in clinical trials: The nursing summaries. *Cancer Nursing, 19*, 343–347.

McEvoy, M.D., Cannon, L., & MacDermott, M.L. (1991). The professional role for nurses in clinical trials. *Seminars in Oncology Nursing, 4*, 268–274.

Meili, L. (1991). The community hospital perspective of clinical trials and the role of the nurse educator. *Seminars in Oncology Nursing, 4*, 280–287.

Melink, T.J., & Whitacre, M.Y. (1991). Planning and implementing clinical trials. *Seminars in Oncology Nursing, 4*, 243–251.

Smith, R., & Buscemi, C.K. (2005). The missing link in nursing orientation: Introducing clinical research trials [Abstract]. *Oncology Nursing Forum, 32*, 464.

Spilker, B. (1991). *Guide to clinical trials*. New York: Raven Press.

Wheeler, V.S. (1991). Preparing nurses for clinical trials: The cancer center approach. *Seminars in Oncology Nursing, 4*, 275–279.

CHAPTER 11
Clinical Research/Interdisciplinary Team

Carolyn R. Schmidt, RN, MSHA, OCN®

Introduction

The key component of a successful clinical research program is the team of individuals who are committed to advancing patient care through the conduct of high-quality clinical trials. This team of individuals is responsible for the selection of good scientific protocols to meet the needs of their specific patient populations. At the same time, they must ensure the protection of the rights, interests, and safety of these patients, which remains the number-one priority in clinical research.

Key attributes of a highly successful clinical research or interdisciplinary team have been identified as "devotion of adequate time and energy, conscientious acceptance of significant responsibilities, availability of suitably trained and committed staff with sufficient time allowances, and access to adequate facilities which support the conduct of clinical research activities" (Christian, Abrams, & Parkinson, 2004, p. 390). These attributes can be viewed as crucial across the board—whether for the principal investigator, physician subinvestigators, clinical trials office (CTO) staff, clinical staff who perform patient assessment and treatment administration, pharmacy personnel, laboratory personnel, etc.—as all play a pivotal role and all must possess the integrity, knowledge, and expertise necessary to conduct high-quality cancer clinical trials.

Team Members

For purposes of this discussion, the "team" will be divided into two components, one being the *clinical research team* (i.e., principal investigator, physician subinvestigators, and CTO personnel), and the other being the *interdisciplinary team* (i.e., all individuals involved in clinical research activities inclusive of the clinical research team). Numbers and types of individuals may vary per clinical setting, but the primary functions needed to support good clinical practice across the board remain the same.

The team leader for any clinical trial is the designated *principal investigator* (PI). This individual assumes full responsibility for the overall conduct of the trial. In addition to having a clear appreciation of the ethical issues involved in the clinical research process, the PI must have

- A working knowledge of institutional review board (IRB) and regulatory requirements
- A thorough understanding of the protocol
- The enthusiasm and desire to participate and motivate others
- The ability to ensure that eligible patients are enrolled
- The ability to ensure that the protocol treatment is appropriately administered
- The ability to maintain a high level of protocol compliance with ongoing submission of prompt and accurate data (Cassidy, 2002; Lader et al., 2004).

Likewise, other participating physician subinvestigators must incorporate the same standards and display the same level of scrutiny as is expected of the PI. Designated CTO personnel are very important to the physician investigators and function to ensure compliance mandated by federal, institutional, and sponsor regulations.

The primary tasks associated with the CTO irrespective of its composition fall into three categories: administrative tasks, case management tasks, and data management tasks (see Figure 11-1). Depending upon the research environment (e.g., number of patients enrolled, type of clinical practice), these functions may be handled collectively by an individual clinical research coordinator or associate who, in the opinion of this author, should be an RN because of the direct patient care services provided. Conversely, the tasks could be handled by a staff of individuals, each of whom would have a very select menu of job responsibili-

The author would like to acknowledge Beverly Meadows, RN, MS, OCN®, and Suzanne Fioravanti, RN, BSN, OCN®, for their contribution that remains unchanged from the first edition.

ties (Christian et al., 2004). When the latter model is used, distinct administrative, data management, and case management functions would primarily be divided among the staff as indicated in Figure 11-1. Regardless of which type of program is established, both institutional and cancer program support need to exist at the senior administrative level as well as being part of the cancer program's goals and institution's strategic plans.

Figure 11-1. Categories of Interdisciplinary Team Tasks

Administrative Tasks
- Staff supervision
- Institutional review board requirements
- Regulatory requirements
- Team education/support
- Contracts/budgets/grants/invoicing
- Quality assurance
- Information flow
- Program development
- Protocol review processes
- Supplies management

Case Management Tasks
- Patient screening/recruitment
- Nursing assessments
- Eligibility verification
- Informed consent process
- Protocol compliance
- Patient safety and monitoring
- Patient education/support
- Clinical staff education
- Source documentation
- Specimen handling

Data Management Tasks
- Data abstracting
- Data submission
- Study start-up tasks
- Serious adverse event reporting
- Database input
- Auditing processes
- Long-term follow-up
- Affiliate oversight
- Data collection forms
- Pathology submission

This latter model further lends itself to the development of clinical trial specialists who have the capability of becoming experts in their job responsibilities and very knowledgeable in their area of oversight. However, to be a truly well-functioning team, it is imperative that provisions be made for each member of the team to have exposure to all facets of the clinical research process. This will provide for a well-rounded understanding of all functions and will support cross-coverage of assignments if occasions arise. The challenge with this model, however, is to make sure that the "gray area" (i.e., responsibilities that cross boundaries and have the potential for duplication or neglect) is kept to a minimum. To do so, each individual must make a commitment to work and communicate closely with other members of the CTO and to ensure that critical knowledge is shared

with respect to a particular protocol and/or patient. It also means that for quality assurance purposes, a mechanism must be in place to capture and share information regarding protocol deviations and/or opportunities for improvement. An example of a tool used to track protocol deviations is shown in Figure 11-2. Quality assurance processes are best handled by one individual. Having one designee allows for frequent and current feedback to staff and clinicians on an individual basis and also supports a more sophisticated mechanism for predetermined updates (e.g., quarterly) as may be required by programmatic, institutional, sponsor, and federal guidelines. It truly can be very impressive to sponsors if quality assurance issues, along with process improvement mechanisms, are presented to them before they identify any deficits.

Some clinical research models are designed so that all individuals involved in the protocol-specific tasks are part of the CTO team. In other models, individuals involved in these tasks are employed by other departments, which may occur, in particular, with case management or nursing personnel. When staff members from other departments are involved, the administrative, data management, and clerical personnel generally are part of the CTO personnel. When CTO personnel are limited in number, these individuals usually will fall under the direction of the PI or the oncology services manager. When the CTO personnel are larger in number and have more selective responsibilities, a designated *clinical research manager* likely will oversee the entire operation. The responsibilities of the clinical research manager are outlined in Figure 11-3.

In defining a highly effective clinical research team, it generally is one that demonstrates a high educational background and has personnel that are well trained, cohesive in their appreciation of good clinical research practices, and able to demonstrate flexibility and autonomy while displaying a willingness to standardize processes. Other criteria would include individuals who are detail oriented, self-motivated, computer literate, and well organized and have an understanding of research methodology, statistics, and tumor registry and staging (Cassidy, 2002).

The interdisciplinary team, as a whole, plays an integral role in the performance of specific requirements of designated clinical trials. These individuals are key to the overall success of the clinical trial. Without their support, it would be extremely difficult, if not impossible, to ensure protocol compliance.

For any protocol in which an investigational agent is supplied, the PI is held accountable for ensuring its appropriate distribution and for meticulous recordkeeping with respect to storage, shipping, and distribution (Nesbitt, 2004). Although these responsibilities may be handled by anyone licensed to distribute medications, a designated *research pharmacist* has the capability, knowledge, and expertise to handle these responsibilities in the most efficient and thorough manner. In addition, a research pharmacist can be instrumental in the initial review of the protocol

Figure 11-2. Protocol Deviations Log

QUALITY ASSESSMENT LOG

Date	MRN	Study	Clinic	Deviation w/ Explanation	Status	Attribution

Deviations

C = Consent
E = Eligibility
L = Labs
PE = Physical
QOL = Quality of life
RE = Receptionist/appt. staff
RC = Reconsent
AD = Administrative staff
T = Tests
U = Unknown
TX = Treatment
V = V/S, P/S, H or W
Other = Explain

Status

1 = Done variation
2 = Not done, w/ explanation
3 = Not done, no explanation
4 = Noncompliant patient

Attributed to

MD = Physician
CM = Case manager
TN = Treatment nurse
PH = Pharmacist

Note. Designed in conjunction with Rose Ermete, RN, BSN, CCRP, Quality Assurance Specialist, Henry Ford Health System, Detroit, MI.

and can be a tremendous resource with respect to staff education and training.

Depending upon the nature of the protocol, other interdisciplinary team members may include physician investigators from other departments (e.g., other specialties such as radiation therapy, surgery, urology, nuclear medicine), physicians within a specialized training program (e.g., residents, fellows), nurse practitioners, physician associates, and designated clinical support staff. These individuals will be able to coordinate protocol-required procedures and provide treatments that are specific to their area of expertise. Appropriate protocol information must be shared to ensure that all aspects of the protocol, with respect to the procedures and/or treatments, can be administered appropriately.

Nurses working in either the inpatient unit or the ambulatory treatment center are invaluable resources because of their direct involvement with each patient. Not only are they called upon to deliver protocol treatments (which can be extremely complicated and challenging), but they also may be asked to conduct patient assessments, ensure schedule adherence, support completion of patient surveys, provide for patient educational opportunities, and so on. It generally is expected that these individuals have a comprehensive understanding of oncology and the research process and maintain excellent communication, organizational, and

time management skills (Cusack, Jones, & Chisholm, 2004; Cusack, Jones-Wells, & Chisholm, 2004; Jones, Cusack, & Chisholm, 2004). It is imperative that these clinicians receive all of the necessary protocol information prior to a patient encounter, with the optimal method being a one-on-one interaction with clinical research personnel (Thompson, Pickler, & Reyna, 2005).

Diagnostic radiology frequently is part of the multidisciplinary team because of the ongoing disease assessments that are critical to the evaluation of the protocol treatment. For many clinical trials, it is necessary to identify both a designated and a back-up *radiologist* who will assume responsibility for all diagnostic evaluations at the site. These individuals need to be kept abreast as to potential clinical trial candidates and the status and required evaluations for previously registered patients.

Central *laboratory services personnel* (e.g., pathologists, laboratory directors, technicians) provide protocol support at the time of biopsies, tumor resections, and specimen collections. Before an institution decides whether to participate in a clinical trial requiring laboratory services, the protocol must be reviewed by a laboratory representative to ensure that the services involved can be provided. Because of the support they provide with respect to equipment and facilities, they often are called upon to collect and prepare specimens, centrifuge body fluids, provide for specimen

---

Figure 11-3. Clinical Research Manager Responsibilities

- Day-to-day work flow
- Staff training
- Staff supervision and coaching
- Quality assurance
- Coordination of clinical trial processes with sponsor
- Incorporation of standard operating procedures
- Program development
- Site marketing
- Clinical trials marketing (e.g., television, radio, Web site, newspapers, community events, tumor boards)
- Financial and contractual processes
- Ongoing team communication
- Team education and development (e.g., continuing education units, certification)
- Patient care support (e.g., patient overload, staff absence, unit support)

Note. Based on information from Pierre, 2005.

---

storage (e.g., –20°C or –70°C freezer space), handle or assist with specimen shipping, or provide necessary supplies (e.g., International Air Transport Association–approved containers, dry ice, packing materials, shipping labels). All protocol-specific instructions and supplies (e.g., containers, collection devices) must be given to the appropriate laboratory personnel either in bulk or on a per-patient basis, whichever is most suitable to meet their needs and ensure protocol compliance. Pharmacy staff members also need to be involved from the start so that they know what is expected in regard to drug preparation and storage, mixing, and drug accountability.

Other key team members, who work somewhat behind the scenes but play a vital role in the overall undertaking of clinical research, include social workers, marketing and public relations staff, and clerical personnel. *Social workers* are called upon to provide emotional support, as well to support the patient's physical needs associated with protocol treatments (e.g., meal and parking tickets, treatment assistance, transportation). *Marketing and public relations staff* support the overall clinical research program or individual trials by means of advertising, brochure design, and other promotional activities. *Clerical personnel* directly support the CTO team members. Their responsibilities are associated with the overall functioning of the office (e.g., information flow, meeting and site-visit coordination, supplies maintenance). Clerical personnel also may be instrumental in appointment scheduling and patient triaging.

How to Keep a Good Team Functional

Both the clinical research team and the interdisciplinary team must individually and collectively establish a positive team approach and maintain a conscientious effort toward effective communication patterns. Given the hectic schedules of most clinicians and the never-ending challenges of clinical research personnel, maintaining open and thorough communication channels is not always easy to accomplish.

However, *good communication* and *knowledgeable team members* are the two most important attributes in clinical trial success and thus must be given priority. It is critical that the clinical research manager ensure that information received both externally and internally becomes available to either the entire staff or designated individuals as appropriate. For example, when a protocol amendment is received, not only should the IRB administrative staff have access, but also the PI, designated case manager, data manager, and possibly other team members must receive a copy, as it may have current implications for patients, thus making the timeliness of IRB approval more critical. This communication flow should also be documented; a suggestion would be to indicate on the top of the original copy (which may be kept with the master protocol file or regulatory binder).

In addition, an ongoing effort is needed to promote cohesiveness among team members and the establishment of consistent standards of processes and practice. Examples of how this might be accomplished could be a team lunch or an after-work get-together; these prove to be very successful in helping team members to get to know one another at a more personal level. A weekend retreat for CTO staff and other clinical personnel (e.g., treatment nurses, pharmacists, laboratory personnel, patient schedulers) with a focus on team-building and quality initiatives has proved to be an extraordinary opportunity for both professional and personal growth.

Last, but certainly not least, is the need to show appreciation for a job well done and to ensure that members of the team are receiving positive rewards, both personal and professional. As positive contributions are made, they need to be acknowledged individually and collectively. Presenting a complete listing at the time of yearly review reinforces the importance of each and every contribution. Individuals can be acknowledged at specific times; a birthday or work anniversary cake or celebration goes a long way in letting individuals know that they are valued and appreciated. It also is important that staff do not feel that they are in a "dead-end position"; employees need to be able to support their professional growth through meeting attendance and perhaps certification wherein there is acknowledgement of the same. Becoming stagnant in a role can bring down not only the individual but also the team. Everyone needs to be stimulated with new ideas and challenges, and this needs to happen continually and consistently.

Team development is an ever-evolving concept with respect to clinical research because changes are constantly evolving in the clinical research environment. As a means of keeping the team abreast of current events and issues, it is important to have *regularly scheduled meetings* or *networking opportunities* during which individuals can share information, ideas, experiences, and concerns. Being creative in bringing physicians together can be challenging. Perhaps taking 15–20 minutes in an already scheduled staff meeting, teleconferencing, communicating electronically, or inviting team members to monthly or bimonthly (rather than weekly) meetings at a central location might facilitate the protocol decision making and education that needs to transpire. Having regularly scheduled events (whatever the format) gives physicians the opportunity to provide necessary input and remain abreast of currently available protocols and issues. Including all members of the interdisciplinary team who need to be part of protocol decision making is critical, as is including them in protocol compliance issues, establishment of protocol processes, and educational opportunities, such as site initiation and auditing visits.

Ongoing training of clinical research personnel and other members of the interdisciplinary team is imperative to ensure the safety of research participants and the scientific integrity of the clinical research activities. Regulations mandate special educational requirements for investigators receiving federal funding. Many institutions have site-specific policies in place, which are considered obligatory for those involved in clinical research activities (Califf et al., 2003). Per the American Society of Clinical Oncology (ASCO) guidelines, training programs for physician investigators and clinical research personnel should include ethical and scientific standards for the conduct of research, protection of human participants, communication techniques with patients during the informed consent process, and potential issues with conflicts of interest (ASCO, 2003).

Teams function most effectively when consistent guidelines exist to provide direction. The most comprehensive of those guidelines should be in the context of standard operating procedures (SOPs), which are a requirement of the U.S. Food and Drug Administration. It is important to standardize SOPs so they are specific to the site, as each site will have its own nuances. See Chapter 46 for a detailed discussion of SOPs.

Encouraging participation in professional organizations is another opportunity for strengthening the team and increasing their skill level. The Oncology Nursing Society (ONS, www.ons.org), as well as more clinical-research–based organizations, such as the Society of Clinical Research Associates (SoCRA, www.socra.org) and the Association of Clinical Research Professionals (www.acrp.org), provide educational programs and opportunities for certification testing and networking opportunities. In addition to the programs and Web sites available through these entities, the National Cancer Institute Web site (www.cancer.gov) provides links to many other educational opportunities (Christian et al., 2004). Although oncology nurses and other clinical research personnel listed here are not required to be certified, these professional organizations provide a mechanism wherein individuals have the opportunity to become certified and obtain professional credentials through testing initially and with continuing education credits for recertification (e.g., ONS Oncology Certified Nurse [OCN®], SoCRA Certified Clinical Research Professional [CCRP]). These certifications reflect a standard of education and a

Figure 11-4. Point System for Clinical Trials Office Workload Management		
Administrative Staff		
Tasks	Yearly Activities	Points
New Application		
High complexity	80	1.5
Moderate complexity	120	1.0
Low complexity	240	0.5
Renewal w/ consent	800	0.15
Renewals w/o consent	1,200	0.1
Amendment w/ consent	800	0.15
Amendment w/o consent	1,200	0.1
Investigator's brochure	2,400	0.05
Safety report w/ consent	2,400	0.05
Safety report w/o consent	4,800	0.025
Protocol review committee review	480	0.25
Study start-up	37	3.25
Grants monitoring	2,000	0.06
Protocol invoicing	2,000	0.06
Screening log submission	6,000	0.02
Supplies inventory and maintenance	3,000	0.04
Budgeting	400	0.3
Regulatory submission	120	1.0
Regulatory maintenance	240	0.5
Administrative team yearly standard = 120 points		
Case Management		
Tasks	Yearly Activities	Points
Protocol patients		
High complexity	40	1.5
Moderate complexity	60	1.0
Low complexity	120	0.5
Long-term follow-up with physical examination	600	0.1
Long-term follow-up without physical examination	1200	0.05
Drug inservice	600	0.1
(Continued on next page)		

Figure 11-4. Point System for Clinical Trials Office Workload Management *(Continued)*

Tasks	Yearly Activities	Points
Serious adverse event	600	0.1
Specimen handling (pharmacokinetics)	1,200	0.05
Special monitoring	1,200	0.05
Randomization screening	600	0.1
Case management yearly standard = 60 points		

Data Management

Tasks	Yearly Activities	Points
Case report form (CRF) completion		
High complexity	40	1.5
Moderate complexity	60	1.0
Low complexity	120	0.5
Cooperative Group Outreach Program affiliates	1,200	0.05
Long-term follow-up	2,400	0.025
Pathology submission	2,400	0.025
Radiation support	2,400	0.025
Database management	2,400	0.025
CRF design (per study)	60	1.0
Multisite study initiation (per study)	150	0.4
Multisite study coordinator (per site)	75	0.8
Multisite patient monitoring (per patient)	300	0.2
Data management yearly standard = 60 points		

Note. Designed in conjunction with Tiffany Pearce, BA, RHIT, Grant Specialist, Clinical Trials Office, Henry Ford Health System, Detroit, MI.

validation of knowledge and experience achieved. A strong clinical research program supports and encourages the certification of its team members (Meldrum, 2005).

A Model for Clinical Research Staffing Ratios

One of the greatest challenges within a clinical research program is the provision for a sufficient, but not surplus, number of clinical research personnel. Staffing ratio models have been designed based on certain indicators. One such model utilizes the two indicators of protocol acuity score and total acuity number per the clinical research associate/clinical research coordinator (CRA/CRC). Using this methodology, protocols are evaluated based on "x" number of procedures, each with an associated time requirement and level of difficulty (e.g., outpatient versus inpatient, protocol requirement complexity, other staffing support required, sponsor driven) for one patient. The score then is multiplied by the number of anticipated patients, which provides an overall protocol acuity score (e.g., total procedural/tasks value of 65 times 5 patients equals protocol acuity score of 325). The CRA/CRC acuity score is primarily based on that individual's percentage of involvement with all aspects of protocol operations and the percentage of effort handled by other staff. For purposes of this model, an acuity score of 500–650 generally is considered to be manageable without causing a constant feeling of being overloaded and overwhelmed. Thus, if one CRA/CRC were handling 100% of the clinical trial responsibilities, he or she could manage a maximum of two trials if each had an acuity score of 325 (Fowler & Thomas, 2003).

Another methodology is a budgeting tool that helps to calculate the cost of a CRA/CRC's time. Based on low, medium, and high activity assignments (i.e., the number of study visits and daily, weekly, and monthly tasks based on an hourly comparison), the estimated amount of time per CRA/CRC per protocol is obtained. A staffing ratio then can be determined based on the total number of protocols (Johnson, 2003).

SoCRA has established a standard wherein 1.0 full-time equivalent CRA/CRC handling basically all responsibilities (i.e., regulatory, IRB, patient monitoring, data management, sponsor encounters/audits) could effectively manage approximately 30 new patients per year. This number could be skewed because of the type of trial (i.e., industry trials tend to be more labor intensive, whereas cooperative group trials are more labor-driven by disease site) and over time because of additional long-term follow-up requirements and increased protocol complexities (Cohen, 2003).

One model, as presented in Figure 11-4, that was developed and instituted by this author in a centralized CTO setting looks at a designated point system for identifying workloads applicable to administrative, case management, and data management functions. The premise of this model is to link a point value to low-, moderate-, and high-complexity protocols based on the specific responsibilities of each group. In addition, certain specific tasks were identified, to which a point value also was given. Each point value was determined based on the number of times that any one activity could be performed by a given individual within a one-year time frame.

To capture the level of workload on an individual basis, each team member would enter a completed activity into a specifically designed database. This allows for a daily calculation of each individual's workload and productivity. It also provides an opportunity to evaluate the workload intensity and to make necessary workload shifts to maintain a balance. The program, when linked with a billing system, allows for each activity cost to be offset against a grant or department. Figure 11-4 displays the tables utilized in this model.

Protocol complexity criteria for the administrative staff were based on factors such as length of the consent form, involvement of other departments, and priority status. Case management and data management criteria were similar with respect to phase of study, length of treatment, sponsor/clinical research organization involvement, patient follow-up requirements, and ancillary studies (e.g., central laboratory submissions).

Immense value exists in having a system in which the workload of CTO personnel can be monitored and adjusted for balance. This type of mechanism will promote quality patient care, efficiencies in protocol activation and continuation, adherence to data submission requirements, and compliance with all regulations. In addition, it will promote a collegial atmosphere and the perspective of a fair work environment among clinical research personnel. (See Chapters 4 and 5.)

Summary

It certainly is a team effort to accomplish the tasks in cancer clinical research. All members of the team must share the common goals of providing patients with opportunities to participate in good, sound, scientific clinical trials and ensuring protocol adherence and patient monitoring, which are critical for the overall well-being of patients. Clinical trial nurses have a professional obligation to patients that information gained from their participation will be handled in an appropriate and efficient manner, that their confidentiality will be maintained, and that the data will be utilized to help to advance the knowledge of cancer therapies. It is imperative that all individuals involved in the clinical trial process be overly conscientious and zealous in their activities. They must have the determination and eagerness to assume whatever individual and collective responsibilities are necessary to uphold the standards to conduct high-quality clinical research. It is not an easy job, but one that is certainly worthwhile for clinical trial nurses as professionals and, more importantly, for the well-being of patients.

References

American Society of Clinical Oncology. (2003). American Society of Clinical Oncology policy statement: Oversight of clinical research. *Journal of Clinical Oncology, 21*, 2377–2386.

Califf, R.M., Morse, M.A., Wittes, J., Goodman, S.N., Nelson, D.K., DeMets, D.L., et al. (2003). Toward protecting the safety of participants in clinical trials. *Controlled Clinical Trials, 24*, 256–271.

Cassidy, J. (2002). Data and data management in clinical trials. In J.I. Gallin (Ed.), *Principles and practices of clinical research* (pp. 69–103). San Diego, CA: Academic Press.

Christian, M.C., Abrams, J.S., & Parkinson, D.R. (2004). Structures supporting cancer clinical trials. In M.D. Abeloff, J.O. Armitage, J.E. Niederhuber, M.B. Kastan, & W.G. McKenna (Eds.), *Clinical oncology* (pp. 383–393). Philadelphia: Elsevier.

Cohen, G.I. (2003). Clinical research by community oncologists. *CA: A Cancer Journal for Clinicians, 53*, 73–81.

Cusack, G., Jones, A., & Chisholm, L. (2004). Patient intensity in an ambulatory oncology research center: A step forward for the field of ambulatory care—part III. *Nursing Economics, 22*, 193–195, 175.

Cusack, G., Jones-Wells, A., & Chisholm, L. (2004). Patient intensity in an ambulatory oncology research center: A step forward for the field of ambulatory care. *Nursing Economics, 22*, 58–63, 55.

Fowler, D.R., & Thomas, C.J. (2003). Protocol acuity scoring as a rational approach to clinical research management. *Research Practitioner, 4*, 64–71.

Johnson, G.P. (2003, August). Budget tool helps investigative sites calculate the costs of coordinator's time for a typical outpatient study visit, part II. *SoCRA Source, 2*(37), 31–37.

Jones, A., Cusack, G., & Chisholm, L. (2004). Patient intensity in an ambulatory oncology research center: A step forward for the field of ambulatory care—part II. *Nursing Economics, 22*, 120–123, 107.

Lader, E.W., Cannon, C.P., Ohman, E.M., Newby, K., Sulmasy, O.F.M., Barst, R.J., et al. (2004). The clinician as investigator. *Circulation, 109*, 2672–2679.

Meldrum, C.A. (2005). An overview of hiring practices and job requirements for CRSs and CRCs. *Monitor, 19*, 61–67.

Nesbitt, L.A. (Ed.). (2004). *Clinical research—what it is and how it works.* Sudbury, MA: Jones and Bartlett.

Pierre, C. (2005). The career pathway to site manager. *Monitor, 19*, 29–31.

Thompson, A., Pickler, R., & Reyna, B. (2005). Clinical coordination of research. *Applied Nursing Research, 18*, 102–105.

SECTION IV.

Legislative and Regulatory Issues

CHAPTER 12

Introduction to Legal and Regulatory Issues

Sally D. Brown, RN, BSN, MGA, OCN®, CCRP,
and Sue Markus, RN, BSN, MS, OCN®, CCRC

Introduction

Knowledge and understanding of research-related laws and regulations is expected of all individuals involved in the conduct of clinical research. Past wrongdoings in the treatment of research participants have led to the development of legal and regulatory systems that scrutinize every aspect of clinical research. Everyone associated with research on humans, regardless of their role, is expected to comply with the standards and rules of conduct that govern research practices. It is important to note that standards for conducting research are not set in stone; they are living documents that change and evolve.

This chapter is intended to introduce and familiarize the reader with the legal and regulatory components of conducting clinical research. This is by no means the totality of the enterprises for overseeing the conduct of human clinical trials. What will be included in this chapter are the principles and sources of standards for practice. The aspects of clinical research to which these principles and standards apply are presented in depth in other chapters of this manual.

The Belmont Report

Laws, regulations, and ethics are closely related but have some distinct differences. The Belmont Report (see Appendix 3), written in 1979, is the standard for the ethical conduct of clinical trials. Most, although not all, human subject research is regulated by the federal government in the United States. Research that receives federal funds or involves obtaining a license for a drug or product is within the scope of federal regulations. The Office for Human Research Protections (OHRP) regulates research that receives federal funds. The U.S. Food and Drug Administration (FDA) regulates research that involves the licensing of a drug or product (Charrow & Goldman, 2004; Kalb & Koehler, 2002; Mathieu, 2005; Wood, 2002).

The culture of research regulation contains expertise from a variety of disciplines. These include law, ethics, finance, medicine, information technology, and others. The organizations and concepts used in regulating clinical research represent the framework for ensuring ethical conduct and scientific integrity of clinical research.

Terminology

Legal, regulatory, and ethical issues should begin with the basic understanding of the meaning of several terms. The terms listed in Table 12-1 provide a basic knowledge of regulatory language.

Regulatory Authority

Several different regulatory and compliance programs are involved in the conduct of clinical trials. These range from regulations, such as 45 CFR 46 and 21 CFR 54, to guidelines, such as good clinical practice guidelines and the Belmont Report (Lanter, 2006). In the United States, the conduct of clinical trials is governed at the federal level by regulations that are enacted by the U.S. Department of Health and Human Services (DHHS). The DHHS agencies involved are the OHRP and the FDA. These agencies obtain their power from Congress. The agencies then develop administrative regulations to explain or carry out the statute and executive orders that govern the agencies (Cornell Law School, 2006).

To obtain the applicable regulatory and compliance information, it is necessary to determine which federal agency has oversight for the individual trial. This will determine the appropriate agency regulations, which may affect the study under consideration. The FDA has oversight for privately sponsored studies. OHRP oversees clinical research that receives federal funding or is conducted by DHHS agencies (Kalb & Koehler, 2002; Mathieu, 2005; Wood, 2002). A limited organizational structure of DHHS is exhibited in Figure 12-1.

Regulations enacted by DHHS appear in Title 45 of the *Code of Federal Regulations*, Public Welfare and Human Services, and those enacted by the FDA appear in Title

Table 12-1. Glossary of Legal Terms	
Terms	**Definitions**
Act	Something done, usually intentionally or voluntarily or with a purpose (Lehman & Phelps, 2005)
Act of Congress	A law that is formally enacted in accordance with the legislative power granted to Congress by the U.S. Constitution (Garner, 2004)
Code	A systematic and comprehensive compilation of laws, rules, or regulations that are consolidated and classified according to subject matter (Lehman & Phelps, 2005)
Code of Federal Regulations (CFR)	Permanent and organized source of federal regulations that is completely revised each year and published by the U.S. Printing Office (Lehman & Phelps, 2005). The code is divided into titles, parts, and sections. Titles are general categories; parts are board topics; and sections are specific areas within the topic. For example, 21 CFR 56.107 translates to: Title 21 (Food and Drugs) of the *Code of Federal Regulations,* part 56 (Institutional Review Boards [IRBs]), section 107 (IRB membership).
Common Rule	45 CFR 46; governs the conduct of human subject research funded through any one of 17 federal agencies (Grady, 2002; Mathieu, 2005) (see Appendix 5)
Ethics	The rules or standards governing the conduct of a person or members of a profession (Pickett, 2000)
Guidelines	Documents that provide directives. Guidelines are not legally binding but contain expectations of conduct. Guidelines must be followed as strictly as regulations because they represent the standard of practice that should be maintained. Breaching them is not punishable by law; however, failure to comply can have disciplinary consequences or can lead to legal liability. Examples of legal liability include breach of protocol, standard operating procedures, and negligence to participants (Jones-Wright, 2006b). Example: U.S. Food and Drug Administration (FDA) documents prepared for FDA staff, applicants/sponsors, and the public that describe the agency's interpretation of, or policy on, a regulatory issue (Zoon & Yetter, 2002).
Law	(1) The regime that orders human activities and relations through systematic application of the force of a politically organized society or through social pressures, backed by force in such a society; the legal system; (2) the aggregate legislation, judicial precedents, and accepted legal principle; the body of authoritative grounds of judicial and administration action, especially the body of rules, standards, and principles of the courts of a particular jurisdiction apply in deciding controversies brought before them; (3) the set of rules and principles dealing with a specific area of a legal system (e.g., copyright law); (4) the judicial and administrative process, legal actions, and proceedings; (5) a statute; (6) common law; (7) the legal profession (Garner, 2004)
Legal	(1) Of or pertaining to law, falling within the province of law; (2) established, required, or permitted by law; (3) of or relating to law as opposed to equity (Garner, 2004)
Negligence	Failure to exercise the standard of care that a reasonably prudent person would have exercised in a similar situation; any conduct the falls below the legal standard established to protect against unreasonable risk of harm except for conduct that is intentionally wanton or willfully disregardful of others' risks (Garner, 2004).
Regulation/rule	(1) A rule of order having the force of law prescribed by a superior and competent authority, relating to the actions of those under the authority's control; (2) are designed to guide the activity of those regulated by the agency and the agency's employees; (3) function to ensure uniform application of the law; (4) issued by various federal government departments and agencies to carry out the intent of legislation enacted by Congress (Lehman & Phelps, 2005)
Statute	A law enacted by or by the authority of the supreme legislative branch of government (Gove, 2002)

21, Food and Drugs (see Table 12-2). Although Titles 21 and 45 regulate different types of research, some issues are addressed in both titles. Table 12-3, compiled from Rozovsky and Adams (2003), illustrates some differences between FDA regulation (Title 21) and the Common Rule (Title 45).

U.S. Food and Drug Administration

The FDA obtains its statutory authority through several acts of Congress and sets of laws. The acts of Congress include the Federal Food, Drug and Cosmetic Act, the Public Health Services Act, the Prescription Drug User Fee Act, the Prescription Drug Marketing Act, and the FDA Modernization Act of 1997. The set of laws on which the FDA received its statutory authority include Interstate Commerce, Foreign Commerce, Comonent Jurisdiction, and Generic Equivalence (Zoon & Yetter, 2002). The organizational structure of the FDA is shown in Table 12-4.

Investigational new drug (IND) applications are submitted to, reviewed by, and overseen by the Center for Drug Evaluation and Research (CDER). The required forms for an IND submission are included on the FDA CDER Web site at www.fda.gov/opacom/morechoices/fdaforms/cder. html. This Web page also contains FDA form 1572 (Statement of Investigator), form 3455 (Disclosure: Financial

Figure 12-1. Partial* Organizational Structure of the U.S. Department of Health and Human Services

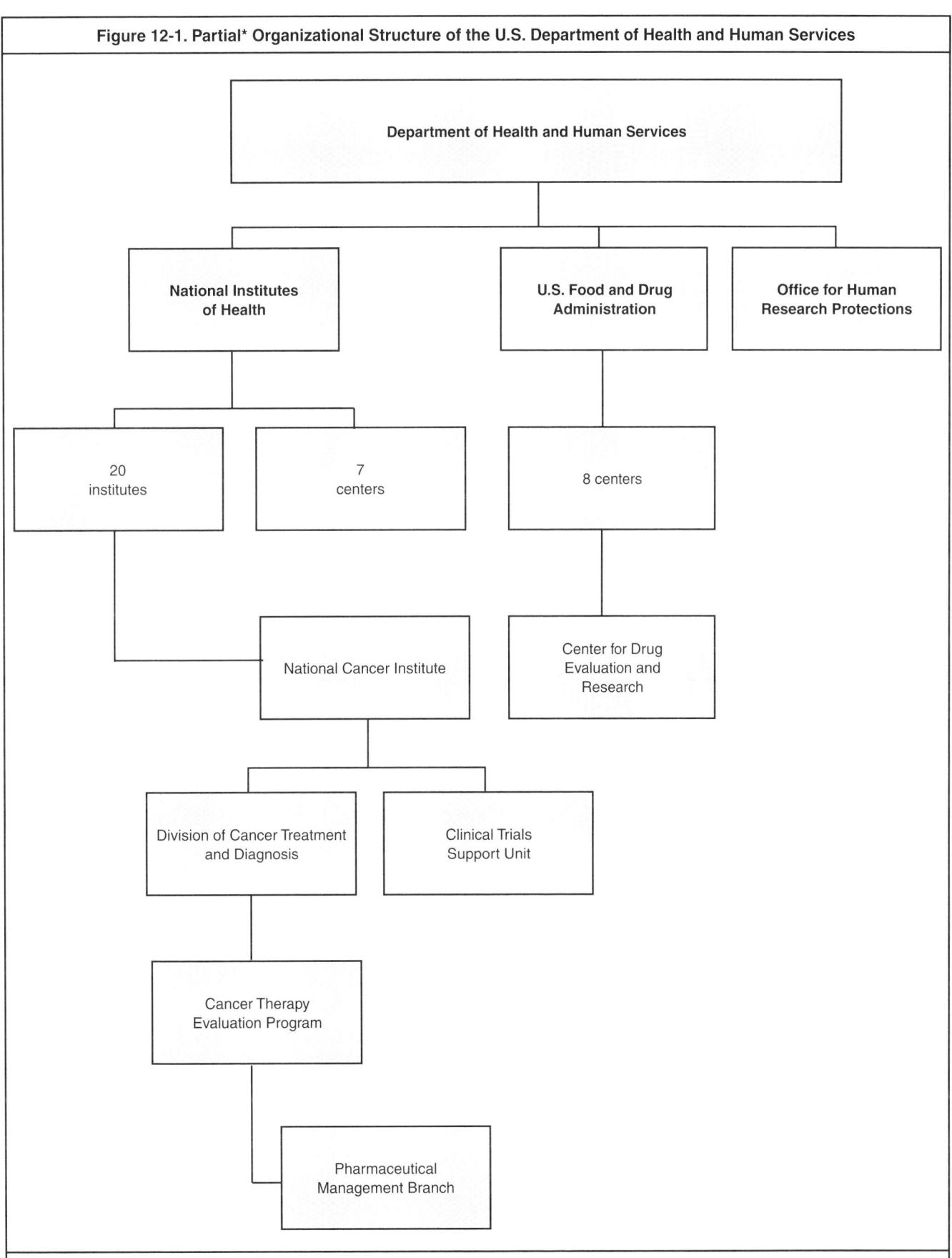

*Entire organizational structure for each agency may be obtained at each agency's Web site (National Institutes of Health: www.nih.gov/icd; U.S. Food and Drug Administration: www.fda.gov/opacom/7org.html; National Cancer Institute: www.cancer.gov/aboutnci/organization; Cancer Therapy Evaluation Program: http://ctep.info.nih.gov/about/index.html; and Division of Cancer Treatment and Disgnosis: http://dctd.cancer.gov/About/programs.htm).

Table 12-2. Comparison of Content of Titles 21 and 45 of the *Code of Federal Regulations*			
Title 21: Food and Drugs		**Title 45: Public Welfare and Human Services**	
Part	**Topic Addressed**	**Part**	**Topic Addressed**
Part 11	Electronic records and signature	Part 46	Protection of human subjects
Part 50	Protection of human subjects	Part 46, subpart A	Basic Health and Human Services policy for protection of human research subjects
Part 54	Financial disclosure by clinical investigators	Part 46, subpart B	Additional protection pertaining to research development and research activities involving fetuses, pregnant women, and human in vitro fertilization
Part 56	Institutional review boards		
Part 312	Investigational new drug application		
Part 314	Application for Food and Drug Administration approval to market a new drug		
Part 600	Biological products		
Part 812	Investigational device exemptions		

Interest and Arrangements of Clinical Investigators), and MedWatch forms. The FDA Web site contains a section titled "Good Clinical Practice in FDA-Regulated Clinical Trials" (www.fda.gov/oc/gcp/default.htm), which provides information about regulations, laws enforced by the FDA, proposed regulations and draft guidances, enforcement information, educational materials, contact information for good clinical practice staff, and upcoming workshops (FDA, 2006).

Office for Human Research Protections

OHRP is an agency within DHHS. This agency is responsible for the conduct of clinical research that is sponsored or conducted by DHHS agencies (Mathieu, 2005). The National Institutes of Health (NIH) is an agency of the DHHS and is composed of 20 institutes and seven centers. Cooperative clinical trial groups conduct many large cancer clinical trials. These groups are funded through the National Cancer Institute (NCI), which is an institute within NIH.

National Cancer Institute

NCI is composed of divisions (see Figure 12-2) that are directly involved with the conduct of clinical trials, both intramural and extramural. Intramural trials are conducted at the NCI campus in Bethesda, MD. Extramural trials are conducted at sites other than NCI's Bethesda campus.

The Division of Cancer Treatment and Diagnosis (DCTD) (see Figure 12-3) is responsible for funding national cancer research and sponsoring clinical trials to evaluate new anti-cancer agents. The Cancer Therapy Evaluation Program (CTEP) is within the DCTD (see Fig-

ure 12-4). The CTEP Web site (http://ctep.info.nih.gov) is an excellent resource. One item provided on the site is *The Investigator's Handbook: A Manual for Participants in Clinical Trials of Investigational Agents Sponsored by DCTD, NCI* (NCI CTEP, 2002). This handbook provides information that is useful for anyone involved in clinical trials in areas such as protocol design and submission, reporting requirements, agent accountability, phases of clinical trials and the associated requirements and responsibilities, responsibilities in multicenter trials, investigator responsibilities, and audit procedures (Kaltman & Isidor, 2006). The CTEP Web site also provides the NCI Common Terminology Criteria for Adverse Events and information for requisition and management of agents.

The Pharmaceutical Management Branch (PMB) is a division within the CTEP. Two functions of the PMB are management of a registry of participating physicians and authorization and distribution of investigational agents. To register physicians for participation in cooperative group clinical trials, FDA form 1572 must be submitted to the PMB. An NCI investigator number will be assigned to the physician; the investigator number is necessary to obtain investigational agents that are supplied through the NCI. The 1572 is an agreement that must be updated *annually*.

The NCI created the Cancer Trials Support Unit (CTSU) to increase participation in phase III cooperative group studies (CTSU, n.d.). The CTSU Web site (www.ctsu.org) supplies regulatory information, including investigator registration information and forms. The Web site has an area for the general public, as well as a members' area. It is necessary to register with CTEP to access the CTSU

Table 12-3. Comparison of U.S. Food and Drug Administration (FDA) Rules (21 CFR) Versus the Common Rule (45 CFR)		
Topic	**FDA Rules**	**Common Rule**
Foreign clinical trials	• FDA Modernization Act of 1997 (Public Law 105-115) and the FDA's participation in the International Conference on Harmonisation of Technical Requirements of Registration of Pharmaceuticals for Human Use approach recognizing drugs developed through clinical trials abroad • Provides criteria for accepting foreign clinical studies that are not done under an investigational new drug application (21 CFR § 812.1; Rozovsky & Adams, 2003) • The FDA does not regulate this type of research unless an emergency treatment provision found in the FDA regulations addresses the issue.	• U.S. department head may approve the procedures of a foreign institution if it provides protection at least equivalent to the U.S. federal regulations (45 CFR § 101[h]; Rozovsky & Adams, 2003). • Permits an institutional review board (IRB) to approve to alter or waive consent requirements in certain cases (45 CFR § 116[d]; Rozovsky & Adams, 2003)
Definitions	• Provisions define terms specific to the type of research covered by the FDA regulations (test article, application for research or marketing permit, and clinical investigation). Includes a definition for emergency use. Adopted the Common Rule (21 CFR).	–
Reporting obligation	• IRBs must have and follow written procedures to ensure that unanticipated problems are reported by the sponsor and clinical investigator (21 CFR).	• Requires prompt reporting of unanticipated problems to the appropriate agency
Confidentiality	• Does not permit an IRB to waive the requirements for signed consent when the principal risk is a breach of confidentiality. (The rationale is that because the FDA does not regulate research protocols that would include this type of research, it need not make provisions for it [21 CFR].)	• Permits an IRB to approve to alter or waive consent requirements in certain cases (CFR § 116[d]; Rozovsky & Adams, 2003)
Behavioral research	• Not regulated by the FDA; no provision made	• Certain types of research can be reviewed using expedited review. This includes certain types of behavioral studies (21 CFR).
IRB membership	• No provision	• Requires IRBs to report changes in membership (21 CFR)
Noncompliance	• Sanctions for regulatory noncompliance	• Allows termination of research support and evaluation of applications and proposals in view of prior noncompliance (21 CFR)
Inspection of records	• Requires that subjects be informed that the agency may inspect the records of the study	• The department or agency has the right to inspect records of the study, but disclosure of this possibility is not a requirement of consent (21 CFR).

members' area. Registration is done on the CTEP Web site. CTEP encourages personnel involved in the conduct of NCI-sponsored clinical trials to register.

NCI has also created a central IRB (CIRB) that reviews phase III cooperative group trials. Participation in the NCI CIRB streamlines the IRB process for the individual site and local IRB. To utilize the CIRB, the local IRB must recognize the NCI CIRB as the IRB of record with OHRP.

NCI made on-site monitoring (auditing) a requirement for the Clinical Trials Cooperative Group Program in 1982. The guidelines require that each institution undergo an audit at least every 36 months (NCI CTEP, 2006).

The conduct of clinical research is also affected by DHHS's Office of Civil Rights regulations. This office regulates national standards to protect the privacy of personal health information (Office of Civil Rights, 2006).

Overlap exists between FDA regulations and OHRP regulations. Cooperative groups receive financial support from industry sources in addition to federal funding. All clinical research governed by federal regulations has overlap with state and local regulations. The investigator and coordinator are held to the most stringent of all the regulations (Kaltman & Isidor, 2006). Numerous additional regulations exist that affect the conduct of clinical trials.

State and Local Regulations

The state laws and regulations must be followed *if they are stricter* than federal regulations (Kaltman & Isidor, 2006). Regulations that affect the conduct of clinical trials are very diverse on the state level (Serio, Tichner, & Dilley, 2004). Although some states do not have specific clinical trial regulations, three states (Maryland, Virginia,

Table 12-4. Organizational Structure of the U.S. Food and Drug Administration

Office	Acronym
Office of the Commissioner	–
Center for Biologics Evaluation and Research	CBER
Center for Devices and Radiological Health	CDRH
Center for Drug Evaluation and Research	CDER
Center for Food Safety and Applied Nutrition	CFSAN
Center for Veterinary Medicine	CVM
National Center for Toxicological Research	NCTR
Office of Orphan Products Development	OOPD
Office of Regulatory Affairs	ORA

and California) have created statutes or regulations that affect the conduct of clinical trials that exceed the federal requirements. Maryland requires that all human subject clinical trials, even those without federal funding, comply with federal regulations in 45 CFR 46 (Kaltman & Isidor, 2006).

Information about state regulations may be difficult to locate. The regulations may not be readily available online. The individual institution's IRB is a source of information because the IRB must be aware of the state regulations. Other sources include healthcare law attorneys, institutional risk management and legal departments, and the legal department of the sponsor or clinical research office (Kaltman & Isidor, 2006). Print sources are available, but discretion must be taken when using print media as a source because of the fluid, evolving nature of laws and regulations. Regulations can change before a composite work may reach distribution.

Good Clinical Practice

The International Conference on Harmonisation of Technical Requirements for Registration of Pharmaceuticals for Human Use (ICH) authored good clinical practice (GCP) guidelines, which are published in the *Federal Register*. This series of documents provides standards that will encourage uniformity in the conduct of research internationally. Although it is not a U.S. regulation, sponsors may require compliance with these guidelines (Woodin, 2004). The ICH GCP is an efficacy guideline and is formatted by topics resembling the *Code of Federal Regulations* format (Jones-Wright, 2006b). These are displayed in Table 12-5 ("Selected Regulations," 2005).

ICH includes representation from the United States, the European Union, and Japan. Health Canada, the World Health Organization, and the European Free Trade Asso-

ciation act as links between ICH areas and non-ICH areas (Jones-Wright, 2006b).

Shipment of Research Specimens

Some clinical studies require that specimens be shipped to central laboratories for review. The shipping of these specimens is subject to federal regulations. Specimens may fall into the hazardous materials category. They often contain dry ice, formalin, and/or body fluids.

The Occupational Safety and Health Administration, the U.S. Department of Transportation, and the International Civil Aviation Organization, which is a multinational

Figure 12-2. Composition of the National Cancer Institute

Offices
- Office of Communications
- Office of International Affairs
- Office of Science Planning and Assessment
- Office of Management
- Office of Centers, Training, and Resources
- Office of Budget and Financial Management
- Division of Cancer Control and Population Sciences

Divisions
- Division of Cancer Prevention
- Division of Extramural Activities
- Division of Cancer Epidemiology and Genetics
- Division of Cancer Treatment and Diagnosis
- Division of Cancer Biology

Centers
- Center for Bioinformatics
- Center to Reduce Cancer Health Disparities
- Center for Cancer Research

Figure 12-3. Composition of the Division of Cancer Treatment and Diagnosis (DCTD)

Programs Within the DCTD
- Radiation Research Program
- Cancer Treatment Evaluation Program
- Developmental Therapeutics Program
- Cancer Diagnosis Program
- Cancer Imaging Program

Figure 12-4. Composition (Branches) of the Cancer Treatment Evaluation Program (CTEP)

Branches of the CTEP
- Investigational Drug Branch
- Pharmaceutical Management Branch
- Regulatory Affairs Branch
- Clinical Investigations Branch
- Clinical Trials Monitoring Branch
- Clinical Grants and Contracts Branch

Table 12-5. List of Relevant ICH Guidelines and Topics

Code	Topic
E1	The Extent of Population Exposure to Assess Clinical Safety for Drugs Intended for Long-Term Treatment on Non-Life-Threatening Conditions
E2A	Clinical Safety Data Management: Definitions and Standards for Expedited Reporting
E2B	Clinical Safety Data Management: Data Elements for Transmission of Individual Case Safety Reports
E2C	Clinical Safety Data Management: Periodic Safety Update Reports for Marketed Drugs
E3	Structure and Content of Clinical Study Reports
E4	Dose-Response Information to Support Drug Registration
E5	Ethnic Factors in the Acceptability of Foreign Clinical Data
E6	Good Clinical Practice: Consolidated Guideline
E7	Studies in Support of Special Populations: Geriatrics
E8	General Considerations for Clinical Trials
E9	Statistical Considerations in the Design of Clinical Trials
E10	Choice of Control Group in Clinical Trials
M3	Nonclinical Safety Studies for the Conduct of Human Clinical Trials for Pharmaceuticals
S6	Safety Studies for Biotechnology-Derived Products

ICH—International Conference on Harmonisation of Technical Requirements for Registration of Pharmaceuticals for Human Use

regulatory organization, regulate the shipment of these materials. The Federal Aviation Administration, the Federal Highway Administration, the Federal Railroad Administration, and the U.S. Coast Guard enforce the regulations within the United States.

In 2005, the International Air Transport Association (IATA), a trade association, provided an exemption for "patient specimens" from IATA's dangerous goods regulations. IATA considers research specimens to be patient specimens. Although research specimens are exempt from more stringent shipping requirements, basic requirements still must be followed. These include the use of the appropriate designation on the outside box. The packages must be marked with "UN3373" surrounded by a diamond and packed according to packing instructions (IATA, 2006a). In October 2006, IATA listed research specimens as Biological Substances Category B. Packages must be marked with UN3373 and Biological Substance, Category B (IATA, 2006b).

The packaging must include a leak-proof primary receptacle, a leak-proof secondary packaging, and an outer packaging of adequate strength for its capacity, mass, and the intended use. The package must contain sufficient absorbent material to absorb all the contents of the primary receptacle, and fragile primary receptacles must be wrapped or separated (Johnson & Goldfarb, 2005).

Retention of Records

All study-related records must be retained after the study is completed. "Completed" in this instance means that the sample size has been met and significant data have been collected so that no additional data are to be obtained or submitted to the sponsor. The ICH GCP, OHRP, and FDA have varying requirements (see Table 12-6). ICH GCP provides recommendations, whereas the OHRP (i.e., 45 CFR 46.115) and FDA (i.e., 21 CFR 56.115) provide regulations (Jones-Wright, 2006a).

Compliance Issues

Regulations and guidelines for the conduct of clinical research are constantly evolving. Compliance with these regulations and guidelines requires awareness of the ongoing changes. The monitoring of clinical research activities for compliance with regulatory measures is an evolving field and has raised awareness of the importance of protection of research subjects. Federal legislation is based on fundamental ethical principles that have been defined in the Belmont Report (Dunn & Chadwick, 2002). These three basic ethical principles are *respect for persons, beneficence,* and *justice* (Khin-Maung-Gyi & Whalen, 2006). Table 12-7 displays definitions of these principles and their application

Table 12-6. Comparison of Duration of Record Retention Among U.S. Governing Bodies

ICH GCP	45 CFR 46.115	21 CFR 56.115
At least 2 years after last approval of marketing application	3 years after completion of study (institutional review board records)	At least 3 years after completion of research
At least 2 years after formal discontinuation if no marketing application is submitted		Records must be accessible for inspection at reasonable times and in a reasonable manners.
Sponsors in United States and Europe must retain records 15 years.		
Sponsors in Canada must retain records 25 years.		

ICH GCP—International Conference on Harmonisation of Technical Requirements for Registration of Pharmaceuticals for Human Use Good Clinical Practice

Table 12-7. Definitions of Ethical Principles and Applications to Clinical Research

Ethical Principle	Definition	Application to Research
Respect for persons	An obligation to respect and not interfere with the self-determined choices and actions of autonomous individuals	Informed consent for enrollment and ongoing participation
Benefi- cence	An obligation to never deliberately harm another person and to maximize benefits and minimize risks	Analysis of risks and benefits; determination that the benefits justify the risks
Justice	An obligation to be fair in the distribution of social goods such as the benefits and burdens of research	Fair procedures and outcomes in the selection of subjects

to research. Table 12-8 provides a list of Web sites that serve as sources for clinical trial regulatory information. *Ignorance of the regulatory requirements of conducting clinical research is not an acceptable defense for noncompliance.*

Research Misconduct

Research misconduct includes "fabrication, falsification, or plagiarism (FFP) in proposing, performing, or reviewing research or in reporting research results as well as unethical treatment of participants" (Jones-Wright, 2006b, p. 31). However, it does not include honest error. It may involve issues of disclosure about the researchers, being forthcoming with information about the conduct of the study or the study findings, or inclusion of appropriate study subjects.

Between 1980 and 2000, at least 10 federal responses were issued concerning research integrity and misconduct (Schechter, 2002). One of these resulted from what was thought to be the scientific community's lack of response to problems of scientific misconduct. As a result, in 1985, first-time recipients of NIH funds were required to have administrative processes in place to address allegations of misconduct. The Public Health Service then issued guidelines that in 1989 became known as the "Final Rule." It provides the federal government with broader legal powers when government funds are involved or when the federal government is conducting the research (Schechter, 2002). Figure 12-5 shows three parts of the "Final Rule" that have been implemented.

In 1992, what had been the NIH Office of Scientific Integrity became the Office of Research Integrity (ORI) under the DHHS. The ORI has taken on more education and oversight duties and has fewer investigative and adjudicative functions than it did initially (Schechter, 2002). Continual consideration is given on how to improve the accountability for those involved in clinical research.

Noncompliance

Noncompliance may be discovered during a sponsor's monitor visit, during a routine, scheduled audit, or by someone involved in the research organization that may later become identified as a whistleblower. The reporting of the event will initiate a more in-depth investigation. The investigation is conducted by the appropriate government agency, such as the FDA or the ORI. *Intent, awareness,* and *regard for what was being done* carry great weight when determining whether misconduct has occurred.

Consequences of Noncompliance

The consequences of noncompliance with federal regulations depend on the severity of misconduct. The FDA can take action against the sponsor of the study, the institution, or the investigator. It can obtain a court order requiring the violation to be stopped, charge the violator with a crime, seize the goods involved, bar the violator from future participation in a new drug application, impose a

Table 12-8. Internet Sources for Clinical Trials Regulatory Information

Government Office	Web Site
U.S. Food and Drug Administration (FDA)	www.fda.gov
Good Clinical Practice in FDA-Regulated Clinical Trials	www.fda.gov/oc/gcp/default.htm
FDA forms	www.fda.gov/opacom/morechoices/ fdaforms/cder.html
Office for Human Research Protections	http://hhs.gov/ohrp
Office of Research Integrity	http://ori.hhs.gov
National Cancer Institute	www.cancer.gov
Cancer Therapy Evaluation Program	http://ctep.info.nih.gov
Cancer Trials Support Unit	www.ctsu.org
Office for Civil Rights Privacy Protection	http://hhs.gov/ocr/hipaa/assist.html
Oncology Nursing Society	www.ons.org
Association of Clinical Research Professionals	www.acrpnet.org
Society of Clinical Research Associates	www.socra.org
Regulatory Affairs Professionals Society	http://raps.org
NCI Central Institutional Review Board Initiative	www.ncicirb.org

Figure 12-5. Key Concepts of the "Final Rule"

Key Concepts
Misconduct in science is defined as fabrication, falsification, or other practices that seriously deviate from those that are commonly accepted within the scientific community for proposing, conducting, or reporting research. It does not include honest error or honest differences in interpretations or judgments of data.

- Created the Office of Scientific Integrity in the Office of the National Institutes of Health Director and the Office of Scientific Integrity Review in the Office of the Department of the Assistant Secretary of Health, Department of Health and Human Services. These have since merged to create the Office of Research Integrity.
- Each institution supported by the Public Health Service must have relevant administrative processes in place for review of allegations of misconduct.

civil monetary penalty, or issue a written notice or warning (Rozovsky & Adams, 2003). Consequences can range from a temporary suspension of the investigator from conducting clinical trials to a lifetime suspension. Names of disqualified or restricted clinical investigators will be listed in the *Federal Register* and on the FDA Internet home page indefinitely, even if the disqualification or restriction is lifted. Penalties also may include fines and prison sentences.

Misconduct can be pursued using federal statutory, criminal, and civil law (Rozovsky & Adams, 2003). The institution also may be affected by noncompliance. The functions of the IRB may be suspended by OHRP for DHHS-funded research if the IRB procedures are found to be deficient (Schechter, 2002). This can result in loss of funding, damaged reputation, and expensive corrective actions (Rozovsky & Adams, 2003).

Financial Fraud and Abuse

Financial fraud and abuse occur when the management of clinical trial funds is not handled honestly and accurately. It occurs when Medicare or any insurance party is billed for services that are to be paid by the sponsor of a clinical trial. Billing more than one source for a service is known as "double dipping"; only one party is to be billed for a service. It is necessary to know which clinical trial activities or procedures are standard of care and which are research related in order to determine the appropriate payer (see Chapter 5). Fraud and abuse occur when a report is filed that indicates additional funding is necessary to conduct the study when, in fact, it is not. It is essential that the fiscal management of clinical trials be done with *knowledge, accuracy, accountability,* and *integrity.*

The Office of Management Assessment (OMA) investigates concerns of fraud and abuse in NIH-sponsored research. Reimbursement fraud can be prosecuted under the False Claims Act (FCA). This requires knowledge that false or fraudulent claims and false statements were made to the government. The FCA primarily is enforced through the Department of Justice (Kalb & Koehler, 2002).

Conflict of Interest

Clinical trials are increasingly being affected by conflict of interest. Conflict of interest may involve financial arrangements and roles of the investigator. As the stakes in clinical testing have increased, so has the risk of conflict of interest. For-profit organizations are willing to provide a larger payment per participant than federally funded studies. The federal government requires disclosure of financial conflicts of the investigator. Institutions are required to manage any conflicts of interest. Disclosures must be made to the institution, the IRB, and the subjects (Nelson, 2006).

A conflict is inherent when the treating physician is the investigator. It is important to be aware of this situation in order to decrease the level of conflict. Morin et al. (2002) suggested that a physician who is involved in a patient's treatment should not be involved in the consenting process. They also suggested that additional staff should be available to answer study-related questions.

Negligence

Several types of negligence exist. These include *contributory negligence, criminal negligence,* and *culpable negligence.* Several elements must be proved to establish negligence. These elements are that the healthcare provider owed a duty to the patient, this duty was breached, damages occurred, and the damages were caused by the breach of duty.

Informed Consent

Courts focus on the quality of *informed consent* (Kvochak, 2002). The predominant legal liability issues in clinical trials involve informed consent. This stems from the common law action of battery, or the right of an individual to be protected from nonconsensual touching. Damages were awarded based on the occurrence of the touching without consent, regardless of whether harm had resulted. Prior to the 1950s, courts viewed consent issues (i.e., failure to obtain proper consent) as battery. Since then, the courts have viewed this as negligence instead (Garner, 2004; Kvochak).

Participating in the Process

It is important to be aware of changes and potential changes to regulations. One way to obtain information is to read the *Federal Register.* The federal government publishes the *Federal Register* daily. It contains information concerning the daily activities of the government, including proposed regulations, executive orders, news from federal agencies, and announcements calling for applications for federal grants (Lehman, 2005). Often there is a request for a response to the proposed regulations. Maintaining a current list of federal representatives and senators, or having the knowledge of how to obtain the current list, can facilitate a response to a proposal. A current list of state representatives also should be maintained. Clinical trial nurses (CTNs) have a responsibility to communicate their opinions to their representatives regarding the effects of proposed regulations and legislation. CTNs provide expertise that the representatives may lack.

Maintaining memberships in professional organizations is a step in legislative education. The Oncology Nursing Society (ONS) maintains an e-mail discussion list that notifies members of important events. ONS members may sign up for ONStat. The ONStat list allows for a quick response if legislation might be influenced by a member's representation. Several organizations have clinical trials research as their primary focus. These organizations are concerned with legislation at all levels, whether it is state, federal, or international. Examples of these organizations are the Society of Clinical Research Associates (SoCRA), the Association of Clinical Research Professionals (ACRP), the Regulatory Affairs Professionals Society (RAPS), and the Society for Clinical Trials. They all have Web sites with contact information and membership requirements. Joining or establishing a government or legislative committee within a local ONS, SoCRA, or ACRP chapter can strengthen an individual's voice.

Reading beyond nursing literature and subscribing to professional journals will provide increased exposure to proposed changes in clinical trial regulatory and compliance issues. These journals include those provided with membership to nursing and clinical trial professional organizations. Other journals are available online and through subscriptions.

Summary

The investigator assumes responsibility for the conduct of the study when he or she signs FDA form 1572. CTNs acting as study coordinators, site managers, clinical research associates, study monitors, regulatory associates, or project managers have an obligation to know the current regulatory and compliance standards and when changes are implemented. The federal government has a number of systems in place to ensure the safety and well-being of research participants. State governments and local healthcare institutions have developed measures to guide the conduct of clinical trials. It is the steadfast commitment of those involved in clinical research to providing for the protection of individual research participants while on the quest for knowledge that will reinforce the public's trust.

References

Charrow, R.P., & Goldman, E.B. (2004). *Regulation of clinical trials by the FDA: A process in search of procedures.* Retrieved March 16, 2006, from http://pubs.bna.com/ip/BNA/mrl.NSF/d166ae8c56b90b3985356d03005ca273/fe4f8239a12fc2d98

Clinical Trials Support Unit. (n.d.). *General information.* Retrieved March 29, 2006, from http://www.ctsu.org

Cornell Law School. (2006, September 27). *Administrative law.* Retrieved March 28, 2007, from http://www.law.cornell.edu/wex/index.php/Administrative_law

Dunn, C.M., & Chadwick, G. (2002). Ethics and federal regulations. In W. Allen (Ed.), *Protecting study volunteers in research—A manual for investigative sites* (pp. 28–43). Boston: Thompson CenterWatch.

Garner, B.A. (Ed.). (2004). *Black's law dictionary* (8th ed.). St. Paul, MN: West.

Gove, P.B. (Ed.). (2002). *Webster's third new international dictionary.* Springfield, MA: Merriam-Webster.

Grady, C. (2002). Ethical principles in clinical research. In J.I. Gallin (Ed.), *Principles and practice of clinical research* (pp. 15–26). Amsterdam: Academic Press.

International Air Transport Association. (2006a). *Packing instruction 650.* Retrieved April 6, 2006, from http://www.iata.org/NR/rdonlyres/F9D6D81A-71FB-46C3-BD6A-DDE849FD8A56/0/PACKINGINSTRUCTION650.pdf

International Air Transport Association. (2006b). *Guidance document: Infectious substances.* Retrieved August 28, 2007, from http://www.uchsc.edu/safety/Downloads/IATAGuidance48thDGR-InfxsSubstncs01-2007.pdf

Johnson, J., & Goldfarb, M. (2005). Ignorance of the shipping regulations may be hazardous to the health of your business. *Journal of Clinical Research Best Practices, 1*(12). Retrieved March 8, 2006, from http://www.firstclinical.com/resources/journal/0512/hazmat.pdf

Jones-Wright, P. (2006a). Documentation. In C.A. Fedor, P.A. Cola, & C. Pierre (Eds.), *Responsible research: A guide for coordinators* (pp. 123–140). London: Remedica.

Jones-Wright, P. (2006b). Guiding principles and regulations. In C.A. Fedor, P.A. Cola, & C. Pierre (Eds.), *Responsible research: A guide for coordinators* (pp. 11–34). London: Remedica.

Kalb, P.E., & Koehler, K.G. (2002). Legal issues in scientific research [Electronic version]. *JAMA, 287,* 85–91.

Kaltman, S.P., & Isidor, J.M. (2006). State law. In E.A. Bankert & R.J. Amdur (Eds.), *Institutional review board management and function* (pp. 304–307). Sudbury, MA: Jones and Bartlett.

Khin-Maung-Gyi, F.A., & Whalen, M. (2006). Ethics and human subject protection. In A. Fedor, P.A. Cola, & C. Pierre (Eds.), *Responsible research: A guide for coordinators* (pp. 35–41). London: Remedica.

Kvochak, P.A. (2002). Legal issues. In J.I. Gallin (Ed.), *Principles and practice of clinical research* (pp. 133–145). San Diego, CA: Academic Press.

Lanter, J. (2006, February). Complexities of starting an industry-sponsored clinical study: Guidance for new investigators. *Monitor, 20,* 25–28.

Lehman, J., & Phelps, S. (Eds.). (2005). *West's encyclopedia of American law* (2nd ed., Vols. 1, 2, & 8). San Diego, CA: Thompson-Gale.

Mathieu, M. (2005, December). GCP compliance and enforcement: A global view. *Monitor, 19,* 15–18.

Morin, K., Rakatansky, H., Riddick, F.A., Morse, L.J., O'Bannon, J.M., Goldrich, M.S., et al. (2002). Managing conflicts of interest in the conduct of clinical trials [Electronic version]. *JAMA, 287,* 78–84.

National Cancer Institute Cancer Therapy Evaluation Program. (2002). *Guidelines for monitoring clinical trials for cooperative groups. CCOP research bases and the Clinical Trials Support Unit (CTSU).* Retrieved August 16, 2007, from http://ctep.cancer.gov/monitoring/guidelines.html

Nelson, D.K. (2006). Conflict of interest: Researchers. In E.A. Bankert & R.J. Amdur (Eds.), *Institutional review board management and function* (pp. 3168–3171). Sudbury, MA: Jones and Bartlett.

Office of Civil Rights. (2006). *HIPAA.* Retrieved March 23, 2006, from http://www.hhs.gov/ocr/hipaa/assist.html

Pickett, J.P. (Ed.). (2000). *American heritage dictionary of the English language* (4th ed.). Boston: Houghton Mifflin.

Rozovsky, F.A., & Adams, R.K. (2003). *Clinical trials and human research: A practical guide to regulatory compliance.* San Francisco: Jossey-Bass.

Schechter, A.N. (2002). Integrity in research: Individual and institutional responsibility. In J.I. Gallin (Ed.), *Principles and practice of clinical research* (pp. 39–46). San Diego, CA: Academic Press.

Selected regulations and guidance for drug studies. (2005). Philadelphia: Clinical Research Resources.

Serio, J.C., Tichner, J.P., & Dilley, M.E. (2004). *State-by-state clinical trial requirements reference guide.* Waltham, MA: Barnett International.

U.S. Food and Drug Administration. (2006). *Good clinical practice in FDA-regulated clinical trials.* Retrieved March 8, 2006, from http://www.fda.gov/oc/gcp/default.htm

Wood, L.S. (2002, November). *Introduction to clinical trials nursing: A primer.* Paper presented at Oncology Nursing Society's Institutes of Learning, Seattle, WA. Retrieved April 6, 2006, from http://www.ons.org

Woodin, K.D. (2004). *The CRC's guide to coordinating clinical research* (p. 36). Boston: Thomson CenterWatch.

Zoon, K.C., & Yetter, R.A. (2002). The regulation of drugs and biological products by the Food and Drug Administration. In J.I. Gallin (Ed.), *Principles and practice of clinical research* (pp. 123–132). Amsterdam: Academic Press.

CHAPTER 13

Institutional Review Boards/Protocol Modifications

Kelly Filchner, RN, MSN, OCN®, CCRC,
and Patricia B. Herman, MSN, RN, AOCN®

Introduction

Research on humans has led to improvements in the prevention and treatment of many diseases. Unfortunately, human experimentation has been abused (see Chapter 1). Such abuse was not always the product of demented or perverted aspirations; rather, it sometimes resulted from well-motivated researchers lacking care and ethical sensitivity and overlooking the rights of human beings in an effort to ensure scientific progress or academic advancement (Ashley & O'Rourke, 1989).

In accordance with the international standard to prevent human rights violations, the U.S. government requires that every institution conducting research projects with public funds establish an institutional review board (IRB). The federal government will not fund research projects unless they have been first approved by an IRB. More information about IRBs can be found online at www.fda.gov/oc/ohrt/irbs.

The IRB has a vital role in the protection of human participants in the clinical trial process, whether it is during the initial review, revisions/modifications, clarification of treatment guidelines, deviations, or consent form revision. This chapter includes definitions, processes, and nursing implications of protocol revisions, modifications, clarifications of treatment guidelines, deviations, and consent form revisions. The information is presented as a general guideline for the clinical trial nurse (CTN). The CTN must apply these guidelines within the standards of his or her own institution and study group(s).

Institutional Review Boards

According to U.S. Food and Drug Administration (FDA) regulations, an IRB is an appropriately constituted group that is formally designated to review and monitor biomedical research involving human subjects. The section of the Code of Federal Regulations (CFR) pertaining to the FDA can be accessed online at www.gpoaccess.gov/cfr/index.html. FDA regulations state that an IRB has the authority to approve, require modification in, or disapprove research (FDA, 2005).

The purpose of IRB review is to ensure, both in advance of and during research, that appropriate steps are taken to protect the rights and welfare of human subjects. To accomplish this, IRBs use a *group process* to review research protocols and related materials (e.g., informed consent documents, investigator's brochures).

Regulations require that an institution's IRB be composed of at least five members with varying backgrounds to promote complete and adequate review of research activities commonly conducted at that institution. The membership should include males and females of various races and cultural backgrounds. At least one member must be a nonmedical professional (e.g., lawyer, clergy member) who possesses the competence to ascertain the acceptability of the proposed research in terms of the institutional commitments and regulations, applicable law, and standards of professional conduct and practice. One person must have no direct affiliation with the institution performing the research (e.g., layperson, community representative). If an IRB regularly reviews research that involves a vulnerable category of subjects (e.g., children, prisoners, pregnant women, handicapped or mentally disabled individuals), one or more people knowledgeable about and experienced in working with these subjects should be considered for inclusion on the board (Office for Human Research Protections [OHRP], 2005). The diversity of an IRB is critical to *maintaining objectivity* in assessing the ethical considerations of human research projects. An IRB can review a protocol at any time. The four types of review are shown in Figure 13-1.

The authors would like to acknowledge Marjorie J. Good, RN, BSN, MPH, OCN®, for her contribution that remains unchanged from the first edition.

Figure 13-1. Types of Institutional Review Board Review

- Initial review
- Continuation or annual review
- Modification review
- Expedited review

Initial Review

To approve research, an IRB must determine that all of the following requirements are satisfied (OHRP, 2005).

- Risks to subjects are minimized by using procedures that are consistent with sound research design and that do not unnecessarily expose subjects to risk and, whenever appropriate, by using procedures already being performed on the subjects for diagnostic or treatment purposes.
- The risks to subjects are to be reasonable in relation to the anticipated benefits to subjects and to the importance of the knowledge that may be expected to result.
- The selection of subjects is to be fair and equal.
- Informed consent is to be obtained from each subject or from the subject's legal guardian and is appropriately documented.
- The research plan should include provisions for monitoring the data collected to ensure the safety, privacy, and confidentiality of subjects.

When a study needs to be approved prior to a full IRB meeting, the study may be reviewed expeditiously. *Expedited review* is a procedure through which certain kinds of research may be reviewed and approved without convening a meeting of the IRB. An IRB may use the expedited review procedure to review either or both of the following: (a) when some or all of the research involves no more than minimal risk to subjects, and (b) when minor changes are proposed in previously approved research during the period covered by the original approval (one year or less) (OHRP, 2005).

Studies involving the collection of biologic specimens by noninvasive means, or the collection of data from voice or video recording, would qualify for expedited review. Under the expedited review procedure, review of research may be performed by the IRB chair or by one or more experienced members of the IRB designated by the chair. The reviewer may exercise all of the authorities of the IRB, except disapproval. *Research may only be disapproved following review by the full board* (FDA, 2005).

An IRB can approve, require modifications in, or disapprove research activities. The IRB then notifies the investigator and the institution in writing of its decision. If the IRB decides to disapprove a research activity, it must include in its written notification a statement of the reasons for its decision and give the investigator an opportunity to respond in person or in writing. An IRB must do these activities according to its own written procedures, sometimes referred to as *standard operating procedures* (SOPs). See Chapter 46 for an in-depth discussion of this topic.

Continuation or Annual Review

Annual reviews of clinical trials are conducted to determine which trials need verification from sources (other than the investigator) that no material changes in the research have occurred since the previous IRB review; to ensure that changes in approved research are promptly reported to and approved by the IRB; and to allow for suspension or termination of approval of research that is not being conducted in accordance with the IRB's requirements (FDA, 2005). The IRB is to conduct a continuing review of research covered at intervals appropriate to the degree of risk but *not less than once per year* (OHRP, 2005).

The FDA's continuing review regulations outline minimum requirements. The FDA does not provide specific instructions to IRBs on how to set up their own rules for continuing review within the framework of the regulations. Therefore, the regulations allow institutions or IRBs to impose greater and more detailed standards of protection for human subjects than those specified by the regulations and permit each IRB to develop procedures according to its needs. By regulation, the IRB has the authority and the responsibility to take appropriate steps to possibly terminate or suspend approval of research that is not being conducted in accordance with the IRB's requirements. The criteria to be met for continuing review are the same as for the initial review.

Continuing review should include IRB review of a written progress report from the clinical investigator (see Figure 13-2). Special attention should be paid to determining whether new information or unanticipated risks were discovered during the research. Any significant new findings that may relate to the subjects' willingness to continue participation should be provided to the subjects.

The IRB must obtain a copy of the consent document currently in use and determine whether its content is still accurate and complete, including whether new information that may have been obtained during the course of the study needs to be added. Obtaining the consent document provides a check on whether the document being used by the clinical investigator has current IRB approval. Verifying the current consent document with the IRB date of approval is accomplished easily and reflects good practice.

Figure 13-2. Progress Report Components

- The number of subjects entered into the research study
- Study status (i.e., is the study recruiting patients or in follow-up only)
- A summary description of subjects' experiences (e.g., benefits, adverse reactions, deaths)
- Number of withdrawals from the research; reasons for withdrawals
- The research results obtained up to that point in time, including any publications resulting from the research
- A current risk-benefit assessment based on study results
- Any new information or protocol changes since the institutional review board's last review
- A copy of the current informed consent document

The purpose of continuing review is to allow a review of the entire study, not just its changes. Continuing review may not be conducted using an expedited review procedure unless (a) the study was eligible for and was reviewed initially using an expedited review procedure, (b) the study has changed such that the only activities remaining are eligible for expedited review, or (c) the study is closed to accrual and patients are followed only for toxicity and survival data (FDA, 2005).

According to the FDA (2005), the continuation of research after the expiration of IRB approval is a violation of regulations. If the IRB has not reviewed and approved a research study before the study's current expiration date (i.e., IRB approval has expired), research activities should be stopped, and no new subjects may be enrolled in the study. If the investigator is actively pursuing renewal with the IRB and the IRB believes that an overriding safety concern or ethical issue is involved, it may stop research activities. However, an IRB may permit currently enrolled subjects to continue the trial for the brief time required to complete the review process.

When the IRB terminates study approval (e.g., because of a lack of compliance with continuing review requirements or when the study is complete), all research activities should be stopped, and remaining subjects should be notified. Procedures for withdrawal of enrolled subjects should take into account the rights and welfare of subjects. If follow-up of subjects for safety reasons is permitted or required by the IRB, the subjects should be informed, and any adverse events or outcomes should be reported to the IRB and the sponsor.

Protocol Revisions and Modifications

Although all clinical trials must have an IRB-approved protocol before they are implemented, these documents are not set in stone once written. During the life of a clinical trial protocol, many revisions or modifications may be made. These revisions can range from changing the pagination or title page, to therapeutic (e.g., drug dosing) or statistical analysis changes, to telephone number changes for contact individuals on the study. Protocol revisions do not necessarily originate with the principal investigator (PI). Many protocol revisions come from those who are administering the protocol, as well as from the study's data safety and monitoring committee. If research staff in the field find items in the protocol that do not "fit" or "make sense," a simple phone call to the contact person for the protocol may initiate the process for revisions. The PI, the protocol staff, or study sponsor where the trial *originated* writes the revisions.

Once the revision is written, the changes are sent to the proper approving agency (e.g., National Cancer Institute, FDA). After the revision has been approved, the changes are distributed to all participating centers. Generally, the study sponsor will outline what steps will be taken. For example, the revision may warrant suspension of the protocol until the IRB can approve the changes. The revision may need expedited or full IRB approval. Each IRB has the authority to determine what type of approval is necessary according to its SOPs. An example of the type of change that would require full approval would be a change in the treatment dosing because of newly reported toxicities or any change that involves patient risk. Conversely, a revision such as a change in the page numbers because of a typographical error would not require full IRB approval.

The person responsible for protocol management must examine the revision for possible consent form changes. These changes must be included in the consent form, which is reviewed by the IRB. The dates of revisions need to be included on the revised consent form.

Once the IRB has approved the revision, the revision pages are placed into the working protocol. Each participating center should keep a master file of the revisions, including the old protocol pages. The working protocol is the most current version of the protocol. The protocol staff uses the updated copy to implement treatment guidelines on a day-by-day basis. If changes to the protocol are substantial, the study sponsor distributes a completely new document. When this occurs, the newly distributed document becomes the working protocol. A separate file containing the protocol and revisions in their original form is maintained to satisfy requirements of regulatory agencies. If the revision requires full IRB approval, the appropriate regulatory forms are completed and submitted to the applicable cooperative group or sponsoring agency (McFadden, 1998).

Clarification of Treatment Guidelines

The sponsoring group of the clinical trial establishes a communication system when the protocol is disseminated to participating institutions. This communication system benefits all people involved in the research. The CTN who is coordinating the protocol treatment may have questions regarding protocol instructions, such as the timing of medications, dosing, or calculation of corrected body surface area. Some protocol instructions are written vaguely to allow for the clinical judgment of the site investigator. However, the protocol may not state clearly when the site investigator is allowed to exercise this judgment. Designated contact people are available to find answers to protocol questions in a timely manner to help to avoid protocol deviations.

A designated contact person usually is identified on the title page of a protocol. For example, some cooperative groups will have one contact number for all clinical questions, whereas others will have one person per protocol. Each protocol must designate who has the authority to make protocol clarifications. A shared authority may exist between the study chair and the sponsoring group. The designated contact person, the study chair, a nurse, and the data manager at the coordinating group are all resources for protocol clarification. A clinical research organization also may be involved in the study, and this would provide additional resources. Knowing these sources is important because study groups vary in how protocol clarifications are made.

Documentation of a clarification given by telephone or e-mail should be put into writing and include the date, time, and names of the people involved in the communication. In most cases, documentation should be kept with the specific patient's records or in a general correspondence file.

Deviations

A *deviation* is defined as "a noticeable or marked departure from accepted norms of behavior" (*Merriam-Webster's Collegiate Dictionary*, 1995, p. 137). In a clinical trial, a deviation is a departure from the printed guidelines of the protocol. Deviations are divided into major and minor categories. A *major deviation* is a protocol variance that makes the resulting data questionable (e.g., factors having a significant impact on eligibility, treatment, toxicity reporting). A *minor deviation* is one that does not affect the outcome or interpretation of the study. Each research group or sponsor has SOPs for classification of deviations.

Most deviations are revealed during the audit process. However, if the site discovers a deviation, the problem should immediately be brought to the PI's attention. If appropriate, the contact person or PI of the sponsoring group should be notified. If patterns of deviations are noted, the site's status in conducting research could be jeopardized.

The site and all personnel involved need to develop a plan for improving data collection. The goal of this plan is to prevent further deviations. The site PI ultimately is responsible for all data (McFadden, 1998). However, all protocol personnel are responsible for good research practices. Established communication patterns between the site investigator and protocol staff are key to quality data gathering and reporting.

Adverse Reaction Review

The IRB's continuing review responsibilities include reviewing reports of adverse reactions and unexpected events involving risks to participants or others. The IRB should establish a procedure for receiving and reviewing these reports. For more information on reporting of adverse events, see Section IX: Quality Improvement.

Informed Consent Review

According to FDA (2005) and Department of Health and Human Services (DHHS) regulations (OHRP, 2005), no investigator may involve a human being as a subject in research unless the investigator has obtained informed consent from the subject or the subject's legally authorized representative in accordance with regulations. A sponsor or those involved in a cooperative group study often develop sample or draft consent documents. However, the approving IRB is responsible for reviewing these consent documents and ensuring that the required elements are addressed adequately, that no exculpatory (i.e., guilt- or fault-like) language is used, and that the subjects can understand the language (it must be written at a sixth-grade reading level). The IRB should inform the investigator that only IRB-approved documents can be used.

The DHHS and the FDA have designated basic elements of informed consent (see Chapter 14). Informed consent documentation requirements permit the use of either a written consent document that contains the elements of informed consent or a "short form" stating that the elements of informed consent have been presented orally to the subject. Whichever document is used, a copy must be given to the person signing the document. Although not specifically mentioned in the FDA guidelines, the signature on the consent document should be dated at the time the subject signs it to verify that consent actually was obtained prior to the subject's participation in the study.

When the short-form method is used, the regulations require IRB review and approval of a written summary of the information that will be presented to the subject. A witness is required to attest to the adequacy of the consent process and to the subject's voluntary consent. The subject or the subject's legally authorized representative must sign the short form. The witness must sign both the short form and a copy of the summary, and the person actually obtaining the consent must sign a copy of the summary. The subject or the representative must be given a copy of the summary, as well as a copy of the short form.

Many IRBs develop standard language or a standard template to be used in portions of all consent documents. Standard language typically is developed for those elements that deal with confidentiality, compensation, answers to questions, and the voluntary nature of participation. Each investigator should determine the local IRB's requirements before submitting a study for initial review.

Consent Forms: Revisions and Addenda

When a revision requires a change to the consent form, the changes are reviewed by the IRB and incorporated into the consent form. The consent form must include dates of the revision. The inclusion of dates in the margin of the consent where a revision exists or at the end of the document reflects an accurate history of required consent form changes (see Figures 13-3 and 13-4).

When a revision is made to an industry-sponsored trial, changes are incorporated into the institutional consent form. Frequently, the sponsor must approve this revised consent before it may be submitted to the local IRB.

Once a consent form is revised, old copies are destroyed to prevent confusion and the signing of the wrong form. Old versions of consent forms are kept only in the site's regulatory files. At some institutions, an identifying stamp is affixed to all consent forms (see Figure 13-5). The purpose of the stamp is to verify that the document is the most

Figure 13-3. Revision Dates in Margin

ATH IRB Rev 4/95   I am deciding whether or not . . .

Figure 13-4. Revision History at the End of the Consent Form

Original 1/03
ATH IRB 1/04-periodic review
ATH IRB 9/04-rev. 1
ATH IRB 1/05-periodic review
ATH IRB 6/05-rev. 2

Figure 13-5. Identifying Stamp

Protocol Approval
Start date:
End date:
Initials:
Any hospital, IRB
Address:

current version of the consent form. The stamp is affixed to the first and last pages of the protocol.

The CTN assesses the impact of a revised consent form on the patient. Because informed consent is an ongoing process, a revised consent form may need to be signed by the enrolled patient. Possible situations for reconsent include treatment dosing or schedule changes, emergence of new information about the treatment, or a change in protocol requirements. The local IRB may dictate how patients are to be reconsented after protocol revisions have occurred (Amdur, 2003).

Nursing Implications

The first thing a nurse must recognize whenever a revision exists is the impact the revision will have on the *patient.* The enrolled patient needs to be informed of the changes that affect him or her and the reason for the changes. Minor revisions will have no impact on the patient. However, new information about the side effects of drugs being used may have a significant impact on the patient.

Patients can be informed about a revision in various ways. A letter with the new information may be sent to patients. The patient may be asked to sign and return a copy of the letter to verify that he or she has been informed. Periodically, a new consent form will need to be signed. How quickly the new consent form needs to be signed varies with the seriousness of the information that required the change. If the information was to change requirements for follow-up care, the consent will not have to be signed as quickly as when the change involves a modification of treatment.

The process of reconsent can increase the patient's anxiety. This is especially true when new side effects are

discovered. The CTN must help the patient to understand how the changes affect him or her. The patient may consider withdrawing from active treatment because of the changes. The CTN must be supportive and offer alternatives if the patient decides to withdraw from the protocol or discontinue therapy because of new information. The nurse should gain consent for continued follow-up should the patient decide to discontinue therapy. A patient may decide to withdraw permission for further follow-up data collection. This usually requires a separate signed statement.

To prevent deviations, the nurse must thoroughly understand the changes mandated in a revision or amendment. A revision in the data submission schedule or study parameter schedule may require a change in the patient follow-up schedule. A protocol may change several times after the patient completes protocol treatment. The CTN needs to apply the revisions to patients who have completed protocol therapy, as well as to patients who currently are receiving therapy.

The CTN also must maintain communication with investigators at the participating institution so that everyone involved is aware of protocol changes. This can be accomplished by establishing a communication system within the institution. A lack of communication between protocol staff and the investigators could result in protocol deviations.

Summary

Protocol revisions begin a cascade of events that affect both the protocol staff and the enrolled patient. The CTN has an important responsibility to assess the revisions and determine the most appropriate course of action. Proper clarification of protocol questions is an important nursing responsibility. Strict adherence to protocol guidelines and seeking clarification when protocol guidelines are unclear will reduce the risk of protocol deviations. Consent form changes caused by revisions may increase patient anxiety. Helping the patient to understand that informed consent is a continuous process involving the site investigator, the CTN, and the patient can reduce his or her anxiety.

The goal of every IRB is to protect human subjects. The IRB reviews clinical trial protocols and informed consent documents for *risk to subjects.* The four types of IRB review are initial review, continuation or annual review, modification review, and adverse reaction review. The CTN's involvement with the IRB may vary greatly from institution to institution. A CTN may be required to submit all protocols and documentation to the IRB or just be available to be contacted regarding protocol questions at an IRB meeting. Working collaboratively with the IRB and adhering to basic concepts in clinical trial management is yet another way that the CTN can improve study outcomes and safeguard the care of patients enrolled in clinical trials.

References

Amdur, R. (2003). *The institutional review board member handbook.* Sudbury, MA: Jones and Bartlett.

Ashley, B.M., & O'Rourke, K.D. (1989). *Healthcare ethics: A theological analysis.* St. Louis, MO: Catholic Health Association of the United States.

McFadden, E. (1998). *Management of data in clinical trials.* New York: Wiley.

Merriam-Webster's collegiate dictionary (10th ed.). (1995). Springfield, MA: Merriam-Webster.

Office for Human Research Protections. (2005). *Code of federal regulations* (Title 45, Vol. 1, Part 46). Retrieved December 30, 2005, from http://www.hhs.gov/ohrp/humansubjects/guidance/45cfr46.htm

U.S. Food and Drug Administration. (2005). *Code of federal regulations* (Title 21, Vol. 1, Part 56, Title 45, Vol. 1, Part 46). Retrieved from December 30, 2005, from www.fda.gov/oc/gcp/regulations.html

CHAPTER 14
Informed Consent

Angela D. Klimaszewski, RN, MSN

Introduction

Human rights in clinical trials (CTs) can be protected only when informed consent (IC) is approached as a process (National Commission for the Protection of Human Subjects of Biomedical and Behavioral Research [National Commission], 1979). That process is central to the recruitment of human subjects in CTs and is stringently regulated (Cumming, Sahni, & McClelland, 2006). And so it should be. This chapter reviews the IC process in CT research that involves human subjects in the United States.

Guiding Principles

The Belmont Report (see Appendix 4) in 1979 established three principles for the ethical conduct of CTs involving human subjects in the United States: (1) respect for persons, (2) beneficence, and (3) justice (National Commission, 1979). *Respect for persons* means recognizing a subject's personal dignity and autonomy, or the right of subjects to act in their best interest, as well as recognizing that subjects with diminished autonomy (e.g., children, older adults) require additional protection. *Beneficence* protects research subjects from harm and ensures their well-being. *Justice* means that benefits and burdens are fairly distributed among all subjects. Klimaszewski (2006) cited an example of justice as "not limiting drug research to one population such as adult males, when it could benefit adult females and children" (p. 493).

The Belmont Report (National Commission, 1979) identified IC as a process derived from the principle of respect for persons. It further delineated three elements of the IC process: (1) information, (2) comprehension, and (3) voluntariness. Part D of the Belmont Report addressed these elements in the subsection of Informed Consent:

- The extent and nature of *information* should be such that persons, knowing that the procedure is neither necessary for their care nor perhaps fully understood, can decide whether they wish to participate in the furthering of knowledge. Even when some direct benefit to them is anticipated, the subjects should understand clearly the range of risk and the voluntary nature of participation.
- Because the subject's ability to understand is a function of intelligence, rationality, maturity, and language, it is necessary to adapt the presentation of the information to the subject's capacities. Investigators are responsible for ascertaining whether the subject has *comprehended* the information. Although there is always an obligation to ascertain that the information about risk to subjects is complete and adequately comprehended, when the risks are more serious, that obligation increases. On occasion, it may be suitable to give some oral or written tests of comprehension.
- An agreement to participate in research constitutes a valid consent only if it has been *voluntarily* given. This element of IC requires conditions free of coercion and undue influence. Coercion occurs when an overt threat of harm is intentionally presented by one person to another to obtain compliance. Undue influence, by contrast, occurs through an offer of an excessive, unwarranted, inappropriate, or improper reward or other overture to obtain compliance.

The U.S. Department of Health and Human Services (DHHS) and its agencies, the Office for Human Research Protections (OHRP) and the U.S. Food and Drug Administration (FDA), revised their regulations on CTs involving human subjects in response to the Belmont Report (National Cancer Institute [NCI], 2006c). It is important for the clinical trial nurse (CTN) to know which agency regulations apply to a given CT, as specific agency regulations may have slight differences.

The OHRP regulates federally funded CTs with regulations in Title 45 of the *Code of Federal Regulations*, Public

The author would like to acknowledge Susan Anderson, RN, BSN, MFA, and Marjorie J. Good, RN, BSN, MPH, OCN®, for their contribution that remains unchanged from the first edition.

Welfare and Human Services, Protection of Human Subjects, Part 46. The FDA regulates trials that involve the licensing of a drug or product. Generally, but not exclusively, these are privately sponsored and thus are governed by regulations in Title 21 of the *Code of Federal Regulations*, Food and Drugs, Parts 50 and 56 (see Chapter 12). The FDA regulations for CTs are found in 21 CFR 312 and 21 CFR 812.

Federal regulations on CTs will share common characteristics with state and local regulations. When this occurs, the investigator and research staff must comply with the regulations that are most stringent (Kaltman & Isidor, 2006). Every institutional review board (IRB) must be aware of state regulations; therefore, the IRB is an excellent resource for the CTN regarding regulatory issues. The reader is referred to Chapter 12 for additional information on regulatory structure and function pertaining to CTs.

The investigator or a person designated by the investigator must obtain IC from the subject or the subject's legally authorized representative (LAR) prior to involving the subject in any aspect of research (International Conference on Harmonisation of Technical Requirements for Registration of Pharmaceuticals for Human Use, 1996; National Commission, 1979). Mackintosh and Molloy (2003) noted that significant physician involvement is required for IC in studies where the science is technologically complicated. The physician will need more time to adequately explain the study requirements and answer questions. CTNs play a pivotal role in ascertaining the subject's understanding of the IC document, clarifying misconceptions, and being the liaison between the patient and the physician regarding IC issues.

A recent FDA (2007) draft guidance titled "Guidance for Industry: Protecting the Rights, Safety, and Welfare of Study Subjects—Supervisory Responsibilities of Investigators" provided an overview of the responsibilities of a person who conducts a CT. Only the portions that pertain to IC will be addressed here. The FDA stated that when an investigator delegates tasks, he or she is responsible for adequately supervising those to whom the tasks were delegated. Consequently, the investigator is accountable for regulatory violations resulting from failure to adequately supervise the conduct of the study. An example of inappropriate delegation by an investigator is when the individuals who obtained IC lacked the medical training, knowledge of the clinical protocol, or familiarity of the investigational product needed to be able to discuss the risks and benefits of a CT with prospective subjects.

Clinical investigators are responsible for protecting the rights, safety, and welfare of subjects under their care during a CT. The investigator must ensure that IC is obtained from each subject in accordance with Title 21, Part 50 of the *Code of Federal Regulations* and that the study is not begun until FDA and IRB approvals have been obtained. Furthermore, the FDA (2007) noted that it is the responsibility of the investigator to ensure that all staff involved in the conduct of the study

- Have a general familiarity with the study and protocol
- Have a specific understanding of the details of the protocol and the investigational product, relevant to the tasks they will be performing
- Are aware of regulatory requirements and acceptable standards for the conduct of CTs, both in respect to the conduct of the CT and human subject protection
- Are competent to perform the tasks that they are delegated
- Are informed of any pertinent changes during the conduct of the trial and are educated or given additional training as appropriate.

Adequate supervision with regard to IC is identified as a procedure for ensuring that the consent process is being conducted in accordance with Title 21, Part 50 of the *Code of Federal Regulations* and that the study subjects understand the nature of their participation, risks, and so on. At the time of publication, this FDA (2007) guidance is only a draft of a recommendation.

Additionally, 45 CFR 46.116 (OHRP, 2005) requires that potential subjects receive complete information about the study in the IC document and have opportunities for the researcher and subject to exchange information and ask questions without coercion or undue influence. Furthermore, the information must be presented in language understandable to the subject or the subject's LAR (45 CFR 46.116).

Of note in 45 CFR 46.116 (OHRP, 2005) is the requirement that no IC, whether oral or written, may include any exculpatory language through which the subject or representative is made to waive or appear to waive any of the subject's legal rights. The IC also cannot include language that releases or appears to release the investigator, the sponsor, the institution, or its agents from liability for negligence.

Required Elements of the Informed Consent Document

Figure 14-1 presents the basic elements of an IC document from OHRP. Additional elements that specifically address issues such as unforeseeable risks to the individual, consequences of withdrawal from the study, and sharing of significant new findings with the individual are delineated in Figure 14-2. The consent document requirements for both OHRP and the FDA may be viewed at http://www.cancer.gov/clinicaltrials/understanding/simplification-of-informed-consent-docs/page4#appendix2.

NCI developed an IC template in 1998 and made it available to investigators. The updated version (NCI, 2006d) is reproduced in Appendix 10 and also may be accessed at www.cancer.gov/clinicaltrials/understanding/simplification-of-informed-consent-docs/page3. The CTN should note that every institution's IRB generally has its own IC template for investigators to use, as well.

The IRB must approve the IC document prior to use. The IC form should be written using terminology that the subject understands. Figure 14-3 presents a checklist of characteristics of easy-to-read IC document text.

Figure 14-1. General Requirements for Informed Consent

1. A statement that the study involves research, an explanation of the purposes of the research and the expected duration of the subject's participation, a description of the procedures to be followed, and identification of any procedures that are experimental
2. A description of any reasonably foreseeable risks or discomforts to the subject
3. A description of any benefits to the subject or to others that may reasonably be expected from the research
4. A disclosure of appropriate alternative procedures or courses of treatment, if any, that might be advantageous to the subject
5. A statement describing the extent, if any, to which confidentiality of records identifying the subject will be maintained
6. For research involving more than minimal risk, an explanation as to whether any compensation and medical treatments are available if injury occurs and, if so, what they consist of or where further information may be obtained
7. An explanation of whom to contact for answers to pertinent questions about the research and research subjects' rights and whom to contact in the event of a research-related injury to the subject
8. A statement that participation is voluntary, that refusal to participate will involve no penalty or loss of benefits to which the subject is otherwise entitled, and that the subject may discontinue participation at any time without penalty or loss of benefits to which the subject is otherwise entitled

Note. From *The Code of Federal Regulations, Title 45: Public Welfare, Part 46: Protection of Human Subjects* [Online], by the U.S. Department of Health and Human Services, 2005. Retrieved January, 11, 2008, from http://www.hhs.gov/ohrp/humansubjects/guidance/45cfr46.htm#46.116

Figure 14-2. Additional Elements of Informed Consent

When appropriate, one or more of the following elements of information shall also be provided to each subject.
1. A statement that the particular treatment or procedure may involve risks to the subject (or to the embryo or fetus, if the subject is or may become pregnant) that are currently unforeseeable
2. Anticipated circumstances under which the subject's participation may be terminated by the investigator without regard to the subject's consent
3. Any additional costs to the subject that may result from participation in the research
4. The consequences of a subject's decision to withdraw from the research and procedures for orderly termination of participation by the subject
5. A statement that significant new findings developed during the course of the research that may relate to the subject's willingness to continue participation will be provided to the subject
6. The approximate number of subjects involved in the study

Note. From *The Code of Federal Regulations, Title 45: Public Welfare, Part 46: Protection of Human Subjects* [Online], by the U.S. Department of Health and Human Services, 2005. Retrieved January, 11, 2008, from http://www.hhs.gov/ohrp/humansubjects/guidance/45cfr46.htm#46.116

Figure 14-3. National Cancer Institute Checklist for Easy-to-Read Informed Consent Documents[a,b,c,d]

Text
- Words are familiar to the reader. Any scientific, medical, or legal words are defined clearly.
- Words and terminology are consistent throughout the document.
- Sentences are short, simple, and direct.
- Line length is limited to 30–50 characters and spaces.
- Paragraphs are short. Convey one idea per paragraph.
- Verbs are in active voice (i.e., the subject is the doer of the act).
- Personal pronouns are used to increase personal identification.
- Each idea is clear and logically sequenced (according to audience logic).
- Important points are highlighted.
- Study purpose is presented early in the text.
- Titles, subtitles, and other headers help to clarify organization of text.
- Headers are simple and close to text.
- Underlining, bold, or boxes (rather than all caps or italics) are used to give emphasis.
- Layout balances white space with words and graphics.
- Left margins are justified. Right margins are ragged.
- Uppercase and lowercase letters are used.
- Style of print is easy to read.
- Type size is at least 12 point.
- Readability analysis is done to determine reading level (should be eighth grade or lower).
- **Avoid:**
  - Abbreviations and acronyms.
  - Large blocks of print.
  - Words containing more than three syllables (where possible).

Graphics
- Graphics are
  - Helpful in explaining the text.
  - Easy to understand.
  - Meaningful to the audience.
  - Appropriately located. Text and graphics go together.
  - Simple and uncluttered.
- Images reflect cultural context.
- Visuals have captions.
- Each visual is directly related to one message.
- Cues, such as circles or arrows, point out key information.
- Colors, when used, are appealing to the audience.
- Avoid graphics that will not reproduce well.

[a] National Cancer Institute, *Clear and Simple,* 23.
[b] National Cancer Institute, *Making Health Communications Programs Work,* 37.
[c] C. Doak et al., *Teaching Patients With Low Literacy Skills,* 2nd ed. (New York: Lippincott, 1996): 3.
[d] C. Meade et al., "Consent forms: How to determine and improve their readability," *Oncology Nursing Forum,* 19 (1992): 1523-8.

Note. From *Simplification of Informed Consent Documents, Appendix 3: Checklist for Easy-to-Read Informed Consent Documents,* by the National Cancer Institute, 2006. Retrieved August 1, 2006, from http://www.cancer.gov/clinicaltrials/understanding/simplification-of-informed-consent-docs/page5#appendix3

Assessing Comprehension and Improving Readability

Assessment of the participant's understanding of the CT and the IC form is vital to the IC process (National Commission, 1979). Cumming et al. (2006) stressed that the IC process needs to ensure a two-way flow of information to address the subject's understanding of the information. Documentation or, preferably, a tape recording of the conversation between the subject and the research team is crucial. Documentation in the medical record must include how the subject's understanding was assessed (e.g., oral question-and-answer session, written post-test) (Jaynes, 2005). Newton (2007) stated, "The best way to validate the effectiveness of the education that patients receive is to have them repeat the information back" (p. 14). Bertie Ford, RN, MS, AOCN® (see Chapter 30), recommends explaining important information first and then having the subject repeat back the information three times. Asking questions that require more than an affirmative or negative response will provide the CTN with a greater appreciation of what the subject truly understands. Hochhauser (2004) maintained that unless comprehension criteria have been established *before* the CT is opened, no benchmark can exist for determining low, average, or above-average comprehension.

While the NCI (2006c) recommends writing consent documents at an eighth-grade level or lower, Rust, Rogers, and Joyce (2007) note that 20% of U.S. adults read below a sixth-grade reading level. Therefore, any medical language, abbreviations, or jargon should be converted to layperson's language written at no higher than a sixth-grade reading level. Evaluating the subject's level of understanding may result in adapting the presentation of information to the subject's capacities (National Commission, 1979). See the "Special Populations" section of this chapter for additional information. Communication methods pertaining to IC are detailed in Figure 14-4.

The Process of Informed Consent

The IC process relies on the basic principles of the Belmont Report (see Appendix 4). Potential subjects may begin the IC process when they read an advertisement or receive a phone call about a specific CT. Once a subject is identified as a potential candidate for a study, physicians or CTNs begin by introducing the CT, including the investigative procedures (e.g., blood and urine collection, biopsies, radiographic procedures) to the subjects (Green & Rickles, 2007). Subjects are encouraged to ask questions and take enough time to critically review their options. Subjects need to fully discuss the treatment plan, adverse reactions, and expected risks and benefits with professionals (i.e., principal investigator, CTN, referring physician) and family members before consenting. It is important to have a relaxed conversation with the potential subject so that he or she has adequate time to review the IC form. The IC form is given to the subject to take home, read, and

---

Figure 14-4. Communication Methods for the Informed Consent Process

Time to Read and Discuss the Form

Researchers should encourage the potential research participant to thoroughly read and re-read the consent form and supplemental materials, if provided, and to discuss the proposed research with others before signing the consent form. This may require a delay between the describing of the study and the signing of the consent document.

Assess Understanding

It may be helpful for the researcher to ask the potential research participant short questions, after the research has been described and the consent form read, in order to assess that the potential research participant has at least a basic understanding of what the research involves.[a] Example questions include

- Tell me in your own words what this study is all about.
- Tell me what you think will happen to you in this study.
- What do you expect to gain by taking part in this research?
- What risks might you experience by participating in the research?
- What are your alternatives (other choices or options to participating in this research)?

Communication Techniques

Videos, audiotapes, interactive computer programs, and discussions with qualified lay individuals may assist in educating the potential research participant about the clinical trial.

---

[a] Titus et al., "Do you understand? An ethical assessment of researchers' description of the consenting process," *Journal of Clinical Ethics, 7* (1996): 60-80.

Note. From *Simplification of Informed Consent Documents, Appendix 4: Communication Methods*, by the National Cancer Institute, 2006. Retrieved August 1, 2006, from http://www.cancer.gov/clinicaltrials/understanding/simplification-of-informed-consent-docs/page2#appendix4

---

consider, away from the clinical setting. This entire process must be documented in the subject's medical record. Table 14-1 outlines the steps in the IC process.

Documenting Informed Consent

Two acceptable ways exist for obtaining written IC from a subject participating in a CT. The first is by the use of a written consent form approved by the IRB prior to obtaining the signature of the subject or the subject's LAR. This consent form must contain all of the required elements and may be read to the subject or the subject's LAR. The investigator is responsible for ensuring that the subject (or his or her representative) has adequate time to read it, has time to ask questions before signing it, and receives a written copy (45 CFR 46.117) (OHRP, 2005).

The second way to document IC involves an oral presentation of consent to the subject or the subject's LAR in the presence of a witness. Before the form can be used, the IRB must approve a short, written form that clearly states that the required elements of the IC have been presented orally to the subject or the subject's LAR. Only then may the subject or the LAR sign the IC form. Whereas the subject

Table 14-1. Steps in the Informed Consent Process	
Step	**Key Elements**
Initial meeting	Provide subject and family with the informed consent (IC) document. Discuss the IC document logically with subject and one or more members of the research team. Encourage subject and family to take notes. Provide adequate time for subject and family members to consider participation and have all questions answered. Provide subject with a video, audiotape, or interactive computer program to help him or her to understand the information in the IC document. Parents will represent subjects under age 18. If subject is between ages 6 and 18, ask for assent to participate, and provide an assent document for signature.
Time to read and consider participation	Subject is afforded adequate time to review the IC document at his or her leisure. Subject discusses the IC document with family, friends, social workers, clergy, a subject representative, or other trusted advisers. Subject records questions and concerns for discussion at next meeting.
Assessment of understanding	Discuss subject's questions and concerns that were recorded at home. Assess subject's understanding with interactive questioning, a written questionnaire, or by having the patient explain specific parts of the IC document in his or her own words. Document assessment of subject's understanding. Answer subject's questions until the patient states that he or she has enough information to make a decision. Document subject's statement regarding his or her decision.
Questions	Encourage subject to ask questions until the participant is satisfied with his or her understanding of the IC document. Encourage subject to record questions while away from the clinic and either bring them to the next meeting or schedule a visit to have the questions discussed.
New information	Assure subject that any new information available will be shared. Follow-up on assurance. Provide subject with an updated IC document for signature (as required). Document subject's understanding of new information in the presence of family. Document subject's signing of the new IC, review of IC, and that all subject's questions were answered. Provide copy of the IC form to subject.
Communication techniques	Videotapes, audiotapes, interactive computer programs, discussions with qualified professional and lay individuals
Supplemental materials	Videotapes, audiotapes, written materials, interactive computer programs
Note. Based on information from National Cancer Institute, 2006a, 2006b.	

(or LAR) signs only the short form, the witness must sign both the short form and the summary. Additionally, the person giving the oral presentation must sign the summary. The subject receives copies of both the short form and the summary (45 CFR 46.117) (OHRP, 2005). It is important to note that each IRB will have its own policies regarding the use of the short-form consent process.

Risks of treatment must be weighed against the benefits before the subject decides to proceed with any treatment for any disease. In a CT, some of the risks and benefits may not be known or may be observed during the course of the study. The principal investigator is responsible for providing subjects with an adequate explanation of expected effects of the treatment on an ongoing basis throughout the study. If unexpected toxicities are observed during the course of the study, the consent form will be amended and re-reviewed by the IRB. Subjects still engaged in therapy or otherwise affected by the new findings must sign an amended consent.

The participant has the right to withdraw from a CT at any time. However, if withdrawal endangers the subject's health, such as withdrawal from a high-dose chemotherapy regimen for bone marrow transplant *before* rescue or stem cell reinfusion, the consent form clearly must state the possibility of serious complications or death.

Procedures for Consent of a Non–English-Speaking Subject

NCI emphasized the need to include diverse populations in cancer research:

This important and complex issue requires cultural sensitivity in developing the informed consent document and communicating with the potential research participant and family members. The standards for valid consent should not be compromised in the face of language, cultural, or physical challenges. (NCI, 2006c, p. 5)

A non–English-speaking subject must be presented with a consent form written in the subject's native language. Alternatively, an oral presentation of IC information by a translator in conjunction with a short-form written consent document (stating that the elements of consent have been presented orally) and a written summary of what is presented orally can be utilized. The short-form written document should be in a language understandable to the subject. In this case, the IRB-approved English-language IC document may serve as the summary, and the witness should be fluent in both English and the subject's language.

At the time of consent, the subject or the subject's LAR should sign the short-form document. The summary (i.e., the English-language IC document) should be signed by the investigator. The witness should sign the short-form document and the summary. When a translator assists the person obtaining consent, the translator may serve as the witness.

Caution should be exercised when selecting an interpreter for IC. Each institution will have its own policy on the type and availability of interpreter services. Becze (2007) reported that several states have developed guidelines and standards regarding the training and certification of medical interpreters. The goal is to ensure that interpreters are proficient in (a) both languages being used and (b) medical terminology.

The IRB must receive all foreign-language versions of the short-form document as a condition of approval. Expedited review of these versions is acceptable if the protocol, the full English-language IC document, and the English version of the short-form document have already been approved by the convened IRB. In any case, each IRB will have its own set of policies on the use of the short-form process.

Source Documentation for the Informed Consent Process

The original signed consent form must be kept in the subject's record for both English- and non–English-speaking subjects. The subject receives a copy, and an additional copy may be kept in the subject's research file. Although not a regulatory requirement, the subject's medical record should include a notation of the *time* that the IC document was signed. This is especially important for verifying that consent was obtained prior to initiation of the study when the date of consent and the date of initiation of study procedures or administration of study drug are the same.

Special Populations

The Belmont Report (National Commission, 1979) noted that involving vulnerable populations in research must be justifiable. Additionally, it stated that special provisions may need to be made if an individual's comprehension is limited by immaturity or mental disability. *Respect* requires giving the individual the opportunity to choose whether to participate in research. Additionally, the report stated that any objections to participation that are made by these individuals should be honored. Federal regulations require that IRBs give special consideration to protecting the welfare of particularly vulnerable subjects, such as children, prisoners, pregnant women, mentally disabled persons, or the economically or educationally disadvantaged (OHRP, 2005).

Procedures for Consent of a Child

Consent (or permission) for a minor subject is two-fold: The subject must provide assent, and the subject's parent(s) must give consent. Parental permission is confirmed with their signature on the consent form. The IRB must determine whether the permission of both parents is necessary and the conditions under which one parent may be considered "not reasonably available" (45 CFR 46.408 (OHRP, 2005). Children do not need parental consent once they are 18 years old, and emancipated minors are consented as adults. In some lower-risk studies, adolescents will not need parental consent, but this must be at the discretion of the institution's IRB (45 CFR 46.4) (OHRP, 2005).

Assent is obtained from all children who are old enough to consider the risks and benefits of their participation. The IRB is key in determining whether a child is capable of providing assent. The IRB must consider the child's age, level of maturity, and current psychological state (45 CFR 46.408). Barrett (2002) noted that a child's ability to assent should not be based exclusively on age, as children with chronic disease and significant experience with hospitals are "more mature than their years" (p. 3).

A child's failure to object does not indicate assent. Children should be provided with an explanation of what the study will involve and any alternatives available to them. Their right to refuse is evaluated based on factors such as their age and the severity of their illness. Although assent is confirmed with the child's signature on the consent form, in cases of younger children who may not understand the implications of signing a legal document, having a third party sign for the child may be necessary to verify that assent was offered voluntarily (45 CFR 46) (OHRP, 2005). A sample of a child participation assent form can be accessed at www.cancer.gov/clinicaltrials/conducting/informed-consent-guide/page5.

Special conditions, such as a child who is pregnant or one who is a ward of the state, may present. If a child is pregnant, the child's assent and parental permission are obtained (45 CFR 46.204.g) (OHRP, 2005). If a child is a ward of the state, the IRB must require the court to appoint an advocate for the child, in addition to anyone else who may be acting on the child's behalf.

Protection of Pregnant Women, Fetuses, and Neonates

The federal government provides additional protection to pregnant women, fetuses, and neonates involved in clinical research. Specific conditions must be met before these individuals may participate in research at all. Essentially, IC must be obtained from each prospective subject or the subject's LAR. However, as the regulations are both detailed and extensive, the reader is referred to 45 CFR 46.204 through 45 CFR 46.207 in Appendix 5 of this publication for specific information.

Older Adult Subjects

Competent older adult participants generally do not require special protections with regard to research. Obstacles to IC, such as hearing impairment and poor vision, can be overcome by using large-print forms and tape-recorded consents (Klimaszewski, 2006). Older adult subjects studied by West, Bondy, and Hutchinson (1991) proved to be more willing to enroll in a CT than their caregivers were for them to enroll. Some older adults, however, may be deemed ineligible for entry into specific CTs because of concurrent health problems.

Two exceptions exist where older adults may need special protection: (a) if they have a cognitive impairment and/or (b) if they are institutionalized. Under those conditions, the same considerations are applicable as with any other subject in the same circumstances, regardless of the participant's age.

Subjects With Mental Disabilities or Dementia

Consent by the subject's LAR is required for a participant who is mentally ill, impaired, or suffering from dementia. These subjects may be institutionalized (voluntarily or involuntarily) in facilities such as psychiatric hospitals, halfway houses, nursing homes, or psychiatric inpatient units in general hospitals. As with minors, the consent form must include a justification for offering the study to the specified subject population or a rationale for not using a less vulnerable group. Specific benefits to the selected group must be cited. Also, the consent form must clearly state what consequences may result from withdrawal, such as transfer to another institution or a discontinuation of previous therapies.

Few subjects document their wishes regarding participation in CTs in advance directives (High & Doole, 1995). Dresser (2001) suggested use of a research advance directive. Such a directive would delineate a person's preference in the event that a particular study would become available after the person develops cognitive impairment. Unlike research involving children, prisoners, and fetuses, however, no additional DHHS regulations specifically govern research that involves participants who are cognitively impaired. Thus, the IRB must make the final determination of who will provide consent.

As a general rule, all adults, regardless of their diagnosis or condition, should be presumed competent to consent unless evidence exists of serious mental disability that would impair reasoning or judgment. Even those who do have a diagnosed mental disorder may be perfectly able to understand the matter of being a research volunteer and may be quite capable of consenting or assenting to or refusing participation (National Commission, 1979). Mental disability alone should not disqualify a person from consenting to participate in research; rather, there should be specific evidence of an individual's incapacity to understand and to make a choice before he or she is deemed unable to consent.

People formally deemed incompetent have a court-appointed guardian who must be consulted and will consent on their behalf. Officials of the institution in which incompetent patients reside (even if they are the patient's legal guardians) generally are not considered appropriate. Family members or others who are financially responsible for the patient also may be subject to conflicting interests because of financial pressures, emotional distancing, or other ambivalent feelings that are common in such circumstances. IRBs should bear this in mind when determining appropriate consent procedures for cognitively impaired subjects.

Because no generally accepted criteria for determining competence to consent to research exist, the role of the IRB in assessing the criteria proposed by the investigator is of major importance. The selection of an appropriate representative to consent on behalf of those unable to consent for themselves must be accomplished without clear guidance from statutes, case law, or regulations.

Prisoners

Protocols that are written for populations in prison must state so in the text of the written protocol. This then is reviewed by the institution's IRB. Prisoner advocates can be consulted to review the protocol and consent form in order to prevent exploitation of a population that may not have full access to resources to guarantee their rights. These safeguards are in place to prevent involuntary or coerced participation of a prisoner. Additionally, if a prisoner enrolled in a CT completes the study and is required to have follow-up examinations, provisions must be made for that to occur. Prior to signing the consent document, the prisoner must be informed of and agree to the follow-up examinations. If a prisoner is being considered for a protocol written for the general population, the IRB must be informed, and an amendment to the consent form may be required (45 CFR 46) (OHRP, 2005).

Gene Therapy and Genetic Testing

Recent developments in gene therapy and genetic testing have raised the ethics of science to a new level, resulting in poignant questions about the use of these procedures. Obtaining consent for a CT involving gene therapy or any form of genetic testing is addressed in Chapter 33.

Exemptions and Waivers

In special circumstances, the legal requirement for IC does not apply. A subject's right to self-determination is not absolute in those cases. The requirement to obtain IC may be waived by an IRB in special circumstances. The OHRP provides graphic aids in the form of decision trees to assist investigators, IRBs, and others with questions regarding whether the IC, its elements, or IC documentation may be waived (OHRP, 2004). These decision charts may be accessed at www.hhs.gov/ohrp/humansubjects/guidance/decisioncharts.htm.

Role of the Clinical Trial Nurse

The CTN should be an advocate to confirm with the investigator that the subject has had an adequate amount of time to review the consent form and that all of the subject's questions have been answered. The CTN must verify that the IC form has been signed, with the original in the medical record and a copy given to the subject, before performing any study tests or administering any study treatments.

Wujcik (2007) compared patient education with the IC process, stating, "Patients and family members need an ongoing assessment of their understanding and willingness to continue with the plan of care" (p. 5). Every time the subject returns for treatment, the CTN should determine if the subject truly wishes to continue. Asking "Are you ready for your treatment today?" may evoke a humorous response from the subject, a serious response, or one that will immediately alert the CTN to the possibility that the subject is considering withdrawing consent. The subject may intimate that his or her spouse wants the subject to continue with the CT, even though the subject admits to being "tired" and "ready to stop." The CTN must notify the investigator if the subject has additional questions or decides to withdraw consent. By taking the additional time to verify consent, the CTN will protect and maintain the rights of the subject and the integrity of the IC.

Additional Information

The CTN may elect to seek additional information regarding IC in this manual and can consult the following chapters.
- Chapter 13 addresses the topic of IRBs and presents a more detailed discussion of IC review and revisions.
- Chapter 32 presents IC as it pertains to pharmacokinetics and genetics.
- Chapter 33 discusses components of IC involving genetic material and testing.
- Chapter 46 addresses the topic of continuing IC.
- Chapter 47 presents discussion on the auditing elements of IC in a CT.

Future Directions

If methodology and ethics drive the design and conduct of multicenter trials (Fazi et al., 2006), then ethics, education of the subject (or the subject's LAR), and documentation drive the IC process. It may be only a matter of time before some of the following become routine in the IC process.
- Participant choice to learn about trial results integrated into the IC document so that participants have the option to decline future contact (Partridge & Winer, 2002)
- Increased comprehension where interactive multimedia presentations are programmed with correctional feedback to the participant's response to questions, creating a loop to review information that was not understood and enabling participants to ask higher-level questions
- Improved documentation of IC where computer software links consent documentation to the participant's electronic medical record, automatically entering information from the IC process onto the correct forms
- Enhanced compliance with regulatory requirements for evidence of the IC process by tape recording the entire process, thus enhancing protection of human subjects
- Enhanced interaction where subjects may enter questions into an IC program, send it to their physician, and have the groundwork laid for discussion at their next encounter (Brady, 2003)

Continual improvements in the IC process and IC document, along with public awareness of the efforts being made to protect the rights of human subjects, will improve participant education and decision making (Brady, 2003) and the public image of CTs as a whole.

Summary

The IC process may begin with an advertisement or a phone call, progress to a frank discussion about the contents of the IC document, and then develop into an ongoing relationship between the subject and the research team. Education must be tailored to the subject's level of understanding, ability, and learning styles and preferences. Reinforcement, updating, and reassessment promote fully informed decisions. Special vulnerable subject populations may require additional advocacy and aids to ensure that fully informed consent is obtained. In every case, it is the subject who must decide whether to participate in a CT. It is the subject's disease and the subject's decision.

The past decade brought significant improvements worldwide in the protection of human rights in human subject research. CTNs can help to protect human participants by being advocates and educators in the process of IC. By protecting a subject's rights, remaining objective, and respecting whatever decisions a subject makes, CTNs will foster ethical and autonomous IC.

References

Barrett, J. (2002, July 1). Why aren't more pediatric trials performed? *Applied Clinical Trials.* Retrieved August 4, 2006, from http://www.actmagazine.com/appliedclinicaltrials/content/printContentPopup.jsp?id=83729

Becze, E. (2007, March). Certified medical interpreters provide better services. *ONS Connect, 22*(3), p. 30.

Brady, J.S. (2003, January 1). Multimedia delivery can enhance the consent process. *Applied Clinical Trials*. Retrieved June 28, 2006, from http://www.actmagazine.com/appliedclinicaltrials/content/printContentPopup.jsp?id=80369

Cumming, J.F., Sahni, A.R., & McClelland, G.R. (2006, March 1). The importance of the subject in informed consent. *Applied Clinical Trials*. Retrieved June 28, 2006, from http://www.actmagazine.com/appliedclinicaltrials/content/printContentPopup.jsp?id=310810

Dresser, R. (2001). Advance directives in dementia research: Promoting autonomy and protecting subjects. *IRB, 23*(1), 1–6.

Fazi, P., Ali, L.C., Luzi, D., Ricci, F.L., Serbanati, L.D., & Vignetti, M. (2006, January 1). A proposed clinical trial model: Analyzing the CT process. *Applied Clinical Trials*. Retrieved June 28, 2006, from http://www.actmagazine.com/appliedclinicaltrials/content/printContentPopup.jsp?id=283029

Green, D., & Rickles, F.R. (2007). Enhancing participation in clinical research: Keys to obtaining informed consent. *Journal of Supportive Oncology, 5*, 48–50.

High, D.M., & Doole, M.M. (1995). Ethical and legal issues in conducting research on elderly subjects. *Behavioral Sciences and the Law, 13*, 319–335.

Hochhauser, M. (2004, April 1). Informed consent: Reading and understanding are not the same. *Applied Clinical Trials*. Retrieved June 28, 2006, from http://www.actmagazine.com/appliedclinicaltrials/content/printContentPopup.jsp?id=90594

International Conference on Harmonisation of Technical Requirements for Registration of Pharmaceuticals for Human Use. (1996). Guidance for industry. E6 good clinical practice: Consolidated guidance. *Federal Register, 62*, May 9, 1997.

Jaynes, T. (2005, June 1). Informed consent: Imparting knowledge or signing a form? *Applied Clinical Trials*. Retrieved June 28, 2006, from http://www.actmagazine.com/appliedclinicaltrials/content/printContentPopup.jsp?id= 165486

Kaltman, S.P., & Isidor, J.M. (2006). State law. In E.A. Bankert & R.J. Amdur (Eds.), *Institutional review board management and function* (pp. 304–307). Sudbury, MA: Jones and Bartlett.

Klimaszewski, A.D. (2006). Psychosocial aspects of experimental therapy: Clinical trials. In R.M. Carroll-Johnson, L.M. Gorman, & N.J. Bush (Eds.), *Psychosocial nursing care along the cancer continuum* (2nd ed., pp. 489–497). Pittsburgh, PA: Oncology Nursing Society.

Mackintosh, D.R., & Molloy, V.J. (2003, May 1). Opportunities to improve informed consent. *Applied Clinical Trials*. Retrieved June 28, 2006, from http://www.actmagazine.com/appliedclinicaltrials/content/printContentPopup.jsp?id=88095

National Cancer Institute. (2006a, March 24). *A guide to understanding informed consent: What to expect*. Retrieved July 5, 2006, from http://www.cancer.gov/clinicaltrials/conducting/informed-consent-guide/page5

National Cancer Institute. (2006b, May 23). *Simplification of informed consent documents: Appendix 2: Code of federal regulations for the protection of human subjects in research*. Retrieved July 5, 2006, from http://www.cancer.gov/clinicaltrials/understanding/simplification-of-informed-consent-docs/page4#appendix2

National Cancer Institute. (2006c). *Simplification of informed consent documents: Recommendations*. Retrieved August 1, 2006, from http://www.cancer.gov/clinicaltrials/understanding/simplification-of-informed-consent-docs/page2

National Cancer Institute. (2006d, May 23). *Simplification of informed consent documents: Templates*. Retrieved August 1, 2006, from http://www.cancer.gov/clinicaltrials/understanding/simplification-of-informed-consent-docs/page3

National Commission for the Protection of Human Subjects of Biomedical and Behavioral Research. (1979, April 18). *The Belmont report: Ethical principles and guidelines for the protection of human subjects of research*. Retrieved June 3, 2007, from http://ohsr.od.nih.gov/guidelines/belmont.html

Newton, S. (2007, May). Patients should be able to repeat key points. *ONS Connect, 22*(5), p. 14.

Office for Human Research Protections. (2004, September 24). *Human subject regulations decision charts*. Retrieved June 28, 2006, from http://www.hhs.gov/ohrp/humansubjects/guidance/decisioncharts.htm

Office for Human Research Protections. (2005, June 23). *Code of Federal Regulations (Title 45, Vol. 1, Part 46)*. Retrieved June 28, 2006, from http://www.hhs.gov/ohrp/humansubjects/guidance/45cfr46.htm

Partridge, A.H., & Winer, E.P. (2002). Informing clinical trial participants about study results. *JAMA, 288*, 363–365.

Rust, D., Rogers, B., & Joyce, M. (2007, May). Materials should be simplified and contain visuals. *ONS Connect, 22*(5), p. 14.

U.S. Food and Drug Administration. (2007, May). *Guidance for industry. Protecting the rights, safety, and welfare of study subjects—supervisory responsibilities of investigators*. Retrieved May 31, 2007, from http://www.fda.gov/cber/gdlns/studysub.pdf

West, M., Bondy, E., & Hutchinson, S. (1991). Interviewing institutionalized elders: Threats to validity. *Image, 23*, 171–176.

Wujcik, D. (2007, May). Human interaction is the key to effective patient education. *ONS Connect, 22*(5), p. 5.

CHAPTER 15

Compassionate Use of Investigational Drugs

Patricia Hentschel, RN, MS, ANP, CCRC

Introduction

Clinical trial nurses (CTNs) often are asked to explore options for patients in need of treatment who have exhausted all standard therapies. Circumstances may arise in which these patients are ineligible for existing clinical trials or where potential therapies are no longer available through clinical trials because of pending U.S. Food and Drug Administration (FDA) approval. Under these circumstances, investigational drugs can be made available on a compassionate (nonresearch) basis through programs sponsored by the National Cancer Institute's (NCI's) Cancer Therapy Evaluation Program (CTEP). This chapter will review these programs in detail and provide access information for drug procurement.

The National Cancer Institute's Compassionate Release of Investigational Drugs

The NCI CTEP can release investigational drugs for compassionate use under defined circumstances. The two mechanisms for obtaining drugs in this setting are Group C and Special Exception. These mechanisms differ in regard to purpose and the reporting and procedural responsibilities of the investigator (NCI CTEP, 2002b). The ultimate purpose of both mechanisms is to make nonapproved agents that are significantly active against specific malignancies available to patients with cancer and their physicians. CTEP's Pharmaceutical Management Branch (PMB) coordinates, authorizes, and processes all requests for Group C and Special Exception investigational agents. Requests can be submitted to CTEP in writing (Clinical Research Pharmacy Section, Pharmaceutical Management Branch, CTEP, 9000 Rockville Pike, Executive Plaza North, Room 804, Bethesda, MD 20892) or by telephone (301-496-5725; fax: 301-402-4870). CTEP also has a Web site (http://ctep.info.nih.gov) that provides a list of resource staff and their e-mail addresses.

Requests for compassionate use of investigational agents via Group C or Special Exception will be considered if the following criteria are met (FDA, 1998; Jenkins & Hubbard, 1991; NCI CTEP, 2002b, 2004).
- The patient is ineligible for a research protocol.
- Standard therapies have been exhausted.
- Objective evidence exists indicating that the investigational agent is active in regard to the disease for which the request is being made (CTEP usually requires published phase II data as objective evidence).
- The drug is likely to benefit the patient.

Group C Drugs
Definition and Purpose

The Group C mechanism was established through an agreement between the FDA and NCI. It is a means for compassionate distribution of investigational agents to oncologists for the treatment of individual patients with cancer under guideline protocols outside the controlled clinical trial. Group C investigational agents are drugs that have shown evidence of reproducible efficacy in treating one or more specific tumor types and have altered or are likely to alter the pattern of treatment of the disease. In recent years, CTEP has considered Group C classification only for agents with well-established activity in the phase III setting and those pending final FDA approval. Generally, trained physicians can administer Group C drugs without the need for specialized supportive-care facilities.

Criteria for Use and Procurement

A list of current Group C drugs can be obtained by contacting the CTEP PMB by telephone at 301-496-5725 on Monday through Friday between 9 am and 4:30 pm EST. This list also can be accessed via the Internet at http://ctep.cancer.gov/requisition/compassion.html (NCI CTEP, 2004). The list is subject to change as drugs receive FDA approval. Group C drugs should be requested to treat patients with an indication specifically authorized for the requested drug. All other nonresearch requests for clinical use are considered Special Exceptions.

The Guideline Protocol

The use of a drug for a Group C–approved indication is fully described in the guideline protocol written by CTEP and approved by the FDA. It describes the indications, dosage, precautions, warnings, and known adverse events for the specific indications. The guideline protocol also contains an FDA-approved informed consent, which must be used if no local institutional review board (IRB) review has occurred.

When requesting Group C treatment from the PMB, the amount of patient information required varies for each Group C drug. The physician ordering the drug must register or be registered with NCI as an investigator (he or she will receive an NCI number) by completing the statement of investigator (FDA form 1572), a supplemental investigator data form, and a financial disclosure form submitted with a current curriculum vitae. All of these should be signed and dated within the past year. Forms can be obtained by contacting the PMB Drug Management and Authorization Section at 301-496-5725 or online at http://ctep.cancer.gov/forms/index.html (NCI CTEP, 2002b). If the request is approved, a supply of the drug will be shipped along with an approval letter, a copy of the guideline protocol, and procedures for reporting adverse drug reactions (ADRs).

Responsibilities and Reporting

The physician requesting a Group C drug accepts clearly outlined responsibilities designed to safeguard the patient, including obtaining informed consent, receiving IRB approval, and maintaining drug accountability, quality assurance, and compliance with the guideline protocol. The physician also is responsible for submitting reports related to ADRs and treatments. NCI mandates compliance with all of the following procedures. Failure to comply could result in suspension of the investigator's status and could prevent further drug shipments.

Informed consent: Written informed consent must be obtained from all patients treated with Group C drugs and kept on file. A model informed consent (FDA-approved), which will arrive with the guideline protocol, may have to be modified for local IRBs.

IRB approval: Because Group C drugs are not administered with a primary research intent, an IRB waiver usually has already been obtained from the FDA. However, some IRBs have a policy that requires their local approval.

Investigational drug accountability: NCI Investigational Drug Accountability Records must be maintained for Group C drugs and kept on file.

ADRs: Because Group C drugs are still investigational agents, physicians are obliged to report ADRs to CTEP. ADR reporting forms and a toxicity rating scale should be included with the guideline protocol. Over the past several years, NCI instituted an electronic system for expedited

submission of adverse events, the Adverse Event Expedited Reporting System (AdEERS). Detailed instructions for reporting ADRs via AdEERS as well as computer-based training can be found on the CTEP home page at http://ctep.cancer.gov (under "Reporting Guidelines") or by telephone at 301-230-2330 (NCI CTEP, 2002b). All reports should be mailed to the Investigational Drug Branch, P.O. Box 30012, Bethesda, MD 20824.

Quality assurance: Medical records confirming that the patient has been treated according to the Group C protocol must be maintained at the site and stored in a confidential manner. The FDA and NCI should be provided with these records for monitoring and audit purposes upon request.

Treatment reports: The physician may be required to provide patient reports if specified in the protocol. If required, patient-specific forms may be sent to the physician separately; samples of these forms would be included in the protocol.

Drug reorders: An additional drug supply may be requested by completing an NCI clinical drug request form (form NIH-986), which also can be accessed online at http://ctep.cancer.gov/requisition. A blank drug request form is enclosed with each drug shipment.

Special Exception Drugs
Definition and Purpose

Physicians with patients who have no other treatment options and have a cancer diagnosis for which an investigational drug has demonstrated activity may request a drug from CTEP as a Special Exception to the policy of administering investigational agents only under a research protocol. If the requested drug is a Group C drug for that indication, it should be requested under the Group C mechanism. Unlike Group C drugs, Special Exception drugs are always part of phase II or phase III trials. Patients treated under the Special Exception mechanism should not be eligible for these ongoing clinical trials (NCI CTEP, 2002b).

The Special Exception mechanism allows NCI to provide a special service to oncologists and patients with cancer. Physicians can obtain investigational agents directly from CTEP instead of having to submit an individual investigational new drug request to the FDA for emergency use of an investigational drug, which can be a lengthy process.

Criteria for Use and Procurement

Requests for Special Exceptions may be made in writing or by telephone to NCI's PMB (see Figure 15-1). Physicians and pharmacists at PMB will review the Special Exception request and make a decision on a case-by-case basis. Considerable evidence should demonstrate that the agent shows activity for the indication requested, and a reasonable expectation should exist that the agent will prolong survival or improve quality of life in a cohort of similar patients so treated. Reports of low response rates or occasional responses are not sufficient to justify approval.

Figure 15-1. Information Required for a Special Exception Request

- Patient's name or identification number, age, and sex
- Diagnosis and date of diagnosis
- Previous cancer therapy
- Current clinical status
- Intended dose and schedule of the requested agent (based on the current literature)
- Potential concomitant therapy
- Pertinent laboratory data
- An explanation of why the proposed use of the investigational drug is more beneficial than a commercially available drug

Note. Based on information from National Cancer Institute Cancer Therapy Evaluation Program, 2002a.

Consideration also will be given as to whether a research protocol exists for which the patient is eligible, whether all standard therapies have been tried, and whether the requested agent is active in the disease for which it is being requested (NCI CTEP, 2002b).

As with the Group C mechanism, the physician ordering the drug must register or be registered with NCI as an investigator and complete the same forms as for Group C Drug procurement. Upon registering, the physician will receive an NCI investigator number.

NCI provides a Special Exception packet that contains the required information for procurement of Special Exception drugs along with all of the necessary forms. Physicians can obtain this packet by telephoning and asking to speak to a pharmacist. The pharmacist will ask for the investigator's NCI number to fulfill this request.

Responsibilities and Reporting

As with Group C drugs, NCI clearly outlines physicians' responsibilities for Special Exception drugs. Required reports are similar to those required for Group C drugs, with the addition of a brief summary protocol for each patient. NCI mandates compliance with all of the following procedures. Noncompliance can result in the suspension of the investigator's status and could prevent further drug shipments.

Protocol: A brief protocol that describes the treatment plan, toxicity, efficacy, and monitoring procedures must be submitted for each patient. NCI provides a standard protocol form, called the Special Exception Protocol, which is included in the Special Exception packet. This form must be completed and returned (the original and three copies) to NCI within 10 working days. It is important to note that the Special Exception mechanism must not be used to obtain agents to treat a series of patients on a protocol or to do pilot work for an intended study (NCI CTEP, 2002b).

Informed consent: Written informed consent must be obtained from the patient or his or her guardian prior to treatment and retained in the patient's medical record. The consent form, written by the investigator, should include

a reasonable statement about the potential side effects of the drug and should address each of the eight elements of informed consent required by the FDA. The Special Exception packet will provide the required elements of informed consent.

IRB approval: IRB approval of the Special Exception Protocol and consent form must be obtained before beginning treatment. Documentation of this approval must be kept in the patient's medical record.

Investigational drug accountability: NCI Investigational Drug Accountability Records must be maintained for Special Exception drugs and kept on file.

ADRs: Because Special Exception drugs are investigational agents, physicians are obliged to report ADRs to CTEP. The Special Exception packet includes guidelines for reporting ADRs, ADR reporting forms, and the NCI Common Terminology Criteria for Adverse Events. Please refer to additional information about ADR reporting described in the Group C Drugs section.

Drug reorders: As with Group C drugs, an additional drug supply may be requested by completing an NCI clinical drug request form. A blank request form is enclosed with each drug shipment. The drug can be reordered only for the patient specifically named on the protocol.

Final patient report: Upon completion of the patient's therapy, the physician must provide NCI with a report of the treatment experience, which describes toxicity and efficacy. The physician records this information on a form called the Report of the Independent Investigator, which is included in the Special Exception packet.

Summary

Procurement of investigational drugs for compassionate use outside of a clinical trial requires knowledge of the available access mechanisms, each of which differs in purpose and procedure. The scope of the CTN's practice often extends to the compassionate use of investigational drugs, which necessitates a thorough understanding of each of the access mechanisms discussed in this chapter.

References

Jenkins, J., & Hubbard, S. (1991). History of clinical trials. *Seminars in Oncology Nursing, 7,* 228–234.

National Cancer Institute Cancer Therapy Evaluation Program. (2002a). *A manual for participants in clinical trials of investigational agents sponsored by DCTD, NCI.* Retrieved December 9, 2007, from http://ctep.cancer.gov/forms/Hndbk.pdf

National Cancer Institute Cancer Therapy Evaluation Program. (2002b). *The treatment referral center and non-research (compassionate) use of investigational agents.* Retrieved December 9, 2007, from http://ctep.cancer.gov/requisition/compassion.html#GC

National Cancer Institute Cancer Therapy Evaluation Program. (2004, January 5). *Non-protocol access to experimental agents.* Retrieved November 23, 2007, from http://ctep.cancer.gov/requisition/compassion.html

U.S. Food and Drug Administration. (1998). *Guidance for institutional review boards and clinical investigators: Treatment use of investigational drugs.* Retrieved November 17, 2005, from http://www.fda.gov/oc/ohrt/irbs/drugsbiologics.html#treatment

CHAPTER 16
Conflicts of Interest

Mary E. Brimer, RN, MSN, OCN®

Introduction

Throughout the years, examples of unethical behavior in research have been exposed, which has led to increased oversight of research practices. The National Commission for the Protection of Human Subjects of Biomedical and Behavioral Research (National Commision, 1979) defined the core principles underlying ethically sound research in the Belmont Report, which is reprinted in Appendix 4. The ethical principles described in the Belmont Report—respect for persons, beneficence, and justice—have guided research ever since. Openness and honesty of the researcher are characteristics that promote ethical research and can only strengthen the research process. In recent years, however, conflict of interest, or the appearance of conflict of interest, has called into question the scientific integrity of scientists and researchers.

Researchers may wear many hats, including clinician, educator, scientist, institutional leader, consultant, businessman, and/or author. The complex and demanding nature of research today gives rise to competing obligations and interests (Steneck, n.d.). Researchers have a conflict of interest when their interests or commitments compromise their judgments, research reports, or communications to research participants, patients, or clients (Office for Human Research Protections, 2001). In a survey of potential research participants, the majority responded that knowing conflict of interest information was "extremely" or "very " important (Kim, Millard, Nisbet, Cox, & Caine, 2004).

What Is Conflict of Interest?

The Association of American Medical Colleges has described conflict of interest in science as "situations in which financial or other personal considerations may compromise, or have the appearance of compromising, an investigator's professional judgment in conducting or reporting research" (DeAngelis, Fontanarosa, & Flanagin, 2001, p. 89). Such conflicts may be potential or actual, perceived or real, and harmful or insignificant. Conflicts of interest represent the potential for biased judgment but are not an indicator of the likelihood or certainty that such judgments or compromises will occur.

For instance, a conflict of interest exists when a member of the research team attempts to occupy dual roles that should not be performed together (Morin et al., 2002). A physician who acts as the principal investigator (PI) and serves on the institutional review board (IRB) is just one example. A conflict of interest also can be defined as a discrepancy between the personal interests and professional responsibilities of a person in a position of trust (Morin et al.). One example of this would be if the PI and the investigative staff owned stock in the pharmaceutical company that was running a clinical trial with the same group.

To understand conflict of interest in the conduct of clinical trials, one must take several objective steps backward from the clinical situation and understand the distinct perspectives of the patient and the physician as a clinical investigator. For the patient, a clinical trial may be the difference between life and death. The trial is the hope of a cure, receiving a few more days to finalize plans, or spending time with family. For the patient, the act of participation in a clinical trial is a uniquely human event in the pursuit of life itself (Jassak & Ryan, 1989).

On the other hand, the perspective of the physician and investigative team may be radically different from, and possibly in opposition to, the view of the patient. It is hoped that the physician/investigator holds the best interest of the patient as the primary goal while participating in a purely academic endeavor—an attempt to understand drug toxicity, disease processes, and novel treatments. This mainstream ethical approach to clinical trials attempts to

The author would like to acknowledge Suzanne Cabriales, RN, BSN, OCN®, for her contribution that remains unchanged from the first edition.

have it both ways: to view the clinical trial as a scientific experiment aimed at producing knowledge that can help to improve the care of future patients and as treatment conducted by physicians who must retain fidelity to the principles of therapeutic beneficence and nonmalfeasance that govern the ethics of clinical medicine (Miller & Brody, 2003).

The clinician/investigator must balance the best interests of the individual patient as the ultimate goal while fully attempting to answer a scientific question, which can be generalized to a larger population. This subtle difference in viewpoint is important when evaluating the conflicts that can arise in the development of a clinical trial, the scientific question being asked, and the use of placebos in randomized trials.

More obvious conflicts can arise when the investigator wishes to enroll patients in order to receive added income for his or her personal use or to support personal projects. Additionally, the goal of involvement may be to become published in an academic journal (Shimm & Spece, 1991). In short, the patient's goal of cure may not be the first issue that the investigator is considering.

Within the scientific community exists an understanding that cancer clinical trials are necessary and that they provide the answers to questions about medical treatment and care (Grady, 1991). Clinical trial nurses (CTNs) may encounter troubling ethical questions during the course of caring for patients who are enrolled in clinical trials.

Ethical Considerations

Clinical trials may be funded by large research centers or by even larger pharmaceutical companies. Physicians and nurses who are involved in these studies may receive financial gain, academic notoriety, publication authorship, and, in some cases, public acknowledgment. Because of these possible advantages, conflict of interest becomes an ethical predicament.

Shimm and Spece (1991) proposed that two major ethical issues exist within the context of clinical trials. The first is found in informed consent, in that experimental subjects are rarely, if ever, informed that their physicians stand to receive substantial payments from pharmaceutical companies for entering patients into studies and that study nurses' salaries may derive from payments for patient accrual. Second, a potential conflict of interest exists because the payment from a drug company can entice physicians (or nurses) to recommend company-sponsored experimental protocols over standard modes of therapy or no treatment at all.

Investigators and participating research teams have several benefits in clinical trials. The first is a positive ability to provide patients with access to new drugs that are not otherwise available. By participating in and publishing clinical research, investigators and research teams will achieve an enhanced academic reputation, which may increase prospects for promotion, tenure, salary increases, or other forms of public or personal recognition. The investigator with the highest accrual of research subjects often is recognized as the first author in the official scientific publication of the research findings. Also of note is the capitation payment of patient enrollment into clinical trials, which typically is $2,000–$5,000 per subject in non–federally funded trials (Spece, Shimm, & Buchanan, 1996). The opportunity for researchers to receive financial rewards from these endeavors is not intrinsically unacceptable, as long as this opportunity does not adversely influence scientific or clinical decision making (Association of American Medical Colleges, 2001).

The California Supreme Court, in a judgment regarding conflict of interest in clinical trials, ruled that a physician must disclose personal interest unrelated to the patient's health and whether research or economics may affect the physician's professional judgment. Furthermore, a failure to disclose such interests may give rise to a cause of action against the physician for performing medical procedures without informed consent (Shimm & Spece, 1991). Because the safety and welfare of human beings are at stake, financial interests in human subject research are rightly the focus of intense scrutiny (Association of American Medical Colleges, 2001).

The core to understanding how a conflict of interest is ethically unsound is to apply that conflict to the standard ethical principles of the Belmont Report: beneficence, justice, and general respect for persons, along with one other vital principle—nonmaleficence (Grady, 1991).

Beneficence

Beneficence is the principle that expresses the research team's obligation to promote the good of others. The availability of pharmaceutical company funding, with the potential for excess payments, introduces the possibility of conflict of interest because it is an enticement for researchers to plan projects that are primarily beneficial to the pharmaceutical company, although alternative projects may be of more benefit to patients or society. This type of behavior manifests with a slight difference when investigators enroll patients into clinical trials that are not necessarily the best medical option for the patients. The U.S. Food and Drug Administration (FDA) reported that some investigators have gone so far as to fabricate patients in order to collect the capitation payment from the pharmaceutical company (FDA Office of Review, personal communication, March 7, 1998).

Justice

Justice is the sense of "fairness in distribution" or "what is deserved." An injustice occurs when some benefit to which a person is entitled is denied without good reason or when some burden is imposed unduly. Therefore, in the area of clinical research, justice demands both that the research is not only available to those who can afford it and that such research should not unduly involve people from groups unlikely to be among the beneficiaries of subsequent applications of the research (National Commission, 1979).

Respect for Persons

Respect for persons implies that both the autonomy of individuals and protection for those incapable of autonomous behavior are respected. One can infer from this that when a person is able, the research team refrains from interfering with that person's choices or actions. If a conflict of interest exists within the investigative team, there may be a tendency to coerce patients into a decision that they would not choose independently. Patients must be made aware of the benefits and risks of the trial and of payment made to the investigator or any other relevant information to freely consent to the clinical trial treatment. See Chapter 14 for a more detailed discussion of informed consent.

Nonmaleficence

Nonmaleficence is the ethical principle and obligation to do no harm. Patients enter clinical trials believing that the doctors and nurses have only the patients' best interests in mind. What may be the truth is that investigators are more interested in answering a scientific question or accruing patients for academic or financial gain. Anthony S. Fauci, MD, director of the National Institute of Allergy and Infectious Diseases, described phase III clinical trials as a method to answer a scientific question, not a mode of delivering therapy, thereby making the question more important than patient treatment and outcome (Spece et al., 1996). Patients must have a clear understanding their right to consent and enroll into a study, as well as their right to leave the study at any time. Patients must be educated about all of their rights.

Role of the Clinical Trial Nurse

Coglianno-Shutta (as cited in Jassak & Ryan, 1989) identified three important factors for oncology nurses working with clinical trials to consider: know thyself, remain objective, and identify your role.

Through self-reflection, one can begin to understand his or her own feelings and beliefs regarding participation in clinical trials. Some questions to consider: Would I want to enroll in a phase I trial? How would I feel if I knew that my physician and nurse were paid for my enrollment? Although it is impossible for people to know how they would feel or what choice they would make unless they are in a similar situation, if CTNs begin to understand their own feelings, they may function better as patient advocates. By remaining objective, CTNs can weigh patients' options and the benefit to patients versus the potential risks, all with the knowledge of what investigators and research teams stand to gain from patients' enrollment.

The CTN's role is varied, and CTNs assume responsibility as patient and family educator, patient advocate, care provider, and research team member (Grady, 1991). Within the scope of these roles, CTNs carefully explain and clarify informed consent to patients. CTNs must be sure that patients not only understand the possible risks and benefits, the drug administration, and the protocol schema but also the conduct of the study and the monetary support received from the pharmaceutical sponsor. The health care that CTNs provide within the practice of clinical trials is not just another commodity on which industry and individuals can earn fortunes. This health care is a social necessity and a social good.

Summary

The potential for conflicts of interest will be present in the course of any type of clinical trial. There is, in the moment between action and reaction, a period that allows CTNs to choose, and the CTN must consider the ethical principles that guide clinical research. The CTN may differ from the investigator in his or her interpretation of what a conflict of interest is. This could lead to a difficult decision about what is revealed to a patient or what information needs to be communicated to the oversight committee at the practicing institution. As an educated nurse committed to ethical principles and personal values, the CTN must be able to choose wisely in that moment.

References

Association of American Medical Colleges. (2001, December). *Protecting subjects, preserving trust, promoting progress: Policy and guidelines for the oversight of individual financial interests in human subjects research.* Washington, DC: Author.

DeAngelis, C.D., Fontanarosa, P.B., & Flanagin, A. (2001). Reporting financial conflicts of interest and relationships between investigators and research sponsors. *JAMA, 286,* 89–91.

Grady, C. (1991). Ethical issues in clinical trials. *Seminars in Oncology Nursing, 7,* 288–296.

Jassak, P.F., & Ryan, M.P. (1989). Ethical issues in clinical research. *Seminars in Oncology Nursing, 5,* 102–108.

Kim, S.Y., Millard, R.W., Nisbet, P., Cox, C., & Caine, E.D. (2004). Potential research participants' views regarding researcher and institutional financial conflicts of interest [Electronic version]. *Journal of Medical Ethics, 30,* 73–79.

Miller, F.G., & Brody, H. (2003). A critique of clinical equipoise: Therapeutic misconception in the ethics of clinical trials. *Hastings Center Report, 33*(3), 19–28.

Morin, K., Rakatansky, H., Riddick, F.A., Jr., Morse, L.J., O'Bannon, J.M., Goldrich, M.S., et al. (2002). Managing conflicts of interest in the conduct of clinical trials. *JAMA, 287,* 78–84.

National Commission for the Protection of Human Subjects of Biomedical and Behavioral Research. (1979). *The Belmont report: Ethical principles and guidelines for the protection of human subjects of research.* Retrieved January 20, 2006, from http://www.nihtraining.com/ohsrsite/guidelines/belmont.html

Office for Human Research Protections. (2001). *NHRPAC recommendations on HHS's draft interim guidance on financial relationships in clinical research.* Retrieved January 20, 2006, from http://www.hhs.gov/ohrp/nhrpac/doc-report.htm

Shimm, D.S., & Spece, R.G. (1991). Conflict of interest and informed consent in industry-sponsored clinical trials. *Journal of Legal Medicine, 12,* 477–513.

Spece, R.G., Shimm, D.S., & Buchanan, A.E. (Eds.). (1996). *Conflicts of interest in clinical practice and research*. New York: Oxford University Press.

Steneck, N.H. (n.d.). *Introduction to the responsible conduct of research*. Retrieved January 6, 2006, from http://ori.dhhs.gov/publications/ori_intro_text.shtml

CHAPTER 17
Legislative Issues

Denise Dearing, RN, BSN, OCN®

Introduction

Failure to comply with investigative new drug (IND) protocol is severe and punishable by law. It can trigger immediate closure of the facility's clinical trial department and a complete U.S. Food and Drug Administration (FDA) investigation of all open and closed clinical trials. This chapter will help clinical trial nurses (CTNs) to understand the laws governing the practice of clinical trials nursing.

Case Study

An adult oncology CTN received a call from the Neonatal Intensive Care Unit for stat nitric oxide for William, a struggling newborn. The supervisor was out of town, and the charge nurse was taking calls for the hospital's clinical trial office. After a prompt phone conversation, the supervisor informed the CTN that nitric oxide made a terrific difference for preemies. There was nitric oxide in the hospital, and the requesting anesthesiologist had used the IND nitric oxide in another premature infant.

The consents were signed, and treatment was begun. William began to get better with the increased perfusion of his circulatory system. His blood gases improved steadily as the ventilator delivered IND nitric oxide. The next morning, he remained stable. Over the next seven days, he was weaned off the nitric oxide, and his parents were able to begin feeding him. After staying in the hospital to gain a few ounces, he went home. The nitric oxide had clearly saved the baby. This outcome of a clinical trial was powerfully imprinted on the CTN's career.

During William's time on the nitric oxide, the CTN documented the appropriate records and faxed them to the FDA. Midway during his treatment, the FDA called the nurse to say that the IND records from the institution were incomplete. For the first baby, there was record of drug dispensed, but no medical or drug follow-up information. Fortunately, the research department had the records that had not been received by the FDA IND division. The appropriate documents were faxed to the FDA, and the conduct of the trial assumed with appropriate legal compliance in place. During that week, the CTN toiled over pages of clinical trial data and proper IND documentation, including physician signatures.

How National Laws Affect Nursing Practice

The day-to-day practice of clinical trials is described in volume 21 of the *Federal Register*. This increasing sum of scientific knowledge requires changes and modifications as part of good clinical practice (GCP) in FDA-regulated trials. When the U.S. Congress enacts new laws, a procedure begins that translates the law into daily clinical practice. A primer of information from the FDA Web site follows, including the preambles to GCP regulation that explain their purpose.

Preambles to Good Clinical Practice Regulations

Each time Congress enacts a law affecting products regulated by the FDA, the FDA develops rules to implement the law. The FDA takes various steps to develop these rules, including publishing a variety of documents in the *Federal Register*. These documents announce the FDA's interest in formulating, amending, or repealing a rule and offer the public the opportunity to comment on the agency's proposal. The *Federal Register* notice explains the legal issues and basis for the proposal and provides information about how interested individuals can submit written data, views, or arguments on the proposal. Any comments that are submitted are addressed in subsequent publications that are part of the agency's decision-making process.

The "preamble" to each of these publications includes all of the printed information immediately preceding the codified regulation (FDA, n.d.). The preamble provides information about the regulation, such as why it is being proposed, the FDA's interpretation of the meaning and impact of the proposed regulation, and, in cases where the agency has solicited public comment, the agency's review and commentary on the public's input. The preamble also can include an environmental impact assessment, an analysis of the cost impact, comments related to the Paperwork Reduction Act, and the effective date of implementation or revocation (as the case may be) of the regulation.

The documents described in the following list include the various publications that contributed to the development of final rules related to the FDA's regulations on GCP and clinical trials (www.fda.gov/oc/gcp/regulations.html) (FDA, n.d.).

- **Advanced notice of proposed rulemaking (ANPRM):** The FDA may publish an ANPRM to gather information about a subject that the FDA may be formulating ideas about to better regulate a specific practice or product.
- **Notice of proposed rulemaking (NPRM):** After reviewing comments from the public from the ANPRM, the FDA may issue an NPRM. An NPRM contains proposed changes to the FDA's rules and seeks public comment on these proposals.
- **Proposed rule:** After reviewing public comments to the NPRM, the FDA may choose to issue a proposed rule regarding specific issues raised in the comments. The proposed rule also may be used to announce the FDA's plans to create or amend a rule. The proposed rule provides a final opportunity for the public to comment on the rule.
- **Interim rule:** The FDA may propose an interim rule. This is similar to a final rule, except that it offers the public an opportunity to submit additional comments. An interim rule may be used to help the agency to meet specific congressionally mandated time frames or to expeditiously address issues of public health concern.
- **Final rule:** After considering comments to the NPRM or proposed rule, the FDA issues a final rule. The *Federal Register* summary provides a summary of contents.

Guidance Documents

The FDA provides guidance documents, which are Internet-based guidelines for fulfilling current FDA rules. The FDA description of guidance documents states that guidance documents represent the Agency's current thinking on a particular subject (FDA, 2007). They do not create or confer any rights for or on any person and do not operate to bind the FDA or the public. An alternative approach may be used if such approach satisfies the requirements of the applicable statute, regulations, or both (FDA, 2007). FDA guidance documents also may be found through the Division of Drug Information Database, available online (see www.fda.gov/cder/dib/dibinfo.htm).

Distinction Between Law and Ethics

Legislative directives (laws) are **minimal** standards. Legislation seeks to dictate ethical behavior, which is in reality beyond legal directive. *Ethical behavior* dictates **high** standards. In the context of clinical trials, the best or highest standards are those that protect the subjects, particularly those who may be easily coerced or manipulated. A danger exists that people desperate for a cure may be exploited in their search for medical treatment offered by clinical trials. Therefore, it is imperative that the clinician adheres to the highest ethical standards. Ethical principles and their application during clinical research are outlined in the Belmont Report (see Appendix 4).

Ethical standards are different from moral standards. Moral standards are based on a specific set of cultural and/or ethnic mores. Because morals vary from place to place on the globe, the *ethical standard* must be used as the goal for clinical trials. For instance, in some countries, women routinely are stoned to death for infidelity to their spouse. In other countries, adultery is looked upon as a moral failing but is not punished by law. In yet another part of the world, adultery may be accepted and not judged at all. The moral opinion of a society dictates the outcome of the event.

Nuremberg Code

During World War II, pseudo-scientific experiments were performed on unwilling and often unwitting prisoners in concentration camps. Nazi doctors performed extraordinarily cruel acts in the name of medical clinical research. These acts were malignant in nature and absolutely unethical. The specific criminal counts are cited in Figure 17-1.

Some limited rules and protocols on human medical experimentation had existed prior to the Second World War. One of these, interestingly enough, was developed in Germany in 1931 in reaction to a failed vaccination experiment. However, none of these carried the force of law or had been subjected to advanced legal scrutiny. This changed during the Nuremberg War Crimes Trials (Weindling, 2001).

These trials were convened in 1946 by the victorious Allies to prosecute German war criminals. One of the groups placed on trial was German doctors who had conducted these experiments on prisoners. In the ruling of the tribunal in the case of USA v. Karl Brandt, et al., the court laid out a list of six (later expanded to 10) characteristics of legitimate human research. The document went well beyond the then-existing American Medical Association directives and became the foundation for the Nuremberg Code (Weindling, 2001).

The Nuremberg Code (1949), and the later, related Helsinki Declaration, have been incorporated into U.S. law in Title 45 of the Code of Federal Regulations. 45 CFR contains the regulations issued by the U.S. Department of Health and Human Services concerning all federally funded research in the United States. These rules cover documentation, informed consent, disclosure, and other issues of concern to anyone conducting clinical trials (Weindling, 2001).

Figure 17-1. Text of Indictment in *USA v. Karl Brandt, et al.*

The Doctors Trial

The Medical Case of the Subsequent Nuremberg Proceedings

The transcription of this document comes from the official trial record: *Trials of War Criminals before the Nuremberg Military Tribunals under Control Council Law No. 10. Nuremberg, October 1946–April 1949.* Washington, D.C.: U.S. G.P.O., 1949–1953. Page numbers corresponding to those in the trial record are provided in brackets [ ].

[page 8] INDICTMENT

The United States of America, by the undersigned Telford Taylor, Chief of Counsel for War Crimes, duly appointed to represent said Government in the prosecution of war criminals, charges that the defendants herein participated in a common design or conspiracy to commit and did commit war crimes and crimes against humanity, as defined in Control Council Law No. 10, duly enacted by the Allied Control Council on 20 December 1945. These crimes included murders, brutalities, cruelties, tortures, atrocities, and other inhumane acts, as set forth in counts one, two, and three of this indictment. Certain defendants are further charged with membership in a criminal organization, as set forth in count four of this indictment.

COUNT TWO — WAR CRIMES

6. Between September 1939 and April 1945 all of the defendants herein unlawfully, willfully, and knowingly committed war crimes, as defined by Article II of Control Council Law No. 10, in that they were principals in, accessories to, ordered, abetted, took a consenting part in, and were connected with plans and enterprises involving medical experiments without the subjects' consent, upon civilians and members of the armed forces of nations then at war with the German Reich and who were in the custody of the German Reich in exercise of belligerent control, in the course of which experiments the defendants committed murders, brutalities, cruelties, tortures, atrocities, and other inhuman acts. Such experiments included, but were not limited to, the following:

(A) High-Altitude Experiments. From about March 1942 to about August 1942, experiments were conducted at the Dachau concentration camp, for the benefit of the German Air Force, to investigate the limits of human endurance and existence at extremely high altitudes. The experiments were carried out in a low-pressure chamber in which atmospheric conditions and pressures prevailing at high altitude (up to 68,000 feet) could be duplicated. The experimental subjects were placed in the low-pressure chamber and thereafter the simulated altitude therein was raised. Many victims died as a result of these experiments and others suffered grave injury, torture, and ill-treatment. The defendants Karl Brandt, Handloser, Schroeder, Gebhardt, Rudolf Brandt, Mrugowsky, Poppendick, Sievers, Ruff, Romberg, Becker-Freyseng, and Weltz are charged with special responsibility for and participation in these crimes.

(B) Freezing Experiments. From about August 1942 to about May 1943, experiments were conducted at the Dachau concentration camp, primarily for the benefit of the German Air Force, to investigate the most effective means of treating persons who had been severely chilled or frozen. In one series of experiments the subjects were forced to remain in a tank of ice water for periods up to 3 hours. Extreme rigor developed in a short time. Numerous victims died in the course of these experiments. After the survivors were severely chilled, rewarming was attempted by various means. In another series of experiments, the subjects were kept naked outdoors for many hours at temperatures below freezing. The victims screamed with pain as their bodies froze. The defendants Karl Brandt, Handloser, Schroeder, Gebhardt, Rudolf Brandt, Mrugowsky, [page 12] Poppendick, Sievers, Becker-Freyseng, and Weltz are charged with special responsibility for and participation in these crimes.

(C) Malaria Experiments. From about February 1942 to about April 1945, experiments were conducted at the Dachau concentration camp in order to investigate immunization for and treatment of malaria. Healthy concentration-camp inmates were infected by mosquitoes or by injections of extracts of the mucous glands of mosquitoes. After having contracted malaria, the subjects were treated with various drugs to test their relative efficacy. Over 1,000 involuntary subjects were used in these experiments. Many of the victims died and others suffered severe pain and permanent disability. The defendants Karl Brandt, Handloser, Rostock, Gebhardt, Blome, Rudolf Brandt, Mrugowsky, Poppendick, and Sievers are charged with special responsibility for and participation in these crimes.

(D) Lost (Mustard) Gas Experiments. At various times between September 1939 and April 1945, experiments were conducted at Sachsenhausen, Natzweiler, and other concentration camps for the benefit of the German Armed Forces to investigate the most effective treatment of wounds caused by Lost gas. Lost is a poison gas which is commonly known as mustard gas. Wounds deliberately inflicted on the subjects were infected with Lost. Some of the subjects died as a result of these experiments and others suffered intense pain and injury. The defendants Karl Brandt, Handloser, Blome, Rostock, Gebhardt, Rudolf Brandt, and Sievers are charged with special responsibility for and participation in these crimes.

(E) Sulfanilamide Experiments. From about July 1942 to about September 1943, experiments to investigate the effectiveness of sulfanilamide were conducted at the Ravensbrueck concentration camp for the benefit of the German Armed Forces. Wounds deliberately inflicted on the experimental subjects were infected with bacteria such as streptococcus, gas gangrene, and tetanus. Circulation of blood was interrupted by tying off blood vessels at both ends of the wound to create a condition similar to that of a battlefield wound. Infection was aggravated by forcing wood shavings and ground glass into the wounds. The infection was treated with sulfanilamide and other drugs to determine their effectiveness. Some subjects died as a result of these experiments and others suffered serious injury and intense agony. The defendants Karl Brandt, Handloser, Rostock, Schroeder, Genzken, Gebhardt, Blome, Rudolf Brandt, Mrugowsky, Poppendick, Becker-Freyseng, Oberheuser, and Fischer are charged with special responsibility for and participation in these crimes.

(F) Bone, Muscle, and Nerve Regeneration and Bone Transplantation Experiments. From about September 1942 to about December 1943, experiments were conducted at the Ravensbrueck concentration camp, for the benefit of the German Armed Forces, to study bone, [page 13] muscle, and nerve regeneration, and bone transplantation from one person to another. Sections of bones, muscles, and nerves were removed from the subjects. As a result of these operations, many victims suffered intense agony, mutilation, and permanent disability. The defendants Karl Brandt, Handloser, Rostock, Gebhardt, Rudolf Brandt, Oberheuser, and Fischer are charged with special responsibility for and participation in these crimes.

(Continued on next page)

Figure 17-1. Text of Indictment in *USA v. Karl Brandt, et al. (Continued)*

(G) Sea-water Experiments. From about July 1944 to about September 1944, experiments were conducted at the Dachau concentration camp, for the benefit of the German Air Force and Navy, to study various methods of making sea water drinkable. The subjects were deprived of all food and given only chemically processed sea water. Such experiments caused great pain and suffering and resulted in serious bodily injury to the victims. The defendants Karl Brandt, Handloser, Rostock, Schroeder, Gebhardt, Rudolf Brandt, Mrugowsky, Poppendick, Sievers, Becker-Freyseng, Schaefer, and Beiglboeck are charged with special responsibility for and participation in these crimes.

(H) Epidemic Jaundice Experiments. From about June 1943 to about January 1945, experiments were conducted at the Sachsenhausen and Natzweiler concentration camps, for the benefit of the German Armed Forces, to investigate the causes of, and inoculations against, epidemic jaundice. Experimental subjects were deliberately infected with epidemic jaundice, some of whom died as a result, and others were caused great pain and suffering. The defendants Karl Brandt, Handloser, Rostock, Schroeder, Gebhardt, Rudolf Brandt, Mrugowsky, Poppendick, Sievers, Rose, and Becker-Freyseng are charged with special responsibility for and participation in these crimes.

(I) Sterilization Experiments. From about March 1941 to about January 1945, sterilization experiments were conducted at the Auschwitz and Ravensbrueck concentration camps, and other places. The purpose of these experiments was to develop a method of sterilization which would be suitable for sterilizing millions of people with a minimum of time and effort. These experiments were conducted by means of X-ray, surgery, and various drugs. Thousands of victims were sterilized and thereby suffered great mental and physical anguish. The defendants Karl Brandt, Gebhardt, Rudolf Brandt, Mrugowsky, Poppendick, Brack, Pokorny, and Oberheuser are charged with special responsibility for and participation in these crimes.

(J) Spotted Fever (Fleckfieber) Experiments. [It was definitely ascertained in the course of the proceedings, by both prosecution and defense, that the correct translation of "Fleckfieber" is typhus. A finding to this effect is contained in the judgment. A similar initial inadequate translation occurred in the case of "typhus" and "paratyphus" which should be rendered as typhoid and paratyphoid.] From about December 1941 to about February 1945, experiments were conducted at the Buchenwald and Natzweiler concentration camps, for the benefit [page 14] of the German Armed Forces, to investigate the effectiveness of spotted fever and other vaccines. At Buchenwald numerous healthy inmates were deliberately infected with spotted fever virus in order to keep the virus alive; over 90 percent of the victims died as a result. Other healthy inmates were used to determine the effectiveness of different spotted fever vaccines and of various chemical substances. In the course of these experiments, 75 percent of the selected number of inmates were vaccinated with one of the vaccines or nourished with one of the chemical substances and, after a period of 3 to 4 weeks, were infected with spotted fever germs. The remaining 25 percent were infected without any previous protection in order to compare the effectiveness of the vaccines and the chemical substances. As a result, hundreds of the persons experimented upon died. Experiments with yellow fever, smallpox, typhus, paratyphus [It was definitely ascertained in the course of the proceedings, by both prosecution ad defense, that the correct translation of "Fleckfieber" is typhus. A finding to this effect is contained in the judgment. A similar initial inadequate translation occurred in the case of "typhus" and "paratyphus" which should be rendered as typhoid and paratyphoid] A and B, cholera, and diphtheria were also conducted. Similar experiments with like results were conducted at Natzweiler concentration camp. The defendants Karl Brandt, Handloser, Rostock, Schroeder, Genzken, Gebhardt, Rudolf Brandt, Mrugowsky, Poppendick, Sievers, Rose, Becker-Freyseng, and Hoven are charged with special responsibility for and participation in these crimes.

(K) Experiments with Poison. In or about December 1943, and in or about October 1944, experiments were conducted at the Buchenwald concentration camp to investigate the effect of various poisons upon human beings. The poisons were secretly administered to experimental subjects in their food. The victims died as a result of the poison or were killed immediately in order to permit autopsies. In or about September 1944, experimental subjects were shot with poison bullets and suffered torture and death. The defendants Genzken, Gebhardt, Mrugowsky, and Poppendick are charged with special responsibility for and participation in these crimes.

(L) Incendiary Bomb Experiments. From about November 1943 to about January 1944, experiments were conducted at the Buchenwald concentration camp to test the effect of various pharmaceutical preparations on phosphorous burns. These burns were inflicted on experimental subjects with phosphorous matter taken from incendiary bombs, and caused severe pain, suffering, and serious bodily injury. The defendants Genzken, Gebhardt, Mrugowsky, and Poppendick are charged with special responsibility for and participation in these crimes.

Note. From *The Public Domain Official Trial Record: Trials of War Criminals Before the Nuremberg Military Tribunals Under Control Council Law No. 10. Nuremberg, October 1946–April 1949,* 1949–1953, Washington, DC: U.S. Government Printing Office. Retrieved June 24, 2006, from http://www.ushmm.org/research/doctors/indiptx.htm

---

International Standards and Laws

The International Conference on Harmonisation of Technical Requirements for Registration of Pharmaceuticals for Human Use (ICH) was established by representatives from the European Union, Japan, and the United States. It is a joint initiative involving both regulators and industry as equal partners in the scientific and technical discussions of testing procedures that are required to ensure and assess the safety, quality, and efficacy of medicines (ICH, n.d.-b). The United States is represented by the FDA and the Pharmaceutical Research and Manufacturers of America.

The focus of ICH has been on the technical requirements for medicinal products containing new drugs (ICH, n.d.-b). The vast majority of those new drugs and medicines are developed in Western Europe, Japan, and the United States; therefore, when ICH was established, it was agreed that its scope would be confined to registration in those three regions. The six parties directly involved in the decision-making process are founding members of the ICH and represent regulatory bodies and research-based industry in the European Union, Japan, and the United States (ICH, n.d.-b).

The Need to Harmonize

Harmonization requires the melding of international regulatory requirements (ICH, n.d.-a). Harmonization of regulatory requirements was pioneered by the European Community (now the European Union) in the 1980s, as it moved toward the development of a single market for pharmaceuticals. The success achieved in Europe demonstrated that harmonization was feasible. At the same time, bilateral discussions were ongoing between Europe, Japan, and the United States on the possibilities for harmonization (ICH, n.d.-a).

It was, however, at the World Health Organization Conference of Drug Regulatory Authorities in Paris in 1989 that specific plans for action began to materialize. Soon afterward, the authorities approached the International Federation of Pharmaceutical Manufacturers and Associations to discuss a joint regulatory-industry initiative on international harmonization, and ICH was conceived (ICH, n.d.-a).

In much of the industrialized world, the history of medicinal product registration has followed a similar pattern, which could be described as *initiation, acceleration, rationalization,* and *harmonization* (ICH, n.d.-a). The realization of the importance of having an independent evaluation of medicinal products before they are allowed on the market was reached at different times in different countries. For example, in the United States, a tragic mistake in the formulation of a children's syrup in the 1930s was the trigger for setting up the product authorization system under the FDA. In Japan, government regulations requiring all medicinal products to be registered for sale started in the 1950s. In many countries in Europe, the trigger was the thalidomide tragedy of the 1960s, which revealed that the new generation of synthetic drugs, which were revolutionizing medicine at the time, had the potential to harm as well as heal (ICH, n.d.-a).

Regardless of whether most countries had initiated product registration controls, the 1960s and 1970s revealed a rapid increase in laws, regulations, and guidelines for reporting and evaluating data on the safety, quality, and efficacy of new medicinal products (ICH, n.d.-a). The industry at the time was becoming more international and seeking new global markets, but the registration of medicines remained a national responsibility. Although different regulatory systems were based on the same fundamental obligations to evaluate the quality, safety, and efficacy, the detailed technical requirements had diverged over time to such an extent that industry found it necessary to duplicate many time-consuming and expensive test procedures in order to market new products internationally (ICH, n.d.-a).

The urgent need to rationalize and harmonize regulation was impelled by concerns over rising costs of health care, escalation of the cost of research and development, and the need to meet the public expectation that there should be a minimum of delay in making safe and efficacious new treatments available to patients in need (ICH, n.d.-a).

U.S. Food and Drug Administration Adopts International Conference on Harmonisation Clinical Good Practices

As published in the *Federal Register* (FDA, 1997) the FDA adopted the ICH GCP guidelines. The basis of the ICH GCP is the World Medical Association (WMA) Declaration of Helsinki Ethical Principles for Medical Research Involving Human Subjects. The document was last updated at the 2004 WMA General Assembly in Tokyo (WMA, 2004).

FDA compliance ensures that the clinical trial is being conducted in such a fashion as to be considered ethical and worthwhile using ICH GCP guidelines. The FDA provides an expectation when applying nursing outcomes to clinical trial conduct. When an institution participates in an FDA-approved clinical trial, appropriate nursing behavior will be defined by industry or institutional protocol.

The Office for Human Research Protections

The Office for Human Research Protections (OHRP) is a national agency reporting to the U.S. Department of Health and Human Services (DHHS). It focuses on the ethical conduct of institutional review boards and independent ethics committees. Registration and assurance are required for any facility performing human subject research that is conducted or supported by an agency of the DHHS.

Institutions that conduct any human subject research are required to register. Registration is provided through OHRP and is accompanied by an assurance. An institution engaged in federally conducted or supported human subject research must provide written documentation of the protection of those subjects, referred to as an assurance of compliance.

For human subject research conducted or supported by the DHHS, the OHRP must approve an institution's assurance before funds can be awarded and human subject research can begin (OHRP, 2005). The federalwide assurance (FWA) is the only type of assurance approved by OHRP. The OHRP-approved assurance of compliance indicates that the institution will conduct human subject research within DHHS regulations (45 CFR 46.103) for the protection of human subjects (OHRP). See Chapter 2 for a more detailed discussion of assurances.

If the institution is a Veterans Health Administration facility under the guidance of the Department of Veterans Affairs, an additional FWA is required (OHRP, 2001, 2005). This assures that human subject research will comply with all requirements of Department of Veterans Affairs regulations at Title 38 of the *Code of Federal Regulations (CFR)* (38 CFR 16) and all other pertinent Department of Veterans Affairs policies and procedures. This includes all policies and procedures of the Office of Research Oversight (formerly the Office of Research Compliance and Assurance) and the Office of Research and Development as issued in manuals, handbooks, and other relevant authorized directives.

Ongoing National Clinical Trial Legislation

Senate Bill 467 (2007), "Fair Access to Clinical Trials Act of 2005" (formally titled "A Bill to Amend the Public Health Service Act to Expand the Clinical Trials Drug Data

Bank," proposes transparency and free and open access to data from all clinical trials. A powerful component of the bill is the mandate to establish a clinical trial results database of all publicly and privately funded clinical trial results regardless of outcome. The scientific community, healthcare practitioners, and members of the public would have access to the database. This is not a law, so it does not affect clinical trials nursing at the time of this writing. At the time of this writing, it has been referred to the Committee on Health, Education, Labor and Pensions. Ongoing information on Senate Bill 467 is available at the Library of Congress Web site, http://thomas.loc.gov. This Web site is a convenient way to check the status of Senate and House of Representatives legislation.

Patients' Open Access to Clinical Trials

Within the United States, two levels of government have the ability to direct patient access to clinical trials. At the national level, clinical trials are regulated by the DHHS, represented by the secretary of Health and Human Services (HHS), a member of the presidential cabinet. The FDA is responsible for regulation of biomedical clinical trials. The commissioner of the FDA reports to the secretary of the HHS. The FDA is the enforcement arm of the agency, which oversees clinical trial conduct as outlined in the *CFR*, Title 21. The *CFR* is a codification of the general and permanent rules published in the *Federal Register* by the executive departments and agencies of the federal government. Title 21 of the *CFR* is reserved for rules of the FDA. Each title (or volume) of the *CFR* is revised once each calendar year. A revised Title 21 is issued on approximately April 1 of each year (FDA, 2002).

Nationally Mandated Clinical Trial Legislation

In 2000, a presidential memorandum introduced access to clinical trials to Medicare subscribers. Even with this increased access, only a small percentage of adults enroll in cancer clinical trials. The National Cancer Institute (NCI) has begun a nationwide effort to ensure clinical trials coverage in a series of collaborative agreements with third-party payers.

In an effort to expand participation, NCI has developed agreements that increase access to clinical trials for the Department of Defense (DoD) and the Department of Veterans Affairs (NCI, 2002). An innovative agreement between NCI and the DoD has given thousands of DoD patients with cancer more options for care and greater access to state-of-the-art treatments. Patients who are beneficiaries of TRICARE/CHAMPUS, the DoD's health program, are covered for NCI-sponsored phase II and phase III clinical treatment trials. An agreement with the Department of Veterans Affairs provides coverage for eligible veterans of the armed services to participate in NCI-sponsored prevention, diagnosis, and treatment studies nationwide (NCI).

NCI also is partnering with private insurers to increase access to cancer clinical trials (NCI, 2002). In Wisconsin and Minnesota, some NCI cooperative groups have reached agreements with several insurers to provide more than 200,000 people there with coverage for patient care costs if they participate in a cooperative group–sponsored trial. The Pediatric Cancer Care Network is a cooperative agreement among the Children's Cancer Group, the Pediatric Oncology Group, and the Blue Cross Blue Shield (BCBS) System Association nationwide. It is designed to ensure that children of BCBS subscribers receive care at designated centers of cancer care excellence. Furthermore, it may encourage the enrollment of children in cooperative group clinical trials (NCI).

State-Mandated Clinical Trial Legislation

More than 20 states have legislated access to clinical trials for life-threatening diseases, such as cancer. Each state's law is unique, requiring assessment on a case-by-case basis. In several states, state legislation addresses third-party reimbursement for clinical trials for the treatment of cancer (Amreican Cancer Society, 2006).

Since 1989, the State Cancer Legislative Database (SCLD), a program of NCI, has monitored and analyzed cancer-related state legislation (NCI, n.d.). In 2005, NCI began offering online access to the searchable database. The SCLD was developed to advance one of NCI's goals: the support of research projects in cancer control. SCLD data allow researchers to examine and compare cancer-related legislation across the United States. The SCLD contains information synthesized from enacted state laws and resolutions addressing selected aspects of cancer control, genetics, and tobacco. Also included are the few relevant state ballot initiatives that have been used to affect tobacco product excise taxes (NCI, n.d.).

As noted in SCLD information describing third-party reimbursement for clinical trials for the treatment of cancer, arrangements for reimbursement for several states fall outside the scope of the SCLD and therefore are not included in the database (NCI, 2005). Among these are Delaware, Maine, and North Carolina, which have laws that provide coverage for clinical trials for life-threatening medical conditions but not specifically for the treatment of cancer. Michigan and New Jersey, for instance, have implemented special nonlegislation agreements in which insurers voluntarily cover routine medical care that is part of a clinical trial. Furthermore, according to Ohio's state employees' benefits handbook, the state provides coverage for cancer treatment clinical trials to employees who are enrolled in the state employee health benefit plan (NCI, 2005).

SCLD records are based on program syntheses (or "abstracts") of relevant laws (NCI, n.d.). These syntheses do not contain the full text of the laws, which can be obtained from state sources and legal research services. The SCLD contains substantive laws and amendments, including "changes to the actions required or prohibited by the law, penalties, repeals of the law or portions of the law, and changes to a law's expiration date. Because of the volume of enacted laws, minor amendments to laws are not reported" (NCI, n.d.). SCLD data have been deemed to be substantive according to program protocols. Users can view either lists of data or detailed abstracts or can download information into PDF documents or Excel spreadsheets. Figure 17-2 provides the most recent information about the capacity of SCLD for information retrieval.

Compliance Tips

CTNs have the resources and knowledge needed to develop expertise for the care of clinical trial patients. CTNs must operate within the state-specific Nurse Practice Act and also must follow institutional nursing procedures and practices. The Oncology Nursing Society (www.ons. org) and the American Society of Clinical Oncology (www. asco.org) offer user-friendly online resources accessible to members and the public. Figure 17-3 summarizes compliance tips for CTNs.

Figure 17-2. State Cancer Legislation Database (SCLD)

What areas of cancer-related policy does the SCLD address?
The SCLD contains records related to
• Access to state-of-the-art treatment
• Breast cancer
• Cancer registries (surveillance)
• Cervical cancer
• Colorectal cancer
• Genetics
• Ovarian cancer
• Prostate cancer
• Skin cancer
• Testicular cancer
• Tobacco control
• Uterine cancer.
The SCLD also maintains limited information about state laws and resolutions addressing general cancer issues, including health-related treatment and access to state-of-the-art treatment.

What kinds of information are not available in the SCLD?
The SCLD does **not** contain
• Federal legislation or regulations
• State bills that have been introduced but not enacted
• State regulations
• Executive orders
• Measures implemented by counties, cities, or other localities
• Decisions of federal, state*, or local courts
• Opinions of attorneys general
• Data addressing the implementation of state laws.

*One exception exists to the omission of state-level court decisions. In the area of Tobacco Use/Clean Indoor Air, a very few state court decisions have affected the application of preemption in the State. In these instances, information regarding case law has been captured in the Notes section of the relevant Year-End Status record.

Note. From *State Cancer Legislative Database: FAQs*, by the National Cancer Institute, n.d. Retrieved September 21, 2007, from http://www.scld-nci.net/DB_Search/Help/HLPFAQ.htm

---

Figure 17-3. Compliance Tips

• Stay in close contact with the legal counsel of the institution and counsel (lawyers) of the clinical trial sponsor.
• Keep consents updated with most recent amendments or information.
• Utilize local institutional review board resources.
• Advocate for the very best for constituents or patients; this is the nursing role.
• Respect the validity of one's personal input at all levels of clinical trial development. The clinical trial nurse has unique and extensive knowledge of the behaviors of patients under his or her care.

Summary

This chapter has discussed the origin, development, and application of laws concerning clinical trials. This is a complex subject that has moral, ethical, and even criminal implications and is an ongoing issue in federal and state legislation.

CTNs should remember that their practice is strongly influenced by both state and federal law, and compliance needs to be strict. Guidance will be supplied by several sources, including the CFR, the Federal Register, as well as legal counsel for the hospital conducting and organization sponsoring the trial. Seek this guidance early and often, and keep up to date with changes.

Federal and state legislation are constantly evolving, and mandated insurance coverage is expanding, albeit slowly. CTNs need to keep abreast of developments in this area.

References

American Cancer Society. (2006). *Clinical trials: State laws regarding insurance coverage.* Retrieved September 21, 2007, from http://www.cancer.org/docroot/ETO/content/ETO_6_2x_State_Laws_Regarding_Clinical_Trials.asp

International Conference on Harmonisation of Technical Requirements for Registration of Pharmaceuticals for Human Use. (n.d.-a). *History and future of ICH: A brief history of ICH.* Retrieved June 20, 2006, from http://www.ich.org/cache/compo/276-254-1.html

International Conference on Harmonisation of Technical Requirements for Registration of Pharmaceuticals for Human Use. (n.d.-b). *Structure of ICH.* Retrieved June 20, 2006, from http://www.ich.org/cache/compo/276-254-1.html

National Cancer Institute. (2002, January 30). *Initiatives to expand coverage.* Retrieved June 22, 2006, from http://www.cancer.gov/clinicaltrials/learning/insurance-coverage/page4

National Cancer Institute. (2005, January). *State law addressing third party reimbursement for clinical trials for the treatment of cancer (enacted as of June 30, 2005).* Retrieved June 23, 2006, from http://www.scld-nci.net/Data/clin_trials_reimbursement_6_30_05.pdf

National Cancer Institute. (n.d.). *FAQ.* Retrieved June 27, 2006, from http://www.scld-nci.net/DB_Search/Help/HLPFAQ.htm

The Nuremberg Code. (1949). In *Trials of war criminals before the Nuremberg military tribunals under Control Council Law No. 10* (Vol. 2, pp. 181–182). Washington, DC: U.S. Government Printing Office. Retrieved June 27, 2006, from http://www.hhs.gov/ohrp/references/nurcode.htm

Office for Human Research Protections. (2001, February). *VA addendum to federalwide assurance for Department of Veterans Affairs Veterans Health Administration facilities.* Retrieved June 20, 2006, from http://www.hhs.gov/ohrp/humansubjects/assurance/vasup.rtf

Office for Human Research Protections. (2005, July). *Assurances.* Retrieved June 23, 2006, from http://www.hhs.gov/ohrp/assurances/assurances_index.html

S. 467, 110th Cong. (2007).

U.S. Food and Drug Administration. (1997, May 9). ICH E6 good clinical practice: Consolidated guidance, Section 5.19–Audit. *Federal Register, 62*(90), 25691–25709E7.

U.S. Food and Drug Administration. (2002, March). *Code of Federal Regulations—Title 21—Food and drugs.* Retrieved June 23, 2006, from http://www.fda.gov/cdrh/aboutcfr.html

U.S. Food and Drug Administration. (2007, August 1). *Guidance documents.* Retrieved August 9, 2007, from http://www.fda.gov/cder/guidance/index.htm

U.S. Food and Drug Administration. (n.d.). *Preambles to GCP Regulations.* Retrieved June 20, 2006, from http://www.fda.gov/oc/gcp/preambles/default.htm

Weindling, P. (2001). The origins of informed consent: The International Scientific Commission on War Crimes and the Nuremberg Code. *Bulletin of the History of Medicine, 75*(1), 37–71.

World Medical Association. (2004, September). *World Medical Association Declaration of Helsinki: Ethical principles for medical research involving human subjects.* Retrieved June 20, 2006, from http://www.wma.net/e/policy/b3.htm

CHAPTER 18

General Publication and Authorship Policies for Nurses

Shanita Williams-Brown, PhD, MPH, APRN-BC, Anne E. Belcher, PhD, RN, AOCN®, CNE, FAAN, ANEF, and Janice Phillips, PhD, RN, FAAN

Introduction

For some clinical nurses, writing for publication may appear to be a daunting task. Or, perhaps, a nurse may feel that the idea of being a published author is reserved exclusively for scholars in institutions of higher learning or the American Academy of Nursing. Yet, in reality, the opportunity to publish is open to any nurse who is willing to acquire the necessary tools to share new knowledge with others in the nursing profession or the larger scientific community. Knowledge that is worthy of sharing through the process of scholarly publication includes newer or more effective clinical strategies and techniques, original research findings, clinical insight and personal experiences, and relevant professional and healthcare issues. Take the example of a nurse clinician who has cared for several patients who each experienced unanticipated side effects to a prescribed drug. The nurse then realizes that other nurses, physicians, and, ultimately, patients could benefit from knowing about the drug's undocumented side effects. This clinician is positioned to become a nurse author.

Indeed, nurses have the opportunity to participate in the authorship process on multiple levels. The nurse clinician can call upon his or her unique practice experiences to contribute a nursing perspective to a published abstract or article describing the results of a clinical trial. Or, perhaps, a nurse may have an opportunity to become the principal investigator and first author of a companion study completed in tandem with a clinical trial. Each of these examples represents opportunities for clinical nurses to get involved in the authorship of scholarly publications. The purpose of this chapter is to provide a beginner's overview of writing for publication. The overview will include a brief summary of the writing process, as well as a discussion of select ethical, legal, and practical considerations related to writing for publication.

Why Write for Publication?

Writing for publication is essential to disseminate knowledge, promote scholarship, improve patient care, advance the nursing profession, and ultimately enhance nursing's credibility and visibility. Therefore, nurses have a professional obligation to write for publication. In addition to the professional obligation to write, personal satisfaction, professional development, and other possible rewards of authorship also motivate individuals to become nurse authors.

Identifying a Topic or Purpose

The choices are vast when it comes to selecting a topic about which to write. The selection of a topic requires careful planning along with ongoing consideration of the target audience. An assessment of the author's own interests, areas of expertise, personal and professional experiences, and current issues and trends in health care can be helpful in identifying topics. Nurse authors report anecdotally that they often have identified topics by talking with other healthcare providers and consumers, by reviewing the literature, or in response to an editor's call for manuscripts. Nurse authors also may be inspired to write about clinical practice or healthcare issues that affect patient care and/or patient outcomes. Published nurse authors often start their writing careers by working with faculty members, mentors, or other seasoned authors in converting completed school projects into publishable papers.

First-time authors benefit not only from working with an experienced writer but also from enrolling in workshops or courses that focus on writing for publication. Although some of these opportunities are available in schools of nursing and in healthcare settings, the aspiring author additionally should look for continuing education courses and workshops offered at community colleges, universities, and community centers, to name a few places.

Literature Review

Every writer needs to conduct a literature review during the initial phases of manuscript development for a variety of reasons. First, a review of the literature will help the author to identify gaps in what is known about the topic and will assist in identifying whether the author should consider a new or expanded focus on the topic. Second, if the topic has been well presented in the literature, the author may wish to provide a critical analysis of what has already been published. Third, a review of the literature will help to identify to what extent the target journal has devoted attention to the topic of choice. A review of the literature usually is required even though the author may be current in his or her field of expertise.

A multitude of resources are available to assist the author in examining what is currently known about a topic. Hospital libraries, regional medical libraries, and university and college libraries all provide excellent electronic and print resources. The Cumulative Index to Nursing and Allied Health Literature (CINAHL®) and the International Nursing Index are the two most comprehensive sources for locating nursing publications. MEDLINE® (Medical Literature Analysis and Retrieval System On-Line), a National Library of Medicine database, is another excellent resource for locating biomedical literature materials. These represent only a small portion of the many databases available at a variety of libraries.

Oermann (2002) suggested that when conducting a literature review, the author should review current literature and work backward. As a rule of thumb, authors are advised to include literature that has been published within the past five years. Authors also must be mindful to include landmark or classic published works (e.g., articles, books, chapters, dissertations) if appropriate, even if the published date is beyond the past five years. After a careful review, authors will need to synthesize the review of the literature to identify relationships between and among the published works, gaps in knowledge, and implications for additional work. Finally, Oermann recommended that authors keep track of all of the search products, including all publications, search terms, and limitations related to the literature search. This will be very helpful to authors as they check for accuracy and completeness of the selected literature.

Writing the Manuscript
To Outline or Not to Outline

Although writers pursue the task of preparing manuscripts differently, Fondiller (1999) suggested that the most effective way to prepare an article is to work from a detailed sentence outline. According to Fondiller, outlines are critical for success because they show clearly and explicitly the logical relation of points and will help the writer in achieving proper emphasis in writing. All outlines should include an introduction, a body, and a conclusion—the exact format to be used in the actual manuscript. Some authors prepare their manuscripts without an outline; although this is not recommended for new authors, every author should select an approach that is comfortable for him or her. Regardless of the method used,

it is essential to get one's ideas written down, seek assistance from an expert or mentor to critique the outline and other content, revise accordingly, and refer frequently to the outline as the manuscript is being developed. It is important to realize that the outline provides the structure, and a mentor provides guidance and support. Many successful authors have emphasized the value of a mentor's guidance and support regardless of how one composes a manuscript.

Even with the best of outlines, authors often develop several drafts before submitting a manuscript. Authors are advised to set their writing aside periodically to acquire a renewed focus and to objectively evaluate the manuscript for overall content, flow, and organization. Be prepared to write, and rewrite, and rewrite, as many authors often do. Passion, persistence, and discipline are critical components from beginning to end during the writing and publication process. Often, authors will have their manuscripts returned from an editor requesting them to make enhancements, clarify content, and add or delete content as a means of improving the document. New authors in particular may find this frustrating initially but should take heart that this is a process that ultimately offers an opportunity to enhance the end result—a scholarly publication.

The Title and Abstract

The title and abstract are two critical components of the manuscript primarily because they are the most frequently read. Therefore, careful attention should be given to the selection of a title and the writing of the abstract. An interesting title and abstract are the primary determinants of whether a reader will make the decision to review the entire manuscript more closely.

The title should capture the reader's attention and contain words that describe the key elements of the manuscript. Similarly, the body of a well-constructed abstract should include a summary of the background, rationale, aims/objectives, and theoretical approaches used. The methods and results should comprise the majority of the abstract, followed by a concluding statement and possible implications for nursing practice and/or research. Finally, the abstract should be reviewed and revised after the manuscript is completed.

Most journals specify word limitations and formatting expectations for abstract submission. It is critical that one follow the guidelines for word limitations, font size, or sentence form and structure established by the journal. If these guidelines are not followed, one's manuscript may be quickly rejected. For example, some journals instruct authors not to write in complete sentences. Other journals may direct the author to emphasize the major findings in the abstract and omit background information. Regardless of the specific criteria, the major "take-home message" is to carefully follow the journal's guidelines.

The Body

The body of a manuscript should begin with an *introduction,* followed by the *main body* and *conclusions.* The introduction section should present the main focus or topic of discussion and serves to stimulate the reader's interest. The main body provides supporting documentation to the main idea, whereas the concluding statements bring the discussion to a close. In the conclusion or summation section of the manuscript, major points are emphasized, and implications for practice, research, education, and/or policy are presented. An important point to remember, however, is that the concluding statements should never contain new information that has not been introduced in the main body of the manuscript.

References

Referencing, or the appropriate selection and accurate documentation of sources, is a critical component of any manuscript. Sources typically include any idea, artwork (photos and diagrams), adapted work (illustrations, charts, graphs), or quotation that did not originate with the author (Buchsel, 2001). Accurate documentation of sources signals to the reader that the author has some knowledge of the existing body of literature; this lends credibility to the manuscript. The age-old rule still applies: There are no original thoughts, meaning that when one has a novel or interesting idea, chances are that someone else has not only already thought of it but has also investigated. Any claim to originality is simply an indication of an insufficient knowledge of the literature. Therefore, a main objective of publishing is not to document original ideas but rather to contribute to an existing body of literature. Appropriate and accurate documentation of references is one way to ensure the adequate development of a body of literature in a field.

Manuscript sources can be documented as primary or secondary references. Primary references refer to the original sources of an idea, quotation, or work. Secondary references cite the ideas, quotations, or works of one author that have been summarized or discussed by another author without consulting the original source. Secondary references should be avoided, because if the secondary reference has cited the original source, then the original source obviously has some credibility and should be read by the author as well. There is no reason, particularly in light of today's technology, that the primary reference cannot be located and referenced appropriately. The use of secondary references signals to the editor and reviewers that the author may not fully grasp the available literature and may raise concerns as to the accuracy and credibility of the manuscript (Buchsel, 2001).

Reference Manager Programs

To assist the author in accurately documenting references, a number of reference/citation manager software programs have entered the market in the past few years. Reference manager software can be a valuable tool to increase the efficiency and accuracy of source documentation. An author can use this software to create reference libraries that are essentially a database of references from other papers, books, or online sources that have been stored in a personal filing cabinet. As one develops a manuscript, he or she can link to references in this filing cabinet. The software formats the references to fit the particular formatting style of the chosen journal. The software also allows one to connect directly to bibliographic databases, such as PubMed or CINAHL, and import references into one's filing cabinet.

The great advantage of a reference manager program is that it allows the author to create a reference list at the same time that he or she is writing the manuscript. Therefore, the laborious task of compiling, sorting, renumbering, and formatting references throughout the manuscript writing process can be avoided, and errors can be reduced in number or eliminated (U.S. National Institutes of Health Library, 2005).

Grammatical Aspects

All writers should keep a grammar book on hand to serve as a guide and resource during the initial development of the manuscript, as well as during revisions. Commonly occurring grammatical errors include (a) being too wordy, (b) turning a verb or adjective into a noun, (c) using a dangling participle, (d) splitting infinitives, (e) personalizing objects (i.e., "This paper identifies . . . "), (f) using the incorrect form of a word (i.e., *principal* versus *principle*), (g) using "trendy" words such as *paradigm* or *plethora*, (h) incorrectly using the apostrophe, colon, comma, hyphen, parentheses, quotation marks, or semicolons, and (i) using sexist language (Gobel, 2001).

Authorship

Identifying authors of a manuscript, determining the order in which they are listed, and generating acknowledgments are important and sometimes controversial aspects of manuscript preparation. For collaborative projects, all participants must agree on authorship early in the process.

The International Committee of Medical Journal Editors (ICMJE) uniform requirements for manuscripts submitted to biomedical journals define an author as someone who has made a significant intellectual contribution to a published study or report. Three key factors that determine authorship include (1) contributing to project conception and design, data collection, analysis, and interpretation, (2) developing intellectual content of manuscript through drafts and critical revisions of the document, and (3) giving final approval of the published work and be willing to take responsibility for the integrity of the work as a whole (ICMJE, 2006).

It is suggested that the group of prospective authors negotiate the relative weight of various activities, such as generating the idea for the project, conducting the project, gathering and analyzing data, interpreting the findings, and writing the manuscript. One interesting criterion that the authors themselves should consider is their individual ability and willingness to defend the content of the manuscript. In other words, if a letter is submitted to the journal editor or to the authors with questions about any aspect of the paper, the authors should be able to explain, clarify, or defend their position.

The status of individuals within the profession or the organization should not dictate either their inclusion or their sequence in the list of authors. The sequencing of names instead should reflect the descending order of contribution. Honorary authorship is discouraged. However, in some instances, the faculty or nursing director/leader wishes to be an author. If possible, offer to cite this individual in the acknowledgments; if this is not possible, place the person's name in the order in which it is most appropriate, not first or last.

Acknowledgment at the end of the manuscript is more appropriate for those who assisted in data collection or analysis, such as research assistants, artists, or audiovisual personnel who provided diagrams or drawings, or an individual/group/organization that provided financial support. One also can acknowledge an individual who was initially involved in the project but who did not follow through on his or her commitment to the manuscript.

If concern exists about the roles and responsibilities of project personnel in the development of one or more manuscripts, a letter of agreement should be created and signed by all authors. As noted by Hanson (1988), inadequate planning for authorship credit in collaborative projects is "a sure way to lose friends and gain professional enemies" (p. 50). King (2001) also addressed issues of authorship, describing that as a "last resort," editorial intervention may be necessary to resolve authorship issues. All authors should be given the opportunity to review the final version of the manuscript that is to be submitted and should sign the letter of transmittal and the copyright release form.

Selecting a Journal for Publication

A variety of factors influence the journal selection for publication. Oermann (2002) suggested that prospective authors consider a number of factors, including whether the targeted journal publishes articles on the proposed manuscript topic, the match between the proposed topic and the types of articles traditionally published by the targeted journal (e.g., research, clinical, case reports), and the match between the manuscript audience and the proposed journal readership. The quality of a journal, its circulation, and frequency of publication also are important factors to consider when selecting a journal for publication. Publishing timetables vary considerably across journals and also may be of concern for some. The turnaround time from submission to actual publication can range from one month to six months or more.

In discussing the five "rights" of publishing (right journal, right topic, right information, right words, right time), Plaisance (2003) encouraged prospective authors to carefully consider the journal's target audience. For example, does the journal target nurses, researchers, clinicians, physi-

cians, administrators, social workers, or clergy? Depending on the answer, the manuscript should be submitted to the appropriate journal that targets the preferred audience.

Some journals target multidisciplinary audiences, whereas other manuscripts are specific to a specialty (e.g., oncology, cardiovascular, renal) or practice area (e.g., administration, research, education, policy). Some authors prefer to target multidisciplinary journals because the proposed manuscript has relevance for a variety of specialties and disciplines. Still other authors select journals that appeal to international audiences and have relevance from a global perspective. In recent years, the number of journals that address a variety of cultural issues has increased. For example, *Hispanic Health Care International* and the *Journal of Multicultural Nursing and Health* specifically address cultural aspects related to healthcare, practice, research, and policy.

Many accomplished authors, particularly researchers and academicians, choose to target a variety of journals throughout their career to enhance the breadth of their dissemination efforts. For example, nurses initially may publish in nursing-related journals and then broaden their dissemination efforts to inform other audiences about nursing and health-related issues.

Peer-reviewed journals are preferable to non-peer-reviewed publication formats. The peer-review process is designed to ensure the quality and integrity of published information and data. A manuscript published in a peer-reviewed journal typically has undergone rigorous scientific scrutiny by at least two to three reviewers who have expertise in the area as well as by the journal's editor.

Regardless of journal selection, a prospective author must adhere to the journal's publication guidelines. Guidelines for publication typically appear in print in the journal or are available online or upon request to the editor. Guidelines detail specific requirements for publication, such as submission and review policies; appropriate permissions and use of illustrations, charts, and graphs; and policies related to author payment and reprints. The *Writer's Guide to Nursing Periodicals* (Daly, 2000) is an excellent reference on writing for publication for 90 nursing journals. This reference highlights specific guidelines for each of the 90 journals and provides a wealth of information on manuscript submission, manuscript preparation guidelines, readership, circulation, journal focus and purpose, and related editorial policies.

Query Letters

Submitting an unsolicited manuscript to a journal can be a huge waste of the author's time. It could be several weeks before acknowledgment of receipt of a manuscript and several more weeks before the manuscript is assessed for suitability for the journal. Therefore, one can easily wait six months for feedback on a manuscript, only to find out that the journal is not interested in the topic.

A query letter is the author's way of determining what interest a journal has in the author's work. The process of querying an editor is an efficient means to target a journal that is most likely to accept one's manuscript for publication. An author query can streamline the review process and is an important time-saving tool, given the extended peer-review processing time. Therefore, it is prudent to assess a journal's interest in one's manuscript by simply asking the editor. It is acceptable to query the journal's editor on a number of points, such as: What is the editor's interest in the research/clinical topic? Are any special editions planned for which the manuscript might be considered?

An author writes a query letter to identify the focus of the manuscript and to promote his or her work. A query letter should include a fairly detailed, to-the-point description of the manuscript, emphasizing the purpose and relevance of content, particularly for the intended audience. The author should provide information highlighting personal qualifications for writing such an article. The author must keep in mind that a favorable response to a query letter does not guarantee publication; however, once the author commits to submitting the work to a journal, he or she is obligated to follow through. Although more than one query letter may be submitted simultaneously to more than one journal, the general rule of thumb is to submit a manuscript to only one journal for review. It is considered unethical to make simultaneous submissions of the same manuscript to different journals.

Electronic/Internet-Based Publications

Internet writing and electronic publication are becoming an increasingly popular means to disseminate research and clinical findings. Electronic publishing has several advantages. It has reduced publication costs. Articles can be published electronically in a fraction of the time it would take to reach print. Another advantage with electronic publication is increased access. The Internet allows authors worldwide reach and provides access to potential professional and lay readers that otherwise would not have been reached (Björk, 2004; Ludwick & Glazer, 2000).

The primary concerns regarding electronic/Internet-based publications include the quality of published materials and a possible breakdown in the peer-review process. The major concern is that potential authors who are not successful in the traditional peer-review process would utilize Internet writing and publishing as a means to publish materials that have been subjected to less-stringent scholarly criteria and thus have reduced scientific quality and merit. However, trend data have shown a gradual and consistent increase in the number of researchers and clinicians who use the Internet as a means to disseminate their work among colleagues and the lay public (Tenopir & King, 2000).

As Internet publishing becomes increasingly popular, prospective authors will need to be aware of any specific guidelines related to electronic/Internet-based publications. For example, the *Oncology Nursing Forum (ONF)* publishes a small number of electronic articles. The editor makes the decision in concert with the author as to the suitability of the article as an electronic publication. Electronic publications appearing in *ONF* undergo the same peer-review process as *ONF* print publications. The main distinction between *ONF* electronic and print publications is that that there is virtually unrestricted access to the electronic manuscript via the Internet (Carroll-Johnson, 2003).

Ethical Considerations

Ethical concerns are important to consider when writing and publishing. According to King (2001), ethical concerns such as etiquette, fraudulent publication, plagiarism, duplicate publication, authorship, and potential conflict of interest warrant discussion in order to maintain ethical integrity. A few ethical concerns are presented here.

First and foremost, adhering to all specific journal guidelines is the first step to good etiquette. A cover letter with complete and accurate contact information addressed to the appropriate contact person is crucial.

Next, single submission of a manuscript is critical. Potential authors must submit a manuscript to only one journal at a time and must not submit the manuscript under review to another journal until a written rejection is received from the initial journal. Editors maintain exclusive rights to the manuscript; therefore, they should be notified if the manuscript or any of its contents have been previously copyrighted. Authors must receive written permission to cite lengthy quotations and to reproduce or adapt material that has appeared elsewhere.

Another area of concern is the number of original manuscripts that can or should be generated from a single research study. This is a gray area that is sometimes referred to as "salami" publishing, whereby the author publishes short papers to build up his or her bibliography for career advancement. Duplicate publication refers to the author's publication of highly similar material in several journals. Blancett (1991) identified the five levels of duplicate publications as

- Identical content
- Very similar articles with superficial modifications
- Publication of multiple manuscripts whose content could have been described in one paper
- Sequential articles about work in development
- Similar manuscripts produced for publication in journals for different disciplines.

The ethical issue, as labeled by Blancett (1991), is "deceit: the editors of journals are not notified of the author's intent" (p. 34). If an author is concerned about the issue of deceit, he or she should seek advice from a reliable source. For a detailed discussion on the ethical topic of publication deceit, the reader is referred to King (2001).

Conflict of interest and financial disclosure also should be addressed. Increasingly, authors are being asked to sign a conflict-of-interest statement and acknowledge any actual or potential conflict of interest related to their manuscript.

Authors are responsible for disclosing any financial interest and compensation associated with their publications. This information may be acknowledged in the actual publication, depending on journal policy and procedures.

Finally, plagiarism, or literary theft, involves presenting previously documented ideas, quotations, artwork, and/or adapted works as the author's original work. Plagiarism may include acts such as the verbatim lifting of sentences or paragraphs from published material or rewording documented ideas or paraphrasing original work without appropriate referencing. To avoid the presumption of plagiarism, Eoyang (1995) suggested that prospective authors (a) become careful note takers, (b) know the available literature, and (c) request permission to use previously documented works. Accurate documentation of references and primary sources is the most important strategy to avoid plagiarism.

Editorial Review and Feedback

After a manuscript has been submitted for review, the amount of time from the publisher's receipt of the manuscript to the author receiving feedback may vary considerably from journal to journal, anywhere from a few weeks to several months. To ensure that each manuscript is given fair consideration, journal editors often conduct blind reviews, either a double- or single-blind review.

A double-blind review is one in which the identities of both the authors and the reviewers are concealed. On the other hand, with a single-blind review, the author's identity is made known to the reviewers, and the reviewers' identities are concealed (Eoyang, 1995). In either case, the journal editor may provide input into the decision-making process. After a manuscript is reviewed, the author will receive written feedback regarding the overall content, as well as the editor's decision regarding acceptance, the need for revisions/resubmission, or rejection.

When responding to reviewers' comments, the author must be careful to address all concerns. In situations where the author disagrees with the reviewers' concerns, the prospective author should tactfully provide sound justification for not closely following the reviewers' suggestions for revision. Most reviewers spend a substantial amount of time and effort to provide a meaningful review to improve the substantive quality of a manuscript (Guyatt & Haynes, 2006).

The outright acceptance of a manuscript with no revisions required is indeed a rare event. Most editors and/ or reviewers will require some revision before agreeing to publish a manuscript. However, in most instances, if the editor believes that the manuscript has merit, the editor will request that the author revise and resubmit the manuscript after making suggested revisions. A written description of the reviewers' comments usually accompanies a request for resubmission. The author will need to review the comments carefully and decide whether resubmitting to the initial journal is worth the time and effort. The author may choose to submit the manuscript

in its original format to another journal (Carroll-Johnson, 2003; Guyatt & Haynes, 2006).

Authors, particularly first-time authors, often are disappointed when they receive a manuscript rejection letter. Key reasons for an editor's rejecting a manuscript include, but are not limited to, the following.

• Poor quality
• Lack of comprehensive coverage
• Lack of clarity
• Incorrect format
• Poor grammar and spelling
• Lack of interest to the target audience

However, these are not the only criteria for rejecting a manuscript. For example, a journal may have accepted a similar manuscript for publication or recently devoted attention to the same topic, or the topic may not be suitable for the journal's audience (Sheridan & Dowdney, 1997). Regardless of the outcome of the review, the prospective author should take time to consider any feedback received from the editor, including a rejection letter. Reviewer and editor feedback can provide valuable insight for refining, rewriting, or resubmitting the manuscript to another source. Putting the manuscript aside for a brief period of time before attempting to resubmit can give the author a fresh perspective. Perseverance certainly is key to successful publication. Figure 18-1 provides some additional tips for success.

Summary

The focus of this chapter is to provide an overview on writing for publication and guidelines regarding identifying a topic/purpose, selecting a journal, preparing the manuscript, and considering ethical and practical issues, all of which contribute to successful publication. Writing for publication, although time consuming, is essential for advancing the nursing profession, improving patient care, and contributing to one's professional development. Clinical trial nurses, as well as other oncology nurses, have the opportunity to share key aspects of their specialty practice and research in published formats, such as peer-reviewed journals, conference abstracts and posters,

---

Figure 18-1. Tips for Success

• Select a topic and journal that targets the appropriate audience.
• Provide a review and synthesis of the literature of published works within the past five years.
• Develop an outline to provide structure and focus while writing.
• Carefully adhere to all specific journal guidelines to ensure proper publication etiquette.
• Select experienced authors to review manuscripts prior to submission to a journal.
• Emphasize format, clarity, and grammar.
• Develop a realistic timetable to allow more time than expected for journal review and feedback.
• Provide accurate and complete information and citations.
• Resolve authorship issues prior to completion of the manuscript, preferably during the manuscript planning process.

and newsletters. The authors' intent is that the readers of this chapter will use the information to begin writing for publication or perhaps to mentor someone else in the process. In the words of a colleague, *"Bon escriber!"* ("Good writing!").

References

Blancett, S.S. (1991). The ethics of writing and publishing. *Journal of Nursing Administration, 21,* 31–36.

Björk, B-C. (2004). Open access to scientific publications—An analysis of the barriers to change? *Information Research, 9*(2), paper 170. Retrieved May 2, 2007, from http://InformationR.net/ir/9-2/paper170.html

Buchsel, P.C. (2001). Researching and referencing. *Clinical Journal of Oncology Nursing, 5,* 7–11.

Carroll-Johnson, R.M. (2003). Writing for publication. In K.S. Oman, M.E. Krugman, & R.M. Fink (Eds.), *Nursing research secrets: Questions and answers reveal the secrets to successful research and publication* (pp. 243–254). Philadelphia: Hanley & Belfus.

Daly, J.M. (2000). *Writer's guide to nursing periodicals.* Thousand Oaks, CA: Sage Publications.

Eoyang, T. (1995). Something borrowed, something new: How to tell the difference. *Nurse Author and Editor, 5*(2), 1–4.

Fondiller, S.H. (1999). *The writer's workbook: Health professional's guide to getting published* (2nd ed.). Sudbury, MA: Jones and Bartlett.

Gobel, B.H. (2001). Getting started. *Clinical Journal of Oncology Nursing, 5,* 3–6.

Guyatt, G.H., & Haynes, R.B. (2006). Preparing reports for publication and responding to reviewers' comments. *Journal of Clinical Epidemiology, 59,* 900–906.

Hanson, S.M. (1988). Collaborative research and authorship credit: Beginning guidelines. *Nursing Research, 37,* 49–52.

International Committee of Medical Journal Editors. (2006, February). *Uniform requirements for manuscripts submitted to biomedical journals: Writing and editing for biomedical publication.* Retrieved August 28, 2007, from http://www.icmje.org/#author

King, C.R. (2001). Ethical issues in writing and publishing. *Clinical Journal of Oncology Nursing, 5,* 19–24.

Ludwick, R., & Glazer, G. (2000). Electronic publishing: The movement from print to digital publication. *Online Journal of Issues in Nursing, 5*(1), 2.

Oermann, M.H. (2002). *Writing for publication in nursing.* Philadelphia: Lippincott Williams & Wilkins.

Plaisance, L. (2003). The "write" way to get published in a professional journal. *Pain Management, 4,* 165–170.

Sheridan, D.R., & Dowdney, D.L. (1997). *How to write and publish articles in nursing* (2nd ed.). New York: Springer.

Tenopir, C., & King, D.W. (2000). *Towards electronic journals: Realities for scientists, librarians, and publishers.* Washington, DC: SLA Publishing.

U.S. National Institutes of Health Library. (2005). *Reference manager.* Retrieved May 2, 2007, from http://nihlibrary.nih.gov/resourcetraining/trainingdescription.htm?id=35

Additional Resources

American Psychological Association (APA), "APA Style": www.apastyle.org

International Committee of Medical Journal Editors, "Uniform Requirements for Manuscripts Submitted to Biomedical Journals: Writing and Editing for Biomedical Publication": www.icmje.org

Junket Studies Tutoring, "11 Rules of Writing": www.junketstudies.com/rulesofw

Oncology Nursing Society, "Resources for Writers": www.ons.org/publications/publishing/resources.shtml

SECTION V.

Promotion and Patient Retention

CHAPTER 19
Psychosocial Considerations

Angela D. Klimaszewski, RN, MSN

Introduction

Before 1970, a social stigma was associated with cancer in the United States. Patients were not told their diagnosis by a physician (Holland, 2003), nor were they able to discuss their diagnosis with family or healthcare professionals. Psycho-oncology has since developed as a science with standards of care and valid assessment instruments for patients with cancer who are experiencing any of a variety of types of distress (Holland, 1999). The focus of this chapter is psycho-oncology as it pertains to clinical trials and the end of treatment. Specific topics that will be presented include

- The reasons why patients participate in clinical trials
- Distress and the meaning of distress
- Why going off-study may cause distress
- How to assess the patient in emotional distress
- Nursing implications for the patient experiencing emotional distress.

Background

The literature reflects an ever-increasing volume of articles and studies of psychosocial issues that patients with cancer confront. Much knowledge is gained from the works addressing meaning (Carroll-Johnson, 2006; National Cancer Institute [NCI], 2004), coping and adaptation (Bush, 2006b; Nail, 2001; NCI, 2004), hope (Cooper, 2006), anxiety (Bush, 2006a; Marrs, 2006; NCI, 2004), fear (NCI, 2004; Smith, 2002), anger (NCI, 2004; Watson, 2006), decision making (Collyar, 2005; Leighl, Butow, & Tattersall, 2004; Smith), depression (Albright & Valente, 2006; NCI, 2004), and spirituality (NCI, 2004; Sloan et al., 2000; Taylor, 2006). These and many other works offer tremendous insight and useable recommendations for addressing each issue. However, routine psychosocial patient assessment and intervention is still a goal—and not the standard of care—in oncology nursing. This oversight may be taking a toll on all patients with cancer and especially on those enrolled in clinical trials.

Reasons to Enroll

The literature reflects an abundance of research exploring the reasons why patients decline to participate in a clinical trial (Harris Interactive, 2001; NCI, 2005; Simon et al., 2004; Townsley, Selby, & Siu, 2005). Therefore, the reader is referred elsewhere for a discussion of the *barriers* to clinical trial participation. The reasons that patients *do* participate in clinical trials involve physician factors, patient factors, and protocol factors (Klimaszewski, 2006). Collyar (2005) noted that patients' "views on clinical trials cover a vast spectrum, from fear and avoidance, to whole-hearted support" (p. 217). The attitude of the patient's physician toward clinical trials, as well as the phase of the trial and the stage of the patient's disease (Crosson, Eisner, Brown, & Ter Maat, 2001), also will affect a patient's decision to participate or not.

Physician Factors

Klimaszewski (2006) noted, "The trust relationship between a physician and patient is generally considered sacrosanct" (p. 490). Aungst, Haas, Ommaya, and Green (2003) ascertained that patients are willing to follow the advice of their physician, including his or her recommendation to participate in a clinical trial. This is echoed by NCI (2005), which cited patients' unwillingness to go against their personal physician's wishes as a barrier to participation in trials for the general public. Patients studied by Schutta and Burnett (2000) revealed that their physician's interpersonal skills and positive attitude increased their own trust and confidence in a clinical trial.

The author would like to acknowledge Maria Karigan, RN, MSN, CCRC, for her contribution that remains unchanged from the first edition.

If a patient trusts the physician, he or she is more likely to follow the advice of the physician who advocates a clinical trial. Conversely, if the patient perceives that the physician does not wholeheartedly support a clinical trial—or clinical trials in general—the patient is less likely to participate.

Patient Factors

Studies show that most people would be willing to participate in a clinical trial if they had cancer (Aungst et al., 2003; Comis, Miller, Aldige, Krebs, & Stoval, 2003). Hope for a therapeutic benefit and a desire to live were cited as reasons to participate in any phase trial (Albrecht, Blanchard, Ruckdeschel, Coovert, & Strongbow, 1999; Schutta & Burnett, 2000).

Simon et al. (2004) questioned 319 women about participation in clinical trials. Their results suggest that more women would participate if they were provided the opportunity. Furthermore, in a study of 1,000 adults aged 18 and older, 32% said they would be very willing to participate in a clinical trial, and another 38% would consider participating in a clinical trial if asked (Comis et al., 2003). This supports a larger survey of patients with cancer by Harris Interactive (2001), which found that 80% of the public would be willing to participate in a clinical trial for their initial treatment if they were ever diagnosed with cancer. Similarly, 90% would participate if their initial treatment failed (Harris Interactive).

Phase I Trial Participation

Phase I trials are designed to determine the toxicity of an agent, not to attain disease control or remission. Phase I trials are offered to patients who have failed all other forms of therapy and whose disease has advanced through all attempts to control it. For some patients, this may be the first time they consider a clinical trial. Meadows (2000) noted, "Information on clinical trials may not be sought unless it becomes a compelling or desperate issue" (p. 54).

Mack (1999) interviewed 20 patients who met the criteria for participating in phase I trials. Interviewees expressed a "quest for treatment," an active process that proceeded along the specific steps of taking charge, deciding, living on a trial, and dealing with uncertainty. Being involved in a research study provided these participants with a sense of meaning at a time when their life was nearing the end (Mack).

Schain (1994) related that patients who enroll in phase I trials feel gratification for contributing to the advancement of science, thus meeting a basic altruistic concern for the improvement of care for others when no hope of cure exists for them. Additionally, the majority of patients studied by Schutta and Burnett (2000) stressed the value and importance of being the one to make the decision to participate in the trial.

Meropol, Weinfurt, and Schulman (2003) reported that patients who enroll in phase I trials may have a *therapeutic*

misconception, that is, perceiving benefit when none is expected. They suggested the possibility that "high expectations of benefit among patients considering phase I trials may be an expression of confidence and hope for personal benefit" (p. 4659) rather than a misunderstanding of the purpose of the trial.

Similarly, Roychowdhury (2003) studied 106 patients with locally advanced or metastatic cancer with no prior chemotherapy or immunotherapy about participation in a phase I trial. Of the 99 patients who responded to the questionnaire, 58% would participate for personal benefit, 38% for the benefit of others, and 5% for reasons unspecified. Sixty-eight percent responded that they would participate in a phase I trial; 32% would not. Additionally, 73% believed there would be physical benefit, and 62% believed they would benefit psychologically.

Protocol Factors

Lack of access to trials is a commonly cited barrier to clinical trials for the general population (NCI, 2005). Patients may find that a lengthy or complicated protocol that requires additional tests is as unacceptable as one that requires an extended admission (Meadows, 2000). In addition, age restrictions in eligibility requirements, lack of protocol therapies in local treatment centers, and an unwillingness to comply with randomization determinations can contribute to the dearth of older adults participating in clinical trials.

Distress

The term *distress* encompasses an array of psychosocial issues that includes anxiety, depression, anger, decreased social skills, family problems, work problems, meaning in life, and spiritual issues (Albright & Valente, 2006; Bush, 2006a; Carroll-Johnson, 2006; Collyar, 2005; Cooper, 2006; Leighl et al., 2004; Marrs, 2006; Nail, 2001; NCI, 2004; Sloan et al., 2000; Smith, 2002; Taylor, 2006; Watson, 2006). The National Comprehensive Cancer Network (NCCN) developed the first set of standards for psychosocial care and management of distress in patients with cancer (Holland, 1999, 2003). NCCN (2007) defined distress as

> A multifactorial unpleasant emotional experience of a psychological (cognitive, behavioral, emotional), social and/or spiritual nature that may interfere with the ability to cope effectively with cancer, its physical symptoms and its treatment. Distress extends along a continuum, ranging from common normal feelings of vulnerability, sadness, and fears to problems that can become disabling, such as depression, anxiety, panic, social isolation, and existential and spiritual crisis. (p. DIS-2).

NCCN uses the word *distress* because it does not have the same implied meaning (i.e., that one is "crazy") as the words *psychiatric, psychosocial,* or *emotional*. Rather, distress is viewed as a normal reaction and one that is socially acceptable. Additionally, distress "can be defined and measured by self-report" (NCCN, 2007, p. DIS-1).

The patient characteristics of psychosocial distress encompass patients who are at increased risk for distress and periods along the cancer continuum when patients are more vulnerable to experience distress (see Figure 19-1). The periods of vulnerability cover a large part of the cancer continuum, from awaiting treatment, through a change in treatment modality and the end of treatment because of

completion or progressive disease, to treatment failure and advanced cancer.

Why Going Off-Study May Cause Distress

Kelly, Ghazi, and Caldwell (2002) noted that psychological distress is "a challenging outcome of cancer clinical trial participation" (p. 13). While in the active treatment phase of a clinical trial, patients receive psychological as well as physical support from physicians and nurses (Carter, 2004). Ending treatment, or going off-study, may cause feelings of isolation and abandonment to emerge (Carter; NCI, 2005). The sense of security that patients feel by participating in a clinical trial and by the continuity of care that is provided (Cox & Avis, 1996) may lead to feelings of loss that require professional intervention.

The reason for ending treatment will affect a patient differently in each of the following situations.
- Treatment completion and movement to follow-up phase
- Treatment ending because of a new research finding
- Treatment ending because of disease recurrence
- Elective withdrawal from treatment for personal reasons
- Elective withdrawal because of family, caregiver, or transportation issues

Carter (2004) compiled a list of the feelings and experiences of patients when treatment has ended (see Figure 19-2). In all cases, the patient will experience a significant change in the frequency of visits to the clinic, which is where healthcare providers have provided support and education.

Figure 19-1. Psychosocial Distress Patient Characteristics

Patients at Increased Risk for Distress
- History of psychiatric disorder/substance abuse
- History of depression/suicide attempt
- Cognitive impairment
- Communication barriers
- Severe comorbid illnesses
- Social problems
  - Family/caregiver conflicts
  - Inadequate social support
  - Living alone
  - Financial problems
  - Limited access to medical care
  - Young or dependent children
  - Younger age; woman
  - Other stressors

Periods of Increased Vulnerability
- Finding a suspicious symptom
- During workup
- Finding out the diagnosis
- Awaiting treatment
- Change in treatment modality
- End of treatment
- Discharge from hospital following treatment
- Stresses of survivorship
- Medical follow-up and surveillance
- Treatment failure
- Recurrence/progression
- Advanced cancer
- End of life

Note. Reproduced with permission from *The NCCN 1.2007 Distress Management Clinical Practice Guidelines in Oncology* (p. DIS-B). Copyright 2007 by the National Comprehensive Cancer Network. Available at http://www.nccn.org. Retrieved August 3, 2007. To view the most recent and complete version of the guideline, go online to www.nccn.org.

These guidelines and illustrations herein may not be reproduced in any form for any purpose without the express written permission of NCCN.

These guidelines are a work in progress that will be refined as often as new significant data becomes available. The NCCN guidelines are a statement of consensus of its authors regarding their views of currently accepted approaches to treatment. Any clinician seeking to apply or consult any NCCN guideline is expected to use independent medical judgment in the context of individual clinical circumstances to determine any patient's care or treatment. The National Comprehensive Cancer Network makes no warranties of any kind whatsoever regarding their content, use, or application and disclaims any responsibility for the application or use in any way.

Figure 19-2. End-of-Treatment Feelings and Experiences

- Isolation and abandonment
- Worry, anxiety, and panic
- Loss of support
- Self-doubt and poor self-image
- Coping with side effects of treatment (both temporary and permanent)
- Depression (mild to suicide)
- Grief and sadness due to losses
- Uncertainty and doubt about future
- Helplessness and hopelessness (loss of power)
- Fear of recurrence
- Lack of memory and concentration ("Have I lost my mind?")
- Residual fatigue up to a year
- Anger
- Family and social issues
- Workplace issues
- Financial and insurance challenges
- Search for the new definition of "normal"
- Difficulty making long-term plans
- Fear of the power and truth of statistics
- Changes to body, self, and sexual images and function

Note. From "End of Treatment: Laugh or Cry?" by S.E. Carter, 2004, *Community Oncology, 1,* p. 180. Copyright 2004 by Elsevier. Reprinted with permission.

Assessing Distress

Bultz and Carlson (2005) recommended that emotional distress be viewed as the "sixth vital sign" that should be regularly screened for, monitored, and treated along with temperature, pulse, and respiration (TPR), blood pressure (B/P), and pain (Berry et al., 2001). Bultz and Holland (2006) stressed the need for distress assessment at every clinic visit for every patient with cancer, much the way TPR, B/P, and pain are assessed at each visit.

The NCCN screening tool for measuring distress (NCCN, 2007) is shown in Figure 19-3. It is a two-part tool that uses (1) a 0–10 scale drawn on a thermometer to assess distress experienced in the past week, and (2) a list of problems experienced in the past week. The problems are grouped as (NCCN, p. DIS-A)

- Practical (child care, housing, insurance/financial, transportation, work/school),
- Family (dealing with children or partner)
- Emotional (depression, fears, nervousness, sadness, worry, loss of interest in usual activities)
- Spiritual/religious
- Physical (appearance, bathing/dressing, breathing, changes in urination, constipation, diarrhea, eating, fatigue, feeling swollen, fevers, getting around, indigestion, memory/concentration, mouth sore, nausea, nose dry/congested, pain, sexual, sleep, tingling in hands/feet)
- Other.

The distress thermometer uses a 0–10 Likert scale that makes the assessment tool easy for patients to use. A score of 4–5 or higher on the scale indicates that a referral is needed

---

Figure 19-3. Screening Tools for Measuring Distress

SCREENING TOOLS FOR MEASURING DISTRESS

Instructions: First please circle the number (0-10) that best describes how much distress you have been experiencing in the past week including today.

Extreme distress — 10

9

8

7

6

5

4

3

2

1

No distress — 0

Second, please indicate if any of the following has been a problem for you in the past week including today. Be sure to check YES or NO for each.

YES NO **Practical Problems**
☐ ☐ Child care
☐ ☐ Housing
☐ ☐ Insurance/financial
☐ ☐ Transportation
☐ ☐ Work/school

Family Problems
☐ ☐ Dealing with children
☐ ☐ Dealing with partner

Emotional Problems
☐ ☐ Depression
☐ ☐ Fears
☐ ☐ Nervousness
☐ ☐ Sadness
☐ ☐ Worry
☐ ☐ Loss of interest in usual activities

☐ ☐ **Spiritual/religious concerns**

YES NO **Physical Problems**
☐ ☐ Appearance
☐ ☐ Bathing/dressing
☐ ☐ Breathing
☐ ☐ Changes in urination
☐ ☐ Constipation
☐ ☐ Diarrhea
☐ ☐ Eating
☐ ☐ Fatigue
☐ ☐ Feeling Swollen
☐ ☐ Fevers
☐ ☐ Getting around
☐ ☐ Indigestion
☐ ☐ Memory/concentration
☐ ☐ Mouth sores
☐ ☐ Nausea
☐ ☐ Nose dry/congested
☐ ☐ Pain
☐ ☐ Sexual
☐ ☐ Skin dry/itchy
☐ ☐ Sleep
☐ ☐ Tingling in hands/feet

Other Problems: _____

for additional psychosocial or supportive care (Bultz & Holland, 2006). Patients are asked to mark the problem list to identify the "nature and source of their distress (physical, social, psychological, or spiritual)" (Bultz & Holland, p. 313). This helps to determine if—and what kind of (e.g., social work, pastoral services, mental health)—referral needs to be made (Bultz & Holland). Figure 19-4 depicts an overview of the NCCN evaluation and treatment process.

Patients and physicians found screening with the distress management tool to be satisfactory (Bultz & Holland, 2006). Jacobsen et al. (2005) completed a study to validate the tool in an ambulatory care environment. Bultz and Holland advised that caregivers be trained to routinely use the distress screening tool at each patient visit. They recommended online training for nurses that uses the distress thermometer, such as that provided by the American Psychosocial Oncology Society (www.apos-society.org).

Robbins (2007) conducted a pilot project that required the use of the NCCN tool at weeks 1 and 5 of radiation therapy. Audits of patients' charts demonstrated that the NCCN tool was used 75% of the time. Written feedback from nursing staff cited two reasons for not employing the tool: (a) nurses were not always comfortable approaching patients and discussing their concerns, and (b) physicians were not always supportive of the time the patient needed to complete the tool. Subsequent staff in-services followed by chart audits showed an increase in use of the tool (Robbins).

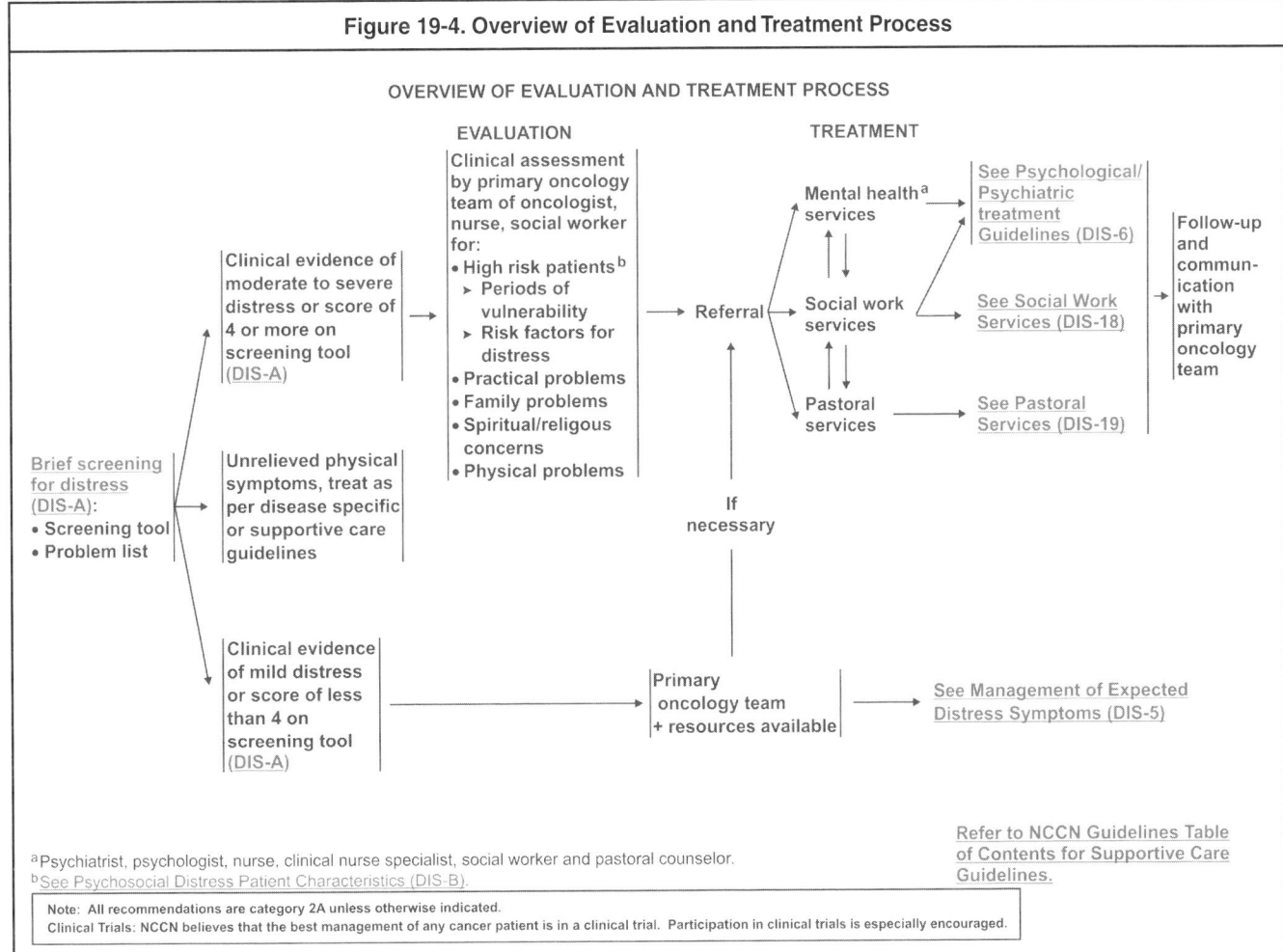

Figure 19-4. Overview of Evaluation and Treatment Process

OVERVIEW OF EVALUATION AND TREATMENT PROCESS
EVALUATION
TREATMENT
Clinical assessment by primary oncology team of oncologist, nurse, social worker for:
• High risk patients b
➤ Periods of vulnerability
➤ Risk factors for distress
• Practical problems
• Family problems
• Spiritual/religous concerns
• Physical problems
Brief screening for distress (DIS-A):
• Screening tool
• Problem list
Clinical evidence of moderate to severe distress or score of 4 or more on screening tool (DIS-A)
Unrelieved physical symptoms, treat as per disease specific or supportive care guidelines
Clinical evidence of mild distress or score of less than 4 on screening tool (DIS-A)
Referral
If necessary
Mental health a services
Social work services
Pastoral services
See Psychological/ Psychiatric treatment Guidelines (DIS-6)
See Social Work Services (DIS-18)
See Pastoral Services (DIS-19)
Follow-up and commun-ication with primary oncology team
Primary oncology team + resources available
See Management of Expected Distress Symptoms (DIS-5)

[a] Psychiatrist, psychologist, nurse, clinical nurse specialist, social worker and pastoral counselor.
[b] See Psychosocial Distress Patient Characteristics (DIS-B).

Refer to NCCN Guidelines Table of Contents for Supportive Care Guidelines.

Note: All recommendations are category 2A unless otherwise indicated.
Clinical Trials: NCCN believes that the best management of any cancer patient is in a clinical trial. Participation in clinical trials is especially encouraged.

Note. Reproduced with permission from *The NCCN 1.2007 Distress Management Clinical Practice Guidelines in Oncology* (p. DIS-4). Copyright 2007 by the National Comprehensive Cancer Network. Available at http://www.nccn.org. Retrieved August 3, 2007. To view the most recent and complete version of the guideline, go online to www.nccn.org.

These guidelines are a work in progress that will be refined as often as new significant data becomes available. The NCCN Guidelines are a statement of consensus of its authors regarding their views of currently accepted approaches to treatment. Any clinician seeking to apply or consult any NCCN guideline is expected to use independent medical judgment in the context of individual clinical circumstances to determine any patient's care or treatment. The National Comprehensive Cancer Network makes no warranties of any kind whatsoever regarding their content, use, or application and disclaims any responsibility for the application or use in any way.

Bruce (2007) stated, "Many healthcare providers do not look for depression or assume that depression is a normal reaction to cancer that does not warrant treatment" (p. 20). Furthermore, McCorkle (2004) reported that nurses are not vigilant in regularly assessing patients' distress because of time constraints, lack of knowledge, and lack of emotional ability. Madden (2006) noted that none of the reasons nurses may have for not assessing a patient's psychological distress are insurmountable. Feeling uncomfortable discussing a patient's feelings, being concerned about upsetting a patient, feeling emotionally "drained" after discussing feelings with a patient, and being under time constraints all may be addressed. Madden stated that "continuing education about psychosocial issues, discussions with peers about why nurses are reluctant to assess for distress, and an honest look inward" (p. 616) will increase a nurse's ability to routinely assess psychosocial distress.

Nursing Implications

Brant and Wickham (2004) edited the Oncology Nursing Society's *Statement on the Scope and Standards of Oncology Nursing Practice*, which addressed psychosocial distress. Specifically, oncology nurses were advised to include an assessment of every patient's coping and comfort. Although standardized tools to assess distress in patients in clinical trials are not on the immediate horizon, the first step is to incorporate a general oncology distress assessment tool into routine nursing practice. If the tool is easy to use and accurate in identifying patients' psychosocial needs, perhaps a tool to specifically assess psychosocial distress of patients enrolled in clinical trials will not be necessary.

The NCCN multidisciplinary panel that developed the standards for psychosocial care and management of distress established minimal quality measures for recognizing and managing distress (Holland & Anderson, 2003). The complete NCCN standards of care for distress management are listed in Figure 19-5.

The implications for nurses, clinical trial nurses (CTNs), and researchers are clear (see Figure 19-5). Patients must be assessed for psychological distress at every visit and receive an appropriate referral, if one is needed. Although this currently may be considered a lofty goal, the result of achieving that goal is astounding. Patients with cancer who are considering, enrolled in, or completing a clinical trial may need psychosocial intervention. Nurses can help patients to cope by identifying and focusing on the components of distress that may be modified (Nail, 2001) and improve the patient's quality of life (Vitek, Rosenzweig, & Stollings, 2007). In any case, distress cannot be treated if it is not identified.

CTNs, by this author's definition, are knowledgeable, skilled, and compassionate. All CTNs need to introspectively assess their own sensitivity with discussing a patient's nonphysical distress and come to terms with it. Vachon (2006) noted that nurses can help patients with cancer to cope with their disease and treatment by "respecting

Figure 19-5. Standards of Care for Distress Management

- Distress should be recognized, monitored, documented, and treated promptly at all stages of disease.
- All patients should be screened for distress at their initial visit, at appropriate intervals, and as clinically indicated especially with changes in disease status (i.e., remission, recurrence, progression).
- Screening should identify the level and nature of the distress.
- Distress should be assessed and managed according to clinical practice guidelines.
- Multidisciplinary institutional committees should be formed to implement standards for distress management.
- Educational and training programs should be developed to ensure that healthcare professionals and pastoral caregivers have knowledge and skills in the assessment and management of distress.
- Licensed mental health professionals and certified pastoral caregivers experienced in psychosocial aspects of cancer should be readily available as staff members or by referral.
- Medical care contracts should include reimbursement for services provided by mental health professionals.
- Clinical health outcomes measurement should include assessment of the psychosocial domain (e.g., quality of life and patient and family satisfaction).
- Patients, families, and treatment teams should be informed that management of distress is an integral part of total medical care and provided with appropriate information about psychosocial services in the treatment center and the community.
- Quality of distress management should be included in institutional continuous quality improvement (CQI) projects.

Note. Reproduced with permission from *The NCCN 1.2007 Distress Management Clinical Practice Guidelines in Oncology* (p. DIS-3). Copyright 2007 by the National Comprehensive Cancer Network. Available at http://www.nccn.org. Retrieved August 3, 2007. To view the most recent and complete version of the guideline, go online to www.nccn.org.

These Guidelines and illustrations herein may not be reproduced in any form for any purpose without the express written permission of NCCN.

These guidelines are a work in progress that will be refined as often as new significant data becomes available. The NCCN Guidelines are a statement of consensus of its authors regarding their views of currently accepted approaches to treatment. Any clinician seeking to apply or consult any NCCN guideline is expected to use independent medical judgment in the context of individual clinical circumstances to determine any patient's care or treatment. The National Comprehensive Cancer Network makes no warranties of any kind whatsoever regarding their content, use, or application and disclaims any responsibility for the application or use in any way.

individual differences and preferences, appreciating patient perspectives, and understanding coping as a process" (p. 28). Carter (2004) identified both helpful and ineffective comments from physicians and nurses to patients ending treatment (see Figure 19-6). CTNs need to seek out ways to make psychosocial distress assessments the "sixth vital sign" (Bultz & Carlson, 2005) and then share those techniques with colleagues. Pilot studies, master's nursing projects, Oncology Nursing Society conference poster and podium sessions, and in-services are ways to help colleagues to appreciate what works and what does not.

Figure 19-6. Helpful Comments From Physicians and Nurses

- "We are not abandoning you; we are changing the focus and frequency of your visits."
- "Tell me what your concerns are."
- "I know someone that can give you the tools and techniques for coping with these emotions and feelings."
- "I hear these concerns often at the end of treatment; they are normal and important to deal with."
- "We want you to live a good quality life; I will refer you to someone who can help you . . ."
- "I am asking you to consider some medication that might help"; or "I can refer you to someone who specializes in emotional and psychological well-being for cancer patients who might be able to help."
- "You will be 'normal,' but it will be a 'new normal' that encompasses all the things that have happened to you since diagnosis."

Dismissive and ineffective comments
- "You'll be fine."
- "It is normal—get over it."
- "Look on the bright side."
- "How could you feel this way when we fought so hard for your life?"
- "Just get back to work; you will feel better."

Note. From "End of Treatment: Laugh or Cry?" by S.E. Carter, 2004, *Community Oncology, 1*, p. 180. Copyright 2004 by Elsevier. Reprinted with permission.

Last, the need to generalize assessments and interventions globally is apparent with the increased number of clinical trials internationally (see the International Section of this manual). The only way to achieve consistency of care worldwide is through the adoption of acceptable and effective standards. This author supports the adoption of NCCN's distress management guidelines and standards by all oncology clinicians as a means to that end.

Summary

Patients with cancer experience an array of personal psychological challenges as they move through the cancer treatment continuum, especially if they are part of a clinical trial. A gap exists in the routine assessment and intervention of psychological distress that needs to be closed before oncology professionals can hope to provide truly holistic care to patients. The first step to accomplish that is to adopt standards for assessment and intervention, such as the NCCN standards. The second step is to incorporate those standards into routine practice and ongoing research. Only then will it be possible to determine whether a psychosocial distress assessment tool that is specific for clinical trial patients is required. There is still a long road ahead.

References

Albrecht, T.L., Blanchard, C., Ruckdeschel, J.C., Coovert, M., & Strongbow, R. (1999). Strategic physician communication and oncology clinical trials. *Journal of Clinical Oncology, 17*, 3324–3332.

Albright, A.V., & Valente, S.M. (2006). Depression and suicide. In R.M. Carroll-Johnson, L.M. Gorman, & N.J. Bush (Eds.), *Psychosocial nursing care along the cancer continuum* (2nd ed., pp. 241–260). Pittsburgh, PA: Oncology Nursing Society.

Aungst, J., Haas, A., Ommaya, A., & Green, L.W. (Eds.). (2003). *Exploring challenges, progress, and new models for engaging the public in the clinical research enterprise: Clinical Research Roundtable Workshop summary.* Washington, DC: National Academies Press. Retrieved November 14, 2003, from http://www.nap.edu/catalog/10757.html

Berry, P.H., Chapman, C.R., Covington, E.C., Dahl, J.L., Katz, J.A., Miaskowski, C., & McLean, M.J. (Eds.). (2001). *Pain: Current understanding of assessment, management and treatments.* Reston, VA: National Pharmaceutical Council, Inc.

Brant, J.M., & Wickham, R.S. (Eds.). (2004). *Statement on the scope and standards of oncology nursing practice.* Pittsburgh, PA: Oncology Nursing Society.

Bruce, S.D. (2007, April). Know how to assess and treat depression in patients with cancer. *ONS Connect, 22*(4), pp. 20–21.

Bultz, B.D., & Carlson, L.E. (2005). Emotional distress: The sixth vital sign in cancer care. *Journal of Clinical Oncology, 23*, 6440–6441.

Bultz, B.D., & Holland, J.C. (2006). Emotional distress in patients with cancer: The sixth vital sign. *Community Oncology, 3*, 311–314.

Bush, N.J. (2006a). Anxiety and the cancer experience. In R.M. Carroll-Johnson, L.M. Gorman, & N.J. Bush (Eds.), *Psychosocial nursing care along the cancer continuum* (2nd ed., pp. 205–221). Pittsburgh, PA: Oncology Nursing Society.

Bush, N.J. (2006b). Coping and adaptation. In R.M. Carroll-Johnson, L.M. Gorman, & N.J. Bush (Eds.), *Psychosocial nursing care along the cancer continuum* (2nd ed., pp. 61–88). Pittsburgh, PA: Oncology Nursing Society.

Carroll-Johnson, R.M. (2006). Life's meaning and cancer. In R.M. Carroll-Johnson, L.M. Gorman, & N.J. Bush (Eds.), *Psychosocial nursing care along the cancer continuum* (2nd ed., pp. 55–60). Pittsburgh, PA: Oncology Nursing Society.

Carter, S.E. (2004). End of treatment: Laugh or cry? *Community Oncology, 1*, 179–181.

Collyar, D.E. (2005). Patient views on clinical trials. *AACR Education Book 2005*, pp. 217–220.

Comis, R.L., Miller, J.D., Aldige, C.R., Krebs, L., & Stoval, E. (2003). Public attitudes in toward participation in cancer clinical trials. *Journal of Clinical Oncology, 21*, 830–835.

Cooper, P.G. (2006). The influence of hope on the psychosocial experience. In R.M. Carroll-Johnson, L.M. Gorman, & N.J. Bush (Eds.), *Psychosocial nursing care along the cancer continuum* (2nd ed., pp. 133–141). Pittsburgh, PA: Oncology Nursing Society.

Cox, K., & Avis, M. (1996). Psychological aspects of participation in early anti-cancer drug trials. *Cancer Nursing, 19*, 177–186.

Crosson, K., Eisner, E., Brown, C., & Ter Maat, J. (2001). Primary care physicians' attitudes, knowledge, and practices related to clinical trials. *Journal of Cancer Education, 16*, 188–192.

Harris Interactive. (2001). *Misconceptions and lack of awareness greatly reduce recruitment for cancer clinical trials.* Retrieved November 9, 2003, from http://www.harrisinteractive.com/news/allnewsbydate.asp?NewsID=222

Holland, J.C. (1999). Update: NCCN practice guidelines for the management of psychosocial distress. *Oncology, 13*, 459–507.

Holland, J.C. (2003). Psychological care of patients: Psycho-oncology's contribution. *Journal of Clinical Oncology, 21*, 253s–265s.

Holland, J.C., & Anderson, B. (2003). Distress management clinical practice guidelines in oncology. *Journal of the National Comprehensive Cancer Network, 1*, 344–374.

Jacobsen, P.B., Donovan, K.A., Trask, P.C., Fleishman, S.B., Zabora, J., Baker, F., et al. (2005). Screening for psychologic distress in ambulatory cancer patients. *Cancer, 103*, 1494–1502.

Kelly, C., Ghazi, F., & Caldwell, K. (2002). Psychological distress of cancer and clinical trial participation: A review of the literature. *European Journal of Cancer Care, 11*, 6–15.

Klimaszewski, A.D. (2006). Psychosocial aspects of experimental therapy: Clinical trials. In R.M. Carroll-Johnson, L.M. Gorman, & N.J. Bush (Eds.), *Psychosocial nursing care along the cancer continuum* (2nd ed., pp. 489–497). Pittsburgh, PA: Oncology Nursing Society.

Leighl, N.B., Butow, P.N., & Tattersall, M.H. (2004). Treatment decision aids in advanced cancer: When the goal is not cure and the answer is not clear. *Journal of Clinical Oncology, 22,* 1759–1762.

Mack, C.H. (1999). *The quest for treatment: Cancer patients' experience of phase I clinical trials* [Oncology Nursing Society Congress Proceedings, Abstract 138]. Retrieved November 14, 2003, from http://www.ons.org

Madden, J. (2006). The problem of distress in patients with cancer: More effective assessment. *Clinical Journal of Oncology Nursing, 10,* 615–619.

Marrs, J.A. (2006). Stress, fears, and phobias: The impact of anxiety. *Clinical Journal of Oncology Nursing, 10,* 319–322.

McCorkle, R. (2004). *Distress management training for oncology nurses: The oncology nurse's role in recognizing distress in patients and family caregivers* [Webcast]. Retrieved June 4, 2007, from http://www.apos-society.org/professionals/meetings-ed/webcasts/webcasts-ican2.aspx#

Meadows, B. (2000). Potential accrual base. In A.D. Klimaszewski, J.L. Aiken, M.A. Bacon, S.A. DiStasio, H.E. Ehrenberger, & B.A. Ford (Eds.), *Manual for clinical trials nursing* (pp. 53–55). Pittsburgh, PA: Oncology Nursing Society.

Meropol, N.J., Weinfurt, K.P., & Schulman, K.A. (2003). Correspondence: In reply. *Journal of Clinical Oncology, 21,* 4659–4660.

Nail, L.M. (2001). I'm coping as fast as I can: Psychosocial adjustment to cancer and cancer treatment. *Oncology Nursing Forum, 28,* 967–970.

National Cancer Institute. (2004). *Life after cancer treatment (facing forward series)* [NIH Publication No. 04-2424]. Bethesda, MD: U.S. Department of Health and Human Services, National Institute of Health.

National Cancer Institute. (2005). *Cancer clinical trials: The in-depth program* [NIH Publication No. 05-5051]. Jenkintown, PA: Author.

National Comprehensive Cancer Network. (2007). Distress management. *NCCN clinical practice guidelines in oncology, version 1.2007.* Jenkintown, PA: Author.

Robbins, M.A. (2007). Barriers to using the National Comprehensive Cancer Network (NCCN) distress management tool: Does it cause more stress [Abstract 2073]? *Oncology Nursing Forum, 34,* 503.

Roychowdhury, D. (2003). Phase I trials: Physician and patient perceptions [Correspondence]. *Journal of Clinical Oncology, 21,* 4658–4659.

Schain, W.S. (1994). Barriers to clinical trials, part II: Knowledge and attitudes of potential participants. *Cancer, 74*(Suppl. 9), 2666–2671.

Schutta, K.M., & Burnett, C.B. (2000). Factors that influence a patient's decision to participate in a phase I cancer clinical trial. *Oncology Nursing Forum, 27,* 1435–1438.

Simon, M.S., Du, W., Flaherty, L., Phillip, P.A., Lorusso, P., Miree, C., et al. (2004). Factors associated with breast cancer clinical trials participation and enrollment at a large academic medical center. *Journal of Clinical Oncology, 22,* 2046–2052.

Sloan, R.P., Bagiella, E., VandeCreek, L., Hover, M., Cassalone, C., Hirsch, T.J., et al. (2000). Should physicians prescribe religious activities? *New England Journal of Medicine, 342,* 1913–1916.

Smith, E.D. (2002). Decision making. In E.G. Gomez & M. Gullatte (Eds.), *Advocacy in health care: Teaching patients, caregivers and professionals* (pp. 28–32). Pittsburgh, PA: Oncology Nursing Society.

Taylor, E.J. (2006). Spirituality and spiritual nurture in cancer care. In R.M. Carroll-Johnson, L.M. Gorman, & N.J. Bush (Eds.), *Psychosocial nursing care along the cancer continuum* (2nd ed., pp. 117–131). Pittsburgh, PA: Oncology Nursing Society.

Townsley, C.A., Selby, R., & Siu, L.L. (2005). Systematic review of barriers to the recruitment of older patients with cancer onto clinical trials. *Journal of Clinical Oncology, 23,* 3112–3124.

Vachon, M.A. (2006). Psychosocial distress and coping after cancer treatment. *American Journal of Nursing, 106*(Suppl. 3), 26–31.

Vitek, L., Rosenzweig, M.Q., & Stollings, S. (2007). Distress in patients with cancer: Definition, assessment, and suggested interventions. *Clinical Journal of Oncology Nursing, 11,* 413–418.

Watson, A.C. (2006). Anger and cancer. In R.M. Carroll-Johnson, L.M. Gorman, & N.J. Bush (Eds.), *Psychosocial nursing care along the cancer continuum* (2nd ed., pp. 223–240). Pittsburgh, PA: Oncology Nursing Society.

CHAPTER 20
Public and Patient Education

David Leos, RN, MBA, OCN®, CCRA

Introduction

Good communication between health professionals and patients is essential for the delivery of high-quality care (Department of Health, 2000). In much the same way, the ability of the clinical trial nurse (CTN) to identify effective public and patient health education methodologies can prove instrumental to ensuring the delivery of adequate healthcare services. It is of great utility to the overall success of clinical trials. The development of new cancer treatments depends on the expedient conduct of clinical trials (Connolly, Schneider, & Hill, 2004).

In today's cancer care setting, the state of the art almost always will incorporate a clinical trial option somewhere along the overall treatment course. Yet, as the traditional purveyors of health information to patients and the public, many healthcare professionals, including CTNs, find themselves with limited knowledge of how to effectively disseminate educational information related to clinical trials. This chapter will review the literature on methods and resources that CTNs can utilize in the challenge to create awareness about clinical trials.

The Clinical Trial Nurse's Role in Education

CTNs must understand and incorporate into their daily practice a philosophy of continually seeking ways to improve lay, and in some cases professional, education about clinical trials. In their pivotal role of overseeing every aspect of the protocol, CTNs are ideally situated to undertake this task. Although CTNs work in unison with other oncology care professionals to provide treatment-related care and information, it is they who focus solely on treatment via clinical trials.

Education Improves Accrual

The CTN must present an increasingly complex array of medical, scientific, and, at times, legal information related to cancer protocols in a form that is appropriate and digestible to the intended audience. The effectiveness with which this is done is a critical yet often underrecognized contributing factor in the overall fate of clinical trials. Along with providing a patient or the public with introductory information about a particular protocol's availability or shedding light on the existence of a clinical trial program within their community, the CTN also must convey certain basic information. This includes the characteristics and expectations that these audiences have for each of the different phases of these protocols. These all will affect the audience's sense of understanding as to the implications of clinical trial participation.

Ultimately, educational efforts can have a significantly positive impact on accrual outcomes. This especially is true if it allays public naiveté, distrust, or outright fear over actual or unfounded accounts of research-related misdeeds or the burdens and risks imposed by participation in clinical trials.

An environment with an overall research-directed mindset realistically can translate into improvements for overall participation in these trials among patients with cancer, which has been approximately 3%–5% of the potentially eligible population (Varrichio, McCabe, Trimble, & Korn, 1996). According to a Harris Interactive (2001) survey of almost 6,000 patients with cancer, 85% of patients reported that they were unaware of the possibility to enroll in a clinical trial for their treatment. Interestingly, a portion of these findings from the Harris Interactive survey pointed out that the fears of nonparticipants in clinical trials generally are inconsistent with the experiences of those who have

The author would like to acknowledge Beverly Meadows, RN, MS, OCN®, for her contribution that remains unchanged from the first edition.

participated in cancer trials. Hence, engaging the testimonials of current participants in clinical trials would provide an insightful source of validation and firsthand experience to pair with information being given to an individual or wider audience about clinical trials.

Recruiting Older Adults

The development of successful advances in the treatment of advanced malignant diseases relies on recruitment of patients into clinical trials of novel agents (Nurgat et al., 2005). However, the expeditious recruitment of an appropriate number of patients that reflects the reality of the population of patients with cancer is a constant challenge. As cancer generally is accepted to be a disease most frequently found in the older adult population, the CTN most likely will find that his or her educational efforts will be directed toward an adult population. Despite the fact that older patients account for the greatest proportion of those with cancer, they are disproportionately underrepresented in many areas of cancer services utilization (Townsley, Selby, & Sui, 2005).

To completely understand how to correctly administer cancer treatment and to increase the utilization of cancer services by this population, clinical trials with an adequate representation of older patients need to be performed. Participation in well-designed clinical trials may afford some older adult patients the optimum treatment (Segelov, Tattersall, & Coates, 1992). Unfortunately, because older patients are not well represented in cancer clinical trials, determining the best treatment for this group becomes difficult (Goodwin, Hunt, Humble, Jey, & Samet, 1988; Tejeda et al., 1996).

The Setting

Armed with these data, the CTN should consider the population and circumstances under which any adult educational activities are carried out, as well as the variables associated with each. Settings for clinical trial education can be divided into two categories: individual and group. Individually oriented education is perhaps the most common example and typically is based at the bedside, in the clinic, or in the medical office setting. The CTN may feel most at home here, but the information recipient may not. The CTN may feel the confidence of being on "home turf" with all the necessary resources close at hand when delivering clinical trial information, but the recipient is less likely to consider this setting to be within his or her comfort zone. Group educational sessions can take place in healthcare facilities or nonhealthcare locations within the community. The healthcare settings outside of that where the CTN practices, such as community clinics and offices, offer a venue to reach study subjects closer to their home turf. The group setting can offer the advantage of a greater audience, which can make individual information recipients feel more comfortable among similarly interested participants. Non-healthcare settings, such as places of employment or worship and other community-based centers, often provide the recipient with the advantage of familiarity, proximity, and convenience. In the non-healthcare group setting, recipients have the opportunity to be exposed to a diversity of perceptions and questions beyond their own about the information being provided. The CTN must consider this as an opportunity to support an open dialogue while at the same time dispelling any misconceptions. This should lead toward a better understanding of the educational message and to more-informed decision making among recipients.

The choice of setting for an educational session is a factor in the public's receptiveness to the message. For example, Linnan et al. (2005) found that beauty shops represent an innovative setting where health promotion interventions may be planned, delivered, and evaluated. Similarly, anecdotal information has suggested that traditional community gathering places for men, such as barbershops, can provide an environment conducive for health education.

Reaching Interested Populations

Studies have shown that opportunities exist to successfully relay information to various populations about clinical trials as a treatment option. Based on the findings of one recent study, approximately 32% of American adults (64 million individuals) indicated that they would be very willing to participate in a cancer clinical trial (Comis, Miller, Aldige, Krebs, & Stoval, 2003). An additional 38% of adults (76 million individuals) scored in a range that indicated that they would be inclined to participate in a cancer clinical trial if asked but would have some questions or reservations about participation (Comis et al.). These findings suggest that perhaps more of the CTN's efforts could be directed toward raising the level of awareness by approaching appropriate patients (and family) with information, both written and verbal, about participation in a trial. The CTN can readily identify patients within his or her healthcare setting for whom clinical trial education would be appropriate. Identifying appropriate patient groups that typically are outside of the CTN's practice setting is more of a challenge but can be achieved by collecting community demographic information (such as census data). This can lead to identification of residential areas and social gathering locations of groups that may be receptive to clinical trial education and who are a population consistent with that being targeted by the protocol. From there, the particular requirements and eligibility criteria of the protocol will be the determining factors in whether a patient is eligible for and indeed consents to registration on the study. Comis et al. also found that the primary problem with accruals is not the attitude of patients but rather the unavailability of an appropriate clinical trial and the ineligibility of a large number of patients.

Further steps that can be taken to educate a patient about a specific clinical trial include an initial assessment of the patient's level of comprehension and emotional-receptive status, especially because this discussion most often coincides with the initial disclosure of a cancer diagnosis. Additionally, the opportunity for the prospective study patient to meet with a patient who is currently on or who has completed the particular study offers valuable insight as to what the patient might expect in terms of side effects, all relayed from a kindred source.

Educating the Public

Opportunities to take clinical trial education to the public audience will vary. One approach involves presenting the information to the audience in a non–protocol-specific manner as a "public service." This effort could involve making an educational presentation to a school or vocational audience, club, or civic organization or to the public at large at health fairs or through the use of radio or television media. A basic approach would be to focus on providing the history of clinical trials and an explanation of key concepts of the clinical trial process, as well as the implications of study participation, all with an emphasis on the audience achieving at least a basic understanding. One should allow time for and invite questions from the audience.

Preparation by the CTN should include creating learning objectives for the presentation and conducting pre- and post-testing to gauge the didactic effect. The CTN should bear in mind that it often is assumed that merely the provision of educational material for patients in an accessible form is sufficient to address informational needs. However, with increasing emphasis on evidence-based practice, an essential element of the patient education process is evaluation of the impact of educational interventions (Templeton & Coates, 2003). An excellent, ready-made, and free (in small quantities) resource for this application is the National Cancer Institute's (NCI's) workbook *Cancer Clinical Trials: The Basic Workbook*, available in the "Publications" section of its Web site, www.cancer.gov.

A public presentation on clinical trials also can be used to bring attention to a specific protocol. Such opportunities come up when the protocol involves a patient population not found within the CTN's typical practice setting. Examples of this would be a cancer prevention study or a study related to the emerging field of proteomics research, wherein prospective study participants need not have a current malignancy. Outside of comprehensive cancer center settings, this healthy population most likely would be limited to family members and visitors of patients at most other clinical practice areas. Therefore, the CTN in this situation would have to seek speaking venues outside of his or her practice setting to reach the necessary audience in meaningful quantities.

Credibility

Potential obstacles that the CTN can face when making a public-wide attempt at either protocol-specific or non–protocol-specific education are the issues of having a credible message and of being a credible messenger. Message credibility can readily be achieved with many audiences through a straightforward, user-friendly presentation of factual and relevant information. It is when the messenger's credibility is either not already established within the audience (i.e., through messenger and/or institution name recognition) or when the presentation fails to establish a credible message that the overall educational objective is not achieved. A preventive action plan for this situation could include first identifying a receptive and appropriate audience for the educational presentation and, second, having the information be presented by or mediated through a known credible messenger, such as a trusted community figure.

Explain the Importance of Eligibility Criteria

As part of public education efforts, the CTN should point out how and why most trials have very specific eligibility criteria that sometimes define a limited patient population. With the advent of targeted and other promising new therapies, this often means that to meet increasingly rigid eligibility criteria, the patient's disease must express specific surface markers. Those patients who do not meet the specific requirements of a study, especially if the trial has received advanced publicity that is encouraging, may very well feel that they have been denied hope. This especially can be true when patients with similar diagnoses exchange health information with each other in treatment settings. This all may contribute to a negative attitude toward the system of clinical trials, which patients may see as arbitrary and favoring scientific principle over patient care.

Formal Sessions for Targeted Groups

More formal approaches to public education on clinical trials have been explored. Ehrenberger, Breeden, and Donovan (2003) examined the implementation of an educational program that included NCI Cancer Clinical Trials Education Program workshops directed toward community-dwelling seniors who, because of their age, were at increased risk for cancer. The study found that these "lunch and learn" educational workshops increased awareness and improved community-dwelling seniors' attitudes toward clinical trials. Identifying an established network of senior health centers clearly facilitated this program's planning (Ehrenberger et al.).

Informational Materials

As limitations in human resources and in program infrastructure often affect the breadth of a clinical trial educational effort, it behooves the CTN to be aware of and take advantage of more simplistic yet readily available resources. Printed materials, such as brochures supplied by the study sponsor, in particular from NCI and some of the cancer cooperative groups, remain a common approach for the delivery of protocol-specific information. These materials represent a peer-reviewed and often no-cost communication tool for the CTN.

The computer and the Internet have both become a worldwide and common means to provide and acquire health information. More than fifty million American adults, or at least 55% of those with Internet access, have used the Web to get health or medical information (Fox & Rainie, 2000; Helft, 2004). A great many are using the Web to gather information on behalf of family or friends (Fox & Rainie). The CTN must recognize the strengths and weaknesses that this medium poses as a source of information for clinical trial education. How best to leverage the Internet's potential as a conduit for valid and forthright information about clinical trials, as well as how to deal with the potential barrage of questions from Internet-savvy patients or members of the public, should provide an impetus for the CTN to acquire and sharpen his or her computer technology skills. Challenges aside, this informational medium should be embraced as a useful tool in the cultivation of today's clinical research landscape.

The CTN must balance the opportunities provided by the Internet with the negative aspects that come with the plethora of health-related information, some of which information is either misleading or outright false. Increasingly, patients and physicians are using the Internet as a source of medical information (Wei et al., 2004). However, concerns exist that access to the Internet is not equivalent for all patients. The observation that minorities and older patients are less familiar with and have less access to the Internet (Metz et al., 2003; Smith et al., 2003) should be considered when planning for education to these populations.

Almost all cancer institutions now provide their own Internet-based information related to cancer care for the public. A mainstay of these Web sites is information related to clinical trials in general and/or about those offered through that institution. Although these sites provide the viewer with information on clinical trials, the availability typically is limited to that vicinity. To reach a wider geographical audience, several publicly or privately sponsored Web sites are available that provide accurate and up-to-date information on all aspects of clinical trial participation, along with registries for listings of actively accruing clinical trials being conducted across the country. Such sites include www.cancer.gov (NCI), www.centerwatch.com (CenterWatch Clinical Trials Listing Service), and http://clinicaltrials.gov (National Library of Medicine, National Institutes of Health). See Chapter 44 for additional information on cancer registries. The CTN should consider registries as a resource when an appropriate protocol is not being offered in his or her local area.

Summary

Educating patients and the public about clinical trials is essential to achieving any further progress in the overall approach to cancer. Oncology nurses play a major role in assessing for and reducing health-related knowledge deficits in patients through teaching. By disseminating information to his or her direct patient population as well as into the general public arena, the CTN can foster a better informed, and conceivably better engaged, healthcare-consuming population. Patient and public outreach education also helps to build a more research-supportive relationship with the CTN's healthcare colleagues through enlightenment and continuous updates on clinical trials. The oncology CTN should expand that role to include devising, implementing, and assessing techniques to effectively present accurate and up-to-date information about cancer clinical trials upon which a patient or the public can base their decision on whether to participate.

References

Comis, R., Miller, J., Aldige, C., Krebs, L., & Stoval, E. (2003). Public attitudes toward participation in cancer clinical trials. *Journal of Clinical Oncology, 21,* 830–835.

Connolly, N.B., Schneider, D., & Hill, A.M. (2004). Improving enrollment in cancer clinical trials. *Oncology Nursing Forum, 31,* 610–614.

Department of Health. (2000). *The NHS cancer plan: A plan for investment, a plan for reform.* London: Author.

Ehrenberger, H.E., Breeden, J.R., & Donovan, M.E. (2003). A demonstration project to increase awareness of cancer clinical trials among community-dwelling seniors [Online exclusive]. *Oncology Nursing Forum, 30,* E80–E83.

Fox, S., & Rainie, L. (2000, November 26). *The online health care revolution: How the Web helps Americans take better care of themselves.* Washington, DC: Pew Internet & American Life Project. Retrieved October 27, 2005, from http://www.pewinternet.org/reports/toc.asp?Report=26

Goodwin, J.S., Hunt, W.C., Humble, C.G., Jey, C.R., & Samet, J.M. (1988). Cancer treatment protocols: Who gets chosen? *Archives of Internal Medicine, 148,* 2258–2260.

Harris Interactive. (2001, January 22). Misconceptions and lack of awareness greatly reduce recruitment for cancer clinical trials. *Health Care News, 1*(3). Retrieved October 30, 2005, from http://www.harrisinteractive.com/news/newsletters/healthnews/HI_HealthCareNews2001Vol1_iss3.pdf

Helft, P.R. (2004). Breast cancer in the information age: A review of recent developments. *Breast Disease, 21,* 41–46.

Linnan, L.A., Ferguson, Y.O., Wasilewski, Y., Lee, A.M., Yang, J., Solomon, F., et al. (2005). Using community-based participatory research methods to reach women with health messages: Results from the North Carolina BEAUTY and Health Pilot Project. *Health Promotion Practice, 6,* 164–173.

Metz, J.M., Devine, P., DeNittis, A., Jones, H., Hampshire, M., Goldwein, J., et al. (2003). A multi-institutional study of Internet utilization by radiation oncology patients. *International Journal of Radiation Oncology, Biology, Physics, 56,* 1201–1205.

Nurgat, Z.A., Craig, W., Campbell, N.C., Bissett, J.D., Cassidy, J., & Nicolson, M.C. (2005). Patient motivations surrounding participation in phase I and phase II clinical trials of cancer chemotherapy. *British Journal of Cancer, 92,* 1001–1005.

Segelov, E., Tattersall, M.H., & Coates, A.S. (1992). Redressing the balance: The ethics of not entering an eligible patient on a randomised clinical trial. *Annals of Oncology, 3,* 103–105.

Smith, R.P., Devine, P., Jones, H., DeNittis, A., Whittington, R., & Metz, J.M. (2003). Internet use by patients with prostate cancer undergoing radiotherapy. *Urology, 62,* 273–277.

Tejeda, H.A., Green, S.B., Trimble, E.L., Ford, L., High, J.L., Ungerleider, R.S., et al. (1996). Representation of African-Americans, Hispanics, and whites in National Cancer Institute cancer treatment trials. *Journal of the National Cancer Institute, 88,* 812–816.

Templeton, H., & Coates, V. (2003). Evaluation of an evidence-based education package for men with prostate cancer on hormonal manipulation therapy. *Patient Education and Counseling, 55,* 55–61.

Townsley, C., Selby, R., & Sui, L. (2005). Systematic review of barriers to the recruitment of older patients with cancer onto clinical trials. *Journal of Clinical Oncology, 23,* 3112–3124.

Varrichio, C.G., McCabe, M.S., Trimble, E., & Korn, E.L. (1996). Quality of life in clinical cancer trials. Introduction. *Journal of the National Cancer Institute, 20,* vii–viii.

Wei, S.J., Metz, J.M., Coyle, C., Hampshire, M., Jones, H.A., Markowitz, S., et al. (2004). Recruitment of patients into an Internet-based clinical trials database: The experience of OncoLink and the National Colorectal Cancer Research Alliance. *Journal of Clinical Oncology, 22,* 4730–4736.

CHAPTER 21

Recruitment and Promotion Strategies for Clinical Trials

Jacquelin Holland, RNC, WHNP-BC

Introduction

Recruiting patients to clinical trials is one of the first roles listed in a clinical trial nurse's (CTN's) job description. Experts warn that with recent advances in biotechnology, the demand for patients to enter clinical trials far exceeds the available supply (Mundell, 2006). This chapter will identify strategies that can be used to increase the recruitment of participants to clinical trials and will discuss the importance of tailoring recruitment methods to meet the needs of special populations. The number of adult participants in clinical trials varies between 3%–5% nationwide (National Cancer Institute [NCI], 2006), with overall accrual estimated to be between 5%–10% of all patients with cancer (Mundell). The low number of adult participants impedes progress toward treatment advances and potential cure of cancer.

Recruitment

Spilker and Cramer (1992) described the stages of recruitment that should be reviewed before starting a clinical trial (see Figure 21-1). The first stage is to *develop a plan on how to contact patients*, which requires an estimate of the pool of patients in the catchment area who would qualify for enrollment. This especially is helpful when initiating a chemoprevention clinical trial, in which the patient does not have a cancer diagnosis. Reviewing the trial requirements is necessary to determine the eligibility criteria that may inhibit recruitment. If a patient has to undergo expensive or invasive tests because of a study requirement, he or she may choose not to enroll in the study. The last item in the development plan is to *estimate the rate of enrollment*. This is one way to determine whether an adequate number of patients will be enrolled and to provide enough time to develop additional strategies for recruitment.

The second stage refers to the *development of a referral base*. This is especially important with chemoprevention trials, in which one must determine at what point the patient will enter the study. For example, in working with a

colorectal cancer prevention study, some patients may see a surgeon, whereas others initially see a gastroenterologist. Therefore, the research staff should meet with both groups, provide information about the study, describe the role of the research staff, and obtain support for the study.

The Health Insurance Portability and Accountability Act Privacy Rule also may affect the process of screening patients. The rule is the first comprehensive federal protection for the privacy of personal health information. Therefore, the prospective participant must be informed about the Privacy Rule Authorization Form and Clinical Research. The research team must explain that questions might be asked regarding the patient's health background,

---

Figure 21-1. Recruitment Steps

1. Develop a plan to reach patients.
2. Review eligibility criteria.
3. Identify criteria that would hinder recruitment.
4. Develop a referral base.
   - Physicians, nurses, healthcare personnel
   - Professional societies
   - Faith-based and community groups
5. Estimate enrollment rate.
6. Market clinical trial.
   - Use media to inform public.
   - Develop institutional table tent cards and payroll inserts.
   - Distribute institutional e-mail announcements.
   - Post listings of open trials on institution Web site with eligibility criteria and schema and research nurse's phone number.
   - Utilize on-hold messages.
7. Use direct mail to patients and public.
8. Educate key players.
   - Nurse colleagues in cancer programs
   - Tumor board
   - Hospital newsletters
   - In-services
   - Community focus groups
9. Screen patients.
10. Initiate informed consent process.

Note. Based on information from Spilker & Cramer, 1992.

The author would like to acknowledge Bertie A. Ford, RN, MS, AOCN®, for her contribution that remains unchanged from the first edition.

social security number, ethnic origin, medical records, and/or notes taken by a doctor or nurse. In certain situations, this could be a deterrent for the participant unless clear, concise, and careful explanations are given regarding the privacy rule.

Referrals for patients who may be potential study participants can come from medical and nonmedical sources, such as family and friends of current patients, professional societies, and lay organizations. The research staff periodically may have difficulty identifying patients for a particular study and will need to rely on others to identify and refer the patients.

According to Spilker and Cramer (1992), the third stage of recruitment is to *use the media* (e.g., radio, television, newspapers) to promote the study. Using advertising for recruitment can be expensive, however, unless the media can promote the trial through a patient interest story or public service announcement that includes a study participant. Additionally, any program to be released to the public must have institutional review board approval.

When marketing clinical trials, marketing departments, in conjunction with research staff, should use a multicustomer approach to inform physicians (who may refer patients) as well as patients themselves. Clinical trial marketing can be taken to the work site by inserting clinical trial information into pay stubs, displaying table tents in the cafeteria, and promoting participation through e-mail broadcasts. Some institutions have a nurse who serves as a recruitment coordinator for specific trials (Ward & Swanson, 1995). Marketing trials to physicians must highlight what would be attractive to physicians who wish to participate. Additionally, the study must address an important research question, be relatively easy to conduct, and employ uncomplicated data collection methods (Macbeth & Stephens, 1996).

The fourth stage in recruitment involves *directly contacting potential participants* (Spilker & Cramer, 1992). Medical records should be screened for potentially eligible patients, and each of the patients should be sent a letter of invitation that describes the available clinical trial. Obtain mailing lists and contact work sites, organizations, specific minority groups, and faith-based organizations to identify potential patients.

The fifth stage of recruitment is *discussing the trial and educating others about it* (Spilker & Cramer, 1992). Educating physicians and nurses, as well as patients, can help recruitment. This can occur within a department, within an institution, in the community (e.g., faith-based or other organizations' meetings), or at professional meetings. Forming focus groups that include key members of the community from whom the CTN wishes to get feedback and ideas about recruiting patients to the trial is important (Paskett, DeGraffinreid, Tatum, & Margitic, 1996). Institutions that participated in the Breast Cancer Prevention Trial, sponsored by the National Surgical Adjuvant Breast and Bowel Project (NSABP), and the Prostate Cancer Prevention

Trial, which was coordinated by the Southwest Oncology Group, used this technique, as they were involved in the discussions (NCI, 2002). The largest breast cancer prevention trial ever conducted is called the STAR trial. Its purpose was to determine which drug, tamoxifen or raloxifene, is more effective in preventing breast cancer with fewer side effects in postmenopausal women at increased risk for developing the disease. The NSABP used several innovative strategies to encourage minority women to participate in STAR. Among these was the STAR Community Outreach Program for Education (known as SCOPE), which took place in several cities in the United States. The effort to increase the participation of women from racial and ethnic minority groups resulted in 93.4% of the participants being white (18,446 women) and 6% being from racial and ethnic minority groups, showing 2.5% African American (488 women), 2% Hispanic (394 women), and 2.1% of other ethnicities (419 women). These figures represent an improvement over the 4% that participated in the Breast Cancer Prevention Trial. These statistics were based on self-identification by the women. In addition to this effort, the National Medical Association, a network of more than 20,000 African American physicians, worked closely with NSABP, resulting in the first year showing slightly increased participation of African American women (NCI, 2006).

The sixth and seventh stages involve *determining patient interest* and *conducting the initial screenings of interested patients* (Spilker & Cramer, 1992). Initial screenings can be conducted in person, over the telephone, or by completing pre-enrollment questionnaires that are mailed to the person's home. The eighth and ninth stages of recruitment involve *performing detailed screening* to *determine patient eligibility.* The last stage of recruitment is to obtain patients' *informed consent* (Spilker & Cramer).

Barriers to Recruitment

Barriers to participation were identified in an evidence report (Ford et al., 2005) and divided into (a) patient barriers, (b) study design barriers, (c) provider barriers, and (d) healthcare system barriers. Examples of barriers included lack of education about trials by patients and healthcare providers, lack of knowledge about origins of cancer, lack of culturally relevant education about clinical trials, limited education or low literacy of potential participants, and lack of dissemination of study opportunities to providers and patients.

The Coalition of Cancer Cooperative Groups reported at the 2006 Annual Meeting of the American Society of Clinical Oncology that 40% of patients with cancer either enrolled or tried to enroll in a clinical trial when informed about one by their doctor (Tam-McDevitt et al., 2007). However, provider barriers, such as increased costs to their practice for the infrastructure to support clinical trials, hinder enrollment. The result is that approximately 70% of patients enrolled are enrolled by 30% of physicians (Mundell, 2006).

Barriers to Recruitment of Special Populations

Specific cultural barriers were delineated in a study involving African Americans (Adams-Campbell et al., 2004). The enrollment was done at Howard University Cancer Center in Washington, DC. The study showed an overall eligibility rate of 8.5% (20 out of 235 patients); however, the enrollment rate among the eligible population was 60% (12 out of 20 patients). Comorbidities rendered 17.1% of the patient population ineligible for the trials. Comorbidities included advanced disease stage, respiratory failure, HIV, anemia, cardiovascular diseases, and renal insufficiency. The researchers determined that comorbidity is a major issue in recruitment of this population in trials (Adams-Campbell et al.).

Murthy, Krumholz, and Gross (2004) analyzed the ethnic distribution of patients enrolled in trials and found that it varied significantly across racial/ethnic and age groups. Older adults and racial and ethnic minorities were less likely to enroll in cooperative group cancer trials than were whites. The identification of barriers in this study showed that the federal policy to expand Medicare coverage for cancer clinical trials most likely would not increase the level of older adult participants (Lewis et al., 2003). Other roadblocks to accrual were older patients being less likely to seek out clinical trials, transportation problems with distant providers, comorbidities, and the reluctance of some investigators to enroll older adult patients. Some trials may even require that patients have a life expectancy of 5 or 10 years.

Recruitment Strategies

Physicians play a critical role in enrolling patients in clinical trials. After a physician expresses interest in supporting a clinical trial, key strategies may enhance his or her willingness to participate (see Figure 21-2). First, physicians should be assured that an infrastructure is available to support them in their research endeavors. If one does not exist, participation may be withheld. Second, incentives for physicians to participate should be provided (e.g., increased funding for grants, per-patient reimbursement, money for travel to educational meetings, recognition).

Additionally, small gifts for participants (e.g., certificates, mugs, pens, free lunch certificates, free parking passes) demonstrate the gratitude of the staff and institution. Recognition is a powerful tool, especially if participants in a clinical trial can help to recruit other participants. Some institutions provide recognition or thank-you dinners to their participants in large chemoprevention trials. This is an excellent idea because current participants can refer potential participants to future trials. Patients may receive thank-you notes after they complete their clinical trial as further confirmation of

---

Figure 21-2. Key Recruitment Strategies

Provider
1. Provide infrastructure to support clinical trial activities.
2. Provide incentives.
   - Increased funding for grants
   - Per-patient reimbursement
   - Funding for educational travel
   - Professional and public recognition

Participants
1. Give recognition.
   - Thank-you notes
   - Thank-you dinners
2. Offer gifts.
   - Certificates
   - Mugs
   - Key chains
   - T-shirts
   - Pens
   - Free lunch pass
   - Free parking pass

---

their importance to clinical research. As CTNs increase efforts to educate the public about clinical trial participation, reference to the improvement of cancer treatment for future generations may serve as a strong incentive to individuals.

A project directed toward the education of oncology nurses regarding minority recruitment, the Oncology Nursing Society Clinical Trials Education Project webcast "Clinical Trials: Opening Doors for the Underserved 2005," identified the need for knowledge of underserved groups, reasons for low accrual among these groups, why inclusion in trials is critical, and development of strategies for increasing accrual. The webcast is available online at http://onsopcontent.ons.org/Education/Webcasts/ClinicalTrials/. The general public appears to have little knowledge of the cancer clinical trials process (Harris Interactive, 2001), and education programs are necessary to meet this need. It is important that healthcare professionals receive education to support their role in the process.

An institutional effort is in place at the Ohio State University Medical Center's James Cancer Hospital and Solove Research Institute in Columbus. The hospital created a department called the Diversity Enhancement Program for the sole purpose of raising awareness of cancer clinical trials in the community, targeting minority and underserved populations. This department is hospital-funded and was created from recommendations from a previous hospital committee called Women and Minorities. The committee had the responsibility of reviewing accrual data, examining recruitment strategies, and recommending solutions to the hospital administrative staff to improve accrual. The department replaced the work of that committee. This program focuses internally on educating staff, increasing the diversity of the staff, and implementing cultural competency programs. Externally, the department reaches thousands of community residents with cancer and clinical trial information by working with individuals at the grassroots level, other healthcare organizations, businesses, faith-based organizations, and educational institutions. To assist with these efforts, the department has applied for and received numerous grants to continue the work. An example is a grant renewed for three years that is funded by Susan B. Komen for the Cure to educate older minority women about clinical trials and participation with the expectation that they would assist with reaching members of the community and their families. Institutions must evaluate their goals and objectives to increase accrual of the ethnic and minority population and decide whether the funding of a department dedicated to this task is feasible.

Efforts also are being directed toward recruitment of minority medical faculty and funded clinical investigators. Although academic physicians usually are involved in the development of clinical research protocols, the percentage of racial and ethnic minority physicians choosing to pursue careers in academic medicine is disproportionately low (Christian & Trimble, 2003). Staff is needed to help to design studies that are relevant to minority communities. Major academic cancer centers need minority investigators who are active members of clinical trial cooperative groups. NSABP's diversity strategic planning committee has spearheaded travel grants for young minority investigators to attend their national meetings. NSABP also provides grant funding for young investigators in support of their research efforts.

Summary

Patients participate in clinical trials for multiple reasons (see Chapter 19 for a more in-depth discussion). Spilker and Cramer (1992) identified 10 stages of recruitment that can be used to increase clinical trial enrollment. The CTN may be responsible for recruitment regardless of whether a marketing department is available to develop a recruitment plan. Involving the media, increasing physician referrals, and using incentives to encourage physicians and patients are a few of the many strategies that may be employed when faced with this challenging task.

Program designs should incorporate information geared toward minority, underserved, and older adult populations. Ongoing continuing education for the CTN, as well as for other members of the oncology team, will ensure consideration of needs of special populations in recruitment strategic plans. The special efforts required for recruiting minority, disadvantaged, and/or older adult patients might result in achieving the patient accrual required for successful clinical trials.

References

Adams-Campbell, L., Ahaghotu, C., Gaskins, M., Dawkins, F.W., Smoot, D., Polk, O.D., et al. (2004). Enrollment of African Americans onto clinical treatment trials: Study design barriers. *Journal of Clinical Oncology, 22*, 730–734.

Christian, M.C., & Trimble, E. (2003). Increasing participation of physicians and patients from underrepresented racial and ethnic groups in National Cancer Institute-sponsored clinical trials. *Cancer Epidemiology, Biomarkers and Prevention, 12*, 277S–283S.

Ford, J., Howerton, M., Bolen, S., Gary, T., Lai, G., Tilburt, J., et al. (2005, June). *Knowledge and access to information on recruitment of underrepresented populations to cancer clinical trials* [AHRQ Publication No. 05-E019-2]. Rockville, MD: Agency for Health Research and Quality.

Lewis, J., Kilgore, M., Goldman, D., Trimble, E., Kaplan, R., Montello, M., et al. (2003). Participation of patients 65 years of age or older in cancer clinical trials. *Journal of Clinical Oncology, 21*, 1383–1389.

Macbeth, F., & Stephens, R. (1996). Marketing clinical trials. *Lancet, 348*, 111–112.

Mundell, E.J. (2006, July 10). *Clinical trials for cancer running out of volunteers.* Retrieved September 1, 2007, from http://prostatecancer.about.com/b/a/257608.htm

Murthy, V.H., Krumholz, H.M., & Gross, C.P. (2004). Participation in cancer clinical trials: Race-, sex-, and age-based disparities. *JAMA, 292*, 2720–2726.

National Cancer Institute. (2002, September). *Cancer clinical trials: The basic workbook.* Retrieved March 10, 2007, from http://www.cancer.gov/clinicaltrials/resources/basicworkbook

National Cancer Institute. (2006, June 21). *The Study of Tamoxifen and Raloxifene (STAR): Questions and answers.* Retrieved March 26, 2007, from http://www.cancer.gov/cancertopics/factsheet/STARresultsQandA

Paskett, E.D., DeGraffinreid, C., Tatum, C.M., & Margitic, S.E. (1996). The recruitment of African-Americans to cancer prevention and control studies. *Preventive Medicine, 25*, 547–553.

Spilker, B., & Cramer, J.A. (1992). *Patient recruitment in clinical trials.* New York: Raven Press.

Tam-McDevitt, J., Balducci, L., Hauser, R.S., Gura, D., Paraghamian, A.L., Thomas, H., et al. (2007). Has demand for clinical trial participants outpaced supply? Correspondence. *Journal of the National Cancer Institute, 99*, 86–87.

Ward, A.J., & Swanson, G.M. (1995). Recruiting minorities into clinical trials: Toward a participant-friendly system. *Journal of the National Cancer Institute, 87*, 1947–1959.

Additional Resource

National Institutes of Health. (2007, February 2). *HIPAA privacy rule: Why should researchers be aware of the HIPAA privacy rule?* Retrieved August 14, 2007, from http://privacyruleandresearch.nih.gov/pr_03.asp

CHAPTER 22
Eligibility

Susan Anderson, RN, BSN, MFA

Introduction

Screening and eligibility criteria identify the patient group to be studied in a clinical trial. The eligibility criteria are stated clearly in each study and establish the parameters and guidelines that define the appropriate patient population. The parameters might limit the participants to patients with a specific type of cancer at a particular stage. The eligibility criteria should include requirements that the patient must have the capacity to give informed consent, general health parameters to protect the patient from untoward effects, and the exclusion of certain comorbidities to determine if effects, both good and bad, are related to the cancer or to an underlying disease.

The clinical trial nurse (CTN) plays a key role in identifying eligible patients, teaching patients and medical staff the importance and purpose of eligibility criteria, and ensuring that appropriate patients are enrolled into studies.

Eligibility Screening

When a study is being designed, much thought is given to the patient population. Ideally, patients enrolled will be those that will best answer the hypothesis of the study. The protocol must, through the eligibility requirements, specify a clearly defined patient group, thereby minimizing any unnecessary or confounding variables in reaching the goals of the study. For example, if the study is measuring the efficacy of a standard adjuvant treatment regimen in breast cancer and comparing it to a higher dose or different schedule of chemotherapy, all patients must be free of metastatic disease. However, the histologic category, estrogen status, or other variables may need to be limited to answer a specific or additional research question. This particularly is true of phase II studies (Hageman & Reeves, 2001).

Phase I trials are less concerned with histology or the extent of disease because the main goal is to establish a safe dose level (Simon, 2001). Organ function, however, plays an important part in testing drug tolerability and the extent of toxicities in these studies. Therefore, parameters of hepatic and renal function may be outlined in the eligibility requirements. Histology and the extent of disease become much more crucial in defining eligibility in phase II studies, where the response to the drug is being tested in a specific disease site. A staging work-up completed within a specified time frame (e.g., two weeks) may be required prior to registration or randomization to ensure that the desired extent of disease has not changed.

Eligibility is written in a format that defines inclusion and exclusion criteria (see Figure 22-1). Inclusion criteria are the elements that must be satisfied before a patient can enter into a trial, whereas exclusion criteria identify elements that, if met, will keep the patient from participating in the trial. Once determined, eligibility criteria must be adhered to. For example, if a platelet count of more than $100,000/mm^3$ is required, then a patient with a platelet count of $101,000/mm^3$ can be enrolled, and a patient with a platelet count of $99,000/mm^3$ cannot be enrolled. Similarly, if a hemoglobin level below 10 g/100 ml is identified in the exclusion criteria, then a patient with a hemoglobin level of 9.8 g/100 ml will not be eligible to participate in the trial. Sometimes a study chair will grant an exception if it would not affect study data or patient safety, such as if a patient had a laboratory test that is one day out of the acceptable window.

Prior to enrolling a patient in a study, the CTN is responsible for confirming that all of the criteria have been met. This is accomplished by interviewing the patient, reviewing the medical record, and obtaining documentation of all required data prior to registering the patient (see Figure 22-2).

Required Testing

All laboratory testing and scans must be completed and documented *before* the patient is enrolled. All studies must have been completed within the time frame specified in the protocol. Most studies are very specific; however, if no time frame is identified, a good rule of thumb is to

Figure 22-1. Example of Eligibility/Pretreatment Worksheet

Protocol	Primary Nurse:
Name:	
Unit #:	Pts Home Phone:
SS #:	Patient Medical Record Number:
DOB:	Attending Physician:
Sex:	
Race:	Fellow:
Primary Tumor Site:	
Stage of Disease:	

Eligibility Criteria	Comments
Older than age 18	
Path confirmed breast ER/PR status +	
Progressive disease after 2 or more cytotoxic regimens for metastatic cancer	
CBC/Chemistries suitable for treatment	
No investigational agent within 3 weeks prior to treatment	
Karnofsky ≥ 50	
Measurable or evaluable disease by RECIST criteria	
Signed informed consent	
HIPAA authorization	
No pregnancy/lactation; effective birth control	
Another uncured malignancy	
History CHF	
Sign/Sym CHF	
Consent signed/dated	
Date of confirmed metastasis	
Prior treatment for metastasis/date	

Prestudy Evaluation (Within 1 Month)	Result	Date	Remarks
Complete H&P			
Height & weight			
BSA			
Vital signs			
CXR			
EKG			
MUGA/echo			
Tumor measurements			
Performance status—Karnofsky			
Beta HCG			
Performed within 5 days			
WBC (4.0–10.0)			
ANC			
Hgb (M 14–18, F 12–16)			
Hct (M 40–52, F 37–47)			
Segs/Bands			
Lymphs			
Platelets (150–350)			
PT/PTT (< 13; < 1 sec contr/25–38)			
Glucose (70–105)			
BUN (8.0–18)			
Creatinine (0.5–1.2)			
CO_2 (22–30)			
Chloride (96–106)			
Sodium (135–145)			
Potassium (3.5–5.0)			
Calcium (9.1–10.6)			
Phosphorus (3.1–4.5)			
T. Protein (6.0–8.0)			
Albumin (3.5–5.0)			
Bili D/Total (< 0.2/< 1.2)			
SGPT/SGOT (0–35)			
LDH (118–242)			
Alk Phos (30–114)			

Figure 22-2. Basic Components of Eligibility Criteria

- Evidence of a specific oncologic or hematologic histology
- Level of overall health of the patient (usually measured by Karnofsky or Eastern Cooperative Oncology Group performance status)
- Age limits
- Major organ system functioning
- Prior medical history, especially related to other malignancies
- Establishment of a baseline disease state from which to measure disease response
- Allowance of concomitant illnesses/medications
- Protection for future offspring of patients of childbearing age
- Establishment of a psychological or mental status that presumes compliance with the study

have all laboratory testing completed within seven days of initiating the experimental therapy. Erroneously entering a patient with outdated laboratory tests or results that do not meet eligibility criteria will render the patient inevaluable and will compromise the study data and data analysis, thus resulting in a major protocol violation.

Financial Screening

The financial aspects of treatment on a research study can be a complicated process within the current economic atmosphere. The nurse should understand the economic considerations for study patients prior to any discussion with a patient about participating in a study. The patient must obtain approval for coverage by his or her insurance payer prior to enrolling in a study. The nurse can play a key role in the development of a study by monitoring unnecessary expenses and streamlining patient visits that might drive up costs needlessly. Caution must be exercised, however, to not dilute the findings of the study simply to make it less costly. Each protocol should have a section addressing this issue, and the nurse needs to know the particulars of each study. The range of costs and reimbursement policies vary and need to be verified in each individual case.

Sponsors (such as pharmaceutical companies) may pay for everything associated with the study, including all lab tests, treatments, doctor visits, and even parking or transportation costs. Drugs obtained from the National Cancer Institute are provided free of charge to the patient. However, doctor visits and tests, such as blood work and scans, may not be covered. Some third-party payers will reimburse patients' costs if they are equal to standard therapy costs, depending on individual state regulations, whereas others will not provide reimbursement if a research drug or treatment is involved.

The following Web pages provide guidelines for Medicare and Medicaid clinical trial coverage: www.cms.hhs.gov and www.cms.hhs.gov/MLNGeninfo

Compliance Screening and Plan

During the CTN's initial encounters with the patient and his or her family, the CTN should perform a *compliance*

assessment. The CTN should consider the following questions: Is the patient capable of following the instructions necessary to comply with all aspects of the study? Is the patient capable of traveling to the facility when necessary? Does the patient fully understand the dangers or risks involved with the study? Will the patient be responsible in reporting symptoms and warning signs to the appropriate medical personnel? If serious concerns develop regarding the patient's ability to fulfill the necessary steps in the study, the nurse must discuss them with the principal investigator. These are important factors to consider in developing a plan for the patient and family and in establishing a calendar for tests and treatments. Patients and family members need to know who to call and what to do if a serious toxicity or problem develops while the patient is on-study. See Chapter 30 for additional information about compliance in clinical trials.

Pathology Review

Pathology reports are crucial in determining patient eligibility, particularly in phase II and III studies. Some institutions require a special review if the original pathology was performed at another facility. Cooperative groups and sponsors sometimes require a centralized review of pathology specimens to ensure consistency. Generally, these requirements are delineated clearly within the text of the protocol. Some special pathology studies may require additional consent from the patient, such as receptor status (e.g., estrogen receptor [ER] and progesterone receptor [PR] status, HER2 expression for patients with breast cancer) or tumor samples for vaccines or genetic studies. Additional consent is required when an extra procedure is required or when analyses are added at a later date. If the original consent includes studies to be performed on blood or tissue, then additional consent for ER/PR or HER2 is not required.

Staging Guidelines

Protocol eligibility criteria identify patients with a specific stage of disease for enrollment. The purpose of staging systems is to classify or describe the extent of disease to provide the physician with enough information to determine treatment options and prognostic indicators. The most common system for staging or categorizing the extent of disease is the tumor, node, metastasis (TNM) system, in which T is the primary tumor size, N indicates the regional lymph node involvement, and M represents distant metastasis (Greene et al., 2002). The TNM system is based on a clinical assessment and work-up. The criteria for evaluating each component of the TNM system were developed by the American Joint Committee on Cancer and are specifically outlined for each disease site in the *AJCC Cancer Staging Manual* (Greene et al.). TNM staging is essential to phase II and III studies, in which the primary goal of the study is to determine response in a specific stage of a specific disease.

The physician is responsible for assessing the stage of the patient's disease, clinical and/or pathologic, depending upon the study end points. Staging is discussed frequently at tumor board meetings or in consultation with physicians from related disciplines, such as pathology and radiology. The CTN must confirm that the staging has been completed *before* enrolling the patient into the study.

Patient, Family, and Professional Education

Patient education begins when the CTN first meets the patient and his or her family. Education, like informed consent, is an ongoing process that requires repetition, patience, and reinforcement. The CTN plays a major role because of his or her familiarity with the concepts of research, basic knowledge of treatments and healthcare delivery, and expertise in the purpose and details of the specific protocol. The CTN designs tools to help the patient to understand the study and his or her responsibilities as a participant. Calendars and pamphlets are study-specific and should be helpful for individual patient situations. An identification card for patients, citing the particular study and a contact person, provides an effective way to help them to communicate with healthcare workers involved in the study.

Professional education is provided to all professionals who will be involved with the patient during the study. Medical, nursing, pharmacy, and support staff all need an orientation appropriate to their level of understanding and degree of involvement with the study. A protocol abridgment (a brief synopsis of the study) and in-service programs should be planned and presented prior to the opening of the study. See Chapter 10 for additional information about staff education.

Registration/Randomization

Patients usually are registered with the study sponsor or centralized registry within the institution responsible for gathering data. Forms for registration include demographics and specific information regarding eligibility. All information must be gathered and documented before registration. Off-site registries usually will accept telephone, fax, or online registrations and will return a confirmation document.

Randomization to a specific treatment arm is performed to avoid unconscious or systematic bias for study outcomes. Patients sometimes are stratified into defined prognostic groups and then randomized to allow bias-free statistical comparison. However, this must be accomplished in a way that minimizes the influence on study end points. A computer, at a centralized location away from the institution providing the treatment, frequently is used to do the randomization. Prior to beginning a study, a research team member is responsible for registration and for obtaining the randomization arm assignment. The treatment assignment is documented in the patient's medical record. Occasionally,

a study chart is kept in addition to the medical record for study-specific clerical documents that do not pertain to the patient's medical condition. During audits, however, both charts must be made available.

Documentation/Forms Submission

All documentation related to the patient's medical condition during the study must be kept in the patient's medical record. These data then are entered into computer or paper research files for analysis. These research files are known as case report forms. They are designed specifically for each study to organize data consistent with the study-specific end points.

Nothing can be entered into the research file that does not exist in the patient's medical record. The maintenance of the medical record is extremely important. The research team and the staff involved with the patient must perform meticulous note-taking and documentation. All physician notes, laboratory reports, and other pertinent information must be filed in the medical record, as well as any communication among the physician, CTN, and study personnel.

The quality of the data is related directly to the accuracy and thoroughness of the documentation. The CTN expedites the study process by developing well-organized, clearly stated documentation.

Summary

Screening and confirming a patient's eligibility is an early, crucial step in managing a successful trial. All criteria must be met and documented in the patient's medical record. Patients must not be started on any clinical trial until all of these criteria have been met. Using a checklist is the most efficient and secure way to establish this information. The level of accuracy and compliance at this point in the study establishes the baseline by which all effects and responses of the treatment being tested will be measured.

References

Greene, F.L., Page, D.L., Fleming, I.D., Fritz, A.G., Balch, C.M., Haller, D., et al. (2002). *AJCC cancer staging manual* (6th ed.). New York: Springer-Verlag.

Hageman, D., & Reeves, D. (2001). Research data management. In V.T. DeVita, S. Hellman, & S.A. Rosenberg (Eds.), *Cancer: Principles and practice of oncology* (6th ed., pp. 539–545). Philadelphia: Lippincott Williams & Wilkins.

Simon, R. (2001). Design and analysis of clinical trials. In V.T. DeVita, S. Hellman, & S.A. Rosenberg (Eds.), *Cancer: Principles and practice of oncology* (6th ed., pp. 521–538). Philadelphia: Lippincott Williams & Wilkins.

Additional Resources

Daugherty, C.K., Ratain, M.J., & Siegler, M. (2001). Ethical issues in clinical research of cancer. In V.T. DeVita, S. Hellman, & S.A. Rosenberg (Eds.), *Cancer: Principles and practice of oncology* (6th ed., pp. 3126–3134). Philadelphia: Lippincott Williams & Wilkins.

Friedman, M.D. (1995). Clinical trials. In G. Murphy, W. Lawrence, & R.E. Lenhard (Eds.), *American Cancer Society textbook of clinical oncology* (2nd ed., pp. 194–197). Atlanta, GA: American Cancer Society.

CHAPTER 23
Designing a Computerized Tool to Verify Eligibility

Vilma Lopez, RN, MSN, OCN®

Introduction

Few computer-based systems exist that match subjects with clinical trials. An extensive search failed to reveal an evidence-based practice tool in CINAHL®, Ovid, PubMed, or the Cochrane Library for verifying eligibility. This chapter will guide the reader through the development of a computerized tool to verify eligibility. The author acknowledges that a variety of software programs may be used to construct an eligibility verification tool. It is the reader's choice to select one that is most appropriate in his or her setting.

Review of the Literature

Tu, Kemper, Lane, Carlson, and Musen (1993) designed a quantitative and probabilistic model and a computer program to help physicians to find potentially eligible patients. This program is neither trial-specific nor based on eligibility criteria. The National Cancer Institute (2007) has its Physician Data Query (PDQ) comprehensive cancer database, which allows Web-based searches for available clinical trials in the database. Fink et al. (2003) have developed a system using logical expressions that determines a patient's eligibility for each trial. It is based on the cost of tests, whether an immediate decision can be made, and a number of related clauses. It is not based on eligibility criteria but on the probability that the answer will lead to a trial for which the patient would be eligible. OncoDoc is a decision support system designed to provide therapeutic recommendations for patients with breast cancer. Used as a computer-based eligibility screening, it matches patient parameters to available clinical trials. Seroussi and Bouaud (2003) analyzed reasons for nonenrollment of potentially eligible patients and found that 30.5% were not recruited because they did not completely match the eligibility criteria of the recommended clinical trials. Seroussi and Bouaud's sample is too small to draw general conclusions based on the results. However, it emphasizes the importance of verification prior to enrollment.

Significance and Background

Selecting eligible subjects is one of the main roles of the clinical trial nurse (CTN). In the clinical setting, screenings are done to determine eligibility prior to enrollment (see Chapter 22: Eligibility). Verifying eligibility also is an important part of monitoring and auditing clinical trials. Enrolling ineligible subjects is a protocol violation. Therefore, finding eligible subjects is basic for compliance. Trials are approved with a limit in the number of subjects that can be accrued. Increasing the accrual number usually requires a protocol amendment. In most situations, ineligible subjects are not evaluable for trial results (i.e., are not included in the data analysis). Ensuring that proper screening is performed to enroll eligible subjects is not only important for trial results but also is cost and time effective.

The screening process requires auditing the subject's medical history and reviewing test results and demographics to ensure that the subject meets the eligibility criteria. The review is time intensive, but it needs to be completed quickly.

All protocols share commonalities, but eligibility criteria for each one are unique. The use of an eligibility verification tool offers many benefits. It simplifies the process by keeping all the required information available at one's fingertips. It provides a list of tests and evaluations, acceptable dates for each one, and acceptable values. Furthermore, it facilitates or eliminates most of the decisions for eligibility screening. With a uniform system, data entry is easier, and the rate of errors decreases. If the protocol manager is not available, any other person can complete the screening, even if the individual is not familiar with the protocol.

The eligibility tool presented later in this chapter does not require purchasing specialized software. It uses Microsoft® Excel®, with which the majority of research workers are familiar. Preparing an automated eligibility tool requires an in-depth review and understanding of the eligibility criteria (see Chapter 22), as well as some preparation. Preparing the criteria is comparable to preparing an eligibility checklist. Once the CTN completes the preparatory process, the tool can be built easily.

The main steps in the preparatory process include

- Reviewing the eligibility criteria
- Simplifying complex criteria
- Determining which source documents are required
- Determining time frames for the documents
- Establishing types of answers for each criterion
- Setting validation parameters.

These steps are necessary for eligibility screening even if the CTN is not going to use the tool described herein. The final result of the process is determination of the patient's eligibility status.

Nursing Preparatory Process

Review the Eligibility Criteria

The eligibility criteria are predefined requirements that the subject should meet before enrolling or registering in a clinical trial or protocol. Inclusion criteria allow the subject's enrollment, whereas exclusion criteria prevent it. The majority of protocols contain a special section for the eligibility criteria. The examples presented in this document have been selected for didactic purposes and may or may not be found within one protocol.

Simplify Complex Criteria

Eligibility criteria need to be differentiated between simple and complex. "Signed informed consent" or "platelets equal to or higher than 100,000" are examples of *simple criteria*. A simple criterion does not require any extra work. A *complex criterion* contains several items. It is necessary to identify all complex criteria and separate each one into its lowest level elements. Each item needs to be answered independently or sorted out for determining eligibility. For example, "adequate bone marrow function (hemoglobin equal to or higher than 10, platelets equal to or higher than 100,000, and absolute neutrophil count equal to or higher than 1,500)" is a complex inclusion criterion because it needs three different values for a positive answer. "Patients with NYHA class III/IV congestive heart failure, unstable angina, or MI in the last 6 months, or evidence of active myocardial ischemia on ECG" (Mathew, 2004) also is a complex criterion. If any of the four elements is answered positively, the patient is excluded from the protocol. See an example of the simplified criterion in Figure 23-1.

Simplifying complex criteria is a key concept for the successful implementation of an eligibility tool. The CTN must follow the same process for each criterion until *all* of them are simplified. The original criteria in the protocol may have five inclusion criteria and five exclusion criteria. The list after simplifying the complex criteria may result in 20 or 30 items each for inclusion and exclusion criteria. Preparing the simplified list may take one to three hours,

Figure 23-1. Simplified Criterion

Criterion Number	Simple Criterion
3	Patients with NYHA class III/IV congestive heart failure (CHF)
3	Unstable angina
3	MI in the last 6 months
3	Evidence of active myocardial ischemia on electro-cardiogram (ECG)

The complex criterion was "patients with NYHA class III/IV congestive heart failure, unstable angina, or MI in the last 6 months. Evidence of active myocardial ischemia on ECG." Right column shows the same criterion after it has been simplified.

depending on the CTN's experience and criteria length. This process may appear labor intensive but saves time because it does not need to be repeated for every subject and is transferable if a different CTN works in the same protocol.

Determine the Documents Required

The CTN determines the source documents that will be used to support each criterion answer and writes the name of each document next to the criterion. A single document will support some criteria, such as a laboratory report that documents hemoglobin level. Other criteria, such as "disease progression evidenced by an increase by 25% of the product of bi-dimensional disease," may require two radiology reports or one radiology report and the history and physical note (H&P).

One source document may contain several items and support different criteria. For example, the H&P includes performance status, current or concomitant medications, prior history, and toxicities. An example of exclusion criteria and related source documents are presented in Figure 23-2.

The CTN then prepares a summary list of source documents from the list in the eligibility criteria section. Each component of the H&P should be considered as separate documents. The same type of document may be repeated for different criteria. If the list includes more than one radiology report, specify each type of radiologic exam separately (e.g., computed tomography scan, bone scan, chest x-ray). The same process should be applied for each different laboratory report.

The CTN must determine whether any labs or exams are optional. The physician may order additional tests, such as an echocardiogram to determine NYHA cardiac staging. If the echocardiogram is not required by the study, it is considered an optional evaluation. ***Do not include optional exams in the final source document list***; otherwise, they will show as missing if they were not done. An example of a source document list appears in Figure 23-3.

Figure 23-2. Exclusion Criteria and Their Source Documents

Criterion Number	Exclusion Criteria	Source Document
1	Patients with severe intercurrent infection	H&P, CXR
1	Or history of diverticulitis in the last 6 months.	H&P
2	Patients with small cell or sarcomatoid cancers.	H&P
3	Patients with NYHA class III/IV congestive heart failure,	H&P, Echo
3	MI in the last 6 months,	H&P
3	Or evidence of active myocardial ischemia on ECG.	ECG
4	CNS metastases that are uncontrolled	H&P
5	Oxygen-dependent lung disease,	H&P, CXR,
5	Chronic liver disease,	H&P
5	Grade 2 (or worse) peripheral neuropathy,	H&P, Res toxicities
5	Or HIV infection.	H&P, Con meds
6	Contraindications to corticosteroids.	H&P
7	Uncontrolled severe hypertension,	H&P
7	Warfarin therapy,	H&P, Con meds
7	Uncontrolled diabetes mellitus.	H&P
8	Second malignancies (except nonmelanoma skin cancer) unless disease-free for 2 years.	H&P
9	Overt psychosis,	H&P
9	Mental disability, or incompetent to give informed consent,	H&P
9	History of noncompliance with medical regimens,	H&P
9	Considered potentially unreliable.	H&P

CXR—chest x-ray; Con meds—concomitant medications; ECG—electrocardiogram; Echo—echocardiogram; H&P—history and physical; Res toxicities—residual toxicities

Note. Criteria are copied directly from the protocol without editing.

Figure 23-3. Source Document List

List Number	Source Document
1	Pathology report
2	History and physical (H&P)
3	• Performance status (in H&P or dictated note)
4	• Current meds (in H&P or dictated note)
5	• Prior history and treatment (in H&P or dictated note)
6	• Residual toxicities from prior treatment (in H&P or dictated note)
7	Computed tomography scan
8	Bone scan
9	Chest x-ray
10	Electrocardiogram
11	Consent
12	Testosterone lab report
13	PSA lab report (for inclusion criterion No. 5)
14	CBC lab report
15	Chemistry lab report
	Registration date

which all documents will be compared is protocol-specific. The most common comparison date is the registration date. Some protocols, with different requirements for registration and randomization, may need documents to be compared to both registration and randomization dates or might require some of the documents to be compared to the registration date and some to the randomization date.

The eligibility tool begins with the source document list because all exams or evaluations need to be within the required time frame to be acceptable for screening or registration. A "not-acceptable" date for a source document is equivalent to not having a result.

Dates are classified as okay (OK) or not acceptable. OK dates are those that occur within the stipulated time frame. Not-acceptable dates are too old or occurred after the registration date and would result in a protocol violation if used.

Establish the Type of Answers for Each Criterion

To select the appropriate answer, the whole criterion must be examined, not just the simplified criteria. The CTN should consider all possible answers that will establish eligibility. As with eligibility criteria, answers can be either simple or complex. Simple answers usually include "yes" or "no" choices. The criterion "signed informed consent"

Determine Time Frames

The time frames for each test or exam are stipulated in the protocol and can be written next to each document. If no time frames are specified in the protocol, follow institutional regulations or good clinical practice. The date to has two possible answers—yes or no. The criterion "non-pregnant female" has three possible answers: yes, no, and not applicable (if the subject is not a female).

Complex answers are multiple choice and hierarchical. Multiple-choice answers can be further divided into two types: "and" and "or." A *multiple-choice/and* answer requires the same positive or negative answer for all its components. The criterion "adequate bone marrow function (hemoglobin equal to or higher than 10, platelets equal to or higher than 100,000, and absolute neutrophil count equal to or higher than 1,500)" needs three different values for a positive answer. For practical purposes, each criterion must be considered as a separate question, and each component requires an individual answer.

A *multiple-choice/or* answer exists when only one among several options is the answer for a criterion. The simple inclusion criterion "liver disease: hepatitis A, hepatitis B, hepatitis C, hepatitis D" is giving four different eligible types of a particular disease. All answers are acceptable, but only one can be chosen. Prepare a list of all acceptable answers.

Hierarchical answers have several layers or levels. The simplified criterion "PSA progression is defined at an absolute increment of at least 1 ng/ml over four weeks" requires comparing two different test results. The comparison means that values from two different dates must be identified. Is the second value greater than the first? If yes, is the minimum absolute change equal to or greater than 1? For a positive answer, the PSA values should have increased within a four-week period. In this case, PSA progression is one component of a complex criterion that requires a *multiple-choice/or* answer. Because PSA progression

has multiple layers, it is considered a hierarchical answer (see Figure 23-4).

Set Validation Parameters

Validation parameters are used to indicate which type of data is to be entered (e.g., hemoglobin value, a date) and must be set for each answer. They simplify the calculations for the appropriate answer or values (e.g., an increase of 25%, total bilirubin equal to or less than 1.5). For example, the criterion "AST no greater than two times the upper limit of normal" requires the limit to be set in accordance with normal laboratory value. Validation parameters may warn of or prevent data-entry errors based on the level of security set. The most common types are yes/no, numerical, and lists. Numerical values and lists are preferred to yes/no, if possible, because they facilitate confirming eligibility or tracking the cause of ineligibility.

Determine Eligibility Status

Eligibility status is the result of the verification or screening process. It classifies subjects in three groups: eligible, ineligible, and unverified. Eligible subjects have complete documents, had all evaluations performed within the appropriate time frame, and meet all eligibility criteria. A 100% completion is required. Ineligible subjects are those who failed to meet criteria for different reasons, such as tests performed out of the time frame, incomplete testing, or out-of-range values. Unverified subjects are those who cannot be classified immediately. They may have missing documents, pending test or evaluation results, or telephone reports, or they may require repeat testing for a borderline

---

Figure 23-4. Hierarchical Criteria With Multiple Levels

	A	B	C	D	E	F
29	4	Evidence of progression			Y	0
30	4	PSA- progression is defined as 2 consecutive increments in PSA (an absolute change of at least 1ng/mL) over 4 weeks.	Lab report		N	
31	4	PSA 1 value	Lab report	11.8	Y	1
32	4	PSA 2 value	Lab report	160.39		
33	4	PSA 1 date	Lab report	1/1/2004	N	
34	4	PSA 2 date	Lab report	2/3/2004		
35	4	25% increase of bidimensional product	H&P Radiology report			2
36	4	30% increase in maximum diameter	H&P Radiology report			3
37	4	increase in number of metastatic lesions on bone scan	H&P Past Hx	yes	Y	4
38	4	Worsening symptoms attributable to disease progression	H&P			5

This inclusion criterion has five components. Each component is identified with numbers. The answer to each one of these components is in the same level (level 1). Question 1 requires comparing two different test results and the two dates when they were collected (level 2).

result. After the temporary issue is resolved, the subject will be reclassified as either eligible or ineligible.

Conclusion of the Preparatory Process

The nursing preparatory process determines patients' eligibility status and involves multiple steps that are standardized into reviewing and simplifying the eligibility criteria, determining source documents and their time frames, establishing the type of answers for each criteria question, and establishing validation parameters.

Building the Tool
Overview of the Tool

After preparing the information, it is time to build the tool in Excel (see Figure 23-5). The tool has six sections: protocol and patient identification; source documents; inclusion criteria; exclusion criteria; eligibility status; and signature, date, and comments area. The identification section does not appear in the sample. It may include the institution name, protocol title, protocol number, patient name, medical record number, and accession number. The source document section includes all required documents or tests and will generate a list of missing documents, which is repeated in the eligibility status section. The time frames, determined in the preparation phase, are included for easy reference. The inclusion criteria and exclusion criteria sections are protocol-specific and include simplified criteria and their corresponding source documents. Each simplified criterion must be copied into a different cell in the spreadsheet. The eligibility status section presents the results of the eligibility verification.

The signature and date section does not appear in the sample. It includes space for the date when the form was completed and for signatures of the person completing the form, the nurse, and the investigator. It is useful to include an area for comments for changes in data, expected date of missing results, and so on.

The sections are listed in the order they appear in the tool. See Figure 23-6 for a sample tool showing the data flow to calculate eligibility status.

Figure 23-5. Completed Tool for Eligible Patient

	A	B	C	D	E	F	G
1		**Source Document**	Missing	Date Done	Results	**Doc Status**	
2	1	H&P		6/1/2000	Ok	1	1
3	2	Prior Hx/Tx (in H&P or dictated note)		1/27/2004	OK	1	2
4	3	CT Scan		1/28/2004	OK	1	3
5	4	Bone Scan		1/29/2004	OK	1	4
6	5	ECG		1/30/2004	Ok	1	5
7	6	Consent		1/29/2004	Ok	1	6
8	7	Chemistry lab report		1/29/2004	OK	1	7
9		Registration Date		2/3/2004			
10		**Missing Documents:**					
11		**Inclusion Criteria**	Source Document			**Eligible vs Non-eligible**	**No data**
12	4	Patients must have evidence of progression of disease.	Lab report		Y	0	
13	4	PSA- progression is defined as 2 consecutive increments in PSA (an absolute change of at least 1ng/mL) over 4 weeks.			N		
14	4	PSA 1 value	Lab report	5.29	N		0
15	4	PSA 2 value	Lab report	4.85			0
16	4	PSA 1 date	Lab report	12/29/2003	N		0
17	4	PSA 2 date	Lab report	1/29/2004			0
18	4	An increase by 25% of the product of bidimensional disease	H&P Radiology report	50	Y		0
19	4	or 30% in maximum diameter qualifies as progression.	H&P Radiology report				0
20	4	An increase in the number of metastatic lesions on bone scan qualifies as progression.	H&P Past Hx	no	N		0
21	4	Worsening symptoms attributable to disease progression qualifies as progression e.g. worsening malignant bony pain.	H&P				0
22	13	total bili ≤1.5 mg/dl	Lab report	0.3	Y	0	0
23	16	Signed informed consent	Consent	yes	Y	0	0
24							
25		**Exclusion Criteria**					
26	2	Patients with small cell or sarcomatoid cancers.	H&P	no	N	0	0
27	3	Evidence of active myocardial ischemia on ECG	ECG	no	N	0	0
28	4	CNS metastases that are uncontrolled.	H&P	no	N	0	0
29		**Non-eligible and No Data counts:**				0	0
30		**Eligibility Status**					
31		Unverified	Eligible	Non-eligible			
32			**X**				
33							

Note. This reduced sample does not display any identifiers, signatures, or comments, which are part of a complete form. The print area is set up for columns A–E. Cell D21 has no data; however, document is not listed as missing because there is a positive answer in E12.

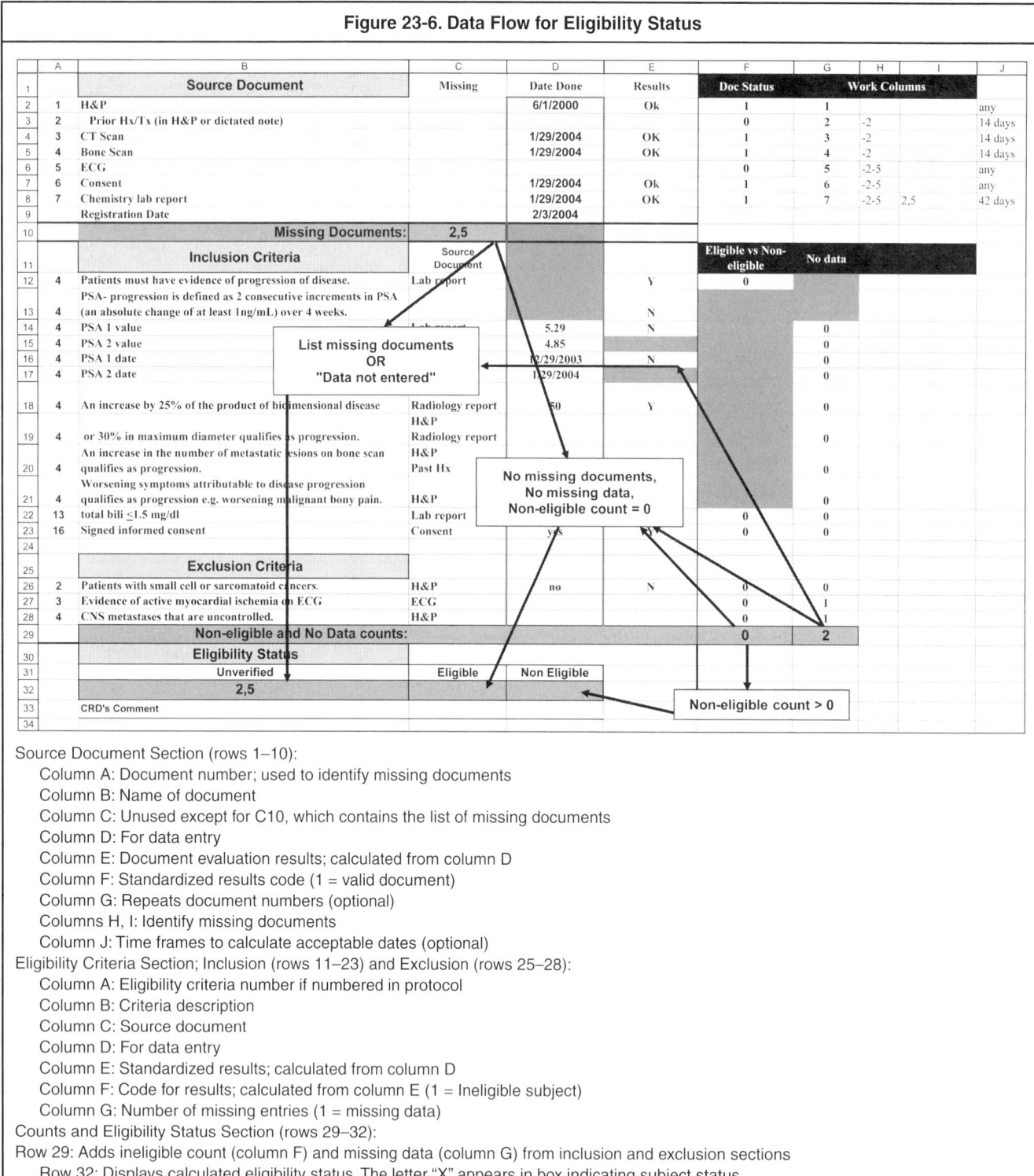

Figure 23-6. Data Flow for Eligibility Status

Source Document Section (rows 1–10):
　　Column A: Document number; used to identify missing documents
　　Column B: Name of document
　　Column C: Unused except for C10, which contains the list of missing documents
　　Column D: For data entry
　　Column E: Document evaluation results; calculated from column D
　　Column F: Standardized results code (1 = valid document)
　　Column G: Repeats document numbers (optional)
　　Columns H, I: Identify missing documents
　　Column J: Time frames to calculate acceptable dates (optional)
Eligibility Criteria Section; Inclusion (rows 11–23) and Exclusion (rows 25–28):
　　Column A: Eligibility criteria number if numbered in protocol
　　Column B: Criteria description
　　Column C: Source document
　　Column D: For data entry
　　Column E: Standardized results; calculated from column D
　　Column F: Code for results; calculated from column E (1 = Ineligible subject)
　　Column G: Number of missing entries (1 = missing data)
Counts and Eligibility Status Section (rows 29–32):
Row 29: Adds ineligible count (column F) and missing data (column G) from inclusion and exclusion sections
　　Row 32: Displays calculated eligibility status. The letter "X" appears in box indicating subject status.

Note. This reduced sample does not display any identifiers, signatures, or comments, which are part of a complete form. The print area is set up for columns A–E.

After the form layout has been completed, it is time to set validation parameters for each data entry cell in the eligibility criteria section. The data validation tool, located in the Excel data menu, checks for numerical values (see Figure 23-7) or looks up the entry in a list (see Figure 23-8).

The final task in preparing the tool is to set up the formulas so that Excel can calculate all required results.

Formulas and Calculations

Two main concepts are used in this tool: "IF" statements and the date calculator. "IF" statements are an Excel func-

Figure 23-7. Data Validation

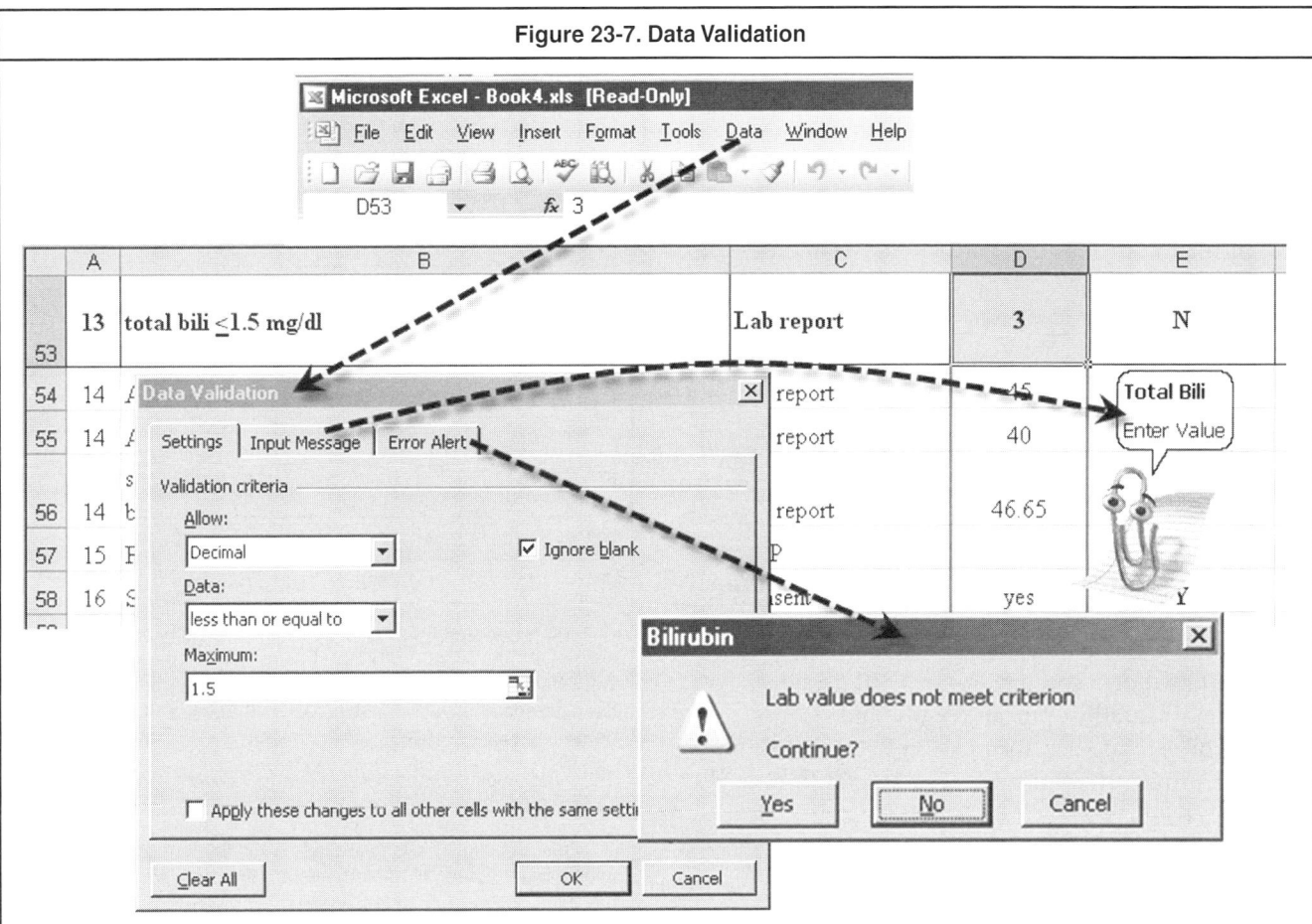

Click the data entry cell where parameters will be set. Validation parameters can be set up from the **Data** menu. Select **Validation** to open the Data Validation window.
- Use **Settings** tab to enter validation criteria.
- Use **Input Message** tab to indicate the type of data to enter
- Use **Error Alert** tab to select the preferred alert style, and type the error message.
The example shows the steps for numerical data validation. Repeat the same steps for every cell where parameters are desired.

Figure 23-8. Data Validation—List

	A	B	C	D	E

79	1	Liver disease:
		  Hepatitis A, Hepatitis B,
		  Hepatitis C, Hepatitis D
			Lab
			report
				B	Y

80				A	
81				B	Select Hepatitis Type
82				C	
83				D	
84					
85					

	A	B	C	D	E

79	1	Liver disease:
		  Hepatitis A, Hepatitis B,
		  Hepatitis C, Hepatitis D
			Lab
			report
				B	=IF(D79="","",
					    IF(OR(D79="A",D79="B",
					        D79="C",D79="D"),
					    "Y",
					    "N"))

Select **List** in the dropdown under **Allow** on the **Settings** tab of the **Data Validation** window as described in Figure 23-7. Type the list.

tion used to determine the appropriate answers for each criterion and to determine eligibility (see Figure 23-9). The simple date calculator compares two or more dates and calculates acceptable dates for a specific criterion or document (see Figure 23-10). The simple calculator will work fine if two dates are present. When one date is missing, a more professional display will be obtained if the date calculator is combined with an "IF" statement (see Figure 23-11).

Sometimes more than one condition exists and all possibilities need to be checked, which requires the use of the compounded "IF" statement (see Figure 23-12). In the eligibility criteria section, the majority of formulas calculate yes and no answers, show eligible versus ineligible results, and count missing data entries (see Figure 23-13). Calculating results for a hierarchical answer requires a more detailed explanation (see Figure 23-14).

This section should not be considered to be a tutorial in Excel but rather a presentation of sample formulas that will allow the CTN to understand the calculations and create a tool based on a specific protocol. All data displayed are for demonstration purposes only and do not refer to any subject. Note that formulas in Excel will show in one long string but are displayed in several lines in the

Figure 23-9. Simple "IF" Statement

Function	Condition	True	False	End
=IF(	B1="",	"",	B2 - B1	)
Note commas:		↑	↑	

The "IF" statement is an Excel function. Users can send data items, separated by commas, to a function, and it returns **one** result (date, number, text, etc.). The IF statement requires three items:
- **Condition:** Cell B1 is blank (indicated by two quotes without a space)
- **True:** What to return if the condition is true (B3 is blank)
- **False:** What to return if the condition is false (days between B2 and B1)

Figure 23-10. Simple Date Calculator

	A	B
1	Chemistry lab report	7/19/2005
2	Registration Date	7/26/2005
3	Days Difference:	7

	A	B
1	Chemistry lab report	7/19/2005
2	Registration Date	7/26/2005
3	Days Difference:	= B2 - B1

The top box shows the number of days between the two dates. The bottom box shows the formula.

Figure 23-11. Date Calculation—A Better Display

	A	B
1	Chemistry lab report	
2	Registration Date	3/1/2006
3	Days Difference:	38777

	A	B
1	Chemistry lab report	
2	Registration Date	3/1/2006
3	Days Difference:	=IF(B1="","",B2 - B1)

	A	B
1	Chemistry lab report	
2	Registration Date	3/1/2006
3	Days Difference:	

The top box shows the results when one date is missing and the simple formula (= B2 – B1) from Figure 23-10 is used. An empty cell defaults to 1/1/1900. Cell B3, formatted as a number, shows the difference between the date March 1, 2006, and the default date of January 1, 1900.

The middle box shows the sample formula used to keep cell B3 blank when the first date is missing.

The bottom box displays the results when the formula in the middle box is used. "IF" statements are explained in detail in Figure 23-9.

examples to facilitate understanding. Be mindful of cell formatting, and select the appropriate format for the type of data to avoid errors in the displayed results.

Tips for Managing the Tool

Create a workbook for each protocol. Keep a tool, *without data,* as a template. The template may be copied, used for each screening, and then saved with the data *for each subject.* These saved forms may serve as documentation for the screening log. When an eligibility criterion changes because of a protocol amendment, the tool must be modified accordingly. The CTN must document in the workbook the changes and the date of when the revised version of the tool will apply.

Summary

The accuracy of the eligibility tool presented has been validated by comparing its results with results from manual forms in use for eligibility verification. The tool organizes data entry, decreases the rate of errors, and decreases processing time in verifying eligibility. By following the steps as presented, the eligibility tool can be adapted or changed for different protocols. To verify eligibility, CTNs must go through the same steps whether in their minds, on a paper checklist, or when designing a tool. The eligibility tool presented in this chapter helps CTNs

Figure 23-12. Compounded "IF" Statement

	A	B	C	D	E
21	15	Chemistry lab report		6/29/2006	Not acceptable
22		Registration Date		7/26/2006	
23		Missing Documents:	1,4,11		

	A	B	C	D	E
21	15	Chemistry lab report		6/29/2006	=IF(D21="","", IF(D22-D21<=7,"OK", "Not acceptable"))
22		Registration Date		7/26/2006	
23		Missing Documents:	1,4,11		

- Users may add more than one condition with different results to create a compounded IF statement (nested IF).
- Construct the condition so that it always returns a value on the "true" result, and add the new IF for the false side.
- The top box shows a document that is not acceptable.
- The bottom box displays the formula used.

Figure 23-13. Eligibility Criteria Results and Missing Entry Counters

	A	B	C	D	E	F	G
53	13	total bili ≤1.5 mg/dl	Lab report	0.3	Y	0	0

	A	B	C	D	E	F	G
53	13	total bili ≤1.5 mg/dl	Lab report	2.9	N	1	0

	A	B	C	D	E	F	G
53	13	total bili <1.5 mg/dl	Lab report	0.3	=IF(D53="","", IF(D53<=1.5,"Y", "N"))	=IF(E53="",0, IF(E53="N",1, 0))	=IF(D53="",1, 0)

Columns E, F and G in the inclusion and exclusion sections contain the standardized result for the entry, one (1) if the entry is ineligible, or one (1) if the entry is missing. If a valid entry is made, both F and G contain zero. The top box shows a valid entry. Y is the eligible value for inclusion criteria; and 0 is the count when eligible. The middle box shows an ineligible entry. N is an ineligible value for inclusion criteria; and 1 is the count when ineligible. The bottom box shows the sample formulas to determine the correct results.

to share the nursing process among each other. Additionally, after preparing tools for several protocols, a criteria bank may be created. Questions, answers, values, and formulas may be recycled from this bank, thus reducing preparation time.

After completing all steps, including reviewing eligibility criteria, simplifying complex criteria, determining the required documents, determining the time frames for each document, establishing the type of answers for each criterion, and setting validation parameters, the CTN can start using the tool with subjects to determine their eligibility status.

The author would like to acknowledge Bill for providing inspiration and support.

References

Fink, E., Hall, L.O., Goldgof, D.B., Goswami, B.D., Boonstra, M., & Krischer, J.P. (2003). Experiments on the automated selection of patients for clinical trials. *Proceedings of the IEEE International Conference on Systems, Man and Cybernetics, 5,* 4541–4545.

Mathew, P. (2004). *Randomized double-blind phase II trial of docetaxel and imatinib versus docetaxel and placebo in metastatic androgen-independent prostate cancer (AIPC) with bone metastases.* Retrieved October 16, 2005, from http://utm-ext01a.mdacc.tmc.edu/dept/prot/clinicaltrialswp.nsf/index/id03-0008

Figure 23-14. Hierarchical Criteria, Multiple-Choice/Or

Top box (data flow)

	A	B	C	D	E	F
29	4	Evidence of progression			Y	0
30	4	PSA- progression is defined as 2 consecutive increments in PSA (an absolute change of at least 1ng/mL) over 4 weeks.	Lab report			
31	4	PSA 1 value	Lab report			
32	4	PSA 2 value	Lab report	160.39		
33	4	PSA 1 date	Lab report			
34	4	PSA 2 date	Lab report	2/3/2004		
35	4	25% increase of bidimensional product	H&P			
36	4	30% increase in maximum diameter	Radiology report	20	N	
37	4	increase in number of metastatic lesions on bone scan	Radiology report	yes	Y	
38	4	Worsening symptoms attributable to disease progression	H&P, Past Hx / H&P			

Bottom box (sample formulas)

	A	B	C	D	E	F
29	4	Evidence of progression	Lab report		=IF(OR(E30="Y",E35="Y",E36="Y",E37="Y",E38="Y"),"Y", IF(OR(E30="",E35="",E36="",E37="",E38=""),"", "N"))	=IF(E29="",0, IF(E29="N",1, 0))
30	4	PSA- progression is defined as 2 consecutive increments in PSA (an absolute change of at least 1ng/mL) over 4 weeks.			=IF(AND(E31="",E33=""),"", IF(E31="N","N", IF(E33="N","N", "Y")))	
31	4	PSA 1 value	Lab report		=IF(D31="","",IF(D32="",,IF(D32>=D31+1,"Y","N")))	
32	4	PSA 2 value	Lab report	160.39	=IF(OR(D33="",D34=""),"",IF(D34>D33+28,"N","Y"))	
33	4	PSA 1 date	Lab report			
34	4	PSA 2 date	Lab report	2/2/2004		
35	4	25% increase of bidimensional product	H&P		=IF(D35="","",IF(D35>=25,"Y","N"))	
36	4	30% increase in maximum diameter	Radiology report	20	=IF(D36="","",IF(D36>=30,"Y","N"))	
37	4	increase in number of metastatic lesions on bone scan	H&P, Past Hx	yes	=IF(D37="","",IF(D37="Yes","Y","N"))	
38	4	Worsening symptoms attributable to disease progression	H&P		=IF(D38="","",IF(D38="Yes","Y","N"))	

The middle connectors are labeled **OR** and **AND**.

The top box shows the data flow for calculating the answer in E29.
One YES answer is required from any of the five criteria in cells E30, E35, E36, E37, or E38 to obtain the final answer in E29. Entries are required in D31 through D34 to determine the result of E30. E31 calculates the difference in values. E33 calculates the difference in dates. The result in E30 is blank if any of those entries are missing. The bottom box displays sample formulas.

National Cancer Institute. (2007, April 27). *PDQ—NCI's comprehensive cancer database.* Retrieved August 15, 2007, from http://www.cancer.gov/cancertopics/pdq/cancerdatabase

Seroussi, B., & Bouaud, J. (2003). Using OncoDoc as a computer-based eligibility screening system to improve accrual onto breast cancer clinical trials. *Artificial Intelligence Medicine, 29,* 153–167.

Tu, S.W., Kemper, C.A., Lane, N.M., Carlson, R.W., & Musen, M.A. (1993). A methodology for determining patients' eligibility for clinical trials. *Methods of Information in Medicine, 32,* 317–325.

CHAPTER 24
Prevention and Control Study Considerations

Marjorie J. Good, RN, BSN, MPH, OCN®

Introduction

Cancer prevention, early detection, and *control* are not new terms in the world of cancer research. The National Cancer Act of 1971 mandated the National Cancer Institute (NCI) to comprehensively and energetically exploit new scientific leads in research that would further the understanding of the cancer process and apply the results to improve methods of cancer prevention, detection, treatment, and control (NCI, 1997). Cancer prevention continues to be depicted as a vital component of the war on cancer. The best treatment of malignant disease is its prevention, and the disease to be prevented is carcinogenesis, not cancer (Hong & Sporn, 1997; Meyskens, 1992).

Controlled clinical trials play a vital role as a means of testing chemopreventive agents as well as nondrug interventions in the realm of cancer prevention and control. However, cancer control and prevention studies have unique characteristics that make promotion and recruitment challenging. This chapter addresses some of those characteristics as well as some of the frustrations and barriers encountered.

Background

Despite advanced technology, by the time a cancer is diagnosed, more than 90% of the biological life of the tumor is over, and the best chance to control the malignant process has been missed (Meyskens, 2004). An extensive analysis conducted more than two decades ago evaluated avoidable causes of cancer and concluded that 50%–70% of all human cancers were preventable (Doll & Peto, 1981). The American Cancer Society (ACS, 2007) stated that all cancer caused by cigarette smoking and heavy use of alcohol could be prevented completely. ACS also suggested that about one-third of the 559,650 cancer deaths expected to occur in 2007 would be related to overweight or obesity, physical inactivity, and nutrition and, thus, also could be prevented. According to Meyskens (2004), major avoidable cancer-related risk factors can be broadly separated into four areas: tobacco, infections, chemical (including hormonal), and diet (see Figure 24-1). Today, cancer prevention strategies are considered at three different levels: *primary,* which addresses normal, asymptomatic individuals; *secondary,* which is directed toward individuals with evidence of preneoplastic disease without frank malignancy; and *tertiary,* which involves decreasing the morbidity of established disease (see Table 24-1) (Meyskens, 2004).

Many researchers today believe that the best approach to making an impact on cancer is the use of successful chemoprevention drugs. The chemoprevention drug development program of NCI's Division of Cancer Prevention began in the early 1980s and has shown considerable growth since that time. Hundreds of compounds have been tested, and the most promising agents currently are being tested in various phases of clinical trials. According to Greenwald (2005), clinical trials will continue to be the

---

Figure 24-1. Major Avoidable Influences on Cancer Development in Humans

Tobacco
- Tobacco smoking has been linked causally with most lung and oropharyngeal cancers and is a significant contributor to the risk for esophageal, pancreatic, bladder, renal, and cervical cancers, as well as for acute myelogenous leukemia.

Dietary
- The role of diet is complex and unproven, but diets high in vegetables and fruits have been consistently protective.

Infectious
- Human papillomavirus and hepatitis have been implicated in the etiology of cervical, hepatic, and some oral cancers, as has the bacterium *Helicobacter pylori* in stomach cancer.

Chemical Carcinogens
- Some examples include aniline dyes (bladder), asbestos (mesothelium), and hormones (breast, prostate, endometrium).

Note. From "Cancer Prevention, Screening, and Early Detection" (p. 428), by F.L. Meyskens, Jr. in M. Abeloff, J. Armitage, J. Niederhuber, and M. Kastan (Eds.), *Clinical Oncology* (3rd ed.), 2004, Philadelphia: Elsevier. Copyright 2004 by Elsevier. Reprinted with permission.

Table 24-1. Levels of Prevention in Cancer Management

Level	Definition	Example
Primary	Decrease risk for normal asymptomatic individuals	Screening[a] Smoking cessation Chemoprevention of breast cancer in asymptomatic women[b] Diet modification
Secondary	Decrease progression of preneoplastic processes	Reverse preneoplastic (cervical intraepithelial neoplasia, leukoplakia) with chemoprevention[c] Early detection
Tertiary	Decrease morbidity of established disease	Chemoprevention of second malignancies

[a] Asymptomatic individuals: If symptomatic, then this would be an example of early detection.
[b] If women had prior breast cancer, this would be an example of tertiary prevention.
[c] Almost all epithelial (solid tumor) cancers have a clinically identifiable precancerous stage known as intraepithelial neoplasia.

Note. From "Cancer Prevention, Screening, and Early Detection" (p. 426), by F.L. Meyskens, Jr. in M. Abeloff, J. Armitage, J. Niederhuber, and M. Kastan (Eds.), *Clinical Oncology* (3rd ed.), 2004, Philadelphia: Elsevier. Copyright 2004 by Elsevier. Reprinted with permission.

gold standard for understanding prevention strategies. To date, more than 70 randomized chemoprevention trials have been reported in the literature. Table 24-2 lists several completed and current NCI-sponsored chemoprevention clinical trials. Based on evidence from the Breast Cancer Prevention Trial, the U.S. Food and Drug Administration (FDA) approved tamoxifen in October 1998 for risk reduction of breast cancer in women who are at increased risk for developing the disease as defined by the Gail model. This was the first FDA approval of an agent for risk reduction and marked a landmark achievement in chemoprevention research (Smith, Tully, & Padberg, 2005). The success of these large-scale chemoprevention clinical trials confirms their usefulness in identifying ways to stop many of the people at risk for cancer from developing cancer (NCI, 2006).

Prevention, Screening, and Early Detection
Prevention

Prevention, screening, and early detection studies assess intervention and screening techniques in people who are at increased risk for developing cancer or, more rarely, in the population at large (primary prevention). These studies may target age groups, socioeconomic levels, or a combination of risk factors. The studies are designed to determine whether cancer mortality is reduced because of the intervention or, as in studies targeting intermediate end points,

to show a delayed onset of disease, which is considered to be a success in the realm of prevention. Cancer prevention studies use drug intervention (chemoprevention), prophylactic therapy, or dietary and lifestyle modification to reduce cancer incidence or delay cancer onset.

Screening and Early Detection

Secondary and/or tertiary prevention may use the phrase "early detection of disease," meaning detecting a disease at an earlier stage than usually would occur in standard clinical practice. This may mean detecting disease at a presymptomatic stage, when the patient has no clinical complaint (i.e., no symptoms or signs) and, thus, no reason to seek medical care for the condition (Gordis, 1996). Studies evaluating screening programs or biomarkers, therefore, play a key role in defining the value of early detection of disease. Cancer screening studies are designed with mechanisms to encourage participants to continue regular screening, such as providing free screening tests, reminder letters, and personal contact with study staff. To assess the effectiveness of screening, follow-up testing is needed to determine the false-negative or false-positive rate for the type of screening used.

In both prevention and screening studies, a control group of participants matched by age, family background, and living habits may be enrolled. Generally, subjects are randomized to guarantee balance between intervention and control groups. The desired end points are a decrease in cancer-related mortality and an increase in overall survival. For screening studies, a reduction in the incidence of advanced cancers is a desired outcome. Intermediate end points, such as serum markers or known cancer precursors, may be used to assess the efficacy of the intervention. Screening studies must look at whether early treatment as a result of early detection actually improves overall or disease-free survival. When evaluating a screening test or tool, Meyskens (2004) reported that beyond the technical issues involved in study design, implementation, analysis, and interpretation, three other requirements also must be met to demonstrate that a screening test is useful (see Figure 24-2).

Chemoprevention

Chemoprevention, the intervention that uses specific agents or drugs to prevent, stop the growth of, or reverse the growth of cancer, has been in progress for more than two decades, but only in the past few years have positive clinical trials been reported to support preclinical data and the use of chemoprevention in humans (Meyskens, 2004). According to Greenwald and Sondik (1986), cancer prevention research seeks to identify preventable causes of cancer, both positive and negative, and to reduce cancer incidence by effective application of prevention strategies in target populations. In 1991, Garewal and Meyskens defined chemoprevention as an intervention with chemical agents, either natural or synthetic, that can prevent, suppress, or

Table 24-2. National Cancer Institute–Sponsored Chemoprevention Clinical Trials

Organ Site	Accrual Period	Agent	Population	Status
Head and neck (Hong et al., 1990)	1983–1990	Isotretinoin 50–100 mg/m²/day versus placebo for 12 months	103 disease-free patients with history of head and neck cancer	Isotretinoin group had fewer second primary tumors. No difference occurred in regard to local, regional, or distant recurrences.
Skin Nutritional Prevention of Cancer (NPC) (Clark et al., 1996)	1983–1991	Selenium 200 mcg daily versus placebo	1,312 residents of eastern United States	Did not affect incidence of nonmelanoma skin cancer. However, did show a significant reduction in total cancer mortality, total cancer incidence, and incidences of lung, prostate, and colorectal cancers.
Lung Alpha-Tocopherol Beta-Carotene Cancer Prevention Trial (ATBC) (Heinonen & Albanes, 1994)	1985–1993	β-carotene (vitamin A) 20 mg/day and α-tocopherol (vitamin E) 50 mg/day alone or in combination versus placebo for 5–8 years	29,133 male smokers	Neither agent reduced lung cancer incidence. In fact, an 18% increase in lung cancer incidence in active smokers in the β-carotene groups was found.
Breast Breast Cancer Prevention Trial (BCPT) (Fisher et al., 1998)	June 1992–September 1997	Tamoxifen versus placebo daily for 5 years	13,388 pre- and post-menopausal women at high risk for breast cancer	Treatment was effective, resulting in 49% fewer diagnoses of invasive breast cancer in women taking tamoxifen. U.S. Food and Drug Administration approved tamoxifen in 1998 for risk reduction of breast cancer in women with increased risk.
Study of Tamoxifen and Raloxifene (STAR) (U.S. Department of Health and Human Services, 2006)	1994–2004	Tamoxifen versus raloxifene daily for 5 years	19,747 high-risk, post-menopausal women, ages > 35	Initial results show raloxifene to be as effective as tamoxifen in reducing the breast cancer risk.
Colon Colorectal Adenoma Prevention Study (CAPS) (Sandler et al., 2003)	1993–2000	Aspirin 325 mg versus placebo	635 men and women diagnosed with early-stage colorectal cancer	Daily aspirin use reduced development of adenomas by 35%.
Celecoxib/Familial Adenomatous Polyposis (FAP) (Steinbach et al., 2000)	December 1996–December 1998	Celecoxib 100 mg or 400 mg twice daily versus placebo for 6 months	77 individuals with diagnosis of FAP	Individuals receiving 400 mg twice daily had significant regression of colorectal adenomas, polyps, and polyp burden.
Adenoma Prevention with Celecoxib (APC) (Solomon et al., 2005)	2000–2002	Celecoxib 200 mg or 400 mg twice daily versus placebo for 3 years	More than 2,000 men and women > age 30	Trial suspended after showing 2.5-fold increased risk of major fatal and nonfatal cardiovascular events in the intervention arm.
Prostate Prostate Cancer Prevention Trial (PCPT) (Thompson et al., 2003)	January 1994–May 1997	Finasteride versus placebo for 7 years	18,882 men with normal digital rectal exam and prostate-specific antigen < 3 ng/ml	Treatment was effective; finasteride reduced the incidence of prostate cancer by 24.8%.
Selenium and Vitamin E Cancer Prevention Trial (SELECT) (Klein et al., 2001)	2001–2004	Selenium 200 mcg versus vitamin E 400 mg versus placebo alone or in combination daily for 12 years	35,534 males age > 55 and African American males age > 50	Results pending

Figure 24-2. Required Elements for a Screening Tool to Be Useful

- A test must be available that will detect cancer earlier than routine methods.
- Evidence must exist that treatment at an earlier stage of disease will result in an improved outcome.
- Evidence must exist of a total health benefit.

Note. Based on information from Meyskens, 2004.

reverse the carcinogenic process. That definition of chemoprevention has remained the same (Smith et al., 2005). The scientific rationale for the use of cancer chemoprevention is based on the fundamental concept of carcinogenesis, which is considered to be a long-evolving, multistep process (up to 20 or more years) leading to the development of invasive cancer (Meyskens & Tully, 2005). Therefore, potential chemoprevention trial participants include people at high risk because of genetic susceptibility, lifestyle, or occupational or accidental exposure to carcinogens; those with detectable precancerous lesions or a clinical history associated with an increased risk of cancer; patients with cancer who are at risk for a new primary cancer; and the general population as well (Greenwald et al., 1990).

Similar to treatment trials, prevention trials may have common study design features, including the randomization of subjects, use of appropriate controls, and blinding (when applicable), as well as use of statistical considerations. Table 24-3 summarizes numerous differences between prevention and treatment trials. Individuals enrolled in chemoprevention trials are referred to as study *participants* rather than *patients* because of their healthy status. Their relative health presents significant challenges for a number of protocol-related issues, such as recruitment, retention, adherence, and long-term follow-up (Smith et al., 2005).

Prevention study populations usually include healthy subjects from the general population or from a defined high-risk group. Because a full-scale prevention trial utilizing an intervention uses cancer incidence as its end point, trial duration often is very long, with an intervention often lasting for five years or more with up to five years of additional follow-up time. Additionally, phase III and IV chemoprevention trials often require large population samples and, for this reason, may cost $10 million to $100 million to fund, amounts considerably more expensive than those associated with standard treatment studies (Meyskens, 2004).

Because chemoprevention agents are administered over long periods of time, dosing the agent at the level of the greatest efficacy with the least risk of adverse side effects is important and challenging. Drop-out rates may increase if even the slightest toxicity is deemed to be intolerable to a healthy individual. Determining the appropriate dose is accomplished by dosing and pharmacokinetic studies in phase I and II chemoprevention trials. Feasibility studies play an important role in chemoprevention research as a

means of determining the financial cost and commitment of resources needed to complete a larger-scale study (Kelloff et al., 1994).

Chemoprevention clinical trials need to be designed around the setting in which the patients normally are seen, which is a challenge for those developing the trials. The chemoprevention treatment and patient monitoring should not interfere with other medications, surgical procedures, or monitoring the patient may be receiving. This discussion then leads to an evaluation of some of the frustrations and barriers associated with recruitment to prevention trials.

Almost all of those involved in the recruitment of subjects to prevention trials agree that they encounter multiple frustrations and barriers in the process. Recruitment to clinical trials involves not only defining eligibility criteria but also determining behavioral and social factors that may affect the validity of the trial (Yeomans-Kinney et al., 1995). Furthermore, the inclusion or eligibility criteria of prevention trials may be viewed as being too strict, thereby limiting the number of subjects that potentially can participate. The screening yield of a prevention trial is related primarily to the inclusion criteria of the protocol in addition to the motivation of patients to enroll. In general, individuals may not be as motivated to take part in a clinical research study if they do not have a diagnosis of cancer or do not perceive themselves to be at risk (Smith et al., 2005). Spilker and Cramer (1992) reported that one can expect approximately 1 in 5 patients to enroll if a trial offers active treatment benefit for a medical problem, whereas one can expect only 1 in 40 screened patients to enroll in a trial that offers the possibility of disease prevention. In the era of limited staff resources and time, this can lead to high frustration and low accrual. Prevention trials generally have a yield of 1%–6% of potential participants screened who actually enroll, whereas treatment trials generally yield 20%–27% (Spilker & Cramer).

Physician barriers to enrolling patients in prevention trials can have a detrimental effect on recruitment efforts. As with treatment trials, reasons exist for physicians not to participate in prevention trials (Cohen, 2002) (see Figure 24-3).

Other reasons for nonparticipation of physicians include a belief that one treatment is superior, a general distrust of "academic medicine," and a dislike of discussing uncertainty with the patient. The embarrassment and personal discomfort in discussing a clinical trial might disturb physicians in private practice settings more than in larger, more impersonal clinics in which a physician or nurse may not see the same patient each time he or she attends the clinic. This especially is important when discussing the possibility of receiving a placebo.

Another important point is that clinical trials require strict adherence to protocol guidelines by physicians as well as participants. The ability to strictly adhere to a protocol is lower in the private physician's practice. Private-practice physician offices rarely have funding for data managers to

Table 24-3. Features of Clinical Prevention Trials Versus Treatment Trials

Variable	Prevention Trial	Treatment Trial

Goal	Cancer prevention
	    Decrease cancer incidence and mortality
	    Prevent or ameliorate precancerous lesions or markers of cancer risk
	    Prevent second primary cancer
		Cancer treatment
		    Increase cure or remission rates
		    Decrease mortality and morbidity

Study population	Noncancerous subjects
	    General population
	    High-risk population
	    People with precancerous lesions
	    Previously treated, disease-free patients with cancer
	    Large scale (thousands of subjects)
	
	Undiagnosed (prevalent) cases may confuse analysis
		Patients with cancer
		
		Small to moderate (hundreds of subjects)
		
		Diagnosis confirmed before therapy

Toxicity of agent	None to moderate, acceptable	Moderate to severe, acceptable

Study protocol	Design
	    Simple (dichotomy)
	    Intervention vs. placebo
	        Factorial
	    Intervention A vs. intervention B vs. intervention AB vs. placebo
	    Multiple simultaneous interventions, including interactions
	
	Pilot study usually required
	
	Placebo run-in considered useful
	
	Study may require 5–10 years or more of intervention and follow-up.
		Design
		    Simple (dichotomy or multiagent)
		    Therapy versus placebo
		    Therapy A versus therapy B
		    Therapy A versus therapy B versus therapy C
		
		Pilot study rarely required
		
		Run-in inappropriate
		
		Study length may be short for aggressive cancers, longer for slower growing cancers or adjuvant studies.

Compliance	Adherence to protocol may be difficult to maintain (i.e., subject-dependent).	Adherence to protocol is easier to maintain (i.e., physician-dependent).

Note. From "Concepts in Cancer Chemoprevention Research," by P. Greenwald, D.W. Nixon, W.F. Malone, G.J. Kelloff, H.R. Stern, and K.M. Witkin, 1990, *Cancer, 65,* p. 1487. Copyright 1990 by Wiley & Sons, Inc. Reprinted with permission.

monitor protocol compliance. Physicians are too busy to verify that protocol guidelines are followed and to ensure that data are submitted. Finally, if primary practice physicians do not feel ownership and involvement in the progress and outcome of the trial, they will not feel the need to enroll or refer patients (Spilker & Cramer, 1992).

Many potential chemoprevention trial participants will be found in the family-practice setting or private physician office. The clinical trial nurse (CTN) will need to keep in mind that many issues related to private-practice or family-practice physicians differ from issues related to an oncologist's participation. Private-practice physicians are more motivated to maintain busy practices than their colleagues in academia. If the physician in private practice has or hopes to establish a long-term medical relationship with the patient, he or she does not want to send the patient elsewhere.

With these difficulties, why attempt to access the population of patients in family-practice or private-practice settings? Some patients desire and even "need" to have a physician whom they trust (i.e., their private physician) make authoritative decisions about their medical care. That physician then plays a key role in a patient's participation. Yeomans-Kinney, Richards, Vernon, and Vogel (1998) reported that primary care physicians (PCPs) played an important role in influencing preventive health behavior when enrolling participants in the Breast Cancer Prevention Trial and recommended enlisting the support of PCPs. One

Figure 24-3. Reasons Physicians Do Not Participate in Prevention Trials

- Insufficient data management support
- Burdensome regulatory requirements
- Strict eligibility requirements
- Lack of interest/motivation
- Lack of time
- Inadequate reimbursement
- Resistance of third-party payers
- Patient/participant refusal

Note. Based on information from Cohen, 2002.

explanation given for the unsuccessful recruitment of African American men into prostate cancer screening included the failure of the physician to inform patients that prostate testing was necessary (Yeomans-Kinney et al.). In a community focus group (Woods, Montgomery, & Herring, 2004), African American males reported that they were not comfortable accessing prevention services in public settings (e.g., health fairs). They preferred to receive screening examinations on a one-on-one basis with a trusted physician with whom they felt comfortable. Respondents felt that when the physician listened to them, talked to them, took time with them, made eye contact, made a connection, and showed personal interest in them and their healthcare needs, it provided them with an impetus to take action with regard to their personal health (Woods et al.). Additionally, Kaluzny et al. (1995) reported that Community Clinical Oncology Programs that were able to accrue participants to cancer prevention and control trials developed links with primary care community physicians with access to potential subjects. Those who did not develop links were not as successful.

Potential subjects for participation in cancer prevention and control studies also experience barriers. The most important reason for not participating is the time and inconvenience involved, including time spent waiting and traveling to and from the clinic or prevention center. Subjects are influenced by negative personal and family attitudes as well as the belief that the evidence of benefit from participation is inadequate. The possibility of experiencing unacceptable toxicities is an issue that must be addressed in the development of a prevention trial. In treatment trials, a certain amount of toxicity is acceptable. Because subjects in prevention trials are healthy, however, significant adverse effects must be avoided.

The cost related to participation is an important issue that needs to be addressed when considering recruitment strategies. Participant-related costs can be associated with study-required medical tests, procedures, and examinations. However, transportation, lost wages because of time off work, and lack of income also are important cost issues. Insurance coverage for prevention trials is, at this time, uncertain and may depend on state regulations. Some studies, such as the Study of Tamoxifen and Raloxifene (known as STAR), had economic funds for women with limited means to obtain the study-required physical examinations and laboratory and radiology tests. Insurance companies are increasingly becoming aware of clinical trials and their related costs. Physicians practicing in managed-care environments may resist referring participants. In addition, populations with low socioeconomic levels may consider health maintenance and disease prevention to be of little importance in their day-to-day survival, offering another challenge to recruitment strategies for cancer control studies. A study conducted by Gross, Filardo, Mayne, and Krumholz (2005) suggested that low socioeconomic status is a more likely mediator in trial enrollment disparities than in willingness to enroll.

Social contacts and social support can play an important role in the use of preventive care services. People with fewer social contacts are less likely to have had medical or dental check-ups than those with more social contacts. Social "pressure" from family and friends may provide the necessary encouragement, information, or logistic means for individuals to seek and maintain screening practices.

Other issues that may influence an individual's participation in a prevention trial include anxiety, fatalism, fear, misconceptions, and availability of and accessibility to the study center (Swanson & Ward, 1995). Increased anxiety levels have been directly related to poor attendance at clinical breast exams and poor adherence to monthly breast self-examinations (McCance, Mooney, Field, & Smith, 1996). Fatalism, a belief that death is inevitable when cancer is present, is a common phenomenon in populations with lower socioeconomic and educational levels. Fatalism is more common in African Americans than in Caucasians and is more common in females than in males. As a result of fatalism, African Americans often avoid seeking medical care for 3–12 months after experiencing symptoms (Swanson & Ward, 1995). Accessing health care at a relatively late stage (i.e., being reluctant to visit doctors, accessing health care only when pain is no longer bearable, and using emergency services as a portal to health care) is an acknowledged health-seeking behavior of African American males; this also has been referred to as the *black male health behavior phenomenon* (Braithwaite, 2001). Fear of the unknown and the possibility of being used as a "guinea pig" also are common reactions when discussing possible participation in prevention trials (NCI, 1997). Some common misconceptions reported are that an illness can be caused by witchcraft or evil spirits or that an illness is a punishment for disobeying God and, therefore, medical treatment will be of little benefit.

Perhaps human behavior is the most important aspect in addressing cancer prevention and early detection. According to the literature, the failure of a participant to place importance on evaluation is a significant barrier, as are cultural bias, language barriers, and denial. McCance et al. (1996) confirmed this, stating that human behavior is crucial in the early detection of cancers. Use of self-examination and participation in screening procedures are vital for the effective detection and treatment of cancer.

Morrow and Bellg (1994) reported that to make effective interventions, one needs to examine the human processes involving an understanding of the sociocultural context of the interaction so that the culture and values of the medical world interact successfully with the culture and values of the patient's world. Second, one should examine the processes involving respect for and cooperation with the patients, so that clinicians can understand what patients want and experience as individuals, and both parties are motivated to do what is necessary to implement change. The third consideration is a healthy respect for the difficulties in implementing behavioral change.

Morrow, Hickok, and Burish (1994) described four health belief concepts. The first belief is *probability*, the perceived likelihood or perception of a patient that he or she has or is expected to have that health condition. This includes the presence of risk factors (e.g., smoking, family history) as well as the patient's knowledge level of the disease and its treatment. The second belief is *severity*, which refers to the individual's perception of the severity of the outcome, whether in the presence of illness or side effects. *Effectiveness*, the third concept, refers to the patient's or physician's idea of the probable success or usefulness of the various arms or components of the trial. The patient, in this case, may be influenced by trust in the medical care or physician and social support system. The patient-physician relationship, again, plays a significant role. The fourth concept, *perceived costs*, includes all of the burdens or barriers to entry into the trial. The concepts of disease probability and severity have minimal influence on accrual to any phase of treatment trials; however, they are of considerable importance in accrual to cancer control trials, particularly prevention, screening, and early detection trials.

Similarly, theories such as the Health Belief Model (HBM) and the Transtheoretical Model (TTM) have allowed healthcare professionals to tailor interventions to individuals using new technologies (Rosenstock, 1974). The HBM provides guidance for tailoring messages according to beliefs shown to influence screening. It includes three constructs: perceived benefits and barriers, perceived risk of contracting a health problem, and confidence in the ability to take action (self-efficacy). According to the TTM, health behavior change can be viewed on a continuum wherein the individual moves from not considering an action or health behavior to maintaining adoption of the behavior. The model considers the individual's past history of the targeted behavior and intention regarding future behavior (Champion & Rawl, 2005). Other models also have been utilized to assess human behavior as it relates to health care, such as the Continuum of Cancer Care Model, the PRECEDE-PROCEED Model, and the Behavioral Model of Utilization.

Continued behavioral science studies will provide more insight into these issues in the future and will lead to an increased understanding of future directions to be taken. Until then, these concepts and beliefs will need to be kept in mind when implementing and recruiting for cancer control and prevention trials.

Paskett, Katz, Degraffinreid, and Tatum (2003) described recruitment strategies that were found to be successful. These strategies were reported to be directed at minority populations but also could be considered for nonminority populations (see Figure 24-4). The potential trial participant's availability and accessibility to the trial also are among the many barriers to consider when recruiting to a prevention trial. If a center is large and confusing, a participant will be less likely to want to participate than if a smaller, community-based center were available. Pro-

---

Figure 24-4. Recruitment Strategies for All Populations

- Characterize the target population.
- Involve members of the population in planning.
- Take the message to the population.
- Give something back to the community.
- Enhance credibility with a community spokesperson.
- Identify and remove barriers.
- Improve staff sensitivity.
- Educate the population about the trial.

Note. Based on information from Paskett et al., 2003.

---

viding transportation to and from the center or providing drive-up service, if appropriate, are other thoughts to keep in mind.

Initial planning strategies for the recruitment of participants to prevention trials should include staffing issues. Recruitment to prevention trials often will require certain marketing and public relations skills or the possible involvement of a marketing department. Prevention trial staff members are required to be dedicated, with a willingness to see the long-term benefits of cancer control in comparison to the shorter-term benefits of treatment trials. The time requirement per participant for a prevention trial can be considerably longer than for that of a treatment trial participant, an issue that needs to be taken into account when considering staffing needs. Recruitment to and maintenance of a prevention trial requires effective time management skills, as well. Many participants may be employed and will be unable to miss work to meet with the prevention trial nurse. The nurse may have to consider changing or fluctuating work hours to meet the needs of trial participants.

Recruitment to prevention trials will require a change of focus of CTNs who have previously only recruited patients to treatment trials. Patients no longer will come unsolicited. The prevention message must be brought to the communities by the CTN and physicians through outreach education. NCI has found that lack of public awareness and knowledge about cancer clinical trials is a major reason for insufficient accrual. Surveys have shown that overall awareness and understanding of clinical treatment and prevention trials is low (NCI, 2001). A positive message related to prevention must therefore be conveyed.

Positive messages to present regarding prevention trials are shown in Figure 24-5. These messages need to be taken to local faith-based organizations, advocacy groups, other civic community health centers and community groups, and outreach physicians who have patients in these trials.

NCI's (2001) *Clinical Trials Education Series* is a collection of resources designed to educate patients with cancer, advocacy groups, healthcare professionals, and the general public about cancer clinical trials. The series includes 13 educational resources in a variety of media, which can be used with several adult education approaches. The resources include workbooks, booklets/brochures, videos, slide programs, and a Web-based course. Organizations, as well as

---

Figure 24-5. Positive Messages to Present Regarding Prevention Trials

- They can offer the participant medical follow-up by experienced staff.
- An illness could be prevented.
- The participant can experience the satisfaction of becoming involved in research.
- The participant may experience an improvement in quality of life.
- The participant could be helping future generations.

---

individual CTNs, can use the materials to educate a variety of audiences by using the suggested agendas and training programs for targeted audiences and settings, as well as the goals and objectives, planning guides, and knowledge evaluation questionnaires. The series includes four sample training programs aimed at audiences needing basic information about clinical trials to a train-the-trainer program. All resources, except the Web-based course, can be ordered individually by calling NCI's Cancer Information Service at 800-4-CANCER (800-422-6237). Most are also available on the Internet at www.cancer.gov. The Web-based course can be accessed at http://cme.cancer.gov.

Adequate funding for prevention trial recruitment and maintenance can be a challenge for the CTN. Additional grants or funds may be needed to cover the costs of a prevention trial. Developing a relationship with a foundation or a separate funding source is essential. Negotiating for lower "research" rates for study-specific tests, examinations, and other participant-related costs through local institutions also can improve accrual to prevention trials.

Recruitment to prevention trials entices the CTN and staff to conduct regular meetings (preferably weekly) to evaluate current strategies and discuss needed modifications. Other discussions can take place regarding current accrual, increased education needed, and plans for new protocols. Graphing accrual progress can offer a visual effect for staff members as well as give a visual goal to be attained.

Recognizing community involvement in prevention trial recruitment can increase current needed accrual. Physician and staff recognition certificates or plaques can reinforce positive recruitment efforts. Continued communication with community physicians and their staff members can be invaluable in maintaining an interest level and willingness to assist with recruitment efforts. Obtaining information from research bases and study centers, as well as having the specific protocol on site, can improve recruitment. Brochure development may be necessary for certain studies. Study-specific brochures should be shared with office staff and made available in patient waiting rooms and exam rooms.

Summary

Recruitment to cancer control and prevention studies can be challenging in many ways. Many factors need to be considered prior to recruitment and during the study phase and follow-up. This chapter shares some of these factors, as well as steps to assist the CTN in his or her efforts to improve accrual to these important studies. As history has shown, it often is the nurse who makes the difference when it comes to patient and family care. The CTN has that opportunity, again, when promoting and supporting cancer control and prevention research.

References

American Cancer Society. (2007). *Cancer facts and figures, 2007*. Atlanta, GA: Author.

Braithwaite, R.L. (2001). The health status of black men. In R.L. Braithwaite & S.E. Taylor (Eds.), *Health issues in the black community* (2nd ed., pp. 62–80). San Francisco: Jossey-Bass.

Champion, V.L., & Rawl, S.M. (2005). Secondary prevention of cancer. *Seminars in Oncology Nursing, 21*, 252–259.

Clark, L.C., Combs, G.F., Turnbull, B.W., Slate, E.H., Chalker, D.K., Chow, J., et al. (1996). Effects of selenium supplementation for cancer prevention in patients with carcinoma of the skin. *JAMA, 276*, 1957–1963.

Cohen, G. (2002). Cancer clinical trials: A primer for participation of community physicians. *American Society of Clinical Oncology 2002 Educational Book*, pp. 283–289.

Doll, R., & Peto, R. (1981). The causes of cancer: Quantitative estimates of avoidable risks of cancer in the United States today. *Journal of the National Cancer Institute, 66*, 1191–1308.

Fisher, B., Costantino, J.P., Wickerham, D.L., Redmond, C.K., Kavanah, M., Cronin, W.M., et al. (1998). Tamoxifen for prevention of breast cancer: Report of the National Surgical Adjuvant Breast and Bowel Project P-1 Study. *Journal of the National Cancer Institute, 90*, 1371–1388.

Garewal, H.S., & Meyskens, F.L., Jr. (1991). Chemoprevention of cancer. *Hematology/Oncology Clinics of North America, 5*, 69–77.

Gordis, L. (1996). *Epidemiology*. Philadelphia: Saunders.

Greenwald, P. (2005). The future of cancer prevention. *Seminars in Oncology Nursing, 21*, 296–298.

Greenwald, P., Nixon, D.W., Malone, W.F., Kelloff, G.J., Stern, H.R., & Witkin, K.M. (1990). Concepts in cancer chemoprevention research. *Cancer, 65*, 1483–1490.

Greenwald, P., & Sondik, E.J. (1986). Cancer control objectives for the nation: 1985–2000. *National Cancer Institute Monographs, 2*, 1–105.

Gross, C.P., Filardo, G., Mayne, S.T., & Krumholz, H.M. (2005). The impact of socioeconomic status and race on trial participation for older women with breast cancer. *Cancer, 103*, 483–491.

Heinonen, O.P., & Albanes, D. (1994). The effect of vitamin E and beta carotene on the incidence of lung cancer and other cancers in male smokers. *New England Journal of Medicine, 330*, 1029–1035.

Hong, W.K., Lippman, S.M., Itri, L., Karp, D.D., Lee, J.S., Byers, R.M., et al. (1990). Prevention of second primary tumors with isotretinoin in squamous-cell carcinoma of the head and neck. *New England Journal of Medicine, 323*, 795–801.

Hong, W.K., & Sporn, M.B. (1997). Recent advances in chemoprevention of cancer. *Science, 278*, 1073–1077.

Kaluzny, A.D., Warnecke, R., Lacey, L.M., Johnson, T., Gillings, D., & Ozer, H. (1995). Using a community clinical trial network for treatment, prevention and control research: Assuring access to state-of-the-art cancer care. *Cancer Investigation, 13*, 517–525.

Kelloff, G.J., Boone, C.W., Steele, V.E., Crowell, J.A., Lubet, R., & Sigman, C.C. (1994). Progress in cancer chemoprevention: Perspectives on agent selection and short-term clinical intervention trials. *Cancer Research, 54*, 2015–2024.

Klein, E.A., Thompson, I.M., Lippman, S.M., Goodman, P.J., Albanes, D., Taylor, P.R., et al. (2001). SELECT: The next prostate cancer prevention trial. *Journal of Urology, 166*, 1311–1315.

McCance, K.L., Mooney, K.H., Field, R., & Smith, K.R. (1996). Influence of others in motivating women to obtain breast cancer screening. *Cancer Practice, 4*, 141–146.

Meyskens, F.L., Jr. (1992). Strategies for prevention of cancer in humans. *Oncology (Williston Park), 6*(Suppl. 2), 15–24.

Meyskens, F.L., Jr. (2004). Cancer prevention, screening, and early detection. In M. Abeloff, J. Armitage, J. Niederhuber, & M. Kastan (Eds.), *Clinical oncology* (3rd ed., pp. 425–472). Philadelphia: Elsevier.

Meyskens, F.L., & Tully, P. (2005). Principles of cancer prevention. *Seminars in Oncology Nursing, 21*, 229–235.

Morrow, G.R., & Bellg, A.J. (1994). Behavioral science in translational research and cancer control. *Cancer, 74*(Suppl. 4), 1409–1417.

Morrow, G.R., Hickok, J.T., & Burish, T.G. (1994). Behavioral aspects of clinical trials: An integrated framework from behavior theory. *Cancer, 74*(Suppl. 9), 2676–2682.

National Cancer Institute. (1997). *Cancer clinical trials education program.* Bethesda, MD: Author.

National Cancer Institute. (2001). *The National Cancer Institute clinical trials education series.* Bethesda, MD: Author.

National Cancer Institute. (2006). *The nation's investment in cancer research: A plan and budget proposal for fiscal year 2008* [NIH Publication No. 06-6090]. Bethesda, MD: Author.

Paskett, E.D., Katz, M.L., Degraffinreid, C.R., & Tatum, C.M. (2003). Participation in cancer trials: Recruitment of underserved populations. *Clinical Advances in Hematology and Oncology, 1*, 607–613.

Rosenstock, I.M. (1974). The Health Belief Model and preventive health behavior. *Health Education Monograph, 2*, 354–386.

Sandler, R.S., Halabi, S., Baron, J.A., Budinger, S., Budinger, S., Paskett, E., et al. (2003). A randomized trial of aspirin to prevent colorectal adenomas in patients with previous colorectal cancer. *New England Journal of Medicine, 348*, 883–890.

Smith, J.J., Tully, P., & Padberg, R.M. (2005). Chemoprevention: A primary cancer prevention strategy. *Seminars in Oncology Nursing, 21*, 243–251.

Solomon, S.D., McMurray, J.V., Pfeffer, M.A., Wittes, J., Fowler, R., Finn, P., et al. (2005). Cardiovascular risk associated with celecoxib in a clinical trial for colorectal adenoma prevention. *New England Journal of Medicine, 352*, 1071–1080.

Spilker, B., & Cramer, J.A. (1992). *Patient recruitment in clinical trials.* New York: Raven Press.

Steinbach, G., Lynch, P.M., Phillips, R.K., Wallace, M.H., Hawk, E., Gordon, G.B., et al. (2000). The effect of celecoxib, a cyclooxygenase-2 inhibitor, in familial adenocarcinomatous polyposis. *New England Journal of Medicine, 342*, 1946–1952.

Swanson, G.M., & Ward, A.J. (1995). Recruiting minorities into clinical trials: Toward a participant-friendly system. *Journal of the National Cancer Institute, 87*, 1747–1759.

Thompson, I.M., Goodman, P.H., Tangen, C.M., Lucia, M.S., Miller, G.J., Ford, L.G., et al. (2003). The influence of finasteride on the development of prostate cancer. *New England Journal of Medicine, 349*, 215–224.

U.S. Department of Health and Human Services, National Institutes of Health. (2006). *Study of Tamoxifen and Raloxifene (STAR) trial.* Retrieved August 22, 2007, from http://www.cancer.gov/clinicaltrials/digestpage/STAR

Woods, V.D., Montgomery, S.B., & Herring, R.P. (2004). Recruiting black/African American men for research on prostate cancer prevention. *Cancer, 100*, 1017–1025.

Yeomans-Kinney, A., Richards, C., Vernon, S.W., & Vogel, V.G. (1998). The effect of physician recommendation on enrollment in the breast cancer chemoprevention trial. *Preventive Medicine, 27*(5 Pt. 1), 713–719.

Yeomans-Kinney, A., Vernon, S.W., Frankowski, R.F., Weber, D.M., Bitsura, J.M., & Vogel, V.G. (1995). Factors related to enrollment in the breast cancer prevention trial at a comprehensive cancer center during the first year of enrollment. *Cancer, 76*, 46–56.

SECTION VI

Active Treatment

CHAPTER 25
Investigational Agents and Procurement of Research Study Drugs

Siu-Fun Wong, PharmD, FASHP, FCSHP, and Joan G. Westendorp, RN, MSN, OCN®

Introduction

During the past century, as new drug developments evolved, the treatment of previously fatal diseases was converted into routine therapeutic interventions. The process of drug development has improved since the 1950s but remains timely and costly. The first step in development is the discovery of a potential new drug molecule, which used to be highly empiric and has since evolved to be more focused to test rationally designed molecules for activity against well-characterized human cancer cell lines, molecular targets, or both. Preclinical testing in animals is essential as the second step of development. This provides essential information about toxicity and pharmacokinetics and is a basis for rational schedule development for the drug in humans. Clinical testing of the drug involves humans going through the phases of clinical trials (see Chapter 1). Discovering and developing safe and effective new drugs is a long, difficult, and expensive process.

Discovery of Drugs

Most new drugs are identified through one of three approaches: (a) chemical modification of a known molecule, (b) random screening for biologic activity of large numbers of natural products such as herbal remedies, poisons, or plants, or (c) rational drug design based on an understanding of biologic mechanisms and chemical structure (Katzung, 2001). Approximately 30% of current effective antineoplastic drugs are from natural sources or are derivatives of natural products (Mann, 1994). Regardless of the method used to develop a drug, an initial sequence of drug screening occurs. This is a variety of biologic assays at the molecular, cellular, organ, and whole animal levels to define the activity and selectivity of the drug. The type of drug screening depends on the pharmacologic goal of the drug (Katzung). After screening and animal testing are completed, an investigational new drug (IND) application can be filed with the U.S. Food and Drug Administration (FDA). The IND becomes effective if the FDA does not reject it within 30 days (FDA, n.d.). The IND application must indicate the results of the previous experiments, including any toxic effects found in the animal studies. After this process, the drug moves to clinical testing.

Clinical testing goes through the three phases of clinical trials. Once the drug's actions, safety, dosage, and toxicities are established, and if effectiveness is found, the pharmaceutical company will file a new drug application (NDA) or biologic license application (BLA) with the FDA. The NDA must contain all of the scientific data that have been collected. Along with the scientific data, all marketing and educational materials relating to the NDA must be included. The FDA is allowed 180 days to review an NDA, but it can take up to two-and-one-half years. The BLA covers specified biotechnology and synthetic biologic products regulated under the Public Health Service Act, and the application process is very similar to that of the NDA. Under a plan implemented by the FDA in early 1989, the Expedited Process, phase II and III protocols may be combined for drugs that indicate sufficient promise in early testing and that are targeted against serious or life-threatening diseases, such as cancer. This may reduce the total number of years of the development process by two to three years (FDA, n.d.).

Once the FDA approves the NDA, the drug becomes available for physicians to prescribe. At this time, phase IV protocols may be undertaken that involve postmarketing surveillance. These are intended to develop "field" information on efficacy and toxicity. The process of drug discovery is extensive and costly, but measures have been developed in the past five years to expedite drug availability for oncology treatment. The new Office of Oncology Drug Products at the FDA and the Rapid Access to Intervention and Development program at the National Cancer Institute (NCI) are examples of the improvement process put forth by the FDA (FDA, n.d.).

Procurement of Research Study Drugs

Prior to the initiation of a research protocol at an institution, the protocol coordinator must ensure that all of the appropriate documents have been filed to facilitate the acquisition of study medications in a timely manner. The following section provides the guidelines for this preparatory stage and for the procurement of research study drugs with various contract sponsors.

When a protocol is approved by all of the governing bodies at an institution, the principal investigator or his or her designee should be identified to initiate the study drug(s) ordering, as indicated. Any investigator who receives and administers an investigational agent supplied by NCI must be registered with NCI by filing the FDA 1572 form (see Figure 25-1), a curriculum vitae, a completed and signed supplemental investigator data form (see Figure 25-2), and a completed financial disclosure form (see Figure 25-3) with an original signature. The investigator must renew this registration annually. Investigational drugs provided by NCI to a registered investigator are the direct responsibility of the investigator. Secondary distribution to other registered investigators does not relieve the primary investigator to whom the original shipment was made from his or her responsibility (NCI Cancer Therapy Evaluation Program [CTEP], 2002).

Research study drugs that are supplied by CTEP for NCI's Division of Cancer Treatment and Diagnosis must be shipped from the Pharmaceutical Management Branch (PMB) directly to the institution or site where the agent will be prepared and administered. Direct shipment of research study drugs to the preparation site simplifies mail and drug-handling tracking for investigators and the PMB, minimizes delays in correspondence in emergencies, ensures drug shipment integrity, reduces administrative workload (i.e., maintenance of additional accountability records, drug transfer forms, and correspondence), and eliminates secondary shipping expenses (NCI, 2002b).

Research study drugs from NCI must not be redistributed or transferred to another institution or site, with the exception of satellite or affiliated facility distribution. Satellite or affiliated facilities are defined as institutions that are located on the same campus or in proximity to the control pharmacy service when transportation of the drugs can be conducted by an institution employee. However, the centralized (control) pharmacy service ultimately is responsible for all investigational agents received and must provide copies of all accountability records during any NCI- or FDA-directed audit (NCI, 2002c).

To order research study drugs, the principal investigator or designee must refer to the drug information section of the protocol to identify the supplier of the study drugs. For research study drugs that are available through NCI, the NCI clinical drug request form must be completed with the following information (NCI, 2002a , 2002d) (see Figure 25-4). Orders must be typed. Incomplete, illegible, or inaccurate clinical drug request forms will be denied and faxed back to the sender; therefore, a return/reply telephone or fax number of the designee must be included on the order form.

1. Investigator name (Identify the principal or lead investigator on the front cover of the protocol or the designated institutional principal investigator at the study institution for cooperative group trials.)
2. NCI investigator number (NCI-designated investigator number)
3. Designee/requester name (investigator or designee identified on the NCI investigator registration form)
4. Title (e.g., physician, pharmacist, nurse, data manager)
5. Telephone number (telephone number of the requester)
6. Fax number (facsimile number of the requester)
7. Investigator signature (investigator or designee must sign the form)
8. Date (date the order was sent)
9. NCI protocol number (Use the NCI-designated protocol number. Do not use an institution-assigned protocol number.)
10. Number of patients currently being treated (number of patients enrolled and active on protocol)
11. Patient or special code (Only if applicable. List of patients' initials or ID numbers for certain protocols is required for drug ordering.)
12. Institution's current inventory (amount of drugs on hand)
13. National Service Center number (six-digit number assigned to a particular drug that can be located either on the cover page or in the "Drug Information" section of the protocol)
14. Drug name (Use the same name as indicated on the protocol. Note that only one agent may be entered in each line; if there is more than one protocol per agent, use a separate line for each protocol.)
15. Strength and dosage form (Such as xx mg vials, ampules, tablets, etc. Note that only one strength/package size may be entered in each line; if there is more than one strength per protocol, use a separate line for each strength/package size.)
16. Quantity ordered (It is recommended to order six- to eight-week supplies.)
17. Date needed (According to the 2002 CTEP Policy and Guidelines for Investigational Agent Ordering (NCI, 2002d), normal PMB processing time is two working days after the order is faxed to 301-480-4612. The orders are shipped by U.S. Postal Service Priority Mail. Agents with special storage or shipping requirements, such as refrigerated or frozen materials, are shipped Monday through Thursday for next-day delivery. For emergency or urgent needs, the drug order must be faxed by 2 pm Eastern Standard Time for next-day delivery. The investigator must provide an express courier account number in the order located in the mid-section at the bottom of the form. A telephone follow-up is highly recommended to ensure receipt of the faxed order.)
18. Shipping address (Located at the lower left-hand corner. Use the address where drugs will be stored [e.g.,

Figure 25-1. Statement of Investigator Form

DEPARTMENT OF HEALTH AND HUMAN SERVICES
FOOD AND DRUG ADMINISTRATION

STATEMENT OF INVESTIGATOR
(TITLE 21, CODE OF FEDERAL REGULATIONS (CFR) PART 312)
(See instructions on reverse side.)

Form Approved: OMB No. 0910-0014.
Expiration Date: May 31, 2009.
See OMB Statement on Reverse.

NOTE: No investigator may participate in an investigation until he/she provides the sponsor with a completed, signed Statement of Investigator, Form FDA 1572 (21 CFR 312.53(c)).

1. NAME AND ADDRESS OF INVESTIGATOR

2. EDUCATION, TRAINING, AND EXPERIENCE THAT QUALIFIES THE INVESTIGATOR AS AN EXPERT IN THE CLINICAL INVESTIGATION OF THE DRUG FOR THE USE UNDER INVESTIGATION. ONE OF THE FOLLOWING IS ATTACHED.

☐ CURRICULUM VITAE   ☐ OTHER STATEMENT OF QUALIFICATIONS

3. NAME AND ADDRESS OF ANY MEDICAL SCHOOL, HOSPITAL OR OTHER RESEARCH FACILITY WHERE THE CLINICAL INVESTIGATION(S) WILL BE CONDUCTED.

4. NAME AND ADDRESS OF ANY CLINICAL LABORATORY FACILITIES TO BE USED IN THE STUDY.

5. NAME AND ADDRESS OF THE INSTITUTIONAL REVIEW BOARD (IRB) THAT IS RESPONSIBLE FOR REVIEW AND APPROVAL OF THE STUDY(IES).

6. NAMES OF THE SUBINVESTIGATORS *(e.g., research fellows, residents, associates)* WHO WILL BE ASSISTING THE INVESTIGATOR IN THE CONDUCT OF THE INVESTIGATION(S).

7. NAME AND CODE NUMBER, IF ANY, OF THE PROTOCOL(S) IN THE IND FOR THE STUDY(IES) TO BE CONDUCTED BY THE INVESTIGATOR.

FORM FDA 1572 (5/06)   PREVIOUS EDITION IS OBSOLETE.   **PAGE 1 OF 2**

PSC Graphics (301) 443-1090   EF

(Continued on next page)

Figure 25-1. Statement of Investigator Form *(Continued)*

8. ATTACH THE FOLLOWING CLINICAL PROTOCOL INFORMATION:

☐ FOR PHASE 1 INVESTIGATIONS, A GENERAL OUTLINE OF THE PLANNED INVESTIGATION INCLUDING THE ESTIMATED DURATION OF THE STUDY AND THE MAXIMUM NUMBER OF SUBJECTS THAT WILL BE INVOLVED.

☐ FOR PHASE 2 OR 3 INVESTIGATIONS, AN OUTLINE OF THE STUDY PROTOCOL INCLUDING AN APPROXIMATION OF THE NUMBER OF SUBJECTS TO BE TREATED WITH THE DRUG AND THE NUMBER TO BE EMPLOYED AS CONTROLS, IF ANY; THE CLINICAL USES TO BE INVESTIGATED; CHARACTERISTICS OF SUBJECTS BY AGE, SEX, AND CONDITION; THE KIND OF CLINICAL OBSERVATIONS AND LABORATORY TESTS TO BE CONDUCTED; THE ESTIMATED DURATION OF THE STUDY; AND COPIES OR A DESCRIPTION OF CASE REPORT FORMS TO BE USED.

9. COMMITMENTS:

I agree to conduct the study(ies) in accordance with the relevant, current protocol(s) and will only make changes in a protocol after notifying the sponsor, except when necessary to protect the safety, rights, or welfare of subjects.

I agree to personally conduct or supervise the described investigation(s).

I agree to inform any patients, or any persons used as controls, that the drugs are being used for investigational purposes and I will ensure that the requirements relating to obtaining informed consent in 21 CFR Part 50 and institutional review board (IRB) review and approval in 21 CFR Part 56 are met.

I agree to report to the sponsor adverse experiences that occur in the course of the investigation(s) in accordance with 21 CFR 312.64.

I have read and understand the information in the investigator's brochure, including the potential risks and side effects of the drug.

I agree to ensure that all associates, colleagues, and employees assisting in the conduct of the study(ies) are informed about their obligations in meeting the above commitments.

I agree to maintain adequate and accurate records in accordance with 21 CFR 312.62 and to make those records available for inspection in accordance with 21 CFR 312.68.

I will ensure that an IRB that complies with the requirements of 21 CFR Part 56 will be responsible for the initial and continuing review and approval of the clinical investigation. I also agree to promptly report to the IRB all changes in the research activity and all unanticipated problems involving risks to human subjects or others. Additionally, I will not make any changes in the research without IRB approval, except where necessary to eliminate apparent immediate hazards to human subjects.

I agree to comply with all other requirements regarding the obligations of clinical investigators and all other pertinent requirements in 21 CFR Part 312.

INSTRUCTIONS FOR COMPLETING FORM FDA 1572
STATEMENT OF INVESTIGATOR:

1. Complete all sections. Attach a separate page if additional space is needed.

2. Attach curriculum vitae or other statement of qualifications as described in Section 2.

3. Attach protocol outline as described in Section 8.

4. Sign and date below.

5. FORWARD THE COMPLETED FORM AND ATTACHMENTS TO THE SPONSOR. The sponsor will incorporate this information along with other technical data into an Investigational New Drug Application (IND).
    INVESTIGATORS SHOULD NOT SEND THIS FORM DIRECTLY TO THE FOOD AND DRUG ADMINISTRATION.

10. SIGNATURE OF INVESTIGATOR	11. DATE

(**WARNING:** A willfully false statement is a criminal offense. U.S.C. Title 18, Sec. 1001.)

Public reporting burden for this collection of information is estimated to average 100 hours per response, including the time for reviewing instructions, searching existing data sources, gathering and maintaining the data needed, and completing reviewing the collection of information. Send comments regarding this burden estimate or any other aspect of this collection of information, including suggestions for reducing this burden to:

| Department of Health and Human Services
Food and Drug Administration
Center for Drug Evaluation and Research (HFD-143)
Central Document Room
5901-B Ammendale Road
Beltsville, MD 207052-1266 | Department of Health and Human Services
Food and Drug Administration
Center for Biologics Evaluation and Research (HFM-99)
1401 Rockville Pike
Rockville, MD 20852-1448 | "An agency may not conduct or sponsor, and a person is not required to respond to, a collection of information unless it displays a currently valid OMB control number." |

Please DO NOT RETURN this application to this address.

FORM FDA 1572 (5/06)   PAGE 2 OF 2

Figure 25-2. National Cancer Institute Supplemental Investigator Data Form

SUPPLEMENTAL INVESTIGATOR DATA FORM

Date (MM/DD/YYYY): ___ / ___ / ___

Sections 1 – 11: REQUIRED INFORMATION (Collected for all investigators participating in NCI-sponsored clinical trials.)

1. Investigator Name (Last, First, Middle, Suffix):

2. Degree(s):

3. NCI Investigator No.:

4. Date of Birth (MM/YYYY): ___ / ____

5. Provider No. (UPIN):

6. Are you currently licensed to practice medicine? ☐ YES ☐ NO

7. Primary Specialty Practice(s): Check all that apply.

Specialty	Board Eligible:	Board Certified:	Specialty	Board Eligible:	Board Certified:
Anatomic and/or Clinical Pathology	☐	☐	Obstetrics and Gynecology	☐	☐
Clinical Genetics	☐	☐	Orthopedic Surgery	☐	☐
Colon and Rectal Surgery	☐	☐	Otolaryngology	☐	☐
Dermatology	☐	☐	Pediatric Hematology-Oncology	☐	☐
Diagnostic Radiology	☐	☐	Pediatrics	☐	☐
Family Practice	☐	☐	Psychiatry	☐	☐
Gastroenterology	☐	☐	Public Health and General Preventative Medicine	☐	☐
Gynecological Oncology	☐	☐	Radiation Oncology	☐	☐
Hematology	☐	☐	Surgery	☐	☐
Internal Medicine	☐	☐	Surgical Oncology	☐	☐
Medical Oncology	☐	☐	Thoracic Surgery	☐	☐
Neurological Surgery	☐	☐	Urology	☐	☐
Neurology	☐	☐	Other _____	☐	☐

8. Have you received training in: *Completion of this training is mandatory for all NCI-registered investigators.*

"Protection of Human Research Participants"?   ☐ YES   DATE COMPLETED (MM/YYYY): ___ / ____

In sections 9 – 11, use this side to either enter new information or view current information.

In sections 9 – 11, use this side to make changes to current information only.

9. Office Address: The office address will be used for receipt of all official correspondence.

Institution: _____	Institution: _____
Internal Office: _____	Internal Office: _____
Street Address: _____	Street Address: _____
Street Address: _____	Street Address: _____
City: _____	City: _____
State/Province: _____	State/Province: _____
Zip/Postal Code: _____	Zip/Postal Code: _____
Country: _____	Country: _____
Office Phone No.: _____	Office Phone No.: _____
Office FAX No.: _____	Office FAX No.: _____
Office E-mail: _____	Office E-mail: _____

(Continued on next page)

Figure 25-2. National Cancer Institute Supplemental Investigator Data Form *(Continued)*

10. Primary Shipping Address: The primary shipping address will be used for receipt of all CTEP-supplied agents.

Institution: _____	Institution: _____
Internal Office: _____	Internal Office: _____
Street Address: _____	Street Address: _____
Street Address: _____	Street Address: _____
City: _____	City: _____
State/Province: _____	State/Province: _____
Zip/Postal Code: _____	Zip/Postal Code: _____
Country: _____	Country: _____

Shipping Designee: Provide name of shipping designee (preferably a pharmacist) approved to order and receive CTEP-supplied agents.

Shipping Designee Name: _____	Shipping Designee Name: _____
Shipping Designee Phone No.: _____	Shipping Designee Phone No.: _____
Shipping Designee FAX No.: _____	Shipping Designee FAX No.: _____
Shipping Designee E-mail: _____	Shipping Designee E-mail: _____

NCI USE ONLY: ☐ PSD   ☐ SD   ☐ IA

11. Ordering Designee(s): Provide name(s) of ordering designee(s) approved to order CTEP-supplied agents. **Note that a "Clinical Drug Request (CDR) Form" for a CTEP-supplied agent must be signed by either the investigator, the authorized shipping designee (from item #10), or an ordering designee (from item #11). An ordering designee must use the primary shipping address (from item #10).**

A. Ordering Designee Name: _____	A. Ordering Designee Name: _____
Ordering Designee Phone No.: _____	Ordering Designee Phone No.: _____
Ordering Designee Fax No.: _____	Ordering Designee Fax No.: _____
Ordering Designee E-mail: _____	Ordering Designee E-mail: _____
B. Ordering Designee Name: _____	B. Ordering Designee Name: _____
Ordering Designee Phone No.: _____	Ordering Designee Phone No.: _____
Ordering Designee Fax No.: _____	Ordering Designee Fax No.: _____
Ordering Designee E-mail: _____	Ordering Designee E-mail: _____
C. Ordering Designee Name: _____	C. Ordering Designee Name: _____
Ordering Designee Phone No.: _____	Ordering Designee Phone No.: _____
Ordering Designee Fax No.: _____	Ordering Designee Fax No.: _____
Ordering Designee E-mail: _____	Ordering Designee E-mail: _____

Please be sure you have also included:
1. Completed FDA Form 1572 with original signature.
2. Current Curriculum Vitae (CV).
3. Completed Financial Disclosure Form with original signature.

I certify that the information on this "Supplemental Investigator Data Form" is true and correct to the best of my knowledge.

Investigator: _____   Date: _____
(Signature)

(Continued on next page)

Figure 25-2. National Cancer Institute Supplemental Investigator Data Form *(Continued)*

Section	INSTRUCTIONS FOR COMPLETING THE SUPPLEMENTAL INVESTIGATOR DATA FORM
1.	**Investigator Name:** Provide legal last name, first name, middle initial or name, and suffix (if applicable).
2.	**Degree(s):** Provide degree(s) (e.g., M.D., D.O., foreign M.D. equivalent).
3.	**NCI Investigator No.:** Provide the unique NCI investigator number assigned to the investigator by the Pharmaceutical Management Branch (PMB), CTEP, DCTD, NCI at the time of initial registration. *(If an investigator has never registered to participate in NCI-sponsored clinical trials, leave field blank. An NCI Investigator No. will be assigned by the PMB as part of the registration process.)*
4.	**Date of Birth:** Indicate the investigator's date of birth (in MM/YYYY format).
5.	**Provider No. (UPIN):** Indicate the investigator's Unique Physician Identification Number (UPIN). *This information is optional and is for internal reporting only.*
6.	**Medical License:** Indicate if the investigator is currently licensed to practice medicine.
7.	**Primary Specialty Practice(s):** Indicate the investigator's primary specialty practice(s). **Board Eligibile:** Indicate if the investigator is eligible for Board Certification in the primary specialty practice selected. **Board Certified:** Indicate if the investigator is Board Certified in the primary specialty practice selected.
8.	**Investigator Training:** Indicate if the investigator has completed the NIH-mandated training in the protection of human research participants, including date completed (in MM/YYYY format). If needed, additional information and online training are available at http://cme.cancer.gov/c01/. The online training takes approximately one hour to complete. *Completion of protection of human research participants training is mandatory for ALL NCI-registered investigators.*
9.	**Office Address:** The office address will be used for receipt of all official correspondence (e.g., annual registration and protocol documents). Include institution, internal office, street, city, state/province, zip/postal code, and country. **Office Phone No.:** Provide daytime phone number at which the investigator can be reached during normal business hours, including area code. Investigators from outside the United States should also include the country code. **Office Fax No.:** Provide Fax number at which the investigator usually receives faxes, including area code. Investigators from outside the United States should also include the country code. **Office E-mail:** Provide E-mail address at which the investigator usually receives e-mail. This address will be used to send information regarding protocols and general information for the investigator.
10.	**Primary Shipping Address:** The primary shipping address will be used for receipt of all CTEP-supplied agents. Include institution, internal office, street, city, state/province, zip/postal code, and country. **Shipping Designee:** Provide name of shipping designee (preferably a pharmacist) approved to order and receive CTEP-supplied agents for the investigator. *Note that a "Clinical Drug Request (CDR) Form" for a CTEP-supplied agent must be signed by either the investigator, the authorized shipping designee (from item #10), or an ordering designee (from item #11).* **Shipping Designee Phone No.:** Provide daytime phone number at which the shipping designee can be reached during normal business hours, including area code. Shipping designees from outside the United States should also include the country code. **Shipping Designee Fax No.:** Provide Fax number at which the shipping designee usually receives faxes, including area code. Shipping designees from outside the United States should also include the country code. **Shipping Designee E-mail:** Provide E-mail address at which the shipping designee usually receives e-mail. This address will be used to send information regarding protocols and general information for shipping designees.
11.	**Ordering Designee(s):** Provide name(s) of ordering designee(s) approved to order CTEP-supplied agents for the investigator. *Note that a "Clinical Drug Request (CDR) Form" for a CTEP-supplied agent must be signed by either the investigator, the authorized shipping designee (from item #10), or an ordering designee (from item #11). An ordering designee must use the primary shipping address (from item #10).* **Ordering Designee Phone No.:** Provide daytime phone number at which the ordering designee can be reached during normal business hours, including area code. Ordering designees from outside the United States should also include the country code. **Ordering Designee Fax No.:** Provide Fax number at which the ordering designee usually receives faxes, including area code. Ordering designees from outside the United States should also include the country code. **Ordering Designee E-mail:** Provide E-mail address at which the ordering designee usually receives e-mail. This address will be used to send information regarding protocols and general information for ordering designees.

Figure 25-3. Financial Disclosure Form

DEPARTMENT OF HEALTH AND HUMAN SERVICES
Food and Drug Administration

Form Approved: OMB No. 0910-0396
Expiration Date: April 30, 2009

DISCLOSURE: FINANCIAL INTERESTS AND ARRANGEMENTS OF CLINICAL INVESTIGATORS

TO BE COMPLETED BY APPLICANT

The following information concerning _____ , who participated
Name of clinical investigator

as a clinical investigator in the submitted study _____
Name of

_____ is submitted in accordance with 21 CFR part 54. The
clinical study

named individual has participated in financial arrangements or holds financial interests that are required to be disclosed as follows:

> *Please mark the applicable check boxes.*

☐ any financial arrangement entered into between the sponsor of the covered study and the clinical investigator involved in the conduct of the covered study, whereby the value of the compensation to the clinical investigator for conducting the study could be influenced by the outcome of the study;

☐ any significant payments of other sorts made on or after February 2, 1999 from the sponsor of the covered study such as a grant to fund ongoing research, compensation in the form of equipment, retainer for ongoing consultation, or honoraria;

☐ any proprietary interest in the product tested in the covered study held by the clinical investigator;

☐ any significant equity interest as defined in 21 CFR 54.2(b), held by the clinical investigator in the sponsor of the covered study.

Details of the individual's disclosable financial arrangements and interests are attached, along with a description of steps taken to minimize the potential bias of clinical study results by any of the disclosed arrangements or interests.

NAME	TITLE
FIRM/ORGANIZATION	
SIGNATURE	DATE

Paperwork Reduction Act Statement

An agency may not conduct or sponsor, and a person is not required to respond to, a collection of information unless it displays a currently valid OMB control number. Public reporting burden for this collection of information is estimated to average 4 hours per response, including time for reviewing instructions, searching existing data sources, gathering and maintaining the necessary data, and completing and reviewing the collection of information. Send comments regarding this burden estimate or any other aspect of this collection of information to:

Department of Health and Human Services
Food and Drug Administration
5600 Fishers Lane, Room 14-72
Rockville, MD 20857

FORM FDA 3455 (4/06)

PSC Graphics: (301) 443-1090   EF

Figure 25-4. Clinical Drug Request Form

CLINICAL DRUG REQUEST
PHARMACEUTICAL MANAGEMENT BRANCH
CANCER THERAPY EVALUATION PROGRAM
DIVISION OF CANCER TREATMENT AND DIAGNOSIS
NATIONAL CANCER INSTITUTE, NIH

Return by FAX to the Pharmaceutical
Management Branch at:

(301) 480-4612

The drugs listed below are requested for the use of (please type or print):

Dr. _____ NCI Investigator Number: _____
Designee/Requester (if other than investigator) (please type or print):
Name _____ Title: _____
Telephone Number: _____ FAX Number: _____
Email address _____

COMMENTS:

NCI USE ONLY
Order number: _____
Date: _____
Authorizing Official Signature _____

Investigator/Designee Signature _____ Date _____

NCI Protocol Number	No. of Pts. Currently Being Treated	Patient or Special Code (if applicable)	Your Current Inventory	NSC Number	Drug Name	Strength & Dosage Form (Specify vials, tablets, etc.)	Quantity Ordered (Specify vials, bottles, etc.)	Date Needed
A								
B								
C								
D								
E								

SHIPPING ADDRESS:

MISCELLANEOUS: Urgent shipments must be accompanied by an express courier account number.

Express Courier Name: _____
Express Courier Acct. No.: _ _ _ – _ _ _ – _ _ _
Reference No.: _____
Express Courier Acct. No. (if other format): _____

INSTRUCTIONS:

1. TYPE ALL INFORMATION - One item or protocol per line.
2. Order using NCI protocol numbers only. Local protocol numbers will cause a delay.
3. Fill in all sections completely including the official shipping address.
4. Limit drug request to an eight (8) week supply.
5. Sign and date the order (must be investigator or designee signature only).
6. Do not mark box labeled FOR NCI USE ONLY.
7. Return to PMB (see above).

NIH Form 986
02/2007

control pharmacy]. The shipping address must be the same as indicated in the investigator's registration form. Any changes in the address must be accompanied by a written explanation with the investigator's or designee's signature.)

In accordance with guidelines set forth by the American Society of Health-System Pharmacists (1991), whenever possible, the pharmacy department should be responsible for drug receipt, storage, accountability, and preparation. All participating investigators at an institution should use the same shipping address.

In some protocols where the drug supply is limited or slow patient accrual is expected, a starter supply of the drug may not be available. Upon enrollment of a patient, use the procedure for emergency supply of drugs to order drugs, or refer to the drug transfer procedures if the circumstance does not allow for timely delivery of the drugs via the emergency ordering procedure. Telephone approval must be obtained from PMB prior to the transfer, and the transfer forms must be submitted within 72 hours of the actual transfer. In cases of emergency transfer during weekends and holidays, PMB must be notified by the next working day (NCI, 2002c).

For pharmaceutical company-sponsored protocols, always refer to the protocol under the "Drug Handling" section for specific instructions.

In protocols where commercially available agents are being used for the study, acquisition of the drugs can be handled as other nonprotocol drugs. However, always refer to the protocol or check with the study coordinator to determine whether a drug accountability form should be kept for tracking the commercially available drugs used for the protocol patients.

Summary

By following the guidelines provided in this chapter, investigators should be able to obtain research study drugs with minimal chance of delay. Accurate documentation is critical in the conduct of clinical trials. Becoming familiar with these requirements will allow investigators to move one step closer to the efficient execution of clinical trials.

References

American Society of Health-System Pharmacists. (1991). Guidelines for the use of investigational drugs in organized health care settings. *American Journal of Health-System Pharmacy, 48,* 315–319.

Katzung, B.G. (2001). Introduction to pharmacology. In B.G. Katzung (Ed.), *Basic and clinical pharmacology* (8th ed., pp. 1–8). San Francisco, CA: Lange & McGraw-Hill.

Mann, J. (1994). Steps to a successful synthesis. *Nature, 367,* 594.

National Cancer Institute. (2002a). *CTEP: Requisition and management of agents. Investigational drug accountability. Forms and instructions.* Bethesda, MD: Author.

National Cancer Institute. (2002b). *CTEP: Requisition and management of agents. Policy and guidelines for investigational agent distribution.* Bethesda, MD: Author.

National Cancer Institute. (2002c). *CTEP: Requisition and management of agents. Policy and guidelines for the transfer of DCTDC supplied investigational agents.* Bethesda, MD: Author.

National Cancer Institute. (2002d). *CTEP: Requisition and management of agents. Policy and guidelines for investigational agent ordering.* Bethesda, MD: Author.

National Cancer Institute Cancer Therapy Evaluation Program. (2002). *Investigator's handbook: A manual for participants in clinical trials of investigational agents sponsored by DCTD, NCI.* Bethesda, MD: Author.

U.S. Food and Drug Administration. (n.d.). *Approvals of FDA-regulated products.* Retrieved October 22, 2007, from http://www.fda.gov/opacom/7approvl.html

CHAPTER 26
Administration of Protocol Agents

Carol Anne Bales, RN, MSN, CCRP, AOCN®,
and Denise Dearing, RN, BSN, OCN®

Introduction

Protocol treatment is a pivotal point in a patient's clinical trial participation. All study procedures up to this point are considered to be preparation for the administration of the investigational treatment. Pre-entry lab work and data obtained before protocol treatment do not contribute to advancing oncology practice. These data serve as a baseline against which to compare the subjects' clinical response to the study treatment. Because of the critical nature of protocol agent administration, the nurse must understand the conditions under which the treatment is administered. This chapter will address the understanding of the knowledge of physical and clinical eligibility criteria, monitoring of critical lab values, and protocol-defined dosage adjustments.

Drug Dosage

Once the planning and evaluation of the protocol are complete and a baseline assessment of the participant has been performed, the first appointment is made to administer the protocol agent or regimen (frequently referred to as "investigational product," "drug," or "study drug"). Prior to administering the protocol-defined agent, the chemotherapy nurse, study coordinator, and investigator must measure the patient's height, weight, and vital signs and evaluate all laboratory parameters required for dose calculation or adjustment. Ongoing review of these criteria will ensure proper dosing in compliance with the study protocol. Dose modifications often have to be made during the course of a study because of a change in the patient's condition. When comparing a patient's laboratory values with the protocol criteria regarding toxicities, the nurse or investigator may discover that an adverse event or patient toxicity has occurred. Each protocol has specific guidelines for dose modification. If a dosage change is required because of an adverse event, the study sponsor or the sponsor's representative (usually called a clinical research associate) or monitor should be contacted. For oncology studies, most protocols contain guidelines for dose adjustments made secondary to the patient's experiencing adverse events.

Calculating Drug Dosage

Several methods are used to determine the dosage of protocol agents. Body surface area (BSA) is widely accepted in determining the dosage of a drug. BSA is measured in square meters (m^2) and is calculated using the patient's height (in centimeters or inches) and weight (in kilograms or pounds). BSA can be determined using a chart called a nomogram. Published nomograms are available, but some have proved to be erroneous. Consequently, mathematical formulas have been developed for the computation of BSA (see Figure 26-1); a calculator with a square root key and the patient's height and weight values are all that is needed. Devices similar to slide rules and calculators that automatically compute BSA are available. Furthermore, online BSA calculators are readily available on the Internet. These tools serve two purposes: to calculate the BSA and to document the calculation via a printout.

Consistency is needed in calculating doses for patients who are overweight. The protocol treatment guidelines should specify whether the BSA is determined using values for ideal body weight or actual body weight. Investigators have suggested that the patient's actual weight be used to determine initial chemotherapy doses in most phase III

Figure 26-1. Equations Used to Calculate Body Surface Area (BSA)

$$BSA\ (m^2) = \sqrt{\frac{Ht\ (in) \times Wt\ (lb)}{3,131}}$$

$$BSA\ (m^2) = \sqrt{\frac{Ht\ (cm) \times Wt\ (kg)}{3,600}}$$

Note. Based on information from Gehan & George, 1970; Mosteller, 1987.

studies, with the exception of high-dose studies (e.g., bone marrow transplant studies) (Gelman et al., 1987). If ideal body weight is used, the study sponsor should identify which tool is used to calculate BSA to ensure correct data and dosing. In some phase III protocols, actual body weight is used, but drug doses may be capped at a BSA of 2 m².

Laboratory Studies
Urine

Studies have shown that the kidney is the major route of drug excretion and clearance for most chemotherapeutic agents. Renal function tests will be required as baseline data for most studies involving investigational agents. Platinum-based chemotherapy can cause permanent changes in the glomerular filtration rate (GFR). Patients with renal dysfunction or those who have received previous chemotherapy have slower carboplatin clearance (Egorin et al., 1985). Creatinine clearance is a measure of kidney function that is based on serum and urine creatinine values and urine volume. A specific protocol might state which method for determining creatinine clearance is acceptable. One formula used for calculating creatinine clearance is based on total urine volume over a specified period of time:

$$\text{creatinine clearance} = \frac{\text{urine creatinine}}{\text{serum creatinine}} \times \frac{\text{urine volume}}{\text{time}}$$

The classic collection time is 24 hours; however, shorter periods have been shown to be equally accurate (Baumann, Staddon, Horst, & Bivins, 1987). Creatinine clearance also can be calculated using the subject's age, weight, and serum creatinine level. The formulas for men and women (Cockroft & Gault, 1986) and for pediatric patients (Knoben, Anderson, & Troutman, 2002) are presented here.

$$\text{creatinine clearance (for men)} = \frac{(140 - \text{age}) \times \text{lean body weight (LBW)}}{\text{serum creatinine} \times 72}$$

$$\text{creatinine clearance (for women)} = 0.85 \times \text{creatinine clearance (men)}$$

$$\text{creatinine clearance (pediatric)} = \frac{0.48 \times \text{height} \times \text{BSA}}{\text{serum creatinine} \times 1.73}$$

When urine cannot be collected, the following formula by Jelliffe (1971) can be used:

$$\frac{\text{creatinine clearance}}{1.73} = \frac{100}{\text{serum creatinine} - 12}$$

Units used for all of these calculations are as follows: creatinine clearance (ml/min); age (yr); serum creatinine (mg/dl); time (minutes); urine creatinine (mg/dl); weight (kg); height (cm); and urine volume (L) (Fischer, Knobf, & Durivage, 2003). Creatinine clearance is a value that can be found on slide calculators that often are provided with study materials.

The following formulas can be used for calculating LBW:

(men)
$$\text{LBW in kg} = [1.10 \times \text{weight (kg)}] - 128 \{\text{weight}^2 [100 \times \text{height (m}^2)]\}$$

(women)
$$\text{LBW in kg} = [1.07 \times \text{weight (kg)}] - 148 \{\text{weight}^2 [100 \times \text{height (m}^2)]\}$$

Blood

Doses of some protocol agents may be substantially modified based on changes in the complete blood count (CBC), as well as other factors. Certain chemotherapeutic agents can cause profound suppression of bone marrow function. A decrease in the blood counts usually occurs within 7–15 days after the therapy is started. The day the blood counts were the lowest is called the *nadir*. Other factors that contribute to myelosuppression are age, nutritional status, and overall health (Sparks & Camp-Sorrell, 1997). The stem cells in the bone marrow, which divide rapidly, are more affected by chemotherapy than the mature cells in circulation. Most protocols specify that the white blood cell (WBC) and red blood cell (RBC) counts and platelet count must be at a certain level prior to dosing (Doyle, 1995).

The absolute neutrophil count (ANC) considers the number of immature cells as well as the WBCs available to generate an immune response to infection. This is a measure of the cells that will mature and become WBCs. The following formula is used to compute the ANC:

$$\text{ANC} = (\% \text{ segmented neutrophils} + \% \text{ band neutrophils}) \times \text{WBC (cells/mm}^3)$$

ANC is described in some literature as the absolute granulocyte count. If this value is below 1,500, the patient is at risk for infection if treated with chemotherapy. Online ANC calculators are available via the Internet. These tools will accurately determine the subject's ANC, thus decreasing the possibility of human error.

RBCs and platelets commonly are affected by chemotherapy. These values are used when determining the degree of myelosuppression and dosage modifications. RBC levels are reflected by hemoglobin and hematocrit measurements, which are components of the CBC. When the hemoglobin is less than 10 g/dl, the patient is considered to be anemic. Platelet levels below 50,000/mm³ predispose the patient to petechiae and bruising. Gastrointestinal bleeding and central nervous system bleeding can occur if platelet levels fall below 20,000/mm³ (Doyle, 1995). Both platelet and

RBC values are evaluated before administering each dose of the protocol agent. Blood counts are assessed any time that evidence of infection or bleeding is present.

Secondary causes of myelosuppression also exist. One of these is that myelosuppression is the primary toxicity of carboplatin, as it is a potent platinum-based compound, like cisplatin. Previous chemotherapy may cause decreased kidney function, resulting in a decreased GFR. A decrease in GFR results in a longer circulating time for carboplatin. Because the GFR affects the degree of myelosuppression, a specific formula is used to calculate carboplatin dosage. O'Dwyer and Johnson (2005) noted that platelet counts reach their nadir 17–21 days following a single dose of carboplatin, and recovery usually occurs by day 28. The effect is dose dependent but is most closely related to the drug exposure in an individual as measured by the area under the concentration-time curve (AUC), as shown by Calvert et al. in 1989:

$$\text{dose (mg)} = \text{target AUC (mg/min/ml)} \times (\text{GFR ml/min} + 25)$$

Although carboplatin is not significantly toxic to the kidneys, pretreatment renal function markedly affects the severity of carboplatin-induced thrombocytopenia (Ratain, 2004). Administration of carboplatin in the pediatric population is based on a formula that uses GFR and body weight (BW) (Newell et al., 1993):

$$\text{dose (mg)} = \text{target AUC} \times \{\text{GFR [ml/min]} + [0.36 \times \text{BW (kg)}]\}$$

Dosing with carboplatin may include pretreatment hydration. The protocol must be reviewed carefully, with special attention given to the sequence of drug administration. Some protocols involve a number of drugs that are given in a designated sequence over a specified time.

Documentation

As soon as treatment is administered, documentation of patient response begins. The protocol may require accurate documentation of the start and stop times for each IV fluid and chemotherapy infusion, as well as premedications given to prevent adverse effects. Documentation during the administration of the protocol agent is very important to evaluate administration-related side effects. Therefore, baseline patient observations as defined by the clinical trial must be made prior to dosing with study agents. Next, prophylactic medications should be administered to prevent expected treatment-related side effects, such as nausea and vomiting. With the patient's cooperation, the nurse should identify and record a follow-up plan in a format that the patient can easily understand. The patient should receive written follow-up guidance, including the name of the study coordinator or nurse assigned to the patient. The study file should

include the patient's correct address and telephone number in addition to an emergency contact. Monitoring the patient after administration of the protocol agent (e.g., calling the patient a day or two following the protocol therapy) helps to ensure patient safety as well as protocol compliance. If chemotherapy is administered in a location other than the research office, copies of the chemotherapy administration records and any updates to the patient contact information need to be sent to the study's principal investigator or study coordinator.

Complete and accurate treatment data are essential in clinical research. Therefore, thorough documentation before, during, and after the administration of the drug is critical. When audited, the medical record should include all the information required by the protocol. Flow sheets and study-specific worksheets further enhance the documentation of treatment. Many times, these tools can be developed by the nurse and can be used as source documentation if the information is not already provided in the medical record.

Guidelines

The following guidelines will ensure that protocol treatment proceeds in a safe and orderly fashion.

- Always double-check the dosage calculations with another chemotherapy-certified nurse, as well as with the research pharmacist.
- Prepare in advance treatment packets that contain patient education materials regarding side effects of the protocol agent, compliance tools (e.g., calendars, diaries), and instructions regarding the reporting of side effects.
- Provide in-service education to nursing and pharmacy staff to enhance team performance. If possible, be present during the initial dose calculations and administration of protocol agents. This support of the patient and nursing staff allows potential problems to be identified and corrected before a protocol deviation occurs.
- Remain in close contact with the principal investigator for each patient. Notify the physician if any toxicities or adverse events occur, especially those that require dose modification or discontinuation or interruption of the drug infusion.
- Before each treatment, assess the patient's desire to continue on the protocol. Patients have the right to withdraw at any time when participating in clinical research. If the patient declines further participation in the trial, the study coordinator should be contacted so that the study sponsor can be notified appropriately.
- The study sponsor and/or his or her representative can be a resource and ally in the clinical research process. Discuss problems and concerns with the sponsor's representative. Experiences occurring at other study sites may be significant as well, both to the nurse and to the patients.
- Sign, date, and note the time on all sources of information to provide source documents.

Policy and Procedure

Nurses who practice in the ambulatory setting and administer chemotherapy drugs are increasing in number. The results of the Oncology Nursing Society Ambulatory Office Nurse Survey were published in 2004 (Ireland, DePalma, Arneson, Stark, & Williamson, 2004). Of the 325 survey respondents, "86% reported that clinical trials were conducted in their practice settings with 75% reporting that clinical trial nurses were available" (Ireland et al., p. E153). The staff nurses who responded to the survey described their role as one that primarily followed protocols and collected data through documentation and collection of blood specimens. Other roles described in 50% of the clinical settings were managing investigational drugs and monitoring clinical trial subjects. Other tasks related to clinical research included helping to develop protocols for submission to funding agencies and the institutional review board, keeping case report forms up to date, providing patient education, performing symptom management, providing toxicity description, and determining dose modification (Ireland et al.). Considering the large numbers of oncology nurses who are involved in such roles, it becomes very important to have standards, policies, and procedures to guide their practice.

The American Society of Clinical Oncology (2003) published a policy statement on the oversight of clinical research. The purpose of the policy was to improve public trust of investigational/research drug development and testing. In recent years, public interest in the safety of clinical trials has been increasing, along with interest in the safety of newly developed drugs approved by the U.S. Food and Drug Administration. The Infusion Nurses Society (2006) published the *Infusion Nursing Standards of Practice*, which includes a chapter on the administration of investigational drugs. Infusion nurses who administer investigational products in the setting of clinical trials should take the time to refer to their institution's policies, as well as these national policies and procedures.

Summary

Research is a unique opportunity to improve the care that patients with cancer receive. Research holds hope for the development of less toxic and more effective treatment and increased comfort for cancer survivors. Nursing roles in clinical research provide job satisfaction and the opportunity to become a ready resource, not only to patients but to colleagues, as well.

References

American Society of Clinical Oncology. (2003, April 29). *American Society of Clinical Oncology policy statement: Oversight of clinical research.* Retrieved October 2, 2007, from http://www.asco.org/asco/downloads/OversightofClinicalResearch.pdf

Baumann, T.J., Staddon, J.E., Horst, H.M., & Bivins, B.A. (1987). Minimum urine collection periods for accurate determination of creatinine clearance in critically ill patients. *Clinical Pharmacy, 6,* 393–398.

Calvert, A.H., Newell, D.R., Gumbrell, L.A., O'Reilly, S., Burnell, M., Boxall, F.E., et al. (1989). Carboplatin dosage: Prospective evaluation of a simple formula based on renal function. *Journal of Clinical Oncology, 7,* 1748–1756.

Cockcroft, D.W., & Gault, M.H. (1976). Prediction of creatinine clearance from serum creatinine. *Nephron, 16,* 31–41.

Doyle, M.A. (1995). Oncologic therapy. In J. Terry, L. Baranowski, R.A. Lonsway, & H. Hedrick (Eds.), *Intravenous therapy: Clinical principles and practices* (pp. 254–255). Philadelphia: Saunders.

Egorin, M.J., Van Echo, D.A., Olman, E.A., Whitacre, M.Y., Forrest, A., & Aisner, J. (1985). Prospective validation of a pharmacologically based dosing scheme for the cisdiammin-edichloroplatinum(II) analogue diamminecyclobu-tanedicarboxylatoplatinum. *Cancer Research, 45,* 6502–6506.

Fischer, D.S., Knobf, M.T., & Durivage, H.J. (2003). *The cancer chemotherapy handbook* (6th ed.). St. Louis, MO: Mosby.

Gehan, E.A., & George, S.L. (1970). Estimation of human body surface area from height and weight. *Cancer Chemotherapy Report, 54,* 225–235.

Gelman, R.S., Tormey, D.C., Betensky, R., Mansour, E.G., Falkson, H.C., Falkson, G., et al. (1987). Actual versus ideal weight in the calculation of surface area: Effects on dose of 11 chemotherapy agents. *Cancer Treatment Reports, 71,* 907–911.

Infusion Nurses Society. (2006). Infusion nursing standards of practice. *Journal of Infusion Nursing, 29*(Suppl. 1), S1–S92.

Ireland, A.M., DePalma, J.A., Arneson, L., Stark, L., & Williamson, J. (2004). The Oncology Nursing Society ambulatory office nurse survey [Online exclusive]. *Oncology Nursing Forum, 31,* E147–E156.

James, W.P.T. (1976). *Research on obesity.* London: Her Majesty's Stationery Office.

Jelliffe, R.W. (1971). Estimation of creatinine clearance when urine cannot be collected. *Lancet, 1,* 975–976.

Knoben, J.E., Anderson, P.O., & Troutman, W.C. (2002). *Handbook of clinical drug data* (10th ed.). Kansas City, MO: Marion Merrell Dow.

Mosteller, R.D. (1987). Simplified calculation of body-surface area [Letter to the editor]. *New England Journal of Medicine, 317,* 1098.

Newell, D.R., Pearson, A.D., Balmanno, K., Price, L., Wylie, R.A., Keir, M., et al. (1993). Carboplatin pharmacokinetics in children: The development of a pediatric dosing formula. *Journal of Clinical Oncology, 11,* 2314–2323.

O'Dwyer, P.J., & Johnson, S.W. (2005). Cisplatin and its analogues. In V.T. DeVita, S. Hellman, & S.A. Rosenberg (Eds.), *Cancer: Principles and practice of oncology* (7th ed., pp. 307–422). Philadelphia: Lippincott Williams & Wilkins.

Ratain, M.J. (2004). Pharmacokinetics and pharmacodynamics. In V.T. DeVita, S. Hellman, & S.A. Rosenberg (Eds.), *Cancer: Principles and practice of oncology* (6th ed., pp. 335–344). Philadelphia: Lippincott Williams & Wilkins.

Sparks, S., & Camp-Sorrell, D. (1997). Assessing the myelo-suppressed patient. *American Journal of Nursing, 97*(Suppl. 5), 4–8.

CHAPTER 27
Symptom Management in Clinical Trials Nursing

Michelle A. Brand, RN, OCN®

Introduction

One of the most challenging and rewarding areas of clinical trials nursing is that of symptom management. The Oncology Nursing Society (1997) position on quality cancer care describes symptom management as interventions that include control of physical symptoms and psychosocial care as a key element of quality cancer care. The goals of this chapter are not to provide specific symptom-related interventions but rather to focus on identifying barriers to effective symptom management and interventions to develop an effective symptom management plan. Although symptom management–focused clinical trials have gained popularity in the past several years, these will be addressed in Chapter 31: Quality-of-Life Studies.

Goals of Symptom Management
Improved Patient Satisfaction and Quality of Life

One of the three goals of symptom management is to make patients feel less like a "research subject" and more like a part of the treatment team. With this sense of well-being and empowerment come *greater compliance* to trial regimens and faster reporting of adverse effects.

Early Identification of Side Effects and Prevention of Serious Complications

In achieving early identification of side effects and preventing serious complications, lower grade toxicities can be more readily managed so that *dose delays are avoided.*

Improved Data Integrity and Patient Safety

When patients experience toxicities, dose reductions, treatment delays, and withdrawals occur. Preventing avoidable dose reductions is important. Less evaluable data is available when patients are removed from a study because of side effects. The total accrual for the study may need to be increased, thus delaying study completion. *Effective symptom management contributes to the success of a clinical trial.*

Barriers to Effective Symptom Management

Communication is now recognized as a core clinical skill in medicine in general and in cancer care in particular (Merckaert, Libert, & Razavi, 2005). Clinical trials can be difficult to understand even for the most experienced clinician. Symptom management information is sparse, and dose modification guidelines often are difficult. A patient with little experience with cancer may be overwhelmed by the information provided. Despite attempts to make research consents readable, patients often are confronted with patient education material they do not understand and medical jargon that is confusing. Patients' comprehension of this material often is limited by their psychological adjustment to cancer, stress, and any physical symptoms they may be experiencing. Previous psychosocial experiences also may play a role in how the patient adapts to new information.

Many patients entering a clinical trial feel that it is their last or only option for treatment. Moore (2001) described the participants' desire to "try anything and everything at any cost" (p. 742). As a result of these fears, participants may minimize symptoms so that they will not be deemed too sick to participate and barred from receiving life-extending therapy.

The average age of clinical trial participants is getting older. Older patients often have multiple comorbidities, making it difficult to delineate what has been caused by the trial and what has been caused by their medical condition. Doorenbos, Given, Given, and Verbitsky (2006) showed

The author would like to acknowledge Barbara L. Harkins, RN, MN, for her contribution that remains unchanged from the first edition.

that patients aged 31–87 with a mean age of 60 who have three or more chronic medical conditions have lower physical functioning when surveyed at 20 weeks into treatment. This study looked at the effect of a behavioral intervention for symptoms primarily among individuals with breast or lung cancers.

Economics can render the best symptom management strategies ineffective if the patient cannot afford them. With the prohibitive cost of growth factors, antiemetics, and antibiotics, clinicians need to be keenly aware of a patient's insurance limitations and coverage.

Developing a Symptom Management Plan

Effective symptom management begins before a patient is even enrolled in a trial. The first step in any symptom management plan should be to know the drug and potential side effects and to review the protocol for any symptom management guidelines (see Figure 27-1). For many drugs that are not approved by the U.S. Food and Drug Administration, the first item the clinical trial nurse (CTN) should review is the investigator's brochure. This document will carefully detail the expected side effects of the drug as well as the results of phase I and II trials. The trial protocol and study consent form also should list any potential side effects of the investigational agent (see Figure 27-2).

Whenever possible, the expected side effects should be grouped by body system. Dodd, Miaskowski, and Lee (2004) proposed that clusters of symptoms might have a significant effect on patients' level of functioning. Careful examination of symptom clusters may lead to the development of symptom management interventions that will en-

---

Figure 27-1. Resources for Information About the Expected Side Effects of Study Therapy

Pertinent sections of the research study document or protocol
- Informed consent
- Protocol sections describing toxicities of study therapies
- Protocol treatment instructions
- Dose modification guidelines
- Background information describing previous clinical experience

Investigator's brochure (usually provided by the sponsoring agency when the clinical trial includes an investigational agent)
- Includes information from earlier clinical trials as well as pre-clinical data
- Safety addenda are added when new toxicity information is reported.

Guidelines, other than the protocol, that have been provided by the sponsor
- Summary or fact sheets
- Nursing or other clinical guidelines

Sponsoring agency's resource staff
- Protocol coordinating department staff
- Drug monitor for pharmaceutical trials
- Cooperative groups may have a "hotline" for questions regarding protocol implementation.

Figure 27-2. Materials to Include in a New Protocol Packet

- Pertinent sections of the protocol (e.g., toxicity descriptions, dose modifications, treatment guidelines)
- "Fact sheet" listing the expected side effects
- Guidelines for patient assessment, including tools to be used for measuring and quantifying the severity of specific side effects
- Symptom management algorithm or care plan that clearly states the recommended and prohibited management of side effects
- Published reports or other documentation describing expected side effects and recommended treatment
- Patient education materials that include the expected side effects and how to prevent or minimize them
- Names and telephone numbers of the principal investigator, research nurse, and other resource people for each study
- Cards or stickers to attach to patients' records or care plans to alert staff that the patient is enrolled in the designated study

---

compass many areas. An example of this would be a patient who has food aversions, ascites, hypoalbuminemia, and peripheral edema. The treatment team could work with the patient to devise food and supplement options that appeal to the patient and increase his or her dietary protein.

During patient education, the CTN can review the disease the study is treating and list the common symptoms by body system. By grouping the potential side effects with the common symptoms, one will have a "snapshot" of potential problems that patients entering the clinical trial will face.

It is useful to determine whether the study will be using the National Cancer Institute's Common Terminology Criteria for Adverse Events (and which version) or a different toxicity grading system. Once the list of side effects and symptoms is established, a worksheet for assessing patients based on the toxicity criteria can be developed. This will save the CTN time and allow the CTN to more accurately assess the severity of patients' symptoms. Allow space on the form to record the duration of the symptom, interventions the patient has tried, and other related problems the patient may be having. Using visual analog scales and other assessment tools can help the patient to quantify symptoms. An example of this would be pictures of the various stages of palmar-plantar erythrodesia, which the CTN can use to compare with the patient's skin.

Many clinical trials lack symptom management information. The absence of guidelines does not mean that certain symptom management strategies are allowed or that symptoms should go unmanaged. The CTN should collaborate with the physician, treatment nurse, and anyone involved in the treatment team and formulate a plan for managing patient symptoms and side effects. If possible, the team should devise "care maps" for common symptoms. These care maps are information sheets for patients and caregivers that serve as a reference when a symptom occurs. The care maps should include pro-

---

Figure 27-3. Selected Resources for Symptom Management Information

Books
- Camp-Sorrell, D., & Hawkins, R.A. (Eds.). (2006). *Clinical manual for the oncology advanced practice nurse* (2nd ed.). Pittsburgh, PA: Oncology Nursing Society.
- Cope, D.G., & Reb, A.M. (Eds.). (2006). *An evidence-based approach to the treatment and care of the older adult with cancer.* Pittsburgh, PA: Oncology Nursing Society.
- Moore-Higgs, G.J. (Ed.). (2000). *Women and cancer: A gynecologic oncology nursing perspective* (2nd ed.). Sudbury, MA: Jones and Bartlett.
- Yarbro, C.H., Frogge, M.H., & Goodman, M. (Eds.). (2004). *Cancer symptom management* (3rd ed.). Sudbury, MA: Jones and Bartlett.
- Yarbro, C.H., Goodman, M., & Frogge, M.H. (Eds.). (2005). *Cancer nursing: Principles and practice* (6th ed.). Sudbury, MA: Jones and Bartlett.

Guidelines
- National Comprehensive Cancer Network. (2007). *NCCN clinical practice guidelines in oncology.* Retrieved October 22, 2007, from http://www.nccn.org/professionals/physician_gls/default.asp

Oncology Nursing Periodicals
- *Cancer Nursing*
- *Clinical Journal of Oncology Nursing*
- *Community Oncology*
- *The Journal of Gynecologic Nurse Oncologists*
- *Oncology Nursing Forum*

Online Cancer Information Services
The following are a few of the many Web sites providing abstracts, articles, patient education materials, resources, and other oncology-related information that may be helpful:
- American Cancer Society—www.cancer.org
- American Society of Clinical Oncology, People Living With Cancer—www.plwc.org
- CancerQuest—www.cancerquest.org
- CancerSource—www.cancersource.com
- National Cancer Institute—www.cancer.gov
- Oncology Nursing Society—www.ons.org
- Society of Gynecologic Nurse Oncologists—www.sgno.org
- Women's Cancer Network—www.wcn.org

Organizations for Specific Cancer Types
- American Brain Tumor Association—www.abta.org
- Colon Cancer Foundation—www.coloncancerfoundation.org
- Gynecologic Cancer Foundation—www.thegcf.org
- Leukemia and Lymphoma Society—www.leukemia-lymphoma.org
- Leukemia Research Foundation—www.leukemia-research.org
- Lung Cancer Alliance—www.alcase.org
- National Breast Cancer Foundation—www.nationalbreastcancer.org

---

phylactic interventions, such as antiemetics to prevent nausea, oral hypothermia to prevent stomatitis, cytokines to prevent anemia and neutropenia, and use of cooling measures to prevent palmar-plantar erythrodesia. All symptom management plans should be reviewed with the study sponsor to ensure that they will not violate the terms of the study. An example of this would be a care map for a drug that causes palmar-plantar erythrodesia.

The care map should include preventive strategies, such as avoiding heat and treatment strategies if the skin becomes red, such as when using a specific cream. The patient will feel more informed, and greater compliance will result (see Figure 27-3).

Patients entering a clinical trial should receive very thorough education related to the action of the drug, potential side effects, and symptom management strategies. The CTN should provide written guidelines to patients, as well as an emergency contact number for problems that they may experience.

Encourage patients to keep a side effect diary (a checklist) as outlined in the study. Patients often feel overwhelmed when they come to their appointments and may forget or minimize problems they experienced between visits. Consider making telephone assessments at key points in the patient's treatment cycle, such as at the nadir or 24–48 hours after treatment, when nausea may be at its peak.

Psychological Distress

Psychological and symptom distress should be assessed at every clinic visit. Cancer, combined with its treatment, is viewed as an event that evokes distress and emotional anguish, thereby taxing individuals' ability to cope (Kelly, Ghazi, & Caldwell, 2002). The emotional benefit of psychological interventions to enhance coping, treat depression, and reduce anxiety may even be life-prolonging (Spiegel, Bloom, & Kraemer, 1989). Given et al. (2006) studied the effect of behavioral interventions for symptoms among patients receiving chemotherapy. The goal was to cause behavioral changes by the acquisition of self-management knowledge, skills, and behaviors. The study showed that a strong relationship exists between depression and physical functioning. If depression is treated, symptoms generally improve. CTNs should strive to intervene as early as possible to assist patients with decreased physical functioning and depression. See Chapter 19 for a more in-depth discussion of psychosocial considerations in clinical trials.

Summary

Effective symptom management improves patients' quality of life and sense of well-being, as well as clinical trial compliance and data accuracy. Through collaborative efforts of the treatment team and careful, thoughtful planning, symptom management for patients in clinical trials is an attainable goal.

References

Dodd, M., Miaskowski, K., & Lee, K. (2004). Occurrence of symptom clusters. *Journal of the National Cancer Institute Monographs, 32,* 76–78.

Doorenbos, A., Given, B., Given, C., & Verbitsky, N. (2006). Physical functioning: Effect of behavioral intervention for symptoms among individuals with cancer. *Nursing Research, 55,* 161–171.

Given, B., Given, C.W., Sikorskii, A., Jeon, S., Sherwood, P., & Rahbar, M. (2006). The impact of providing symptom management assistance on caregiver reaction: Results of a randomized trial. *Journal of Pain and Symptom Management, 32,* 433–443.

Kelly, C.B., Ghazi, F., & Caldwell, K. (2002). Psychological distress of cancer and clinical trial participation: A review of the literature. *European Journal of Cancer Care, 11,* 6–15.

Merckaert, I., Libert, Y., & Razavi, D. (2005). Communication skills training in cancer care: Where are we and where are we going? *Current Opinion in Oncology, 17,* 319–330.

Moore, S. (2001). A need to try everything: Patient participation in phase I trials. *Journal of Advanced Nursing, 33,* 738–747.

Oncology Nursing Society. (1997). Oncology Nursing Society position paper on quality cancer care. *Oncology Nursing Forum, 24,* 951–953.

Spiegel, D., Bloom, J., Kraemer, H.C., & Gottheil, E. (1989). Effect of psychosocial treatment on survival of patients with metastatic breast cancer. *Lancet, 2,* 888–891.

Additional Resources

Anastasia, P., & Blevins, M. (1997). Outpatient chemotherapy: Telephone triage for symptom management. *Oncology Nursing Forum, 24*(Suppl. 1), 13–22.

Given, C., Given, B., Rahbar, M., Jeon, S., McCorkle, R., Cimprich, B., et al. (2004a). Does a symptom management intervention affect depression among cancer patients: Results from a clinical trial. *Psycho-Oncology, 13,* 818–830.

Given, C., Given, B., Rahbar, M., Jeon, S., McCorkle, R., Cimprich, B., et al. (2004b). Effect of cognitive behavioral intervention on reducing symptom severity during chemotherapy. *Journal of Clinical Oncology, 22,* 507–516.

Kelly, C.B., Ghazi, F., & Caldwell, K. (2002). Psychological distress of cancer and clinical trial participation: A review of the literature. *European Journal of Cancer Care, 11,* 6–15.

Mock, V. (2001). Fatigue management: Evidence and guidelines for practice. *Cancer, 92*(Suppl. 6), 1699–1707.

CHAPTER 28
Adverse Events

Laura S. Wood, RN, MSN, OCN®

Introduction

Nursing assessment is critical to the management of patients who are actively receiving protocol treatment. This chapter focuses on the assessment, documentation, and reporting of toxicities and adverse events.

Adverse Events

The terms *adverse event* (AE) and *toxicity* frequently are used interchangeably; however, they really describe two different concepts. A *toxicity* implies a relationship to a treatment, whereas an *adverse event* is any unfavorable and unintended diagnosis, symptom, sign (including an abnormal laboratory finding), or disease that occurs during a study, if absent at baseline, or, if present at baseline, appears to worsen, and may or may not be considered related to the medical treatment or procedure. A *serious adverse event* is any untoward medical occurrence that (National Cancer Institute Cancer Therapy Evaluation Program [NCI CTEP], 2005)

- Results in death
- Is life-threatening
- Requires or prolongs hospitalization
- Causes persistent or significant disability or incapacity
- Results in congenital anomalies or birth defects
- Is any other condition that investigators judge as representing a significant hazard.

AEs associated with the use of a drug are those for which a reasonable possibility exists that the experience may have been caused by the drug (*Electronic Code of Federal Regulations [e-CFR]*, 2007, Title 21, Part 312.21). Title 21 of the CFR includes legal regulations in place to ensure compliance with principles of research and good clinical practice.

Clinical trials are dependent on the collection of accurate and timely information. These data are derived from a variety of sources, such as the patient, significant other,

clinical trial nurse (CTN), staff nurse, physician, and clinical research associates (Allaster, Frayne, Malpage, Smuck, & Studzienny, 1996). A crucial role of the CTN is to assess the patient for actual and potential AEs and to document these findings. These data are used for investigational new drug (IND) safety reports that may lead to revisions in the investigator's brochure and/or the informed consent and IND annual reports (*e-CFR*, 2007, Title 21, Parts 312.22 and 312.32). These data also are used to amplify, validate, and quantify adverse side effects, to compare them to the expected occurrence in a population, and to monitor risk management efforts to reduce the occurrence of known adverse drug reactions (Trontell, 2001).

AEs experienced by the patient are primarily determined by the treatments administered, such as chemotherapy, radiation therapy, surgery, biologic response modifiers, targeted therapies, gene therapy, vaccine treatment, or a combination of treatments. More specifically, the patient's treatment-related AEs are influenced by a variety of factors (see Figure 28-1).

Informational Resources

The CTN, whether caring for a patient in the hospital or the clinic, needs to be knowledgeable regarding the potential short-term and long-term complications resulting from

---

Figure 28-1. Factors Influencing Treatment-Related Reactions

- The regimen, frequency, and dosage of protocol therapy
- The use of concomitant therapies
- The patient's underlying disease
- Comorbid illnesses
- The patient's performance status
- Previous chemotherapy or radiation treatment
- The phase (I, II, or III) of the clinical trial

The author would like to acknowledge Kimberly Power, RN, MSN, for her contribution that remains unchanged from the first edition.

the study therapy. A detailed assessment of the patient's baseline symptoms and an understanding of both the malignancy and comorbid conditions of each patient facilitate accurate identification of AEs and their relationship to the study treatment, the classification/mechanism of action of all of the agents and all modalities of the study treatment (e.g., radiation therapy, surgery). By being familiar with the expected or known AEs of the study treatment, the nurse is able to accurately identify, monitor, and report these data. The protocol, the investigator's brochure (which is usually with the investigator and institutional review board), and published literature are excellent resources that describe expected toxicities. They should be available to all healthcare professionals involved in the patient's care.

The consent form is another document that can help the nurse to review more about the possible complications of a particular regimen; however, it is not the most detailed source. Many cooperative study groups have developed nursing guidelines or nursing summaries to serve as complements to a research protocol. The package insert provides the research nurse with information regarding a particular commercial agent. The pharmaceutical company manufacturing the investigational agent compiles a list of all the expected AEs and continuously revises the investigator's brochure with newly reported information.

The CTN or protocol coordinator, physician, and other members of the healthcare team serve as resources when learning about the expected and unexpected toxicities of a study treatment. They must observe *any* changes in the patient's condition and determine whether the study treatment is the cause. Cooperative groups and pharmaceutical companies usually have specific phone numbers that people can call with questions regarding AE reporting or for general information so that a multi-institutional protocol is conducted uniformly. In addition, the sponsor of the study (e.g., the pharmaceutical company) provides up-to-date information about the expected and unexpected toxicities of a study treatment. Newsletters provide an ongoing source of communication regarding protocol implementation, management, toxicity assessment, and intervention. Teleconferences involving the sponsor, site investigators, and their research staff include discussions regarding AEs and serious AEs. Any AE that may be reasonably regarded as caused by, or probably caused by, the drug must be reported to the U.S. Food and Drug Administration (FDA) within 24 hours of learning of the AE, with a completed reporting of the event within 10 days of the notification (*e-CFR*, 2007, Title 21, Part 312.64).

Patient Information

Before initiating treatment on a clinical trial, the nurse must collect the following patient information: (a) baseline physical assessment and preexisting conditions, (b) a past medical history, including illnesses, (c) a list of current medications, and (d) a description of current symptoms resulting from the disease process or previous therapy. This information is helpful in assessing the attribution of AEs. A *comprehensive* list of preexisting conditions is critical to the ongoing monitoring of AEs.

The patient and family are better able to identify and report AEs resulting from study treatment early if they are educated regarding the expected treatment-related toxicities. Communicating this information directly to the patient and family and providing written patient-education materials for them to take home reinforces the teaching instructions. Family members' observations of changes in the patient's behavior are important and, in certain circumstance (e.g., with a pediatric patient), may be the most reliable source of toxicity-related information. Whenever possible, the patient's perception of the problem and severity are ascertained.

Any unanticipated problems involving risks to subjects or others or any serious or continuing noncompliance must be reported (*e-CFR*, 2007, Title 21, Part 312.32). It is important for patients and family members to understand that even if a problem does not seem to be related to therapy, it should be reported to the physician or nurse. The need to report all new signs and symptoms, even on a weekend or if they "do not want to bother the physician," are vital for the reporting of all events with the study treatment. The healthcare team determines whether the problem is expected or unexpected and related or unrelated to the study treatment and implements appropriate management strategies.

Patients sometimes have difficulty accurately remembering the onset, severity, and duration of symptoms experienced while on therapy. Medications taken to treat disease and study treatment–related toxicities must be recorded on study case report forms (CRFs). The patient should be given a diary sheet to record the administration of medications as part of the investigational therapy, noting the date and time of dosing (see Figure 28-2). Changes in the time of day that the dose is taken may change the toxicity profile, especially for an oral therapeutic strategy. Additional diary sheets should be given to the patient to record side effects and medications taken to treat treatment-related side effects, disease-related symptoms, or other concurrent medical conditions. Patients must be reminded to bring their diary sheets to every appointment.

Patient- and treatment-specific factors must be considered in evaluating AEs. Phone calls initiated by the nurse to assess the onset, severity, and management of side effects may be appropriate. Factors that may influence a patient's reporting of toxicities via telephone are summarized in Figure 28-3.

Early identification and intervention can minimize the severity of the toxicity, as well as the risk of treatment interruption and/or dose reduction. A goal of patient education is the reporting of treatment-related symptoms. Rapid reporting of symptoms will increase the likelihood of success with symptom management strategies and adherence to protocol treatment for that specific patient.

Figure 28-2. Side Effect Diary Sheet				
Date	Time	Temperature	Side Effect	Medication Taken to Treat Side Effect

Nursing Observations

The nurse relies not only on communication skills to gather information from the patient but also on astute observations. The crucial toxicity information that needs to be collected and recorded includes a complete description of the event experienced, the onset date, duration, severity, and interventions that made the condition better or worse. Individuals may be at increased risk for experiencing side effects, or for having a lower tolerance of side effects, because of comorbid conditions or disease-related symptoms such as pain, fatigue, anorexia, or other gastrointestinal symptoms affecting caloric intake. The nurse must assess physical findings, such as lab work, x-rays, physical examinations, and intake and output, and compare them to the patient's baseline. The nurse's observations determine whether a patient is experiencing an expected toxicity, an unusual reaction, or complications related to the disease process.

The nurse is responsible for gathering initial information, discussing findings with the physician, and collaborating on further assessments to determine the severity of the AE and its attribution to the investigational therapy. Although the CTN often is the individual identifying AEs, the physician determines the toxicity grade and attribution.

Identification of unexpected AEs may change the toxicity profile for a therapy, leading to the incorporation of additional side effect or risk information into the informed consent and investigator's brochure.

Assessment of Adverse Events

According to the Oncology Nursing Society's (2004) *Statement on the Scope and Standards of Oncology Nursing Practice*, "The oncology nurse analyzes assessment data to determine nursing diagnoses" (p. 19). Therefore, it is vital that the

CTN utilize the appropriate terminology for AEs that occur with the study treatment. A variety of resources are available for the CTN to use with assessment of the patient.

Each AE is a term that is a unique representation of a specific event used for medical documentation and scientific analyses. The online Medical Dictionary for Regulatory Activities (MedDRA, 2007) is a "pragmatic, medically valid terminology with an emphasis on ease of use for data entry, retrieval, analysis, and display." This terminology applies to all phases of drug development, not including animal toxicology, and also applies to the health effects and malfunction of devices (MedDRA).

The Common Terminology Criteria for Adverse Events (CTCAE version 3.0) was published by the National Institutes of Health (NIH) in July 2003 and includes the descriptions and grading scales of AEs. This booklet incorporates toxicity assessment descriptions associated with chemotherapy, immunotherapy, radiation therapy, bone marrow transplant, and pediatric oncology. The CTCAE can be accessed on CTEP's Web site (http://ctep.info.nih.gov) and is available as a spiral-bound booklet by calling 800-4-CANCER.

An additional resource is the Comprehensive Adverse Events and Potential Risks (CAEPR) list, which provides a single complete list of reported and/or potential AEs associated with an agent using a uniform presentation of events by body system. The CAEPR does not include any frequency data but does include a comprehensive list, the Agent Specific Adverse Event list (ASAEL), which is a subset of AEs that are considered "'expected' for expedited reporting purposes only" (NCI CTEP, n.d., p. 1). Assessment of an AE involves the determination of (a) grade, (b) expectedness, and (c) attribution—association to the study treatment.

Adverse Event Grading

In clinical trials, the severity or intensity of AEs is graded according to the CTCAE by using a numerical scale ranging from 0 to 5. These generally are summarized as follows.

Grade	Severity/Intensity
0	No toxicity or within normal limits
1	Mild
2	Moderate
3	Severe
4	Life-threatening
5	Fatal

Figure 28-3. Factors Influencing a Patient's Willingness to Report Adverse Effects by Telephone
• The patient's access to a telephone • The patient's home situation • The patient's distance from the medical community • The patient's personality • The treatment regimen • The potential side effects • The patient's basic understanding of the protocol and protocol requirements

Under each numerical grade, the CTCAE lists a brief description of symptoms that pertain to that category (see Table 28-1 for the CTCAE category of upper aerodigestive tract mucositis). This assists in standardizing the grading of toxicities among all AEs among all therapies internationally. Detailed and specific documentation of AEs experienced by patients should be in the medical record as the primary source. The toxicity grading determines the dose interruptions, modifications, or discontinuations that must be implemented according to the protocol. The CTN, working in collaboration with other members of the healthcare team, observes, assesses, evaluates, and documents the patient's treatment- and disease-related symptoms. Study documentation and completed CRFs are audited by monitors, sponsors, and the FDA to ensure that toxicity assessments are accurate and that guidelines regarding treatment are followed according to the protocol. This includes dosing, dose modifications, and changes in treatment or study procedures according to protocol amendments. These AEs are reported to the IND sponsors and are used to develop the package insert, sometimes referred to as the toxicity profile.

Adverse Events Expectedness

AEs can be *unexpected* or *expected*. When reviewing the AE, the CTN needs to determine with the clinical trial team whether the event is unexpected or expected. Expected AEs for approved and marketed drugs or devices

Table 28-1. Common Terminology Criteria for Adverse Events (Version 3.0) for Upper Aerodigestive Tract Mucositis

GASTROINTESTINAL

Adverse Event	Short Name	Grade				
		1	2	3	4	5
Mucositis/stomatitis (clinical exam) *Select:* Anus Esophagus Large bowel Larynx Oral cavity Pharynx Rectum Small bowel Stomach Trachea	Mucositis— clinical exam —Select	Erythema of the mucosa	Patchy ulcerations or pseudomembranes	Confluent ulcerations or pseudomembranes; bleeding with minor trauma	Tissue necrosis; significant spontaneous bleeding; life-threatening consequences	Death

Remark: Mucositis/stomatitis (functional/symptomatic) may be used for mucositis of the upper aerodigestive tract caused by radiation, agents, or GVHD.

Adverse Event	Short Name	1	2	3	4	5
Mucositis/stomatitis (functional/symptomatic) *Select:* Anus Esophagus Large bowel Larynx Oral cavity Pharynx Rectum Small bowel Stomach Trachea	Mucositis— functional/ symptomatic – Select	<u>Upper aerodigestive tract sites:</u> Minimal symptoms, normal diet; minimal respiratory symptoms but not interfering with function <u>Lower GI sites:</u> Minimal discomfort, intervention not indicated	<u>Upper aerodigestive tract sites:</u> Symptomatic but can eat and swallow modified diet; respiratory symptoms interfering with function but not interfering with ADL <u>Lower GI sites:</u> Symptomatic, medical intervention indicated but not interfering with ADL	<u>Upper aerodigestive tract sites:</u> Symptomatic and unable to adequately aliment or hydrate orally; respiratory symptoms interfering with ADL <u>Lower GI sites:</u> Stool incontinence or other symptoms interfering with ADL	Symptoms associated with life-threatening consequences	Death

ADL—activities of daily living; GVHD—graft-versus-host disease

Note. From *Common Terminology Criteria for Adverse Events, Version 3.0* (p. 24), by National Cancer Institute Cancer Therapy Evaluation Program, 2006, Bethesda, MD: Author. Retrieved November 26, 2007, from http://ctep.cancer.gov/forms/CTCAEv3.pdf.

are described in the approved package insert. Expected AEs with the investigational new drugs or devices are described in the FDA investigator's brochure. In clinical research studies, information on expected AEs also is in the protocol and the consent form. AEs that are not described in the package insert, investigator's brochure, published medical literature, protocol, or informed consent document are considered to be unexpected AEs (NCI CTEP, 2005).

Adverse Events Attribution

Attribution is the relationship or association between the study treatment and the AE. An AE may be considered by the physician to be unrelated or unlikely to be related to the study treatment. However, if a causal relationship is established between the AE and the study treatment, then the attribution is described as either possibly, probably, or definitely related. The best estimate of the principal investigator at the time of reporting of the causal relationship between an intervention and an AE, the attributions, and the degree of certainty of the causality are graded as in Table 28-2.

Reporting of Adverse Drug Experiences

Vital to the reporting of AEs is ensuring that all individuals involved in caring for patients during and following completion of clinical trials have adequate information regarding the potential risks associated with a drug therapy or device. The responsibilities of the institution and the research team are to (a) complete the appropriate AE form, (b) gather the supporting documentation for the event, (c) complete the additional paperwork for reporting a serious AE to the cooperative study group or pharmaceutical corporation, and (d) notify the local institutional review board.

The FDA and the U.S. Department of Health and Human Services define in the CFR the procedures and requirements governing the use of investigational new drugs and the monitoring of AEs. NCI's CTEP sponsors an extensive national program of cancer research as both an IND application sponsor and/or funding sponsor and is responsible for ensuring that the research is conducted in accordance with federal regulations. These regulations guide the CTN in the area of reporting of the AEs that occur. Clinical investigators and ultimately the protocol principal investigator have the primary responsibility for AE identification, documentation, grading, and assignment of attribution. The CTEP and CTCAE are designed as instruments to be used to document AEs identified through a combination of clinical and laboratory evaluations. The CTEP AE reporting requirements and timing of expedited reports of an AdEERS (the Adverse Event Expedited Reporting System) (see Figure 28-4) include established criteria based upon phase of trial, AE as listed in the CTCAE, whether expected or unexpected as determined by the CTEP agent-specific AE list, attribution, and protocol-specific requirements (NCI CTEP, 2005).

Commercial agents are those agents not provided under an IND application but obtained instead from a commercial source. NCI, rather than a commercial distributor, may on some occasions distribute commercial agents for a trial. Commercial reporting requirements are provided in Table 28-3.

An investigational agent is a protocol drug administered under an IND application. In some instances, the investigational agent may be available commercially but is being tested for indications not included in the approved package label. When a study includes an investigational agent(s) and a commercial agent(s) on the same study arm, but the commercial agent(s) is given for a period of time prior to starting the investigational agent(s), expedited reporting of AEs that occur prior to starting the investigational agent(s) would follow the guidelines for commercial agents. Once therapy with the investigational agent(s) is initiated, all expedited reporting of AEs should follow the investigational guidelines. The AE reporting requirements for phase I trials utilizing an agent under a CTEP or a non–CTEP IND are provided in Table 28-4. The AE reporting requirements for phase II and III trials utilizing an agent under a CTEP IND application are provided in Table 28-5.

Postmarketing Reporting of Adverse Drug Experiences

AEs associated with the use of a drug must continue to be reported to the FDA following the approval of new drugs (e-CFR, 2007, Title 21, Part 314.80). The investigator using the MedWatch reporting system (see Figure 28-5) must voluntarily report unexpected adverse drug effects that are not listed in the current labeling for the drug product. This includes events that may be symptomatically and pathophysiologically related to an event listed in the labeling but differs from the event because of greater severity or specificity (e-CFR, Title 21, Part 314.80).

Table 28-2. Degree of Certainty About Causality	
Attribution	**Description**
Unrelated	The AE *is clearly NOT related* to the intervention.
Unlikely	The AE *is doubtfully related* to the intervention.
Possible	The AE *may be related* to the intervention.
Probable	The AE *is likely related* to the intervention.
Definite	The AE *is clearly related* to the intervention.

Note. From *CTEP, NCI Guidelines: Adverse Event Reporting Requirements* (p. 5), by National Cancer Institute Cancer Therapy Evaluation Program, 2005, Bethesda, MD: Author. Retrieved November 26, 2007, from http://ctep.cancer.gov/reporting/newadverse_2006.pdf.

Figure 28-4. Adverse Event Expedited Report Forms

Department of Health & Human Services

Adverse Event Expedited Report – Single Agent v4.0

Public Health Service
National Institutes of Health
National Cancer Institute
Bethesda, Maryland 20892

INSTRUCTIONS: Use this form to submit an Expedited Report for an Adverse Event (AE) or Death Unrelated to an Adverse Event for NCI clinical trials using one investigational agent sponsored under an NCI IND. Refer to the protocol to determine if NCI IND agents are utilized on the study and how to submit the Expedited Report. **Use this form only when it is impossible to access the Adverse Event Expedited Reporting System (AdEERS) Web application.** The AdEERS Web application can be accessed at https://webapps.ctep.nci.nih.gov/openapps/plsql/gadeers_main$.startup.

This form must be completed using the AdEERS Template Instructions available from the NCI CTEP Help Desk by phone at (301) 840-8202 or by fax at (301) 948-2242. Information components followed by "1," "LOV," "LOV/FT," or "CTC" must be entered using the special instructions below. Please see the AdEERS Template Instructions for a complete description of all components and instructions developed for this template.

1   Date information must be entered in MM/DD/YYYY format except where "MM/YYYY Only" (month and year only) instruction is given.

LOV   Information must be entered using standardized values from the AdEERS List of Values (LOV) document available from the AdEERS Web site.

LOV/FT Information must be entered using the AdEERS LOV or, if an appropriate value cannot be found, using Free Text (values other than those listed in the LOV).

CTC   Adverse Events are to be reported using the terminology and criteria of the NCI Common Toxicity Criteria (CTC), Version 2.0 (publish date April 30, 1999).

COMPLETING THE REPORT:

1. Complete all MANDATORY COMPONENTS in MANDATORY SECTIONS. Complete all *Requisite Components* in MANDATORY SECTIONS if relevant to the patient.
2. Determine which *Requisite Sections* apply to the patient and complete the MANDATORY COMPONENTS (if any) and *Requisite Components* if relevant to the patient.
3. If additional space is required to complete a report section, copy the page where the section appears, complete your entries, and attach to the final report.
4. Complete the form using black or blue ink and send to the Investigational Drug Branch (IDB), P.O. Box 30012, Bethesda, MD 20824 or fax to 301-230-0159.

1. PROTOCOL INFORMATION – THIS SECTION IS MANDATORY FOR ALL EXPEDITED REPORTS

NCI PROTOCOL NUMBER

IS THIS AN AMENDMENT TO A PREVIOUSLY SUBMITTED REPORT? ☐YES ☐NO

IF YES, CHECK AMENDMENT NUMBER: ☐1 ☐2 ☐3

INITIAL EXPEDITED REPORT TICKET NUMBER (AMENDMENTS ONLY)

PROTOCOL TITLE (Continue below)

2. REPORTER INFORMATION – THIS SECTION IS MANDATORY FOR ALL EXPEDITED REPORTS

REPORT DATE 1	LAST NAME	FIRST NAME	PHONE	FAX	E-MAIL

REPORTER

PHYSICIAN INFORMATION (Physician to be consulted for questions)

Fax is a requisite component for **PHYSICIAN INFORMATION**

3. PATIENT INFORMATION – THIS SECTION IS MANDATORY FOR ALL EXPEDITED REPORTS

A PATIENT ID is a unique identification code associated with each patient entered in the trial.

PATIENT ID

PATIENT'S INSTITUTION NAME, CITY, AND STATE (OR INSTITUTION CODE – Institution where patient is registered on the protocol or is currently being treated, see http://ctep.cancer.gov/guidelines/codes.html)

BIRTH DATE (MM/YYYY Only)   RACE LOV   GENDER LOV   HEIGHT (cm)   WEIGHT (kg)   *Baseline Performance Status at Initiation of Protocol – ECOG/Zubrod Scale* LOV

DISEASE NAME LOV

Disease Name Not Listed (Enter a specific disease name when "Solid Tumor NOS" or "Hematologic unspecified" is entered in the **DISEASE NAME** *component)*

PRIMARY SITE OF DISEASE LOV

Other Primary Site of Disease (Enter only when an appropriate primary site is not found in the LOV)

IS DATE OF INITIAL DIAGNOSIS KNOWN: ☐YES ☐NO   IF YES, ENTER THE DATE OF INITIAL DIAGNOSIS (MM/YYYY Only):

February 12, 2002

Page 1 of 4

(Continued on next page)

Figure 28-4. Adverse Event Expedited Report Forms *(Continued)*

4. COURSE INFORMATION – THIS SECTION IS MANDATORY FOR ALL EXPEDITED REPORTS

A Treatment Assignment Code (TAC) is a unique identification code associated with each arm or dose level of the protocol.
Example: Drug ###mg / m2 IV over X hr D1-3 / every 3 weeks)

Treatment Assignment Code (TAC)
If the appropriate TAC is unavailable from the LOV or is unknown, items A through D (below) are mandatory for the treatment arm or dose level.

A. Agent Name [LOV]   B. Dose   C. Administration Route [LOV]   D. Duration and Schedule [LOV]

START DATE OF FIRST COURSE [1]   START DATE OF COURSE ASSOCIATED WITH EXPEDITED REPORT [1]   START DATE OF PRIMARY AE [1]

End Date of AE [1]   COURSE NUMBER ON WHICH AE OCCURRED   TOTAL NUMBER OF COURSES TO DATE

WAS AN INVESTIGATIONAL AGENT(S) ADMINISTERED ON THIS PROTOCOL? ☐YES ☐NO

CROSSOVER STUDIES
The following information is required if this report is associated with a Crossover Study: a) Enter the date the initial Crossover course started in the START DATE OF FIRST COURSE field (Section 4), b) Check YES to WAS AN INVESTIGATIONAL AGENT(S) ADMINISTERED ON THIS PROTOCOL? (Section 4), c) Enter the date the investigational agent was last administered in the DATE LAST ADMINISTERED field (Section 10), and d) Enter the dose administered for the course in the TOTAL DOSE ADMINISTERED THIS COURSE field (Section 10), zero (0) is acceptable if the actual dose is unknown.

5. DESCRIPTION OF EVENT – THIS SECTION IS MANDATORY FOR ALL EXPEDITED REPORTS

DESCRIPTION AND TREATMENT OF EVENT(S) (Continue below)

HAS PATIENT BEEN RETREATED (TO DATE)? ☐YES ☐NO

PRESENT STATUS [LOV] (If you record Fatal/Death or Recovered/Resolved with or without Sequelae as PRESENT STATUS, then *Date of Recovery or Death* [see right] is mandatory)   *Date of Recovery or Death* [1]

WAS PATIENT REMOVED FROM PROTOCOL TREATMENT (TO DATE)? ☐YES ☐NO
IF YES, ENTER THE *Date Removed from Protocol Treatment* (see right)   *Date Removed from Protocol Treatment* [1]

6. DEATH UNRELATED TO ADVERSE EVENT – MANDATORY ONLY IF DEATH IS UNRELATED TO AN AE

Sections 1, 2, 3, 4, 5, 6, 7, and 10 are mandatory when reporting a death caused by suicide, accident, progressive disease, etc.

CAUSE OF DEATH [LOV] (If you record Progressive Disease as the CAUSE OF DEATH, then PRIMARY ORGAN SYSTEM FAILURE CAUSING DEATH [see right] is mandatory)   PRIMARY ORGAN SYSTEM FAILURE CAUSING DEATH [LOV]

7. PRIOR THERAPIES – THIS SECTION IS MANDATORY FOR ALL EXPEDITED REPORTS

THERAPY [LOV] (FOR THE PRIMARY DISEASE) (If you record any of the following as THERAPY, then PRIOR THERAPY AGENT NAME(S) [in column 6] is mandatory: bone marrow transplant, chemotherapy [NOS], chemotherapy [single or multiple agent systemic], hormonal therapy, or immunotherapy)	THERAPY START DATE (If known) (MM/YYYY only)	*Therapy End Date* (MM/YYYY only)	*Comments* (Enter additional therapies, prior therapy for diseases other than primary disease, or agents not included in LOV, if needed)	PRIOR THERAPY AGENT NAME(S) [LOV] (See note in THERAPY column)

8. Pre-Existing Condition(s) – This section is required if the patient has Pre-Existing Conditions
Identify any medical condition(s) the patient experienced prior to receiving current protocol therapy.

CONDITION A [LOV]   CONDITION B [LOV]   *Pre-Existing Condition Not Listed (Enter only when an appropriate condition is not found in the LOV)*

9. Site(s) of Metastatic Disease – This section is required if the patient has Sites of Metastatic Disease

SITE A [LOV]   SITE B [LOV]   *Sites of Metastatic Disease Not Listed (Enter only when an appropriate site is not found in the LOV)*

(Continued on next page)

Figure 28-4. Adverse Event Expedited Report Forms *(Continued)*

10. PROTOCOL AGENT – THIS SECTION IS MANDATORY FOR ALL EXPEDITED REPORTS

AGENT NAME LOV

DATE LAST ADMINISTERED [1] (This is mandatory for crossover studies if an investigational agent was administered at any time, see Section 4)

TOTAL DOSE ADMINISTERED THIS COURSE (Amount of agent given for current dose or cycle, this is not total dose given to date)   UNIT OF MEASURE LOV

Comments

Agent Adjustment LOV   *Was administration delayed?* ☐*Yes* ☐*No If yes, complete Duration Delay below*

Duration Delay   ☐*sec* ☐ *min* ☐*hrs* ☐*days*
(Enter duration length and check Unit of Measure)

CROSSOVER STUDIES – Instruction is provided in Section 4 regarding required information for reports associated with Crossover Studies.

11. Concomitant Medication(s) – This section is required if any non-protocol medication may have contributed to the event(s)

CONCOMITANT MEDICATION A

CONCOMITANT MEDICATION B

CONCOMITANT MEDICATION C

CONCOMITANT MEDICATION D

12. Other Contributing Cause(s) – This section is required if Other Causes may have contributed to the Adverse Event

OTHER CONTRIBUTING CAUSE A

OTHER CONTRIBUTING CAUSE B

OTHER CONTRIBUTING CAUSE C

OTHER CONTRIBUTING CAUSE D

13. ADVERSE EVENTS (CTC) – THIS SECTION IS MANDATORY FOR ALL EXPEDITED REPORTS <u>EXCEPT</u> DEATH UNRELATED TO AE

CATEGORY CTC	ADVERSE EVENT CTC	If AE is other, Specify: (If an appropriate AE term cannot be identified in the CTC, identify the CTC **CATEGORY** and provide AE information in this column)	**GRADE** CTC (If you record a GRADE 3 or higher, Hospitalization or Prolongation of Hospitalization [in column 5] is mandatory)	Hospitalization or Prolongation of Hospitalization (See note in **GRADE** column)	Comments (Enter other relevant information in this column)
AE A:				☐ Yes ☐ No	
AE B:				☐ Yes ☐ No	
AE C:				☐ Yes ☐ No	

14. ATTRIBUTION FOR ADVERSE EVENT – THIS SECTION IS MANDATORY FOR ALL EXPEDITED REPORTS <u>EXCEPT</u> DEATH UNRELATED TO AE

Attribution is the determination whether an AE is related to a medical treatment or procedure. Evaluate each AE the patient experiences to determine what might have caused the event or what interventions or conditions the event might have been attributed to.

IMPORTANT: Every AdEERS report that includes Adverse Events must include for each Adverse Event at least one attribution of Possible, Probable, or Definite to either the Agent, the Disease, Other Causes, or Concomitant Medications. NCI will not accept reports without at least one attribution of Possible, Probable, or Definite to either the Agent, the Disease, Other Causes, or Concomitant Medications for each Adverse Event.

Write the AE term(s) you used in Section 13 in the heading area of columns 2, 3, and 4 (found on page 4). Complete the AGENT NAME, DISEASE, *Concomitant Medication* and/or *Other Contributing Causes* information in column 1 using the same information you provided in Sections 10, 3, 11, and 12. Circle the ATTRIBUTION CODE in each column for each AE based on its relationship to the AGENT NAME, DISEASE, *Concomitant Medication* and/or *Other Contributing Causes* information provided in column 1. An example is provided below.

Example	Anorexia					Bilirubin					Pain-Other				
	ADVERSE EVENT CTC (AE A from Section 13)					ADVERSE EVENT CTC (AE B from Section 13)					ADVERSE EVENT CTC (AE C from Section 13)				
Drug 1	1	2	③	4	5	1	2	③	4	5	1	②	3	4	5
AGENT NAME LOV (from Section 10)															

ATTRIBUTION CODES are defined as:

1	Unrelated -	The Adverse Event is clearly NOT related to the investigational agent, disease, concomitant medication, or other contributing cause.
2	Unlikely -	The Adverse Event is doubtfully related to the investigational agent, disease, concomitant medication, or other contributing cause.
3	Possible -	The Adverse Event may be related to the investigational agent, disease, concomitant medication, or other contributing cause.
4	Probable -	The Adverse Event is likely related to the investigational agent, disease, concomitant medication, or other contributing cause.
5	Definite -	The Adverse Event is clearly related to the investigational agent, disease, concomitant medication, or other contributing cause.

This section continues on page 4.

(Continued on next page)

Figure 28-4. Adverse Event Expedited Report Forms *(Continued)*

14. ATTRIBUTION FOR ADVERSE EVENT (Continued)

	ADVERSE EVENT CTC (AE A from Section 13)					ADVERSE EVENT CTC (AE B from Section 13)					ADVERSE EVENT CTC (AE C from Section 13)				
AGENT NAME LOV (from Section 10)	1	2	3	4	5	1	2	3	4	5	1	2	3	4	5
DISEASE NAME LOV (from Section 3)	1	2	3	4	5	1	2	3	4	5	1	2	3	4	5
Concomitant Medication (A from Section 11)	1	2	3	4	5	1	2	3	4	5	1	2	3	4	5
Concomitant Medication (B from Section 11)	1	2	3	4	5	1	2	3	4	5	1	2	3	4	5
Concomitant Medication (C from Section 11)	1	2	3	4	5	1	2	3	4	5	1	2	3	4	5
Concomitant Medication (D from Section 11)	1	2	3	4	5	1	2	3	4	5	1	2	3	4	5
Other Contributing Causes (A from Section 12)	1	2	3	4	5	1	2	3	4	5	1	2	3	4	5
Other Contributing Causes (B from Section 12)	1	2	3	4	5	1	2	3	4	5	1	2	3	4	5

15. Abnormal and Relevant Normal Laboratory Results – This section is required if Laboratory Results are relevant to the report

This section is not required if Microbiology information is provided in Section 16.

Lab LOV/FI	Baseline			Nadir/Worst		Recovery/Latest	
	Date[1]	Value	Unit of Measure LOV	Date[1]	Value	Date[1]	Value
Lab A:							
Lab B:							
Lab C:							

16. Lab: Microbiology – This section is required for reporting infections

Do not complete Section 15 if Microbiology information is provided below.

Infection Type: ☐ Bacterial ☐ Fungal ☐ Viral

Site   Date[1]   Infectious Agent

17. Additional Information Attached – This section is required if relevant to the report

Check those you have attached for submission with this report.

☐ Autopsy Report   ☐ Consults   ☐ Discharge Summary   ☐ Flow Sheets/CRFs   ☐ Laboratory Reports   ☐ Other information, specify:

☐ Pathology Report   ☐ Progress Notes   ☐ Radiology Reports   ☐ Referral Letters   ☐ Summary Report Sent to IRB

18. Submitter Signature – This section required if submitter is someone other than reporter (from Section 2)

I certify that this Expedited Report has been reviewed and approved by a physician or the medically certified designee responsible for the care of this patient.

LAST NAME   FIRST NAME   PHONE   Fax   E-MAIL

SUBMITTER SIGNATURE   SIGNATURE DATE[1]

(Continued on next page)

Figure 28-4. Adverse Event Expedited Report Forms *(Continued)*

 Department of Health & Human Services

Adverse Event Expedited Report – Multiple Agents v4.0

Public Health Service
National Institutes of Health
National Cancer Institute
Bethesda, Maryland 20892

INSTRUCTIONS: Use this form to submit an Expedited Report for an Adverse Event (AE) or Death Unrelated to an Adverse Event for NCI clinical trials using one investigational agent sponsored under an NCI IND. Refer to the protocol to determine if NCI IND agents are utilized on the study and how to submit the Expedited Report. <u>Use this form only when it is impossible to access the Adverse Event Expedited Reporting System (AdEERS) Web application.</u> The AdEERS Web application can be accessed at https://webapps.ctep.nci.nih.gov/openapps/plsql/gadeers_main$.startup.

This form must be completed using the <u>AdEERS Template Instructions</u> available from the NCI CTEP Help Desk by phone at (301) 840-8202 or by fax at (301) 948-2242. Information components followed by "1," "LOV," "LOV/FT," or "CTC" must be entered using the special instructions below. Please see the <u>AdEERS Template Instructions</u> for a complete description of all components and instructions developed for this template.

1   Date information must be entered in MM/DD/YYYY format except where "MM/YYYY Only" (month and year only) instruction is given.
LOV   Information must be entered using standardized values from the AdEERS List of Values (LOV) document available from the AdEERS Web site.
LOV/FT   Information must be entered using the AdEERS LOV or, if an appropriate value cannot be found, using Free Text (values other than those listed in the LOV).
CTC   Adverse Events are to be reported using the terminology and criteria of the NCI Common Toxicity Criteria (CTC), Version 2.0 (publish date April 30, 1999).

COMPLETING THE REPORT:

1.   Complete all MANDATORY COMPONENTS in MANDATORY SECTIONS. Complete all *Requisite Components* in MANDATORY SECTIONS if relevant to the patient.
2.   Determine which *Requisite Sections* apply to the patient and complete the MANDATORY COMPONENTS (if any) and *Requisite Components* if relevant to the patient.
3.   If additional space is required to complete a report section, copy the page where the section appears, complete your entries, and attach to the final report.
4.   Complete the form using black or blue ink and send to the Investigational Drug Branch (IDB), P.O. Box 30012, Bethesda, MD 20824 or fax to 301-230-0159.

1. PROTOCOL INFORMATION – THIS SECTION IS MANDATORY FOR ALL EXPEDITED REPORTS

IS THIS AN AMENDMENT TO A PREVIOUSLY   IF YES, CHECK AMENDMENT

NCI PROTOCOL NUMBER   SUBMITTED REPORT? ☐YES ☐NO   NUMBER: ☐1 ☐2 ☐3   **INITIAL EXPEDITED REPORT TICKET NUMBER (AMENDMENTS ONLY)**

PROTOCOL TITLE (Continue below)

2. REPORTER INFORMATION – THIS SECTION IS MANDATORY FOR ALL EXPEDITED REPORTS

	LAST NAME	FIRST NAME	PHONE	FAX	E-MAIL
REPORT DATE 1					
REPORTER					
PHYSICIAN INFORMATION (Physician to be consulted for questions)				*Fax is a requisite component for* **PHYSICIAN INFORMATION**	

3. PATIENT INFORMATION – THIS SECTION IS MANDATORY FOR ALL EXPEDITED REPORTS
     A PATIENT ID is a unique identification code associated with each patient entered in the trial.

PATIENT ID   **PATIENT'S INSTITUTION NAME, CITY, AND STATE (OR INSTITUTION CODE** – Institution where patient is registered on the protocol or is currently being treated, see http://ctep.cancer.gov/guidelines/codes.html)

BIRTH DATE (MM/YYYY Only)   RACE LOV   **GENDER** LOV   **HEIGHT (cm)**   **WEIGHT (kg)**   *Baseline Performance Status at Initiation of Protocol – ECOG/Zubrod Scale* LOV

DISEASE NAME LOV   *Disease Name Not Listed (Enter a specific disease name when "Solid Tumor NOS" or "Hematologic unspecified" is entered in the* **DISEASE NAME** *component)*

PRIMARY SITE OF DISEASE LOV   *Other Primary Site of Disease (Enter only when an appropriate primary site is not found in the LOV)*

IS DATE OF INITIAL DIAGNOSIS KNOWN: ☐YES ☐NO   **IF YES, ENTER THE DATE OF INITIAL DIAGNOSIS (MM/YYYY Only):**

(Continued on next page)

Figure 28-4. Adverse Event Expedited Report Forms *(Continued)*

---

4. COURSE INFORMATION – THIS SECTION IS MANDATORY FOR ALL EXPEDITED REPORTS

A Treatment Assignment Code (TAC) is a unique identification code associated with each arm or dose level of the protocol.
Example: Drug ###mg / m2 IV over X hr D1-5 / every 3 weeks)

_____

Treatment Assignment Code (TAC)

If the appropriate TAC is unavailable from the LOV or is unknown, items A through D (below) are mandatory for the treatment arm or dose level.

A. Agent Name(s) LOV	B. Dose	C. Administration Route LOV	D. Duration and Schedule LOV

START DATE OF FIRST COURSE [1]   **START DATE OF COURSE ASSOCIATED WITH EXPEDITED REPORT [1]**   **START DATE OF PRIMARY AE [1]**

End Date of AE [1]   **COURSE NUMBER ON WHICH AE OCCURRED**   **TOTAL NUMBER OF COURSES TO DATE**

WAS AN INVESTIGATIONAL AGENT(S) ADMINISTERED ON THIS PROTOCOL? ☐YES ☐NO

CROSSOVER STUDIES
The following information is required if this report is associated with a Crossover Study: a) Enter the date the initial Crossover course started in the START DATE OF FIRST COURSE field (Section 4), b) Check YES to WAS AN INVESTIGATIONAL AGENT(S) ADMINISTERED ON THIS PROTOCOL? (Section 4), c) Enter the date the investigational agent was last administered in the DATE LAST ADMINISTERED field (Section 10), and d) Enter the dose administered for the course in the TOTAL DOSE ADMINISTERED THIS COURSE field (Section 10), zero (0) is acceptable if the actual dose is unknown.

5. DESCRIPTION OF EVENT – THIS SECTION IS MANDATORY FOR ALL EXPEDITED REPORTS

DESCRIPTION AND TREATMENT OF EVENT(S) (Continue below)

HAS PATIENT BEEN RETREATED (TO DATE)? ☐YES ☐NO

PRESENT STATUS LOV (If you record Fatal/Death or Recovered/Resolved with or without   *Date of Recovery or Death [1]*
Sequelae as PRESENT STATUS, then *Date of Recovery or Death* [see right] is mandatory)

WAS PATIENT REMOVED FROM PROTOCOL TREATMENT (TO DATE)? ☐YES ☐NO
IF YES, ENTER THE *Date Removed from Protocol Treatment* **(see right)**   *Date Removed from Protocol Treatment [1]*

6. DEATH UNRELATED TO ADVERSE EVENT – MANDATORY ONLY IF DEATH IS UNRELATED TO AN AE

Sections 1, 2, 3, 4, 5, 6, 7 and 10 are mandatory when reporting a death caused by suicide, accident, progressive disease, etc.

CAUSE OF DEATH LOV (If you record Progressive Disease as the CAUSE OF DEATH, then PRIMARY ORGAN   **PRIMARY ORGAN SYSTEM FAILURE CAUSING DEATH** LOV
SYSTEM FAILURE CAUSING DEATH [see right] is mandatory.)

7. PRIOR THERAPIES – THIS SECTION IS MANDATORY FOR ALL EXPEDITED REPORTS

THERAPY LOV (FOR THE PRIMARY DISEASE) (If you record any of the following as THERAPY, then PRIOR THERAPY AGENT NAME(S) [in column 6] is mandatory: bone marrow transplant, chemotherapy [NOS], chemotherapy [single or multiple agent systemic], hormonal therapy, or immunotherapy)	THERAPY START DATE (If known) (MM/YYYY only)	*Therapy End Date (MM/YYYY only)*	*Comments (Enter additional therapies, prior therapy for diseases other than primary disease, or agents not included in LOV, if needed)*	PRIOR THERAPY AGENT NAME(S) LOV (See note in THERAPY column)

8. Pre-Existing Condition(s) – This section is required if the patient has Pre-Existing Conditions
Identify any medical condition(s) the patient experienced prior to receiving current protocol therapy.

CONDITION A LOV   **CONDITION B** LOV   *Pre-Existing Condition Not Listed (Enter only when an appropriate condition is not found in the LOV)*

9. Site(s) of Metastatic Disease – This section is required if the patient has Sites of Metastatic Disease

SITE A LOV   **SITE B** LOV   *Sites of Metastatic Disease Not Listed (Enter only when an appropriate site is not found in the LOV)*

(Continued on next page)

Figure 28-4. Adverse Event Expedited Report Forms *(Continued)*

10. PROTOCOL AGENT(S) – THIS SECTION IS MANDATORY FOR ALL EXPEDITED REPORTS

AGENT NAME(S) LOV

| AGENT NAME A LOV | AGENT NAME B LOV | AGENT NAME C LOV | AGENT NAME D LOV |

DATE LAST ADMINISTERED [1]

(This is mandatory for crossover studies if an investigational agent was administered at any time, see Section 4)

TOTAL DOSE ADMINISTERED THIS COURSE

UNIT OF MEASURE LOV   UNIT OF MEASURE LOV   UNIT OF MEASURE LOV   UNIT OF MEASURE LOV
(Amount of agent given for current dose or cycle, this is not total dose given to date)

Comments

Agent Adjustment LOV

Was administration delayed?

| ☐Yes ☐No | ☐Yes ☐No | ☐Yes ☐No | ☐Yes ☐No |
| *If yes, complete Duration Delay below* | *If yes, complete Duration Delay below* | *If yes, complete Duration Delay below* | *If yes, complete Duration Delay below* |

Duration Delay

| ☐sec ☐min ☐hrs ☐days | ☐sec ☐min ☐hrs ☐days | ☐sec ☐min ☐hrs ☐days | ☐sec ☐min ☐hrs ☐days |

(Enter duration length and check Unit of Measure)

CROSSOVER STUDIES – Instruction is provided in Section 4 regarding required information for reports associated with Crossover Studies.

11. Concomitant Medication(s) – This section is required if any non-protocol medication may have contributed to the event(s)

| CONCOMITANT MEDICATION A | CONCOMITANT MEDICATION B |
| CONCOMITANT MEDICATION C | CONCOMITANT MEDICATION D |

12. Other Contributing Cause(s) – This section is required if Other Causes may have contributed to the Adverse Event

| OTHER CONTRIBUTING CAUSE A | OTHER CONTRIBUTING CAUSE B |
| OTHER CONTRIBUTING CAUSE C | OTHER CONTRIBUTING CAUSE D |

13. ADVERSE EVENTS (CTC) – THIS SECTION IS MANDATORY FOR ALL EXPEDITED REPORTS <u>EXCEPT</u> DEATH UNRELATED TO AE

CATEGORY CTC	ADVERSE EVENT CTC	If AE is other, Specify: (If an appropriate AE term cannot be identified in the CTC, identify the CTC **CATEGORY** and provide AE information in this column)	GRADE CTC (If you record a GRADE 3 or higher, Hospitalization or Prolongation of Hospitalization [in column 5] is mandatory)	Hospitalization or Prolongation of Hospitalization (See note in GRADE column)	Comments (Enter other relevant information in this column)
AE A:				☐Yes ☐No	
AE B:				☐Yes ☐No	
AE C:				☐Yes ☐No	

14. ATTRIBUTION FOR ADVERSE EVENT – THIS SECTION IS MANDATORY FOR ALL EXPEDITED REPORTS <u>EXCEPT</u> DEATH UNRELATED TO AE

Attribution is the determination whether an AE is related to a medical treatment or procedure. Evaluate each AE the patient experiences to determine what might have caused the event or what interventions or conditions the event might have been attributed to.

IMPORTANT: Every AdEERS report that includes Adverse Events must include for each Adverse Event at least one attribution of Possible, Probable, or Definite to either the Agent, the Disease, Other Causes, or Concomitant Medications. NCI will not accept reports without at least one attribution of Possible, Probable, or Definite to either the Agent, the Disease, Other Causes, or Concomitant Medications for each Adverse Event.

Write the AE term(s) you used in Section 13 in the heading area of columns 2, 3, and 4 (found on page 4). Complete the AGENT NAME, DISEASE, *Concomitant Medication* and/or *Other Contributing Causes* information in column 1 using the same information you provided in Sections 10, 3, 11, and 12. Circle the ATTRIBUTION CODE in each column for each AE based on its relationship to the AGENT NAME, DISEASE, *Concomitant Medication* and/or *Other Contributing Causes* information provided in column 1. An example is provided below.

Example	Anorexia					Bilirubin					Pain–Other				
	ADVERSE EVENT CTC (AE A from Section 13)					ADVERSE EVENT CTC (AE B from Section 13)					ADVERSE EVENT CTC (AE C from Section 13)				
Drug 1	1	2	③	4	5	1	2	③	4	5	1	②	3	4	5
AGENT NAME LOV (from Section 10)															

ATTRIBUTION CODES are defined as:

1   Unrelated - The Adverse Event is clearly NOT related to the investigational agent, disease, concomitant medication, or other contributing cause.

2   Unlikely - The Adverse Event is doubtfully related to the investigational agent, disease, concomitant medication, or other contributing cause.

3   Possible - The Adverse Event may be related to the investigational agent, disease, concomitant medication, or other contributing cause.

4   Probable - The Adverse Event is likely related to the investigational agent, disease, concomitant medication, or other contributing cause.

5   Definite - The Adverse Event is clearly related to the investigational agent, disease, concomitant medication, or other contributing cause.

This section continues on page 4.

(Continued on next page)

Figure 28-4. Adverse Event Expedited Report Forms *(Continued)*

14. ATTRIBUTION FOR ADVERSE EVENT (Continued)

	ADVERSE EVENT CTC (AE A from Section 13)					ADVERSE EVENT CTC (AE B from Section 13)					ADVERSE EVENT CTC (AE C from Section 13)				
AGENT NAME LOV (AGENT NAME A from Section 10)	1	2	3	4	5	1	2	3	4	5	1	2	3	4	5
AGENT NAME LOV (AGENT NAME B from Section 10)	1	2	3	4	5	1	2	3	4	5	1	2	3	4	5
AGENT NAME LOV (AGENT NAME C from Section 10)	1	2	3	4	5	1	2	3	4	5	1	2	3	4	5
AGENT NAME LOV (AGENT NAME D from Section 10)	1	2	3	4	5	1	2	3	4	5	1	2	3	4	5
DISEASE NAME LOV (from Section 3)	1	2	3	4	5	1	2	3	4	5	1	2	3	4	5
Concomitant Medication (A from Section 11)	1	2	3	4	5	1	2	3	4	5	1	2	3	4	5
Concomitant Medication (B from Section 11)	1	2	3	4	5	1	2	3	4	5	1	2	3	4	5
Concomitant Medication (C from Section 11)	1	2	3	4	5	1	2	3	4	5	1	2	3	4	5
Concomitant Medication (D from Section 11)	1	2	3	4	5	1	2	3	4	5	1	2	3	4	5
Other Contributing Causes (A from Section 12)	1	2	3	4	5	1	2	3	4	5	1	2	3	4	5
Other Contributing Causes (B from Section 12)	1	2	3	4	5	1	2	3	4	5	1	2	3	4	5
Other Contributing Causes (C from Section 12)	1	2	3	4	5	1	2	3	4	5	1	2	3	4	5
Other Contributing Causes (D from Section 12)	1	2	3	4	5	1	2	3	4	5	1	2	3	4	5

15. Abnormal and Relevant Normal Laboratory Results – This section is required if Laboratory Results are relevant to the report
This section is not required if Microbiology information is provided in Section 16.

Lab LOV/FT	Baseline			Nadir/Worst		Recovery/Latest	
	Date ¹	Value	Unit of Measure LOV	Date ¹	Value	Date ¹	Value
Lab A:							
Lab B:							
Lab C:							

16. Lab: Microbiology – This section is required for reporting infections
Do not complete Section 15 if Microbiology information is provided below.

Infection Type: ☐ *Bacterial* ☐ *Fungal* ☐ *Viral*

Site   Date ¹   Infectious Agent

17. Additional Information Attached – This section is required if relevant to the report
Check those you have attached for submission with this report.

☐ *Autopsy Report* ☐ *Consults* ☐ *Discharge Summary* ☐ *Flow Sheets/CRFs* ☐ *Laboratory Reports* ☐ *Other information, specify:*

☐ *Pathology Report* ☐ *Progress Notes* ☐ *Radiology Reports* ☐ *Referral Letters* ☐ *Summary Report Sent to IRB*

18. Submitter Signature – This section required if submitter is someone other than reporter (from section 2)

I certify that this Expedited Report has been reviewed and approved by a physician or the medically certified designee responsible for the care of this patient.

LAST NAME	FIRST NAME	PHONE	Fax	E-MAIL

SUBMITTER SIGNATURE	SIGNATURE DATE ¹

Note. From *CTEP Forms, Templates and Documents,* by National Cancer Institute Cancer Therapy Evaluation Program, n.d., Bethesda, MD: Author. Retrieved November 26, 2007, from http://ctep.cancer.gov/forms.

Table 28-3. Adverse Event Reporting Requirements for Commercial Reporting Requirements

Expedited reporting requirements for adverse events experienced by patients on arm(s) with commercial agents only—Arm X

Attribution	Grade 4		Grade 5[a]		ECOG and Protocol-Specific Requirements
	Unexpected	Expected	Unexpected	Expected	See footnote (b) for special requirements.
Unrelated or Unlikely			7 calendar days	7 calendar days	
Possible, Probable, Definite	7 calendar days		7 calendar days	7 calendar days	

7 Calendar Days: Indicates a full AdEERS report is to be submitted within 7 calendar days of learning of the event.

[a] This includes all deaths within 30 days of the last dose of treatment regardless of attribution. **NOTE: Any death that occurs > 30 days after the last dose of treatment and is attributed possibly, probably, or definitely to the treatment must be reported within 7 calendar days of learning of the event.**

[b] Protocol-specific expedited reporting requirements: The adverse events listed below also require expedited reporting for this trial:

Serious Events: Any event following treatment that results in *persistent or significant disabilities/incapacities, congenital anomalies, or birth defects* must be reported via AdEERS within 7 calendar days of learning of the event. For instructions on how to specifically report these events via AdEERS, please contact the NCI Medical Help Desk at 301-897-7497.

AdEERS—Adverse Event Expedited Reporting System; ECOG—Eastern Cooperative Oncology Group; NCI—National Cancer Institute

Note. From *CTEP, NCI Guidelines: Adverse Event Reporting Requirements,* by National Cancer Institute Cancer Therapy Evaluation Program, January 2005. Retrieved November 25, 2007, from http://ecog.dfci.harvard.edu/ecoginst/adeers/commercial.pdf.

Table 28-4. Reporting Requirements for Adverse Events That Occur Within 30 Days[1] of the Last Dose of the Investigational Agent on Phase I Trials

	1	2	2	3		3		4 & 5[2]
	Unexpected and Expected	Unexpected	Expected	Unexpected		Expected		Unexpected and Expected
				With Hospitalization	Without Hospitalization	With Hospitalization	Without Hospitalization	
Unrelated Unlikely	Not required	Not required	Not required	10 calendar days	Not required	10 calendar days	Not required	24-hour; 5 calendar days
Possible Probable Definite	Not required	10 calendar days	Not required	24-hour; 5 calendar days	24-hour; 5 calendar days	10 calendar days	Not required	24-hour; 5 calendar days

[1] Adverse events with attribution of possible, probable, or definite that occur greater than 30 days after the last dose of treatment with an agent under a CTEP IND require reporting as follows:

AdEERS 24-hour notification followed by complete report within 5 calendar days for:
• Grade 3 unexpected events with hospitalization or prolongation of hospitalization
• Grade 4 unexpected events
• Grade 5 expected and unexpected events

[2] Although an AdEERS 24-hour notification is not required for death clearly related to progressive disease, a full report is required as outlined in the table.

AdEERS—Adverse Event Expedited Reporting System; CTEP—Cancer Therapy Evaluation Program; IND—investigational new drug

Note. From *CTEP, NCI Guidelines: Adverse Event Reporting Requirements* (p. 13), by National Cancer Institute Cancer Therapy Evaluation Program, December 2004, Bethesda, MD: Author. Retrieved November 26, 2007, from http://ctep.cancer.gov/reporting/newadverse_2006.pdf

Table 28-5. Reporting Requirements for Adverse Events That Occur Within 30 Days[1] of the Last Dose of the Investigational Agent on Phase II and III Trials

	1	2	2	3		3		4 & 5[2]
	Unexpected and Expected	Unexpected	Expected	Unexpected		Expected		Unexpected and Expected
				With Hospitalization	Without Hospitalization	With Hospitalization	Without Hospitalization	
Unrelated Unlikely	Not required	Not required	Not required	10 calendar days	Not required	10 calendar days	Not required	24-hour; 5 calendar days
Possible Probable Definite	Not required	10 calendar days	Not required	24-hour; 5 calendar days	24-hour; 5 calendar days	10 calendar days	Not required	24-hour; 5 calendar days

[1] Adverse events with attribution of possible, probable, or definite that occur greater than 30 days after the last dose of treatment with an agent under a CTEP IND require reporting as follows:

AdEERS 24-hour notification followed by complete report within 5 calendar days for:
• Grade 4 and Grade 5 unexpected events

AdEERS 10 calendar day report:
• Grade 3 unexpected events with hospitalization or prolongation of hospitalization
• Grade 5 expected events

[2] Although an AdEERS 24-hour notification is not required for death clearly related to progressive disease, a full report is required as outlined in the table.

AdEERS—Adverse Event Expedited Reporting System; CTEP—Cancer Therapy Evaluation Program; IND—investigational new drug

Note. From *CTEP, NCI Guidelines: Adverse Event Reporting Requirements* (p. 14), by National Cancer Institute Cancer Therapy Evaluation Program, December 2004, Bethesda, MD: Author. Retrieved November 26, 2007, from http://ctep.cancer.gov/reporting/newadverse_2006.pdf

Figure 28-5. MedWatch Form

U.S. Department of Health and Human Services

MEDWATCH

The FDA Safety Information and
Adverse Event Reporting Program

For VOLUNTARY reporting of
adverse events, product problems and
product use errors

Page ____ of ____

Form Approved: OMB No. 0910-0291, Expires: 10/31/08
See OMB statement on reverse.

FDA USE ONLY

Triage unit
sequence #

PLEASE TYPE OR USE BLACK INK

A. PATIENT INFORMATION

1. Patient Identifier	2. Age at Time of Event, or Date of Birth:	3. Sex	4. Weight
In confidence		☐ Female ☐ Male	_____ lb or _____ kg

B. ADVERSE EVENT, PRODUCT PROBLEM OR ERROR

Check all that apply:

1. ☐ Adverse Event   ☐ Product Problem (e.g., defects/malfunctions)
   ☐ Product Use Error ☐ Problem with Different Manufacturer of Same Medicine

2. Outcomes Attributed to Adverse Event
   (Check all that apply)

   ☐ Death: _____ (mm/dd/yyyy)   ☐ Disability or Permanent Damage
   ☐ Life-threatening   ☐ Congenital Anomaly/Birth Defect
   ☐ Hospitalization - initial or prolonged ☐ Other Serious (Important Medical Events)
   ☐ Required Intervention to Prevent Permanent Impairment/Damage (Devices)

3. Date of Event (mm/dd/yyyy)	4. Date of this Report (mm/dd/yyyy)

5. Describe Event, Problem or Product Use Error

6. Relevant Tests/Laboratory Data, Including Dates

7. Other Relevant History, Including Preexisting Medical Conditions (e.g., allergies, race, pregnancy, smoking and alcohol use, liver/kidney problems, etc.)

C. PRODUCT AVAILABILITY

Product Available for Evaluation? *(Do not send product to FDA)*

☐ Yes ☐ No ☐ Returned to Manufacturer on: _____ (mm/dd/yyyy)

D. SUSPECT PRODUCT(S)

1. Name, Strength, Manufacturer *(from product label)*

   #1 _____
   #2 _____

2.	Dose or Amount	Frequency	Route
#1			
#2			

3. Dates of Use (If unknown, give duration) from/to (or best estimate)	5. Event Abated After Use Stopped or Dose Reduced?
#1	#1 ☐ Yes ☐ No ☐ Doesn't Apply
#2	#2 ☐ Yes ☐ No ☐ Doesn't Apply

4. Diagnosis or Reason for Use (Indication)	8. Event Reappeared After Reintroduction?
#1	#1 ☐ Yes ☐ No ☐ Doesn't Apply
#2	#2 ☐ Yes ☐ No ☐ Doesn't Apply

6. Lot #	7. Expiration Date	9. NDC # or Unique ID
#1	#1	
#2	#2	

E. SUSPECT MEDICAL DEVICE

1. Brand Name

2. Common Device Name

3. Manufacturer Name, City and State

4. Model #	Lot #	5. Operator of Device
Catalog #	Expiration Date (mm/dd/yyyy)	☐ Health Professional
Serial #	Other #	☐ Lay User/Patient ☐ Other: _____

6. If Implanted, Give Date (mm/dd/yyyy)	7. If Explanted, Give Date (mm/dd/yyyy)

8. Is this a Single-use Device that was Reprocessed and Reused on a Patient?
   ☐ Yes ☐ No

9. If Yes to Item No. 8, Enter Name and Address of Reprocessor

F. OTHER (CONCOMITANT) MEDICAL PRODUCTS

Product names and therapy dates *(exclude treatment of event)*

G. REPORTER *(See confidentiality section on back)*

1. Name and Address

Phone #	E-mail

2. Health Professional?	3. Occupation	4. Also Reported to:
☐ Yes ☐ No		☐ Manufacturer
5. If you do NOT want your identity disclosed to the manufacturer, place an "X" in this box: ☐		☐ User Facility ☐ Distributor/Importer

FORM FDA 3500 (10/05)   Submission of a report does not constitute an admission that medical personnel or the product caused or contributed to the event.

(Cotinued on next page)

Figure 28-5. MedWatch Form *(Continued)*

ADVICE ABOUT VOLUNTARY REPORTING

Detailed instructions available at: http://www.fda.gov/medwatch/report/consumer/instruct.htm

Report adverse events, product problems or product use errors with:

- Medications *(drugs or biologics)*
- Medical devices *(including in-vitro diagnostics)*
- Combination products *(medication & medical devices)*
- Human cells, tissues, and cellular and tissue-based products
- Special nutritional products *(dietary supplements, medical foods, infant formulas)*
- Cosmetics

Report product problems - quality, performance or safety concerns such as:

- Suspected counterfeit product
- Suspected contamination
- Questionable stability
- Defective components
- Poor packaging or labeling
- Therapeutic failures (product didn't work)

Report SERIOUS adverse events. An event is serious when the patient outcome is:

- Death
- Life-threatening
- Hospitalization - initial or prolonged
- Disability or permanent damage
- Congenital anomaly/birth defect
- Required intervention to prevent permanent impairment or damage
- Other serious (important medical events)

Report even if:

- You're not certain the product caused the event
- You don't have all the details

How to report:

- Just fill in the sections that apply to your report
- Use section D for all products except medical devices
- Attach additional pages if needed
- Use a separate form for each patient
- Report either to FDA or the manufacturer *(or both)*

Other methods of reporting:

- 1-800-FDA-0178 -- To FAX report
- 1-800-FDA-1088 -- To report by phone
- www.fda.gov/medwatch/report.htm -- To report online

If your report involves a serious adverse event with a device and it occurred in a facility outside a doctor's office, that facility may be legally required to report to FDA and/or the manufacturer. Please notify the person in that facility who would handle such reporting.

If your report involves a serious adverse event with a vaccine call 1-800-822-7967 to report.

Confidentiality: The patient's identity is held in strict confidence by FDA and protected to the fullest extent of the law. FDA will not disclose the reporter's identity in response to a request from the public, pursuant to the Freedom of Information Act. The reporter's identity, including the identity of a self-reporter, may be shared with the manufacturer unless requested otherwise.

-Fold Here-   -Fold Here-

The public reporting burden for this collection of information has been estimated to average 36 minutes per response, including the time for reviewing instructions, searching existing data sources, gathering and maintaining the data needed, and completing and reviewing the collection of information. Send comments regarding this burden estimate or any other aspect of this collection of information, including suggestions for reducing this burden to:

Department of Health and Human Services *Food and Drug Administration - MedWatch* *10903 New Hampshire Avenue* *Building 22, Mail Stop 4447* *Silver Spring, MD 20993-0002*	*Please DO NOT* *RETURN this form* *to this address.*	*OMB statement:* *"An agency may not conduct or sponsor, and a person is not required to respond to, a collection of information unless it displays a currently valid OMB control number."*

U.S. DEPARTMENT OF HEALTH AND HUMAN SERVICES
Food and Drug Administration

FORM FDA 3500 (10/05) (Back)   Please Use Address Provided Below -- Fold in Thirds, Tape and Mail

**DEPARTMENT OF
HEALTH & HUMAN SERVICES**

Public Health Service
Food and Drug Administration
Rockville, MD 20857

Official Business
Penalty for Private Use $300

NO POSTAGE
NECESSARY
IF MAILED
IN THE
UNITED STATES
OR APO/FPO

BUSINESS REPLY MAIL
FIRST CLASS MAIL   PERMIT NO. 946   ROCKVILLE MD

MedWatch

The FDA Safety Information and Adverse Event Reporting Program
Food and Drug Administration
5600 Fishers Lane
Rockville, MD 20852-9787

Note. From *MedWatch: The FDA Safety Information and Adverse Event Reporting Program,* by MedWatch, U.S. Department of Health and Human Services, Food and Drug Administration, n.d., Rockville, MD: Author. Retrieved November 26, 2007, from http://www.fda.gov/medwatch/SAFETY/3500.pdf

Summary

Accurate identification, assessment, and intervention for AEs and communication between researchers and clinical trial participants are critical strategies for achieving success in conducting clinical trials (Lengacher et al., 2001). The CTN plays a pivotal role in the comprehensive assessment and reporting of AEs that occur during clinical trial treatments. Adequate knowledge of oncology, of the pathophysiology of malignancies, and of comprehensive assessment skills are critical to ensuring adequate monitoring and reporting of AEs. Ultimately, this ensures the protection of patients participating in clinical trials. Without these skills, patient safety and the future of clinical research are at risk.

References

Allaster, R.M., Frayne, B.K., Malpage, A.S., Smuck, B.L., & Studzienny, L.G. (1996). Development of a comprehensive nursing/toxicity assessment form. *Oncology Nursing Forum, 23,* 1317–1324.

Electronic code of federal regulations. (2007, November 21). Title 21—food and drugs. Retrieved November 26, 2007, from http://ecfr.gpoaccess .gov

Lengacher, C.A., Gonzalez, L.L., Giuliano, R., Bennett, M.P., Cox, C.E., & Reintgen, D.S. (2001). The process of clinical trials: A model for successful clinical trial participation. *Oncology Nursing Forum, 28,* 1115–1120.

MedDRA. (2007). *Welcome to MedDRA and the MSSO.* Retrieved May 26, 2007, from http://www.meddramsso.com/MSSOWeb/index .htm

National Cancer Institute Cancer Therapy Evaluation Program. (2005, January 1). *CTEP, NCI guidelines: Adverse event reporting requirements.* Retrieved November 26, 2007, from http://ctep.cancer.gov/reporting/ newadverse_2006.pdf

National Cancer Institute Cancer Therapy Evaluation Program. (n.d.). *Phase I combination template.* Retrieved November 26, 2007, from http://ctep.cancer.gov/forms/AEcomb1_temp_v1.doc

Oncology Nursing Society. (2004). *Statement on the scope and standards of oncology nursing practice.* Pittsburgh, PA: Oncology Nursing Society.

Trontell, A.E. (2001). How the U.S. Food and Drug Administration defines and detects adverse drug events. *Current Therapeutic Research, 62,* 641–649.

CHAPTER 29
Patient and Family Education

Geri L. Schmotzer, RN, MPH, MSN

Introduction

Assessment of patient and family education needs is a vital process regardless of whether a patient chooses to participate in a clinical trial. The Oncology Nursing Society's *Standards of Oncology Education: Patient/Significant Other and Public* (Blecher, 2004) provides guidelines for developing, implementing, and evaluating patient education programs and can serve as a model for educating patients who are contemplating entering a clinical trial. Figure 29-1 lists the five standards that are used as a resource for achieving quality patient education. Patient education is defined as "a process of influencing behavior to elicit changes in the knowledge level, attitudes, and skills required to maintain and improve health," with the primary goal of providing patients and caregivers the knowledge and skills with which to cope with their disease (Treacy & Mayer, 2000, p. 48).

Assess for Learning Readiness

While caring for or talking with the patient who is experiencing cancer, opportunities are available to assess the patient's readiness to learn (Hagopian, 1996). Readiness to learn can be characterized as "the state of being both willing and able to use the teaching provided" and is affected by the patient's level of comfort—both physical and mental, attention level, energy level, motivation, and capability (Treacy & Mayer, 2000, p. 54). For learning to take place, both the teacher and learner need to feel comfortable physically, psychologically, and in relation to their environment. A patient's interest and energy level determine how and when learning takes place. Everyone has different motivating factors for wanting to acquire information, and the nurse needs to be cognizant of the patient's goals. When talking to patients and families about clinical trials, understanding their motivation for entering a study may provide insight

---

Figure 29-1. Oncology Patient Education Standards

Standard I. The oncology nurse at both the generalist and advanced practice levels is responsible for education of the patient/significant others related to cancer.

Standard II. Adequate resources to achieve the objectives of patient/significant other education related to cancer care are available and appropriate.

Standard III. Knowledge, skills, and attitudes related to the management of human responses to cancer are reflected in the educational activity for the patient and significant others experiencing cancer.

Standard IV. Teaching-learning theories are applied to the development, implementation, and evaluation of learning experiences related to cancer care.

Standard V. The patient and/or significant other apply knowledge, skills, and attitudes to management of actual or potential human responses to the cancer experience.

Note. From *Standards of Oncology Education: Patient/Significant Others and Public* (3rd ed., pp. 3–8), by C.S. Blecher (Ed.), 2004, Pittsburgh, PA: Oncology Nursing Society. Copyright 2004 by the Oncology Nursing Society. Reprinted with permission.

---

into family dynamics and potential compliance issues that may arise in the future. Patients and their significant others may differ in their willingness and capacity to learn. All verbal and written information must be presented at a level that is appropriate for the individual.

Treacy and Mayer (2000) reported that several studies found the information needs of patients to include information related to the diagnosis, prognosis, treatment options and purpose of treatment, side effects, self-care needs, and effects on work and relationships. Assessing the patient's and family's level of comprehension after an office visit with a physician is a dynamic process. Whether at the time of initial diagnosis, recurrence, or a final treatment attempt

---

The author would like to acknowledge Kimberly Power, RN, MSN, for her contribution that remains unchanged from the first edition.

before hospice care, patients and their significant others are inundated with new terminology and *overwhelming* amounts of information (Lake & Jenkins, 1993).

For learning to occur, the patient's and family's stress levels should be minimized. The nurse can help to reduce stress by developing a rapport with the patient and family and can provide reassurance by being a good listener, communicating effectively, and being knowledgeable and available. Teaching is less stressful when performed in a quiet environment and when both parties are able to devote the necessary time to the education process. Barriers to effective learning can consist of internal and external factors. Internal factors include the patient/family members' attention, coping style, culture, emotions, fatigue, hearing/vision impairments, literacy, motivation, pain, readiness, and stress/anxiety levels. External factors include environmental factors, educational media, knowledge and skill of the educator, and timing of instruction (Treacy & Mayer, 2000). When possible, new concepts need to be reinforced either in person or over the phone. Maintaining a realistic level of hope also helps to alleviate the patient's stress. The clinical trial nurse (CTN) needs to assess the patient's age, cultural background, preferred method of learning, desire for information, placement on the healthcare continuum, attitudes toward health care, and other special considerations to determine what style of teaching will be the most effective.

The Adult Learner

The four characteristics of the adult learner are (a) *self-concept,* which implies that people desire to be self-motivated whenever possible, (b) *role of experience,* meaning that previous experiences help in coping with or adapting to the present situation, (c) *readiness to learn,* which is based on the individual's perception of the value of learning to initiate activities of daily life, and (d) *orientation to learning,* which means that once a problem is identified, adults want to immediately acquire the necessary information to solve the problem (Hagopian, 1996).

Another factor to consider is the cultural diversity of the population. Assessing a patient's religious, social, and cultural values are critical when developing patient education material (Meyer, 2000). Social and cultural values influence a patient's knowledge and attitude. An open and trusting communication style is necessary to determine and understand a patient's beliefs.

The Pediatric Learner

Approximately 60% of children with cancer enter into national clinical trials, with an additional 30% being treated on local- or regional-based offshoots of national protocols (Kupst, Patenaude, Walco, & Sterling, 2003). Principles used to determine the educational needs of parents with a child who has cancer are similar to those of the adult learner. The degree to which the parents play a role in decision making depends largely on the child's age and the nature

of the parent-child relationship. The emotional turmoil that parents experience after learning of their child's diagnosis of cancer is a significant obstacle when trying to understand and consider the complex medical information they receive when making treatment choices for their child (Kupst et al.). When providing information to children, educators should ensure that the learning is developmentally appropriate. Jean Piaget (as discussed in Trubowitz, 1998) theorized four stages of cognitive development through which children must progress to develop an understanding of the world around them (see Table 29-1). Comprehending these developmental stages assists the CTN in formulating appropriate learning experiences for children of various ages.

Table 29-1. The Four Developmental Stages of Cognitive Development in Children		
Stage	**Age**	**Level of Development**
Sensorimotor stage	Birth to 2 years old	Child experiences the world through movement and senses and learns object permanence.
Preoperational stage	2–7	Child acquires motor skills.
Concrete operational stage	7–11	Child begins to think logically about concrete events.
Formal operational stage	11 and older	Child develops abstract reasoning.

Challenging Learning Needs

Several patient populations are identified as requiring in-depth and highly individualized assessment. These include some older adult patients; those who are blind, deaf, or mentally deficient; the illiterate; and those who speak a foreign language. Some of these patients may be ineligible for clinical trials because of comorbidities or poor performance status, and for others, informed consent maybe difficult, if not impossible, to obtain (Simon et al., 2004).

When presenting clinical trial information to some older adults, explanations must be simple and clear. Both a verbal and an easily understandable written explanation of the concept should be provided. For patients who are illiterate, patient education videos are useful to facilitate learning. The informed consent document must be read aloud and explained to these individuals, as well as to the blind. Sign-language interpreters and foreign-language translators also are available to assist in communicating with special populations. When many individuals who speak a particular foreign language enroll in a clinical trial, a short, institutional review board–approved consent form written in the appropriate language may be used (Thomas, Saleem, & Abraham, 2005).

Study Phase–Specific Informational Needs

Treatment decisions regarding participation in, continuation of, and completion of clinical trials are made at different points along the healthcare continuum. By identifying where the patient is along this continuum, the nurse is better able to understand the patient's educational needs and use available internal and external resources to meet these needs. For example, at the time of diagnosis, patients with localized disease may be eligible for phase III studies, which compare the standard treatment to a new experimental therapy. Other patients are diagnosed with regional or advanced disease upon the completion of their cancer work-up. For others, participation in a study is contemplated at the time of recurrent or progressive disease.

Phase I Studies

Educating patients and families concerning phase I trials is difficult. Cox and Avis (1996) stated that for patients undergoing early-phase studies, "there are no agreed-upon standards regarding how much information should be disclosed about the nature, risks, benefits, and alternatives of the trial treatment or about the right to withdrawal from the study" (p. 178). A small pilot study conducted by these researchers showed that patients and families initially are inundated with educational materials, but patients appreciate knowing what is going to happen. After the physician explains the protocol, the CTN can be available to serve as an educational resource to answer questions. For parents of a child with cancer, deciding whether to enroll the child into a phase I study is one of the most difficult decisions they will have to make. Information provided by the healthcare team is the most frequently cited factor that influences parents' decision to participate (Hinds et al., 1997). In addition to the informed consent, patients should be given information that reinforces several elements about the phase I study: how the research will be conducted, the risks and benefits of the treatment, the unproven nature of the research, alternatives to participation in research, and the subject's freedom to not participate in the research or to withdraw at any time if they do (Hutchison & Campbell, 2002).

One of the goals of phase I studies is to understand the toxicity profile of the therapy being administered. Usually, the side effects of the investigational treatment are unknown or knowledge is limited because drug testing may have been done only with animals. For this reason, patients and their significant others need to be instructed to report all side effects, whether treatment-related or not, to the healthcare team. Education may include how to document side effects in a daily diary, as well as the importance of notifying the CTN when the patient experiences an unusual symptom.

The patient needs to be aware that safety, not a beneficial response, is the goal in a phase I study. Hutchison and Campbell (2002) reported that most patients participate in phase I studies because they believe they will benefit. A study by Yoder, O'Rourke, Etnyre, Spears, and Brown (1997) revealed that patients participating in phase I studies need to maintain realistic hope but also must be kept informed of their current condition and response to the treatment. Yoder et al. found that when families receive emotional support from the healthcare team, they are better able to meet patients' psychosocial needs. According to Cox and Avis (1996), the patient and family receive less information from the healthcare team as protocol treatment progresses, which causes patients to feel uncertain regarding their future.

Phase II Studies

In phase II studies, additional risks and toxicities are known; therefore, more information is available for the patient and the family. However, uncertainty as to the actual benefit of the treatment still may exist. In phase II studies, similar to phase I studies, patients' expectations may differ from the actual goal of the clinical trial (Ratain, Mick, Schilsky, & Siegler, 1993). From the time the protocol is presented through study completion or being taken off study, the patient and family continue to need educational information and emotional support.

The major end points of phase II studies usually are assessment of tumor shrinkage, duration of response, and the toxicity profile of the therapy (Leventhal, 1988). For these reasons, patients are educated about the importance of following their therapy schedule as well as the testing schedule required to determine tumor response. By establishing a rapport with the patient, the CTN encourages patient compliance. As with phase I studies, the patient and family need instruction on the importance of reporting toxicities in a timely and comprehensive manner.

Phase III Studies

Phase III studies typically require large numbers of participants in an effort to document improvement of a new treatment over the standard therapy. Patients are randomized to receive either the standard therapy for that type and stage of cancer or an investigational treatment that is thought to possibly be better. Patients and families are instructed about the different treatment arms of the study and the various potential side effects attributed to these therapies. If a patient wishes to receive a particular treatment, he or she should not be entered into a study. The concept of randomization must be understood to avoid having patients randomized to receive a treatment they do not consent to have, which compromises the research study.

The treatments being administered in phase III clinical trials have documented toxicities. However, researchers continue to collect toxicity information to determine any unexpected side effects or greater prevalence. Patient education focuses on the expected toxicities and interventions available to alleviate these problems. Teaching reinforces that side effects are not to be endured but rather must be reported so that appropriate medical and nursing actions can be implemented. Skrutkowska and Weijer (1997) documented that patients who are participating in clinical trials are more likely to receive follow-up telephone calls, reassurance, and patient teaching from the nursing staff than are nonprotocol patients. This may be attributed to nurses and physicians wanting to maintain patient compliance and their commitment to being more accessible to patients who are entered on clinical trials.

Completion of Protocol Treatment

Completion of therapy is a celebratory event; however, it also is a time of change and uncertainty for patients and families. To nurses or data managers, the end of treatment may signify that the most difficult part of the recovery process is over. To patients, the final treatment may be viewed as a departure from the support and reassurance of the healthcare team. Patients and families need to receive education at this critical time to outline expectations for the future and as a reminder that follow-up information continues to be obtained according to the protocol. Many clinical trials are introducing study end points that include monitoring of quality of life and long-term toxicities.

Haase and Rostad (1994) examined children's perspectives upon completion of cancer therapy. They discovered that children need assistance in exploring the meaning of treatment completion; understanding the word *remission* and the fears that coincide with the possibility of recurrence; accepting that relationships with peers, family members, and healthcare staff are changing; and identifying life changes and the new normalcy that is to be achieved. For many children, remembering a time when life was "normal" is not possible. When children with cancer receive psychoeducational support, they grow to become adults who are as emotionally stable as their peers (Gray et al., 1992).

Teaching Strategies

Patient teaching presents an ongoing challenge. Some patients and families are more sophisticated and knowledgeable about their health care and treatment choices and desire to understand and want to be involved in their treatment decisions. What a patient with cancer knows about his or her disease can affect the individual's treatment choices and how he or she copes with the illness. Patient information improves treatment compliance and satisfaction with care, lowers anxiety, and improves coping mechanisms (Jones, Nyhof-Young, Friedman, & Catton, 2001). A variety of creative teaching methods are available to CTNs to facilitate patient learning. These include verbal and written information, audiovisual media, and computer-assisted learning. Patients and caregivers want information that is easy for the layperson to understand. They want information that is accurate and individualized to the patient's case. Additionally, patients' needs include information about the

treatment process, side effects, and how the treatment will affect their daily lives (Skalla, Bakitas, Furstenberg, Ahles, & Henderson, 2004). Hietanen, Aro, Holli, and Absetz (2000) conducted a study investigating the communicative needs of patients being asked to participate in a clinical trial and concluded that

- A combination of oral and written information is most effective for patients' decision making on entering a trial.
- Patients have difficulty with the concept of randomization and are unaware that the treatment they will be receiving is one of two alternatives thought to be the best available for them.
- Patients with less education and who are older need more time when making a decision about entering a clinical trial.

Other research has shown that patients want more information earlier in the treatment process (Treacy & Mayer, 2000). Each teaching strategy has advantages and disadvantages. Table 29-2 illustrates the approaches of each.

Verbal Instruction and Written Materials

Verbal instruction is the most common method used in patient education. In discussing clinical trials, the CTN should discuss treatment standards, reasons for the trial, the uncertainty of the experiment drug, and the risks and benefits of the trial. The CTN also should explain the idea of randomization and other terms such as *double-blind* and *placebo-controlled* (Jenkins, Fallowfield, Solis-Trapala, Langridge, & Farewell, 2005). Although patients with cancer prefer to obtain information through discussion, written materials supplement and reinforce the discussion. Written material includes instruction sheets, brochures, pamphlets, booklets, and books and allows the patient to continue learning. However, the readability of written material often exceeds the capabilities of patients' reading level. Therefore, patients should be assessed for literacy, and the patient materials should be assessed for readability (Chelf et al., 2001). Singh's (2003) analysis of 10 cancer brochures from hospitals, clinics, doctors' offices, and cancer organizations found them to be one to seven grades higher than the recommended levels. This meant they were too difficult for average readers.

Audiovisual Media

Telephone, audiotapes, DVDs, CDs, and videotapes are the more common uses of technology-based patient education. Telephone usage can assist patients with obtaining information and support while allowing the CTN to monitor compliance. Audio taping provider-patient encounters assists patients with the retention of verbal information and increases patient satisfaction. Videotapes facilitate patient learning and often result in increased retention. Patients can view the information at their own pace and can review a video as many times as necessary to enhance learning. Use of telephonic-, audio-, and video-based pa-

Table 29-2. The Strengths and Weaknesses of Different Types of Teaching Tools		
Source	**Positive**	**Negative**
Written material	Accessible, inexpensive, easy to use, can be used at learner's pace	Requires literacy, may not be developed at appropriate literacy level, generic content, need to be age and culturally sensitive, not interactive
Verbal instruction	Interactive, can reinforce written material	Low retention, often given at stressful times, time-consuming, reaches smaller numbers of patients
Video/audiotapes	Able to use in own environment, more useful for lower literacy audiences, available for continued use, easy to use, consistent material, available for larger audiences	Not interactive, requires access to audiovisual equipment, expensive to produce
CD-ROM/computer-assisted instruction	Can be interactive, can learn at own pace, may be tailored to individual learning needs	Requires computer and computer literacy, expensive to develop
Internet-based material	Potentially most current information, interactive, personal, anonymity	Credibility of information, computer access necessary

Note. From "Perspectives on Cancer Patient Education," by J.T. Treacy and D.K. Mayer, 2000, *Seminars in Oncology Nursing, 16,* p. 51. Copyright 2000 by Elsevier. Reprinted with permission.

tient education assists with patient compliance, increases patient knowledge and satisfaction, and decreases patient symptoms (Chelf et al., 2001).

Computer-Assisted Learning

Computer-assisted learning (CAL) uses computers to facilitate learning and consists of shared decision-making programs and interactive, computer-based modules. CAL can be interactive and combines several methods of learning into a single program. These can include video, text, animation, graphics, pictures, graphs, and audio. Programs can be self-paced, offer learning and review, and have information print-outs for the patient. Illiterate patients or those with low-level learning abilities can benefit from the multimedia features of CAL (Jones et al., 2001). CAL helps patients with decision making, increases knowledge, provides support, and assists with quality-of-life improvements and improved patient outcome when interactive modules are used (Chelf et al., 2001). Using interactive, multimedia technology (audio, text, graphics, and video) can engage patients in an active learning process that can be done at their own pace (Skalla et al., 2004).

Patients using Internet-based learning can search databases, "chat" with others, view bulletin boards, and get additional patient information. However, Internet sites should adhere to the Health on the Net Foundation code, which has established ethical guidelines for health-related Web sites (Treacy & Mayer, 2000).

Treatment Education

Treatment education combines cognitive, behavioral, and affective components and is defined as "instruction about cancer treatment and the management of side effects" (Chelf et al., 2001, p. 1142).

Available Resource Materials

Organizations such as the American Cancer Society (ACS), the National Cancer Institute (NCI), and the Oncology Nursing Society (ONS) produce a wide variety of informational materials for people with cancer and their families. ACS produces a Web site, www.cancer.org, to provide information to patients and professionals. The site includes an interactive component to assist patients with researching treatment options, locating treatment centers, and finding clinical trials. Additionally, the component for professionals provides a variety of areas to facilitate professional development. Another resource is NCI, which offers many publications for patients about their disease, treatment options, and participation in clinical trials. Also, the site contains an area where patients can find treatment centers that are conducting clinical trials. The Patient Education area of the ONS Web site (www.ons.org/patientEd) has an interactive patient education tool that assists nurses in developing patient education materials.

Many patient teaching materials can be ordered over the Internet or by calling the organization that developed the materials. They usually are free in small quantities and minimally priced for larger quantities. Pharmaceutical companies and cooperative study groups may develop educational information for a particular disease entity, treatment, or clinical trial. Additional resources specific to clinical trials are available through the following Web sites.

- CancerTrials™: A comprehensive online resource for clinical trial information: www.cancer.gov/clinicaltrials
- National Institutes of Health information on clinical trials: http://clinicaltrials.gov
- National Library of Medicine information on clinical trials: www.nlm.nih.gov/medlineplus/clinicaltrials.html
- NCI: www.cancer.gov

• NCI's Web site for education materials: www.cancer.gov/clinicaltrials/learning

Figure 29-2 lists additional organizations that provide patient education resources.

Summary

Providing education to patients and their families is essential in clinical trial participation. Understanding a patient's motivation for entering a study may help to provide insight into the type of education needs the patient has. CTNs should assess the patient's age, cultural background, preferred method of learning, desire for information, placement on the healthcare continuum, attitudes toward health care, and other special considerations to determine what style of teaching will be the most effective. Adult and pediatric learners have different communication needs. Social, cultural, and religious values influence a patient's knowledge and attitude and must be taken into account when developing educational materials. Some populations require in-depth and individualized assessment. These include some older adults; those who are blind, deaf, or mentally deficient; the illiterate; and those who speak a foreign language.

Learning materials should be phase-specific. Understanding the patient's needs will assist the CTN in providing available internal and external education resources. Patients and families desire to understand their options and want to be involved in their treatment decisions. A variety of creative teaching methods are available to CTNs to facilitate patient learning. These include verbal and written information, audiovisual media, and CAL.

Figure 29-2. Patient Education Resources

AIDS*info*
800-448-0440
301-519-0459 (outside the U.S.)
888-480-3739 (TTY)
www.AIDSinfo.nih.gov

American Brain Tumor Association
800-886-2282 (patient line)
847-827-9910
www.abta.org

American Cancer Society
800-ACS-2345
866-228-4327 (TTY)
www.cancer.org

American Foundation for Urologic Disease, Inc.
866-746-4282
410-689-3700 (outside the U.S.)
www.auafoundation.org

Cancer Information Service
800-422-6237
301-496-8664 (outside the U.S.)
http://cis.nci.nih.gov

Candlelighters™ Childhood Cancer Foundation
800-366-2223
301-962-3520 (outside the U.S.)
www.candlelighters.org

Gynecologic Cancer Foundation
800-444-4441
312-578-1439 (outside the U.S.)
www.thegcf.org

Leukemia & Lymphoma Society of America, Inc.
800-955-4572
www.leukemia-lymphoma.org

Susan G. Komen for the Cure
800-462-9273 (national helpline)
972-855-1600
www.komen.org

Note. For more information, see Oncology Nursing Society, n.d.

References

Blecher, C.S. (Ed.). (2004). *Standards of oncology education: Patient/significant other and public* (3rd ed.). Pittsburgh, PA: Oncology Nursing Society.

Chelf, J.H., Agre, P., Axelrod, A., Cheney, L., Cole, D.D., Conrad, K., et al. (2001). Cancer-related patient education: An overview of the last decade of evaluation and research. *Oncology Nursing Forum, 28,* 1139–1147.

Cox, K., & Avis, M. (1996). Psychosocial aspects of participation in early anticancer drug trials: Report of a pilot study. *Cancer Nursing, 19,* 177–186.

Gray, R.E., Doan, B.D., Sherrmer, P., Fitzgerald, A.V., Berry, M.P., Jenkins, D., et al. (1992). Psychologic adaptation of survivors of childhood cancer. *Cancer, 70,* 2713–2721.

Haase, J.E., & Rostad, M. (1994). Experiences of completing cancer therapy: Children's perspectives. *Oncology Nursing Forum, 21,* 1483–1492.

Hagopian, G.A. (1996). Patient and family education. In R. McCorkle, M. Grant, M. Frank-Stromborg, & S.B. Baird (Eds.), *Cancer nursing: A comprehensive textbook* (2nd ed., pp. 1223–1234). Philadelphia: Saunders.

Hietanen, P., Aro, A.R., Holli, K., & Absetz, P. (2000). Information and communication in the context of a clinical trial. *European Journal of Cancer, 36,* 2096–2104.

Hinds, P.S., Oakes, L., Furman, W., Foppiano, P., Olson, M.S., Quargnenti, A., et al. (1997). Decision making by parents and healthcare professionals when considering continued care for pediatric patients with cancer. *Oncology Nursing Forum, 24,* 1523–1528.

Hutchison, C., & Campbell, S. (2002). Evaluation of an information booklet for patients considering participation in phase I clinical trials in cancer. *European Journal of Cancer Care, 11,* 131–138.

Jenkins, V., Fallowfield, L., Solis-Trapala, I., Langridge, C., & Farewell, V. (2005). Discussing randomised clinical trials of cancer therapy: Evaluation of a Cancer Research UK training programme. *BMJ, 330,* 400–403.

Jones, J.M., Nyhof-Young, J., Friedman, A., & Catton, P. (2001). More than just a pamphlet: Development of an innovative computer-based education program for cancer patients. *Patient Education and Counseling, 44,* 271–281.

Kupst, M., Patenaude, A.F., Walco, G.A., & Sterling, C. (2003). Clinical trials in pediatric cancer: Parental perspectives on informed consent. *Journal of Pediatric Hematology/Oncology, 25,* 787–790.

Lake, R., & Jenkins, J. (1993). Cancer chemotherapy: Clinical trials. *Cancer Nursing, 16,* 486–497.

Leventhal, B.G. (1988). An overview of clinical trials in oncology. *Seminars in Oncology, 15,* 414–422.

Meyer, R.M. (2000). Using adult learning concepts to assist patients in completing advanced directives. *Journal of Continuing Education in Nursing, 31,* 174–178.

Oncology Nursing Society. (n.d.). *General patient resource area.* Retrieved October 15, 2007, from http://www.ons.org/patientEd/additional/general.shtml

Ratain, M., Mick, R., Schilsky, R., & Siegler, M. (1993). Statistical and ethical issues in the design and conduct of phase I and II clinical trials of new anticancer agents. *Journal of the National Cancer Institute, 85,* 1637–1643.

Singh, J. (2003). Reading grade level and readability of printed cancer education materials. *Oncology Nursing Forum, 30,* 867–870.

Skalla, K.A., Bakitas, M., Furstenberg, C.T., Ahles, T., & Henderson, J.V. (2004). Patients' need for information about cancer therapy. *Oncology Nursing Forum, 31,* 313–319.

Skrutkowska, M., & Weijer, C. (1997). Do patients with breast cancer participating in clinical trials receive better nursing care? *Oncology Nursing Forum, 24,* 1411–1416.

Simon, M.S., Du, W., Flaherty, L., Philip, P.A., Lorusso, P., Miree, C., et al. (2004). Factors associated with breast cancer clinical trials participation and enrollment at a large academic medical center. *Journal of Clinical Oncology, 22,* 2046–2052.

Thomas, V.N., Saleem, T., & Abraham, R. (2005). Barriers to effective uptake of cancer screening among black and minority ethnic groups. *International Journal of Palliative Nursing, 11,* 562, 564–571.

Treacy, J.T., & Mayer, D.K. (2000). Perspectives on cancer patient education. *Seminars in Oncology Nursing, 16,* 47–56.

Trubowitz, J. (1998). Mental health: Theories and therapies. In E.M. Varcarolis (Ed.), *Foundations of psychiatric mental health nursing* (3rd ed., pp. 29–64). Philadelphia: Saunders.

Yoder, L.H., O'Rourke, T.J., Etnyre, A., Spears, D.T., & Brown, T.D. (1997). Expectation and experiences of patients with cancer participating in phase I clinical trials. *Oncology Nursing Forum, 24,* 891–896.

CHAPTER 30
Adherence in Clinical Trials

Bertie A. Ford, RN, MS, AOCN®

Introduction

The development of exciting new agents for the treatment of cancer has been continuing at a phenomenal rate thanks to clinical trials. The development of vaccines, monoclonal antibodies, and small molecules offers new hope for many patients with cancers for which the standard of therapy has significantly changed in the past couple of years. Oral agents such as capecitabine, erlotinib, imatinib mesylate, cyclophosphamide, prednisone, tamoxifen, exemestane, fulvestrant, and letrozole have provided improvements in survival. However, as these are oral agents, they offer additional challenges for oncologists and nurses to ensure that patients adhere to the treatment regimen. Nonadherence also can occur with IV agents but is much easier to detect.

After a patient has been screened, has been determined to be eligible, has signed the informed consent, has been registered on the protocol, and has started treatment, everything may *seem* easier from this point forward, but that is not the case. In many ways, the difficult part of the process is over, until adherence to the protocol is considered. Adherence with medical treatment is an ongoing issue in managing patients both on and off clinical trials. According to Haynes, Taylor, and Sackett (1979), lack of adherence dates back to Adam and Eve when Eve ate the forbidden fruit. Before discussing nonadherence, however, the definitions of adherence will be addressed.

Definitions

Adherence means to give support, maintain loyalty, be consistent to, or stick to (Gritz, DiMatteo, & Hays, 1989). Adherence assumes a collaboration between the patient and provider toward a mutually agreed-upon end (Bauman, 2000).

Compliance is the extent to which a person's behavior coincides with medical health advice, and *noncompliance* is failure to behave according to medical health advice (Karvonen, Haugew, Levin, & Rubins, 1996).

Some prefer to use *adherence* because they believe *compliance* has a dictatorial tone on the part of the healthcare provider (Gritz et al., 1989) Some have proposed a continuum for describing adherence from fully adherent to partial, overuser, erratic user, partial dropout, and dropout (Partridge, Avorn, Wang, & Winer, 2002). This author prefers to use the term *adherence.*

Nonadherence

Subtypes of nonadherence have been described in the literature (see Figure 30-1). Volitional nonadherence occurs when patients hear and understand the instructions but choose not to comply. Patients are aware that they are not following advice. Patients may or may not acknowledge their nonadherence. Volitional nonadherence occurs when health beliefs and lifestyle interfere with adherence (Bauman, 2000).

Inadvertent, or nonvolitional nonadherence, may be more common. In this situation, patients accept treatment advice and believe that they are adhering well enough to the regimen (Bauman, 2000).

Nonadherence Risk Factors

Is there a way to identify who may be at risk for being nonadherent? The following discussion presents risk

---

Figure 30-1. Types of Nonadherence

Volitional
- Patients are aware they are noncompliant and choose to remain so

Inadvertent or nonvolitional
- Satisfiers who acknowledge missing doses on occasion
- Patients who want to be compliant but face obstacles for adequate adherence, such as illness in the family, loss of job, or any multitude of issues that require them to focus their attention on other issues besides the treatment regimen
- Patients who misunderstood the expectations and follow advice they think they heard or remembered, when it is not what the provider intended

Note. Based on information from Bauman, 2000.

---

factors for volitional nonadherence and nonvolitional nonadherence.

Medical regimen: If the medical regimen is difficult or highly disruptive to a patient's life, a greater risk exists for volitional nonadherence. An example is a medical plan that requires changes in one's lifestyle, such as smoking cessation, diet changes for weight loss, diabetes, or hypertension.

Skepticism about efficacy: A patient may not believe the regimen will be helpful. This type of nonadherence is less likely when therapeutic benefit is experienced soon after initiation of the therapy. If a patient takes pain medication and the pain is diminished, he or she is likely to be adherent. If a physical therapy regimen is implemented in lieu of a more invasive procedure, the patient may not think this treatment regimen is aggressive enough and may not be compliant with an at-home regimen or may miss appointments. Another example is adjuvant therapy given to prevent recurrent disease. If the regimen has side effects and the benefits are not immediately noted, it can be difficult for patients to be compliant (Bauman, 2000).

Cost of treatment: This may or may not be an issue with a clinical trial, as the drugs may or may not be provided free of charge, depending on the phase of the study. If patients go to a center for a trial that is not in their home state, they will bear the costs of travel and housing, and these may be contributors to nonadherence.

Denial of diagnosis: Patients may be in such denial that they have a psychological condition, which drives them to be nonadherent with the regimen. A patient diagnosed with diabetes may not do the blood glucose checks or follow the prescribed diet because he or she is in denial of the diagnosis.

General risk factors for inadvertent nonadherence: A few risk factors exist that, when present, increase the patient's chances of being nonadherent. Patient characteristics such as forgetfulness, poor hearing, poor eyesight, poor mental function, poor quality of life, stress, lack of resources, presence of multiple caregivers, apathy about health, pessimism, poor understanding of provider instructions, low literacy, and language barriers can lead to nonadherence (Bauman, 2002).

Developmental characteristics: If the patient is a child, he or she may refuse to take medications, or an adolescent may be noncompliant to strive for independence and autonomy (Bauman, 2002). Adolescents are the most noncompliant age group (Partridge, 2000).

Provider/system characteristics: This includes poor patient-physician communication, failure of the provider to educate the patient, poor instructions by physicians, long wait time for lab values or treatment, uncomfortable waiting rooms, and an unfriendly staff (Bauman, 2000).

Regimen characteristics: The treatment may have a bad taste or may consist of multiple medications, multiple dosing intervals, or demanding treatment regimens (Bauman, 2000). A good example of this is Desferal® (Novartis Pharmaceuticals Corp.) for the treatment of iron overload in patients who receive transfusions. These patients need to receive a subcutaneous infusion over six to eight hours for five to seven days per week. Nonadherence is common as a result of the complexity of the regimen, the impact on quality of life, and the inability to see the immediate benefits, because iron overload affects the organs negatively over time.

Incidence of Nonadherence

How problematic is nonadherence? An estimated 20%–80% of patients are nonadherent with their treatment regimen (Engstrom, 1991). But, in the clinical trial setting, adherence is *greater than 90%* (Li et al., 2000). Patients who are enrolled in a clinical trial are monitored closely by their clinical trial nurse (CTN). They have frequent visits and communication specifically about trial requirements. U.S. Food and Drug Administration (FDA)-approved therapies for patients are evidence-based, and unless clinical trial patients are compliant with agents/regimens, the patients who use the therapy after FDA approval is granted may not receive the same benefit. Nonadherence can lead to invalid results, inconsistent response rates, and incorrect dosing recommendations (Partridge et al., 2002). In a breast conservation study done by Li et al., 64% of the patients failed to comply with the full course of treatment. Some did not complete the radiation therapy, some were not compliant with the Nolvadex® (AstraZeneca), and some were noncompliant with the follow-up. The noncompliant patients had a higher local failure rate than was seen in the National Surgical Adjuvant Breast and Bowel Project B-06 trial (Li et al.). This could cause an increase in medical costs and an increased need for additional care because of complications, exacerbation, and prolongation of illness and preventable disease. For every noncompliant patient in a trial, another patient needs to be added to the study or the data are inaccurate, at best (Macharia, Leon, Rowe, & Stephenson, 1992).

Assessment

CTNs try to assess how adherent a patient is likely to be during a particular clinical trial before entering the patient into the trial. For example, many chemoprevention trials use a *run-in period*, during which all of the patients initially receive a placebo. This gives the CTN time to perform an as-

---

Figure 30-2. Model of Patient Adherence to Treatment

1. Effective communication of information by the healthcare team
2. A good rapport with the healthcare team
3. Personal beliefs and attitudes
4. Social climate and norms
5. Behavioral intentions
6. Active support system

Note. Based on information from Gritz et al., 1989.

sessment of adherence prior to registration. The nurse needs to assess the patient's ability to come to the clinic and meet the requirements of the study, such as daily treatment or twice-a-day treatment with therapies such as hyperfractionated radiation therapy. If this is not possible, the patient should not be registered for the clinical trial.

Why Are Patients Nonadherent?

Rosenstock (1988) created the Health Belief Model. This model may be applied to problems of explaining, predicting, and influencing behaviors related to health practices. The Health Belief Model, which measures an individual's perception of his or her susceptibility to a disease, describes behaviors related to perceptions (Rosenstock). Gritz et al. (1989) described a six-factor model of adherence (see Figure 30-2). First, an effective communication of information must exist to ensure that the patient understands what is expected of him or her and what the patient can expect from the treatment. Second is the rapport that a patient has with the healthcare team; the quality of the relationship is a primary component of change. The patient must feel that the healthcare provider exhibits behaviors such as trust, warmth, and genuine caring. Third, with the patient's beliefs and attitudes, which are based on the Health Belief Model, the patient must feel that negative health consequences would occur if he or she was noncompliant with a prescribed regimen. Fourth, the patient's social climate and norms affect adherence. The sources of these beliefs and norms are family, friends, social class, and ethnicity. The fifth factor is behavioral intentions. This behavior is strengthened by a written contract (e.g., to lose weight, to perform breast self-exams monthly). Finally, the patient must have active support to decrease any barriers. For example, if the patient cannot afford medications, he or she needs financial assistance; if the patient works during the day, the clinic needs to be open later in the evening; if he or she does not have a vehicle, he or she needs a bus line or other transportation support.

Determining Patient Adherence

What characteristics predict a patient's adherence or nonadherence? Demographic factors such as race, education level, and socioeconomic status do not have a consistent effect on adherence to therapy. How can patient adherence be determined? Self-reporting usually is not reliable because patients may omit information purposefully, or they may forget information and instructions (Gritz et al., 1989). Patients may be compliant only because they know they are being monitored; this is termed the "Hawthorne effect" (Partridge et al., 2002). Many CTNs had a concentrated exposure to reporting of adherence while working with the prevention trials, asking patients if they had missed taking any medications. Some patients denied missing medications, yet based on the actual pill count, they had missed a few days. These can be honest mistakes.

Another way to measure adherence is called the *collateral method*. This method involves documentation of adherence by observations that can be verified by a health professional, family, friends, or others (Gritz et al., 1989). This can be accomplished with pill counts from medications returned after completion of a cycle. Of course, if a patient really wanted to hide his or her nonadherence, he or she could do so by removing the correct number of pills and discarding them.

The best way to measure adherence objectively is by using *pharmacologic markers*, such as serum drug levels or levels of another body element (Gritz et al., 1989). Using multiple measures at different points in time is the most effective method.

Interventions to Promote Adherence

CTNs can employ various interventions to promote adherence. The process model of compliance (adherence) intervention is based on identifying a health problem and prescribing behaviors that are supported organizationally, behaviorally, and educationally (Dunbar, Marshall, & Hovell, 1979). Organizational interventions are described as environmental or system issues. A basic tool that can help patients to be compliant with appointments is a personalized calendar that tells them when their appointments are, when laboratory work is to be performed, or when they need to take special medications, such as steroids or antibiotics. Patients should be provided with reminders about appointments and tests by telephone, postcards, or letters. Giving patients diaries in which they can document taking their medication or any side effects would be ideal. Pillboxes labeled with hours or days of the week are an excellent tool to help patients to maintain compliance (Spilker, 1991).

Patients should have a *supportive environment* within the healthcare system. They should have minimal waiting, adequate parking, and organized and consistent care. They should have health support from a variety of healthcare personnel and continued follow-up.

Many patients on prevention trials like to hear *updates about the trial* to maintain their interest and subsequent compliance. Updates can be provided through newsletters, letters to each patient, or quarterly updates at meetings. Patients who are on a clinical trial should feel that they are special and should receive "perks," such as free parking, lunch vouchers, or other tokens that are given in support and appreciation.

Educational interventions, described as the transferring of information (Dunbar et al., 1979), should be conducted early and on a continuous basis. The *informed consent form* is the initial educational intervention. (See Chapter 14 for more information on the informed consent process.) The informed consent process has undergone changes in the past few years and still is evolving to make the forms easier for patients to understand. Patients should be given a detailed explanation of the trial requirements, treatment, and potential side effects. This can be accomplished through a combination of verbal, written, and video presentations. The most important information should be described first, because people remember what comes first in an explanation. Written information should replicate the oral, and vice versa. The information should be repeated a minimum of three times and should be as specific as possible (McKenney, 1979). The second strategy is organization that focuses on regimen, environmental issues such as wait time and follow-up care, and consistent personnel. According to Dunbar et al., the third intervention focuses on *behavioral aspects*. Several steps can be taken to promote adherence. If the assumption is that the patient simply forgets to take medications or come to appointments, then reminders will be beneficial. If he or she does not want to come in the first place, or appointments are low on his or her priority list, reminders may not be helpful (Spilker, 1991). Other strategies include tailoring the study if allowed, contracts, graduated regimen implementation, self-monitoring, and reinforcement (Dunbar et al.).

Patients should have consistent staff and professionals working with them. This lends *credibility* to what they are accomplishing and to the study. If frequent staffing changes occur, patients may not feel that the study is important (Dunbar et al., 1979).

Developing a *contract* to assist patients in being compliant is helpful. The contract needs to be fair, specific, positive, and consistent. This way, patients are making a commitment to participate in a certain behavior. The *graduated regimen* approach is useful in building up to a certain behavior. If a patient's goal is to be on a 1,000-calorie-per-day diet, begin with a 250-calorie breakfast, and allow the patient to eat the way he or she normally would for the rest of the day. When that is mastered, decrease lunch to 250 calories per day, with normal eating for dinner. When that is mastered, decrease dinner to 500 calories per day. The patient now is consuming the desired amount of calories. This approach is useful for smoking cessation and exercise as well (Dunbar et al., 1979).

CTNs may elect to provide patients with positive reinforcement and consequences that increase the probability of a behavior, such as praise or other perks. For example, if a patient is to decrease the amount of fat in the diet, the CTN may tell the patient that if he or she uses fat-free dressing for dinner, then he or she can have wine that night.

The support of family and friends is essential (Hogue, 1979), whether someone is traveling to radiation appointments or providing child care while the patient is at an appointment. If a patient is on a special diet, the family needs to be especially supportive. A patient can be more compliant if the regimen is tailored to him or her (McKenney, 1979). If the patient has to take medication twice a day, tell the patient to take it after brushing his or her teeth or, if regimens and food do not interfere, with meals. If the patient feels isolated in a weight-loss program, refer him or her to Weight Watchers® or Overeaters Anonymous for group meetings.

When a patient is on a clinical trial, treatment symptoms frequently can lead to noncompliance. If a patient is not taking the required oral medications because of nausea and vomiting, the antiemetic regimen needs to be altered, the dose modified, timing modified, and so on.

All of these strategies should be used as often as appropriate. A multidisciplinary approach is needed among basic scientists, clinicians, behavioral scientists, health educators, and even epidemiologists to maximize patient compliance (Cramer, 1991; Gritz et al., 1989).

Staff Adherence Issues

Armed with all of the knowledge and interventions, a patient's chances of being noncompliant are diminished. Occasionally, a patient will be noncompliant because of a physician error. If the patient calls a physician and is given permission to change his or her next appointment or to take less than the number of pills required to maintain adherence, then the issue is physician education. Educating the physician regarding the protocol and protocol requirements is vital to the successful completion of a study. But, with all of the patients and multiple protocols, mistakes still may occur. To prevent accidental physician nonadherence, patients should be taught to call the CTN if they have problems with making appointments, taking the prescribed treatment, or any other aspect of the clinical trial. Physician nonadherence also may occur as a result of lack of support for the protocol.

The CTN should make physicians aware of required laboratory tests and scans and make sure they are ordered. Chemotherapy orders are written by the CTN at some institutions and reviewed and cosigned by the physician. This provides a "double-check" mechanism to ensure that the treatment dosages and modifications, if required, are correct. The CTN should see each on-treatment patient to ensure that medications, performance status, and side effects are documented and that patients are monitored closely following institutional guidelines.

Research staff members may be noncompliant if the protocol is extremely complicated or if they do not feel that an aspect of the protocol is as important as the primary goal, such as completing a quality-of-life questionnaire. Sadura et al. (1992) described methods to increase compliance with questionnaires, because many clinical trials have quality-of-life components. The quality-of-life assessment should be part of the study. (See Chapter 35 for more information on companion studies.) Clear instructions on how and how often to administer the questionnaire must be documented in the protocol. Some clinical trials offer additional monies to the institution for completing the questionnaire. Principal investigator nonadherence is evidenced by failure to get institutional review board approval, failure to complete end-of-trial reports, failure to report adverse events, or failure to ensure that data are collected promptly (Spilker, 1991).

Sponsors are nonadherent if they do not submit a protocol to the appropriate agencies, such as the FDA or NCI. They may fail to adhere to good manufacturing practices, good laboratory practices, and good clinical practices (Spilker, 1991). Sponsors, most importantly, must report adverse events or major consequences that can occur.

Summary

Maintaining patient adherence with a protocol can be a full-time job in itself. Open communication, understanding, and support from the research team and the institution can assist in achieving patient and physician adherence. The CTN may enhance adherence with early assessment for adherence-related behaviors, assisting patients to overcome obstacles, and educating and working with physicians and multidisciplinary team members. Working together to address adherence will provide timely and accurate completion of a clinical trial. The literature has not changed much with descriptions of adherence. A wealth of literature exists related to diabetes and adherence. However, additional research is needed to evaluate adherence specifically in oncology clinical trials, so that interventions to improve adherence can be evidence-based.

References

Bauman, L.J. (2000). A patient-centered approach to adherence: Risks for nonadherence. In D. Drotar (Ed.), *Promoting adherence to medical treatment in chronic childhood illness: Concepts, methods, and interventions* (pp. 71–93). Mahwah, NJ: Lawrence Erlbaum Associates.

Cramer, J.A. (1991). Identifying and improving compliance patterns: A composite plan for health care providers. In J.A. Cramer & B. Spilker (Eds.), *Patient compliance in medical practice and clinical trials* (pp. 387–392). New York: Raven Press.

Dunbar, J., Marshall, G.D., & Hovell, M.F. (1979). Behavioral strategies for improving compliance. In R.B. Haynes, D.W. Taylor, & D.L. Sackett (Eds.), *Compliance in health care* (pp. 174–191). Baltimore: Johns Hopkins University Press.

Engstrom, P.F. (1991). Specific compliance issues in an antiestrogen trial of women at risk for breast cancer. *Preventive Medicine, 20,* 125–131.

Gritz, E.R., DiMatteo, M.R., & Hays, R.D. (1989). Methodological issues in adherence to cancer control regimens. *Preventive Medicine, 18,* 711–720.

Haynes, R.B., Taylor, D.W., & Sackett, D.L. (Eds.). (1979). *Compliance in health care.* Baltimore: Johns Hopkins University Press.

Hogue, C.C. (1979). Nursing and compliance. In R.B. Haynes, D.W. Taylor, & D.L. Sackett (Eds.), *Compliance in health care* (pp. 247–259). Baltimore: Johns Hopkins University Press.

Karvonen, M.A., Haugew, M., Levin, J.L., & Rubins, H.G. (1996). Issues in clinical trials management: Improving patient compliance in clinical trials. A practical approach. *Research Nurse, 2,* 9–12.

Li, B.D., Brown, W.A., Ampil, F.L., Burton, G.V., Yu, H., & McDonald, J.C. (2000). Patient compliance is critical for equivalent clinical outcomes for breast cancer treated by breast-conservation therapy. *Annals of Surgery, 231,* 883–889.

Macharia, W.M., Leon, G., Rowe, B.H., & Stephenson, B.J. (1992). An overview of interventions to improve compliance with appointment keeping for medical services. *JAMA, 267,* 1813–1817.

McKenney, J.M. (1979). The clinical pharmacy and compliance. In R.B. Haynes, D.W. Taylor, & D.L. Sackett (Eds.), *Compliance in health care* (pp. 260–277). Baltimore: Johns Hopkins University Press.

Partridge, A.H., Avorn, J., Wang, P.S., & Winer, E.P. (2002). Adherence to therapy with oral antineoplastic agents. *Journal of the National Cancer Institute, 94,* 652–661.

Rosenstock, I.M. (1998). Adoption and maintenance of lifestyle modifications. *American Journal of Preventive Medicine, 15,* 349–352.

Sadura, A., Pater, J., Osoba, D., Levine, M., Palmer, M., & Bennett, K. (1992). Quality of life assessment: Patient compliance with questionnaire completion. *Journal of the National Cancer Institute, 84,* 1023–1026.

Spilker, B. (1991). Methods of assessing and improving patient compliance in clinical trials. In J.A. Cramer & B. Spilker (Eds.), *Patient compliance in medical practice and clinical trials* (pp. 37–56). New York: Raven Press.

SECTION VII.

Ancillary Studies

CHAPTER 31
Quality-of-Life Studies

CHAPTER 32
Pharmacokinetics, Pharmacodynamics, and Pharmacogenomics

CHAPTER 33
Genetic Testing and Storage of Genetic Material

CHAPTER 34
Pharmacoeconomic Studies

CHAPTER 35
Nursing Companion Studies

CHAPTER 31
Quality-of-Life Studies

Carol S. Hill, BSN, RN, OCN®

Introduction

Traditionally, end points for randomized clinical trials have focused on toxicity, tumor response, progression-free survival, disease-free survival, or prevention of a disease or toxicity (Roila & Cortesi, 2001). Although data from these trials yield valuable information as to which treatment or prevention strategy is most effective, other factors, such as drug toxicity and the subjective treatment experience of clinical trial participants, may not be considered in such analyses. However, patients and healthcare providers consider all of these factors when choosing therapies; treatment benefits are weighed against side effects, toxicities, duration of treatment, and impact on the patient's lifestyle and activities of daily living. Cella and Tulsky (1990) pointed out the difference between *quantity* of life and *quality* of life (QOL). Traditional end points for clinical trials focus on length of survival (quantity of life), examining the impact that the study treatments have on the patient's well-being (QOL). QOL should be the second most important outcome, with survival being the primary outcome (Frost & Sloan, 2002). Assessment of changes in QOL considers the treatment experience from the perspective of the patient and the patient's willingness to continue treatment. This assessment can help to define the response of treatment in the absence of a quantifiable end point such as tumor progression (Cella, Chang, Lai, & Webster, 2002).

Definition

Researchers have proposed many definitions to describe QOL. Although QOL researchers hail from a variety of disciplines, most of their definitions have two concepts in common: QOL is inherently *subjective* and *multidimensional* (Cella, 1994). According to Cella, "Subjectivity refers to the fact that QOL can only be understood from the patient's perspective" (p. 187). Only the patient can describe and understand the impact that a cancer therapy has upon his or her well-being. Any assessment of QOL requires that the patient be questioned regarding his or her QOL prior to the start of treatment because this could be used as a prognostic factor along with the patient's performance status (Roila & Cortesi, 2001). The second concept, multidimensionality, refers to the various human dimensions that may be affected by the cancer treatment. Ferrans (1990) stated that the multidimensional nature of QOL "covers all areas of life" (p. 252). QOL domains include the physical (ability to conduct activities of daily living), psychological, and social well-being of patients (Varricchio, 1990). Other facets of QOL mentioned in the literature include spiritual, ability to carry out desired activities, economic/financial, sexuality/body image, satisfaction with medical treatment, and family concerns (Cella & Tulsky, 1993; Ferrans; Padilla, Grant, & Ferrell, 1992). Padilla et al. provided a detailed description of four QOL domains: psychological well-being, physical well-being, social and interpersonal well-being, and financial or material well-being. These are outlined in Table 31-1.

Based upon the concepts of subjectivity and multidimensionality, this chapter will adopt the following definition of QOL proposed by Cella and Cherin (1988): "Quality of life refers to patients' appraisal of and satisfaction with their current level of functioning compared to what they perceive to be possible or ideal" (p. 70).

Quality-of-Life Measures

Many efforts have been made in the past few years in oncology to develop a way to assess QOL within clinical trials (Flechtner, 2001). Some researchers have developed single measures (one tool or instrument) (Grant, Padilla,

The author would like to acknowledge Jennifer L. Aikin, RN, MSN, AOCN®, for her contribution that remains unchanged from the first edition.

Table 31-1. Quality-of-Life Attributes

Domain	Examples
Psychological well-being	Satisfaction with life Usefulness Body image Adjustment Emotions (e.g., anxiety) Personal control Recreational/vocational concerns Developing/learning concerns Goal achievement concerns Fulfillment Meaning of life Normality of life Happiness
Physical well-being	Functional ability Activities of daily living Eating/appetite Sex Sleep Strength Fatigue Perceived health/illness Sequelae of diagnosis and treatment
Social and interpersonal well-being	Interpersonal function Social activities Support from significant others Privacy Rejection Role function
Financial/material well-being	Sense of present/future security Housing/shelter concerns Health insurance Job security Mobility/transportation ability

Note. Based on information from Padilla et al., 1992.

of the investigator. Researchers may select established QOL instruments that show reliability, validity, and sensitivity, or they may choose to design their own measures, relying on their clinical knowledge of the problem.

Table 31-2 lists some of the QOL measures commonly used in cancer clinical trials. Use of copyrighted QOL surveys requires permission and may require payment to the initial author of the survey. This will be determined when contacting the author for permission to use the survey. See Cella and Tulsky (1990) for a more comprehensive list of QOL measures.

Quality-of-Life Assessment in Cancer Clinical Trials

In cancer clinical trials, QOL studies may be incorporated into the protocol document or be ancillary studies to larger trials. Although QOL assessments may be conducted by telephone interview from a central office (Kornblith & Holland, 1996), they more commonly are administered via written questionnaires. When the QOL study is incorporated into the protocol itself, baseline questionnaires are required prior to patient registration and at other times as outlined in the protocol. QOL forms are considered required study forms. Aaronson (1992) noted that the most successful QOL studies are those that use short, simple measures, have nondemanding data-collection schedules, and have designated personnel to coordinate the QOL component.

Nursing Roles in Quality-of-Life Studies

Nurses have a key role in QOL research (Hayden et al., 1993), including, for example, serving on committees for cooperative groups or participating in the design of studies. Generally, the research nurse is responsible for ensuring that patients receive QOL questionnaires at the prescribed intervals and that the questionnaires are complete before

Ferrell, & Rhiner, 1990). The single measure may be composed of a single item focusing on one QOL attribute, or it may be a more comprehensive tool addressing factors from general health status to more focused symptom measures (Soni & Cella, 2002). Other researchers advocate using multiple measures (i.e., a number of different tools) to assess QOL from a multitude of perspectives (Jalowiec, 1990). Some measures are specific for patients with cancer. These measures are starting to show an impact in managed care because this information can provide patient satisfaction information regarding the quality of care patients receive (Soni & Cella).

As QOL becomes increasingly important in understanding the overall management of patients with cancer, a number of factors must be considered when selecting QOL measures (Cella et al., 2002). According to Cella and Tulsky (1990), measures should be chosen that will make a clear and important contribution to patient care, will not cause excessive burden to patients or staff, are not perceived as intrusive, and are sufficiently sensitive to address the concerns

Table 31-2. Selective Quality-of-Life Measures Used in Cancer Clinical Trials

Measure	Author
EORTC Quality of Life Questionnaire	Aaronson et al., 1996
Functional Assessment of Cancer Therapy (FACT) questionnaire (includes specific versions for lung, breast, and colon cancers)	Cella et al., 1993
Functional Living Index—Cancer (FLIC)	Schipper et al., 1984
Medical Outcome Study (MOS) short-form General Health Survey	Stewart et al., 1988
Rotterdam Symptom Checklist (RSCL) with added questions	de Haes et al., 1987

Note. Based on information from Cella & Tulsky, 1990.

forwarding them to the study sponsor. Following are some important tips for nurses administering QOL questionnaires.

- When possible, administer the questionnaire in a quiet place and allow sufficient time so that the patient does not feel rushed.
- When giving the QOL questionnaire to the patient, explain that the purpose of QOL research is to learn more about how cancer therapies affect patients. The study is seeking information on how they feel, not how others might think they feel. The patient needs to answer honestly without being influenced by family members or healthcare providers.
- Be available to clarify questions that are confusing to the patient. Do not attempt to interpret the question or influence the patient's response.
- When the patient has finished, check the questionnaire for unanswered questions. If some items are not answered, determine whether the patient intentionally decided not to answer the question (which is his or her prerogative) or if this was an oversight.
- Explain to the patient that his or her decisions about continuing care are not dependent on giving the "right" answers to QOL questions.
- Create tickler files or calendars to serve as reminders for when QOL assessments are due.
- If others are responsible for administering QOL questionnaires (in a physician's office or outpatient setting), offer support by providing them with reminders and a supply of forms.
- In some studies, QOL questionnaires will need to be mailed to study patients at certain intervals. In such cases, send self-addressed, stamped envelopes to the patient so that it is easy for the patient to return the questionnaire. A follow-up telephone call may be necessary to remind the patient and enhance compliance.

Nurse researchers and advanced practice nurses may be involved in the design of QOL studies. Nurse-initiated QOL studies may be conducted at a single institution, or a nurse may participate on a team that develops a QOL study as part of a National Cancer Institute–sponsored clinical trial. Noting that other disciplines are interested in QOL research is important. QOL studies are now being looked at to help to measure general health and the economic evaluation of treatment outcome by managed care (Flechtner, 2001). Nurses may collaborate with psychologists, social scientists, physicians, and statisticians to design large, multi-institutional QOL studies.

Regardless of the scope of the QOL study (single- versus multi-institutional), nurses have a unique perspective when designing such studies. According to Padilla et al. (1992), the purposes of nursing QOL research efforts are to describe patient psychosocial and physical responses to specific diseases, to examine symptom management responses to disease and treatment, to compare patient and/or family responses to treatment, to demonstrate the effect of specific rehabilitative approaches, and to identify vulnerable periods in the health-illness continuum.

When designing a QOL study, nurse researchers should identify the study questions and the target population. Measures that have demonstrated validity and reliability then must be selected. Choosing measures that can be completed in a relatively short period of time (10–15 minutes) is important to avoid putting an unnecessary burden on study participants. Likewise, the schedule for administering the questionnaire should be consistent with already scheduled outpatient visits for patient convenience (Molin & Arrigo, 1995).

Potential Barriers to Quality-of-Life Assessment

A number of barriers may negatively influence the results of QOL research. The first major barrier to QOL research is that of missing data. When a patient fails to complete a QOL questionnaire, data are lost that can never be retrieved (Hayden et al., 1993). If a questionnaire is filled out incompletely, data may be missing for a number of items. To prevent missing data, researchers must design measures that are not burdensome in terms of length or frequency of administration. This increases the likelihood that the patient will answer every item. To comply with the schedule for administering QOL questionnaires, the clinical trial nurse (CTN) must create a reminder system that notifies research staff when assessments are due. After the patient has completed the questionnaire, the questionnaire must be reviewed for completeness while the patient is still in the clinic or physician's office (Molin & Arrigo, 1995). Reminders from the study sponsor may enhance compliance with the completion of questionnaires (Hayden et al.). When conducting cooperative group QOL studies, institutions that fail to submit QOL data should be identified, and failure to correct the problem may affect the institution's standing in the cooperative group. Conversely, institutions that provide timely and complete QOL data should be rewarded.

Other barriers include bias (when patient responses are influenced by family members or healthcare providers), the amount of time required by patients and staff to participate in QOL research, and resistance on the part of some researchers who may not see QOL assessment as a valuable priority. Investigators may minimize bias by training research personnel on how to administer questionnaires without influencing a patient's response. The Eastern Cooperative Oncology Group developed a video to familiarize research staff with QOL research. This video contains role play that demonstrates both inappropriate and appropriate interactions with patients. As previously mentioned, when measures are chosen carefully and questionnaires are brief, the amount of time needed to administer them will not be prohibitive. Financial compensation or "credits" to institutions that participate in QOL research may facilitate research efforts.

CTNs can develop collegial relationships with other QOL researchers that might stand in solidarity when faced with resistance regarding the validity of including QOL end points in a clinical trial. Furthermore, the value of QOL research will be demonstrated when QOL studies yield results that influence clinical decision making.

Summary

Hayden et al. (1993) stated that "involving oncology nurses actively in the research process is critical to the success of QOL research" (p. 1418). QOL end points contribute significantly to an understanding of the treatment experience for patients participating in clinical trials and may provide valuable information when selecting treatment alternatives when other end points are comparable. Thus, CTNs and oncology nurses have the opportunity to have an impact on the future of cancer care by educating patients, nurses, and physicians and by participating in research that involves QOL issues (King & Hinds, 2003).

References

Aaronson, N.K. (1992). Assessing quality of life of patients in cancer clinical trials: Common problems and common sense solutions. *European Journal of Cancer, 28A*, 1304–1307.

Aaronson, N.K., Cull, A.M., Kaasa, S., & Spranger, M.A. (1996). The European Organization for Research and Treatment of Cancer (EORTC) modular approach to quality of life assessment in oncology: An update. In B. Spilker (Ed.), *Quality of life and pharmacoeconomics in clinical trials* (2nd ed., pp. 179–189). Philadelphia: Lippincott-Raven.

Cella, D.F. (1994). Quality of life: Concepts and definition. *Journal of Pain and Symptom Management, 9*, 186–192.

Cella, D.F., Chang, C.H., Lai, J.S., & Webster, K. (2002). Advances in quality of life measurements in oncology patients. *Seminars in Oncology, 29*(3 Suppl. 8), 60–68.

Cella, D.F., & Cherin, E.A. (1988). Quality of life during and after cancer treatment. *Comprehensive Therapy, 14*(5), 69–75.

Cella, D.F., & Tulsky, D.S. (1990). Measuring quality of life today: Methodological aspects. *Oncology (Williston Park), 4*(5), 29–38.

Cella, D.F., & Tulsky, D.S. (1993). Quality of life in cancer: Definition, purpose, and method of measurement. *Cancer Investigation, 11*, 327–336.

Cella, D.F., Tulsky, D.S., Gray, G., Sarafian, B., Linn, E., Bonomi, A., et al. (1993). The Functional Assessment of Cancer Therapy scale: Development and validation of the general measure. *Journal of Clinical Oncology, 11*, 570–579.

de Haes, J.C., Raatgever, J.W., van der Burg, M.E., Hamersma, E., & Neijt, J.P. (1987). Evaluation of quality of life of patients with advanced ovarian cancer treated with combination chemotherapy. In N.K. Aaronson & J. Beckmann (Eds.), *The quality of life of cancer patients* (pp. 215–226). New York: Raven Press.

Ferrans, C.E. (1990). Quality of life: Conceptual issues. *Seminars in Oncology Nursing, 6*, 248–254.

Flechtner, H. (2001). [Quality of life in oncological studies]. *Onkologie, 24*(Suppl. 5), 22–27 (ISSN: 0378-584X).

Frost, M.H., & Sloan, J.A. (2002). Quality of life measurements: A soft outcome—or is it? *American Journal of Managed Care, 8*(Suppl. 18), S574–S579.

Grant, M., Padilla, G.V., Ferrell, B.R., & Rhiner, M. (1990). Assessment of quality of life with a single instrument. *Seminars in Oncology Nursing, 6*, 260–270.

Hayden, K.A., Moinpour, C.M., Metch, B., Feigl, P., O'Bryan, R.M., Green, S., et al. (1993). Pitfalls in quality-of-life assessment: Lessons from a Southwest Oncology Group breast cancer clinical trial. *Oncology Nursing Forum, 20*, 1416–1419.

Jalowiec, A. (1990). Issues in using multiple measures of quality of life. *Seminars in Oncology Nursing, 6*, 271–277.

King, C.R., & Hinds, P.S. (2003). *Quality of life: From nursing and patient perspectives* (2nd ed.). Sudbury, MA: Jones and Bartlett.

Kornblith, A.B., & Holland, J.C. (1996). Model for quality-of-life research from the Cancer and Leukemia Group B: The telephone interview, conceptual approach to measurement, and theoretical framework. *Journal of the National Cancer Institute Monographs, 20*, 55–62.

Molin, C., & Arrigo, C. (1995). Clinical trials and quality of life assessment: The nurses' viewpoint. *European Journal of Cancer, 31A*(Suppl. 6), S8–S10.

Padilla, G.V., Grant, M.M., & Ferrell, B. (1992). Nursing research into quality of life. *Quality of Life Research, 1*, 341–348.

Roila, F., & Cortesi, E. (2001). Quality of life as a primary end point in oncology. *Annals of Oncology, 12*(Suppl. 3), S3–S6.

Schipper, H., Clinch, J., McMurray, A., & Levitt, M. (1984). Measuring the quality of life of cancer patients: The Functional Living Index-Cancer: Development and validation. *Journal of Clinical Oncology, 2*, 472–483.

Soni, M.K., & Cella, D. (2002). Quality of life and symptom measures in oncology: An overview. *American Journal of Management Care, 8*, 560–573.

Stewart, A.L., Hays, R.D., & Ware, J.E. (1988). The MOS short-form general health survey: Reliability and validity in a patient population. *Medical Care, 26*, 724–735.

Varricchio, C.G. (1990). Relevance of quality of life to clinical nursing practice. *Seminars in Oncology Nursing, 6*, 255–259.

CHAPTER 32

Pharmacokinetics, Pharmacodynamics, and Pharmacogenomics

Carol S. Hill, BSN, RN, OCN®

Introduction

An important goal of oncology research is the development of safe and effective new anticancer drugs and the optimal use of existing agents through a better understanding of their clinical pharmacology (Jackson, 1996). During the clinical phase I/II of the drug development process, the pharmacokinetics (PK), pharmacodynamics (PD), and pharmacogenomics (PG) of potential new agents are studied in patients who are treated in clinical trials. PK and PD studies often are important end points in clinical trials of existing anticancer drugs (Grochow, 1998). In recent years, new scientific information has led to new studies of human genes (genome) to help scientists to understand the relationship of the human genome and drugs, especially new drugs, and how the human body responds or does not respond to certain treatments (Rieger, 2001). PG research will require large-scale clinical trials to help to define PG predictive patterns (Vaszar, Cho, & Raffin, 2003). This chapter will provide a basic understanding of PK, PD, and PG studies and will help the reader to know how drugs affect the blood concentration and to describe the role of the clinical trial nurse (CTN) in collecting, processing, and storing samples for these studies.

Role of Pharmacokinetic, Pharmacodynamic, and Pharmacogenomic Studies in Cancer Therapy

PK is the quantitative study of drug disposition (i.e., absorption, distribution, metabolism, and excretion), which represents the effect of drugs within the body (Balis, Holcenberg, & Poplack, 1997; Hicks & Klein, 1996; Tortorice & Hogen, 1997). Table 32-1 defines common PK parameters. Measuring drug concentrations in the plasma, serum, or other body fluids over time are PK studies. Although in most PK studies drug concentrations are measured only in the serum or plasma, the amount of drug in tissue and at the target site can be estimated using PK modeling (Jackson, 1996; Ohning, 1995).

Table 32-1. Pharmacokinetic Terms		
Parameter	**Abbreviation**	**Definition**
Clearance	Cl	The rate of drug elimination; expressed in terms of volume of plasma cleared of drug per unit of time. The sum of renal, metabolic, and biliary (fecal) elimination.
Half-life	$t_{1/2}$	Time required to reduce the drug concentration by 50%
Area under the curve	AUC	The area under the plasma concentration-time curve. A measure of total drug exposure.
Volume of distribution	V_d	The volume required to dissolve the total amount of drug in the body to give the final concentration of drug in the blood
Bioavailability	F	The fraction (percent) of a dose absorbed when administered by some route other than IV
Metabolism	–	Enzymatic alteration to a drug. May result in the activation of a prodrug, conversion to other biologically active intermediates, or inactivation of a drug.

Note. Courtesy of Frank M. Balis, MD, head of the Pharmacology and Experimental Therapeutics Section, Pediatric Branch, National Cancer Institute, 2006.

The author would like to acknowledge Alberta Aikin, RN, BSN, CPON®, and Frank M. Balis, MD, for their contribution that remains unchanged from the first edition.

The focus of PD studies is to quantify a drug's toxic and therapeutic effects, which represent the effect of the drug on the body (Renick-Ettinger, 1993). The information provided by PK, PD, and PG studies is used to determine the optimal drug route, dose, and schedule for administration of a drug (Fitzgerald, 1994; Rieger, 2001). Drug dose and schedule are individualized based on the concentration of the drug in serum or plasma to achieve a therapeutic and nontoxic drug exposure (Reynolds, 1993). Anticancer drug disposition often is highly variable within a group of patients with cancer, and these agents can produce severe toxicity; thus, knowing information about the drug's PK and PD can help to correlate side effects during the peak concentration (Rieger). The recent emphasis in cancer therapy on maximizing dose intensity and the narrow margin between the drug's therapeutic and toxic effects suggest that therapeutic drug monitoring (TDM) should play a role in the management of these drugs (Balis et al., 1997; Egorin, 1998).

Pharmacogenomics

Many clinical trials are adding PG along with PK to determine how investigational drugs respond with certain diseases and conditions. Another goal of PG is to help researchers to find therapeutic drugs that will work on that patient's genetic make-up (Machalek, 2005). As more is known regarding PG, nurses are in need of additional education and training in genetics to help their patients to understand the information (Hetteberg, Prows, Deets, Monsen, & Kenner, 1999). The Human Genome Project, initiated by the National Institutes of Health and the Department of Energy, is in the process of helping schools of nursing to incorporate genetics into their curriculum (Hetteberg et al.; Jenkins, Dimond, & Steinberg, 2001).

New Anticancer Drugs

PK studies play a critical role in the drug development process (see Figure 32-1). Prior to the introduction of a new drug into the clinical setting, extensive preclinical testing is performed in vitro using tumor cell lines and in vivo in animal models. A drug is first tested in the laboratory in human tumor cell lines to determine its spectrum of antitumor activity. It also is administered to tumor-bearing animals to assess antitumor activity in vivo. If evidence of an antitumor effect exists and the drug can be efficiently produced in large quantities, the toxicology and PK are studied in several animal species (usually rodents and dogs) (Jackson, 1996). The toxicology and PK studies in animals are used to determine a starting dose and schedule for the subsequent clinical trial drugs (Balis et al., 1997).

The objectives of a phase I clinical trial are to determine the appropriate route, maximum tolerated dose of a drug, and schedule of administration; to define the spectrum of drug toxicities in human subjects; and to study the PK of the new agent (Tortorice & Hogen, 1997). Because phase I trials are single-agent studies, they provide the best opportunity to identify correlations between PK parameters and the drug's PD (toxicity and response). The results of PK and PD studies are important components of the investigational new drug application that is submitted to the U.S. Food and Drug Administration to gain approval for commercial use of a new drug (Jackson, 1996; Rowland & Tozer, 1989).

Conventional Anticancer Drugs

PK and PD studies have an important impact on the way that conventional anticancer drugs are administered. Carboplatin is an anticancer drug that is used in the treatment of a variety of adult and pediatric cancers. PK and PD studies of the agent demonstrated a relationship between plasma drug exposure and the degree of thrombocytopenia. Carboplatin primarily is excreted by the kidneys, and in PK studies, the rate of drug elimination was proportional to the creatinine clearance, a measure of the glomerular filtration rate (GFR). The recognition of these relationships allowed for the development of adaptive dosing formulas that use each patient's GFR to derive an individualized dose. The use of these formulas to calculate carboplatin dose instead of administering a dose based only on body weight or body surface area results in more uniform and predictable toxicity (Balis et al., 1997; Grochow, 1998). Additionally, TDM plays an important role in the daily management of patients who receive high doses of methotrexate, which requires the administration of a leucovorin rescue after the methotrexate infusion to prevent severe toxicity. The duration of the leucovorin rescue is determined by the individual's plasma concentration of methotrexate (Balis et al.).

Performing Pharmacokinetic Studies

Except for methotrexate, TDM does not play a role in the daily management of anticancer drugs. Therefore, most PK studies of anticancer drugs are performed as part of a research study. In contrast to TDM, in which only peak and

---

Figure 32-1. Steps in the Drug Development Process

In vitro and in vivo screening for antitumor activity
↓
Chemical synthesis or bulk production
↓
Preclinical toxicology
Pharmacology
↓
Formulation
Production
↓
Clinical trials
Phase I, II, III, IV

Note. Figure courtesy of Frank M. Balis, MD, head of the Pharmacology and Experimental Therapeutics Section, Pediatric Branch, National Cancer Institute, 2006.

trough or single steady state plasma or serum samples are drawn, PK research studies use more complex sampling schedules. Research studies often include sampling of other body fluids (e.g., urine, cerebrospinal fluid), feces, or tissues to define the route of drug elimination and to study the drug's distribution (Rowland & Tozer, 1989). The plasma disappearance curve (plasma drug concentration-time profile) for most anticancer drugs is multiphasic; an initial distribution phase occurs, in which the plasma drug concentration declines rapidly as the drug is distributed from the blood into tissues, followed by a more prolonged elimination phase, in which the drug is cleared from the body (Gibaldi, 1977). The timing structure for obtaining PK samples must be established to best describe the plasma concentration-time profile. Several samples must be obtained during each phase of the disappearance curve, and the duration of PK sampling should be at least two to three times longer than the drug's half-life. As a result, PK research studies typically require 6–12 plasma or serum samples.

Study Design

PK research studies that are performed in human subjects must be carefully designed to gain the maximum information about the disposition of the drug while minimizing the risks to patients (Jackson, 1996). The design of the PK study is either included in the primary protocol or is written as a separate protocol. The protocol describes in detail the patients that will be studied, the conditions under which the PK study will be conducted (e.g., fasted subject prior to an oral dose), the dosing of the agent, the sample collection times, the sample processing, and storage conditions. PK research studies frequently require other types of samples, such as urine or cerebrospinal fluid. Urine should be collected quantitatively, the entire specimen should be well-mixed, the total volume should be measured and recorded, and an aliquot should be stored for measurement of the drug or metabolite levels. Cerebrospinal fluid may be obtained via an indwelling ventricular access device, such as an Ommaya® (NeuroCare Group) reservoir, or by lumbar puncture (Patel, Blaney, & Balis, 1998). Most PK studies require that a sample be obtained prior to drug administration. This is used as a control sample in the drug assay. Once the drug is administered, the target times for collecting samples are calculated using the designated times described in the clinical trial and on the PK worksheet (see Figure 32-2). A typical sampling schedule could be prior to the dose, five minutes after completion of the infusion, and 0.25, 0.5, 1, 2, 4, 6, 8, 24, and 48 hours after the end of the drug infusion. Samples should be collected as close to the target times as possible—especially the early samples. The exact time of the collection should be recorded on the tube and on the PK worksheet. If the sample is not drawn at the target time, the exact time that it was collected should be written on the tube because calculations can be made in

the laboratory to accommodate for the difference. When samples have to be drawn by several nurses, synchronizing the time by using one designated clock will help to eliminate time discrepancies. Occasionally, a sample draw time may be missed altogether. If this occurs, a brief explanation should be written on the worksheet and in the source document. Samples then are collected at designated time points after the administration of the drug. In some cases (e.g., with chemically unstable drugs), samples of the actual drug infusate are obtained to confirm the actual dose of drug administered.

The protocol should include a PK worksheet (see Figure 32-2). The worksheet usually includes demographic information about the patient; the patient's weight, height, and body surface area; drug dose and time of administration; exact times that samples were obtained; what time samples were placed in refrigerator or freezer; and comments regarding acute toxicities or problems with dosing or sample collection that may affect the study.

Subject Selection

Because PK is the quantitative study of the effect of a drug on the body, patient selection for PK studies can have a substantial impact on the results. The age, gender, underlying medical conditions, and function of the excretory organs (e.g., liver, kidney), as well as other factors, can directly influence the absorption, distribution, or elimination of a drug (Balis et al., 1997; Hicks & Klein, 1996). The PK of drugs with minimal side effects often is studied initially in healthy volunteers, but for more toxic agents (e.g., anticancer drugs), PK studies usually are performed in patients who have the disease for which the drug is intended (Jackson, 1996). After the PK (including the route of elimination) of an agent is understood in patients with normal liver and kidney function, then PK studies can be undertaken in subjects with varying degrees of liver or kidney dysfunction to define safe doses for these patients (Balis et al.).

Informed Consent

The clinical trial must include an informed consent document signed by the patient that describes the study and its risks and benefits in lay terms to the patient. Patients must understand that the results of these studies will not be made known to them or the clinical site at the end of the study. The samples will not be identified by the patient's name but by the protocol number and the patient's study number. The risks from participation in a PK or PD study usually are minimal and include the loss of a relatively small amount of blood that is collected (usually the total amount of blood is 30–45 ml); the discomfort and small risk of bleeding or infection from blood drawing, Ommaya reservoir puncture, or lumbar puncture; and the time and inconvenience of the collection. Unless PK levels are used in making decisions about the drug dose or schedule during the course of the therapy, the patient receives no

Figure 32-2. Example of a Pharmacokinetic Worksheet

Pharmacokinetic Worksheet

Patient Name: _____   Today's Date: _____

Date of Birth: _____   Dose (mg/m²): _____

Weight (kg): _____   Actual Dose (mg): _____

Height (cm): _____   Dose Start Time: _____

BSA (m²): _____   Dose Completion Time: _____

Sample #	Time Post Dose	Target Time	Actual Time	Comments
1	Pre-Dose			
2	5 min			
3	15 min			
4	30 min			
5	1 hr			
6	2 hr			
7	4 hr			
8	6 hr			
9	8 hr			
10	24 hr			
11	48 hr			

The Target Time in the third column of the table is calculated from the Dose Completion Time (i.e., time at the end of an IV infusion) and the Time Post Dose for each sample. For example, if an infusion ends at 9 am, then the Target Time for Sample #2 is 9:05 am.

Note. Courtesy of Frank M. Balis, MD, head of the Pharmacology and Experimental Therapeutics Section, Pediatric Branch, National Cancer Institute, 2006.

direct benefit from participating. Patients participating in the study know that they are contributing to research that may benefit future patients. Patients have the right to refuse to participate in the PK or PG study without jeopardizing their right to receive treatment on the clinical trial, unless the PK study is necessary to modify the drug dose. The patient or the patient's parent or guardian, along with the nurse and physician, must sign the informed consent form before starting the PK sampling. The patient receives a copy of this signed consent, the original is placed in the patient's medical record, and another copy is kept in the research record.

Drug Administration

Many PK parameters that are calculated from PK studies are dependent on the dose. Therefore, the dose of drug that is being studied must be accurately calculated, prepared, and administered. An incorrect dose could lead to a substantial error in the PK parameters. IV drug infusions should be administered as precisely as possible over the planned duration at a constant rate. Immediately after a drug infusion, the IV line should be flushed at the same rate as the drug infusion. A rapid flush to clear the line will give a mini-bolus of drug that may elevate the peak or end of infusion drug concentration in the blood or may cause an adverse reaction in the patient. For the convenience of the patient and the research staff, the drug should be administered early in the day so that sample collection can be performed during the day rather than after hours or late at night.

Sample Collection

The sample collection procedure starts with careful planning and preparation. This not only enhances patient safety and comfort but also ensures more accurate PK or PD sampling. The nursing staff should be informed about the PK or PD study because they often participate in sample collection. Some studies require that special instructions be communicated to the patient before the study, such as the need to take nothing by mouth prior to administration of the drug. Coordination of drug ordering by the physician and drug preparation by the pharmacy will allow PK studies to start early in the day. It is critical that personnel are available to process these samples in a timely manner, and this requires preplanning to ensure that staff will be able to participate in these studies. Supplies and equipment should be prepared before starting the PK study. The specimen tubes for collecting samples and, if necessary, the cryotubes for freezing samples should be assembled and labeled. Most blood samples are collected in heparinized tubes; however, a serum separator tube or tubes containing other anticoagulants (e.g., edetate disodium) may be required. Special preservatives may need to be added to blood collection tubes for unstable drugs. For example, cytarabine (Ara-C) is metabolized by an enzyme in the blood after the sample is drawn, and this can falsely lower the plasma drug concentration. The inhibitor, tetrahydrouridine, is added to the blood collection tubes to prevent the degradation of cytarabine during the blood drawing and processing procedures. Some drugs adhere to certain materials (e.g., plastics) and may require special tubes to prevent artificial loss of the drug during sample collection. The collection and storage tube labels should include the patient's initials, protocol name, patient's identification number, the drug name, the dose, the date, the time the sample was drawn, and the sample number. The exact time that the sample was collected must be written on the tube label and the PK worksheet after the sample is obtained. Special handling requirements for samples will be explained in the protocol, such as the storage temperature, any requirements to protect them from light, and whether they must be processed immediately or in a batch.

IV access should be established prior to administration of the drug to eliminate delays in obtaining samples. A central venous catheter or a peripheral IV site can be used. If the study drug is administered orally, subcutaneously, intramuscularly, or via another non-IV route, only one IV site for sampling is necessary. If the drug is administered IV, a site other than the drug delivery site must be used for sample collection to prevent contamination, which could artificially increase the plasma drug concentration. When the drug is infused through a multilumen catheter, the alternate lumen should not be used for sampling because of the risk of contamination of the sample. When a steady state level is required during a continuous infusion given through a central venous catheter, the sample must be drawn from a peripheral IV. If achieving peripheral IV access is not possible, the principal investigator (PI) or associate investigator should be contacted. Although not ideal, it may be possible to omit some of the samples, such as those taken during the drug infusion, and still obtain valuable information. If the patient has limited peripheral access, the following should be done: The line should be flushed with at least 10–30 ml of normal saline before drawing a discard (30 ml) according to the clinical trial or institutional policy. Then the sample should be drawn. A smaller size (20 ml) flush and discard can be used in small-lumen or pediatric catheters. If a drug metabolite, and not the drug, is being studied, the IV line through which the drug is infused can be used for drawing a sample because contamination is not an issue. First, the CTN should stop the infusion, flush with normal saline according to the clinical trial or institution policy (usually is 20–30 ml depending on the original catheter size), and draw a discard (20–30 ml) before collecting the sample (or as directed by the protocol). The PI or associate investigator should be consulted prior to sampling from the drug infusion site and must document why the protocol was not followed.

Documentation

Careful and complete documentation is an important part of PK and PD studies. The signed informed consent form must be placed in the patient's medical record, and a copy must be placed in the research record. Nursing notes should include verification that the PK or PD study was explained to the patient, that the consent was signed, that the drug was administered (including dose and time), that samples were collected at specific time points as directed in the protocol, and that the patient tolerated the procedure. The PK worksheet should be completed with the patient's initials or identification number; the patient's weight, height, and body surface area; the date; the dose level and actual dose; and the time the drug was given and the end time. The target times and exact times of collection are recorded along with the site from which the sample was taken (i.e., peripheral IV or central venous catheter). A copy of the PK worksheet is kept in the research folder, and the original copy is sent with the samples for the analysis.

Sample Processing

When PK samples are brought to the laboratory, they are either analyzed immediately, if the drug is unstable, or are prepared for storage. Samples should be handled in a biological safety cabinet and according to universal precautions and laboratory safety guidelines to avoid possible exposure to potentially infectious agents. Plasma or serum must be separated from blood cells by centrifuge. The centrifuge temperature, revolutions per minute, and duration of centrifugation are set according to the directions specified in the protocol. After centrifuge, the plasma or serum can be identified easily as the straw-colored liquid at the top of the tube. If the sample was hemolyzed when it was drawn, the plasma or serum may be pink or reddish in color. Centrifuging the blood sample too rapidly can cause hemolysis. Plasma also may be lipemic if it was drawn after the patient had a meal. The plasma or serum is removed using a pipette and is transferred to labeled cryotubes. Most samples can be transferred using plastic pipettes. However, if the drug adheres to plastic, the protocol will specify the use of glass pipettes. Once the plasma is in the cryotube, it is placed in the freezer. Stored specimens usually are kept in the freezer at –70°C. Cerebrospinal fluid, urine, and the infusate can be transferred directly to the labeled cryotubes and frozen. Cataloging frozen specimens ensures that they can be located when needed. The specific directions for processing the samples should be included in the clinical trial.

Samples may need to be shipped to another facility for analysis. The name, address, and phone number of the person to receive the samples will be specified in the protocol. Federal regulations for shipping body fluids must be followed because they are considered to be a biohazard. Some samples can be shipped at room temperature, but most must be shipped frozen and packed in dry ice. Arrangements are made with a carrier for next-day delivery from Monday through Thursday, unless otherwise specified. The recipients should be informed of the date that the shipment will arrive; this ensures that someone will be available to handle the samples immediately after arrival. A copy of the shipment's tracking number should be kept with the sample forms in the patient's research chart.

Summary

PK and PD studies of anticancer drugs have led to more rational drug administration schedules that have improved patient outcomes. Continued research is needed, especially in determining the role of pharmacogenomics and how drugs affect an individual's management of anticancer drugs, and drugs in general. Patients who participate in research studies make an invaluable contribution to the knowledge base of new and conventional anticancer drugs. The CTN plays an essential role in coordinating and conducting these vital research studies that have a direct impact on the safety and effectiveness of anticancer drugs. It is important that CTNs understand all that they can about PK, PD, and PG so that they can help their colleagues and patients to understand the important roles these studies have in clinical trials.

References

Balis, F.M., Holcenberg, J.S., & Poplack, D.G. (1997). General principles of chemotherapy. In P.A. Pizzo & D.G. Poplack (Eds.), *Principles and practice of pediatric oncology* (3rd ed., pp. 215–258). Philadelphia: Lippincott-Raven.

Egorin, M. (1998). Foreword. In L.B. Grochow & M.M. Ames (Eds.), *A clinician's guide to chemotherapy pharmacokinetics and pharmacodynamics* (p. vii). Baltimore: Williams & Wilkins.

Fitzgerald, M. (1994). Pharmacology highlights and principles of pharmacokinetics. *Journal of the American Academy of Nurses, 6,* 581–583.

Gibaldi, M. (1977). *Biopharmaceutics and clinical pharmacokinetics.* Philadelphia: Lea & Febiger.

Grochow, L.B. (1998). Individualized dosing of anticancer drugs and the role of therapeutic monitoring. In L.B. Grochow & M.M. Ames (Eds.), *A clinician's guide to chemotherapy pharmacokinetics and pharmacodynamics* (pp. 3–11). Baltimore: Williams & Wilkins.

Hetteberg, C.G., Prows, C.A., Deets, C., Monsen, R.B., & Kenner, C.A. (1999). National survey of genetics content in basic nursing preparatory programs in the United States. *Nursing Outlook, 47,* 168–174.

Hicks, F.D., & Klein, D. (1996). Pharmacokinetics in postanesthesia recovery: Implications for nurses. *Journal of Post Anesthesia Nursing, 11,* 97–103.

Jackson, R.C. (1996). *Computer techniques in preclinical and clinical drug development.* Boca Raton, FL: CRC Press.

Jenkins, J.E., Dimond, E., & Steinberg, S. (2001). Preparing for the future through genetics nursing education. *Journal of Nursing Scholarship, 33,* 191–195.

Machalek, A.Z. (2005, September 28). *NIH renews network focused on how genes influence drug responses. Findings will pave the way for individually tailored therapies.* National Institute of General Medical Sciences. Retrieved November 17, 2005, from http://www.nigms.nih.gov/News/Results/20050928PGRN.htm

Ohning, B.L. (1995). Neonatal pharmacodynamics—Basic principles I: Drug delivery. *Neonatal Network, 14*(2), 7–12.

Patel, M., Blaney, S., & Balis, F.M. (1998). Pharmacokinetics of drug delivery to the central nervous system. In L.B. Grochow & M.M. Ames (Eds.), *A clinician's guide to chemotherapy pharmacokinetics and pharmacodynamics* (pp. 67–85). Baltimore: Williams & Wilkins.

Renick-Ettinger, A. (1993). Chemotherapy. In G.V. Foley, D. Frochtman, & M.K. Hardin (Eds.), *Nursing care of the child with cancer* (2nd ed., pp. 81–115). Philadelphia: Saunders.

Reynolds, J.R. (1993). Pharmacokinetic considerations in critical care. *Critical Care Nursing Clinics of North America, 5,* 227–235.

Rieger, P.T. (2001). *Biotherapy: A comprehensive overview* (2nd ed.). Sudbury, MA: Jones and Bartlett.

Rowland, M., & Tozer, T.N. (1989). *Clinical pharmacokinetics: Concepts and applications* (2nd ed.). Philadelphia: Lea & Febiger.

Tortorice, P.V., & Hogen C.M. (1997). Chemotherapy. In S.L. Groenwald, M.H. Frogge, M. Goodman, & C.H. Yarbro (Eds.), *Cancer nursing: Principles and practice* (4th ed., pp. 230–280). Sudbury, MA: Jones and Bartlett.

Vaszar, L.T., Cho, M.K., & Raffin, T.A. (2003). Privacy issues in personalized medicine. *Pharmacogenomics, 4,* 107–112.

CHAPTER 33
Genetic Testing and Storage of Genetic Material

Patricia McLaughlin, RN, MSN, AOCN®

Introduction

In 2003, the Human Genome Project was completed. Although this was a monumental accomplishment in the scientific world, it has had major technical, ethical, legal, and social implications for society as well. Issues such as denial of healthcare insurance, workplace discrimination, interference with patient confidentiality, and potential violations of patients' rights could occur as result of this scientific advancement (National Human Genome Research Institute [NHGRI], 2005c, 2005d). Clinical trial nurses (CTNs) are becoming increasingly involved in treatment protocols that require or request the sampling and storage of genetic material as part of ancillary trials. This chapter will explore the issues surrounding the Human Genome Project and the role of the nurse in responding to the advances in human genomics.

Human Genome Project

The Human Genome Project was based on the results of years of research in genetics dating back to 1911 (NHGRI, 2005c). With funding from the National Institutes of Health and the Department of Energy, the project was formally started in October 1990 (U.S. Department of Energy Office of Science, 2004a). Francis S. Collins, MD, PhD, director of the NHGRI, compared the genome to a book with multiple uses:

> "It's a history book—a narrative of the journey of our species through time. It's a shop manual, with an incredibly detailed blueprint for building every human cell. And it's a transformative textbook of medicine, with insights that will give health care providers immense new powers to treat, prevent, and cure disease." (NHGRI, 2005c, p. 2)

Figure 33-1 details the goals of the Human Genome Project.

Genetic Testing

Several reasons exist for conducting genetic tests. These include to confirm a specific disease; to predict the possibility of developing a disease in the future, known as *predictive testing* (Koliopoulos, 2001); to determine whether an individual is a carrier and could potentially pass the impaired gene on to his or her children; and to predict how well an individual will respond to therapy, known as *pharmacogenomics* (Collins, 2003).

Genetic tests use a variety of techniques to identify genes. Direct testing analyzes the genes of a specific individual. Indirect testing is used when a specific gene cannot be identified and a specific region of a chromosome is analyzed. Indirect testing requires DNA not only from the individual but also from an affected family member (Rice, 2005). As of 2003, approximately 900 specific genetic tests were in existence (Collins, 2003).

Figure 33-1. Goals of the Human Genome Project

- Identify all of the approximately 20,000–25,000 genes in human DNA.
- Determine the sequence of the three billion chemical base pairs that make up human DNA.
- Store information in databases.
- Improve tools for data analysis.
- Transfer related technologies to the private sector.
- Address the ethical, legal, and social issues that may arise from the project.

Note. From *Human Genome Project Information*, by U.S. Department of Energy Office of Science, 2004. Retrieved September 21, 2005, from http://www.ornl.gov/sci/techresources/Human_Genome/home.shtml

---

The author would like to acknowledge Sharon L. Smith, RN, MS, OCN®, for her contribution that remains unchanged from the first edition.

Genetic testing is a very complex process and involves several factors, including reliable lab procedures and the sensitivity of the test to detect mutations. Also to be considered is the possibility of false-positive and false-negative results. Special training is required to analyze and relay the results to individuals and their families. This is the role of specialty-trained physicians, genetic counselors, and the genetics advanced practice nurse (APN) (Rice, 2005).

Six types of tests currently exist.

- *Newborn screening* is used shortly after birth to detect genetic disorders that are treatable. An example of such a test is one that detects phenylketonuria in newborns. If left untreated, this disease can result in mental retardation.
- *Diagnostic testing* is used to identify a genetic or chromosomal disorder when an individual is demonstrating signs and symptoms of a particular genetic disease, such as Down syndrome. This type of test is not available for all genetic diseases.
- The identification of individuals who carry one copy of a gene that, when paired with another copy of the same gene, causes a genetic disorder. This is known as *carrier testing*. This is available for individuals with a family history of a genetic disorder (such as Tay-Sachs disease in the Jewish population) or to one who is a member of an ethnic group with an increased risk of a genetic disorder.
- *Prenatal testing* is done in utero to test the fetus's chromosomes (to detect for diseases such as sickle-cell anemia) before birth. It cannot, however, determine all possible birth or inherited disorders.
- *Predictive* and *presymptomatic testing* are tests used to detect genetic mutations that appear later in life. An example of a predictive test is one that can detect a mutation that may lead to the development of a certain type of cancer. Presymptomatic testing can determine if the individual will develop an inheritable disease, such as Huntington disease, before actual manifestation of symptoms occurs.
- *Forensic testing* uses DNA to identify a specific individual. This type of testing is not used to identify genetic defects but rather is used to identify crime victims and suspects and to establish paternity (U.S. Department of Energy Office of Science, 2004a).

Issues in Genetic Testing

Privacy/Confidentiality

The fear of loss of privacy and confidentiality remains one of the most important concerns of both scientists and the public regarding genetic research. In fact, many individuals refuse testing because of the fear of repercussions should the test results become available to individuals who have no right to the information, which would consequently pose the potential for discrimination.

Little federal legislation is available to protect the privacy of an individual's genetic test results. The only

piece of legislation that currently exists at the federal level is the Health Insurance Portability and Accountability Act (HIPAA) of 1996. The law was implemented in two phases. Phase one, passed in 1996, provides for the standards as listed in Figure 33-2. In April 2003, the law was expanded because Congress failed to pass comprehensive legislation on privacy as required by HIPAA in 1999. The new standards are listed in Figure 33-3 (U.S. Department of Energy Office of Science, 2004b).

Although the NHGRI supported the technologic advances that were being made, researchers were aware of the potential for misuse or abuse of the information that was obtained as a result of the new technology. For this reason, in 1990, the NHGRI created the Ethical, Legal, and Social Implications (ELSI) Research Program (NHGRI, 2005a). The major purpose of this program was to support studies in ethics and policy issues. ELSI also tracks the development of federal and state legislation that protects against misuse of genetic information (NHGRI, 2005a).

Figure 33-2. Elements of Phase 1 of the Health Insurance Portability and Accountability Act

- Prohibits group health plans from using any health status-related factor, including genetic information, as a basis for denying or limiting eligibility for coverage or for charging an individual more for coverage
- Limits exclusions for preexisting conditions in group health plans to 12 months and prohibits such exclusions if the individual has been covered for the previous condition for 12 months or more
- States explicitly that genetic information in the absence of a current diagnosis shall not be considered a preexisting condition
- Does not prohibit employers from refusing to offer health coverage as part of their benefits package

Note. From *Genetics Privacy and Legislation*, by the U.S. Department of Energy Office of Science, 2004. Retrieved September 22, 2005, from http://www.ornl.gov/sci/techresources/Human_Genome/elsi/legislat.shtml#III

Figure 33-3. Current Health Insurance Portability and Accountability Act Standards Regarding Genetic Research

- Limit the nonconsensual use of and release of private information.
- Give patients new rights to access their medical records and to know who else has accessed them.
- Restrict most disclosure of health information to the minimum needed for the intended purpose.
- Establish new criminal and civil sanctions for improper use or disclosure.
- Establish new requirements for access to records by researchers and others.

Note. From *Genetics Privacy and Legislation*, by the U.S. Department of Energy Office of Science, 2004. Retrieved September 22, 2005, from http://www.ornl.gov/sci/techresources/Human_Genome/elsi/legislat.shtml

In addition to federal legislation and the ELSI program, a number of individual states have developed laws against genetic discrimination. The laws, however, are neither comprehensive nor consistent. Laws at the federal and state levels are needed that better protect individuals' rights as they relate specifically to genetic information.

Workplace Discrimination

Genetic discrimination in the workplace does exist. Asymptomatic applicants have been denied jobs based on a predisposition to a genetic illness (NHGRI, 2005b). Many individuals will not take advantage of genetic testing for fear of this type of discrimination. One may question how access to such information can occur. Information may be obtained from medical exams, family history, medical records, or actual genetic test results. Additionally, the lack of specific stringent federal and state laws contributes to the problem.

The Americans with Disabilities Act (ADA) covers individuals who exhibit symptoms or illnesses that are genetically related. What is not clear is whether individuals who are asymptomatic are covered. The Equal Employment Opportunity Commission (EEOC) believes they are covered under the American with Disabilities Act (NHGRI, 1998). Concerns that some will challenge the EEOC's interpretation of the ADA have led to a continued effort by a number of legislators to enact laws to protect individuals from genetics-related discrimination (Miller, 2005). As of 2005, 31 states have adopted laws concerning genetics-related discrimination in the workplace (NHGRI, 1998).

Genetic Discrimination Related to Health Insurance

Genetic information has been used to discriminate against people with a genetic predisposition to an illness and those with actual genetics-related illness by causing them to be denied health insurance. Without insurance, patients often are unable to access health care to treat many diseases. For this reason, many people will refuse genetic testing (NHGRI, 1998, 2005d).

In 1993, the ELSI Working Group of the Human Genome Project made recommendations that people be covered by health insurance no matter what is known about their health status. In addition, the group recommended that "health insurers be prohibited from using genetic information or an individual's request for genetic services to deny or limit health insurance coverage, establish differential rates or have access to an individual's genetic information without the individual's written authorization" (NHGRI, 2005b). It was these recommendations that led to the creation of HIPAA (discussed earlier). Congress introduced nine bills dealing with genetic discrimination in health insurance between 1999 and 2001, and four were introduced between 2001 and 2003. Additionally, 41 states have passed legislation regarding genetics-related health insurance discrimination (NHGRI, 2005b).

Genetic Testing of Children

Genetic testing of children is a very controversial issue. When families have a history of genetics-related illness, it is imperative to consider the potential benefits versus the risks to the child. This is especially true with late-onset illnesses. According to the American College of Medical Genetics (1995b), the impact of potential benefits and harms on decisions about testing should be taken into consideration:

- Timely medical benefit to the child should be the primary justification for genetic testing in children and adolescents.
- Substantial psychosocial benefits to the competent adolescent also may be a justification for genetic testing.
- If the medical or psychosocial benefits of a genetic test will not accrue until adulthood, as in the carrier case of carrier status or adult-onset diseases, genetic testing generally should be deferred.
- If the balance of benefits and harms is uncertain, the provider should respect the decisions of competent adolescents and their families.
- Testing should be discouraged when the provider determines that potential harms of genetic testing in children and adolescents outweigh the potential benefits. (pp. 1233–1234)

Myriad other considerations need to be taken into account; however, the factors listed reflect a general guideline that can be used in making decisions about whether the testing of a child is appropriate.

Genetic Counseling

Because of the great advances made in the field of human genetics, the role of the genetic counselor and genetics APN has become increasingly more important. A genetic counselor/genetics APN helps an individual to understand his or her risk for developing genetic conditions and educates patients and family members (when appropriate) about the specific disease and the risk of passing the disease on to their children. The genetic counselor/genetics APN is part of a healthcare team composed of specialty trained physicians, social workers, and other specialists.

It is the current standard of care that all patients who potentially have a genetic condition meet with a genetic counselor or genetics APN before undergoing any testing. This individual will collect medical information, including family history, and will develop a pedigree (similar to a family tree). The genetic counselor/APN will explain options for testing, implications of genetic testing, and options to prevent the disease if they are available, along with both the risks and benefits of these procedures. The counselor/APN will not perform any procedure (e.g., obtaining a blood sample) without a person's written consent. No patient should ever have a genetic test performed without meeting with a genetic counselor or a genetics APN (Adams, 2003). Similarly, results should not be given to an individual unless the counselor/nurse or specialty-trained physician is present to discuss the findings (Adams).

Storage of Genetic Material

A great number of clinical research trials include a request to store either blood or tissue from a subject for future use. This practice is common both in trials sponsored by the National Cancer Institute and in industry-sponsored trials. DNA can be obtained directly from the patient soon after the specimen is received, or it can be prepared from stored tissues, blood, serum, cytologic preparations, and pathology specimens. Because DNA contains information that is in the form of a code, the code often is entered into a national protected computer database. The database itself is treated in the same fashion as the actual DNA (University of California, San Diego, Human Research Protections Program, 1997).

A human tissue repository collects, stores, and distributes human tissue for research purposes. The *Code of Federal Regulations* (45 CFR Part 46) covers repositories and informed consent. Three areas are involved in human tissue repositories: the collectors of the tissue sample, the repository storage and data management center, and the recipient investigator (Lahl, 2005). Each of these three entities must adhere to specific regulations.

The tissue collector must have institutional review board (IRB) approval to collect the genetic material, informed consent must be obtained from the subject, and there must be a submittal agreement and an assurance of compliance with the regulations. Similarly for the repository storage and methods for data management, the IRB must approve the sample informed consent, a certificate of confidentiality must be obtained, and, again, there must be an assurance of compliance. The recipient investigator must sign a recipient agreement and adhere to all local policies as they relate to research on human genetic material (Office for Protection from Research Risks, 1997).

Informed Consent

Written informed consent regarding genetic material is to protect the individual who is submitting the genetic material. If samples are being used for research purposes or may be associated with or linked to a particular individual, then informed consent must be obtained from the donor unless waived by the IRB. The informed consent requirements stipulate that there must be a clear description of
- The operation of the repository
- The specific types of research to be conducted

- The conditions under which data and specimens will be released to recipient investigators
- Procedures for protecting the privacy of subjects and maintaining the confidentiality of the data (Lahl, 2005),

Specific information addressing these points should be contained in the consent form. This information should be reviewed and discussed in depth with the patient/donor during the consent process. Figure 33-4 includes the required components of informed consent involved with genetic material and testing.

Patients need to understand the potential consequences of genetic testing, such as risks of increased insurance premiums and potential discrimination by employers should the results become known. Another example of a consequence is the possibility that if the results of genetic testing are inaccurate, a false positive or negative regarding paternity may result. Where and for how long samples will be stored, whether the subject may request that samples be destroyed in the future, and whether all personal identifiers will be removed from the sample must be included in the consent. Subjects have the right to know whether test results may be made known to them should they choose to know.

Figure 33-4. Components of Informed Consent Involving Genetic Material and Testing

For genetic screening and testing
- The nature of the disorder
- Reasons for/alternatives to participation
- Risks/benefits of the test
- Description of the test (purpose, limitations [false positive/negative rates])
- Anticipated uses of samples (purpose, disposition/storage)
- Privacy standards and confidentiality mechanisms
- Disclosure to others/third-party access (family members)
- Available support/counseling services
- Subsequent decisions that may be likely after obtaining test results
- The unexpected result (will or will not be disclosed)
- Method of communicating results

For genetic research (in addition to above)
- Possible outcomes/information that could result from test
- Anticipated disposition of samples (destruction, retention [purpose, scope of future testing, anonymity/removal of identifiers, duration of storage, option to withdraw specimen], ownership/designee, death or patient withdrawal)
- Disclosure, conflicts of interest/access to research findings
- Anticipated secondary uses (same or different researchers/purposes, "immortal" cell lines)
- Research findings (publication, access to "discoveries," compensation issues, potential financial gain [test development, profit sharing, commercially valuable products])
- Policy of recontacting (expected/unexpected results, reconsent, future access to information)

Note. Based on information from American College of Medical Genetics, 1995a; American Society of Human Genetics Board of Directors, 1996; Clayton et al., 1995; Scanlon & Fibison, 1995.

In many studies today, genetic material is stored for future use without a specific plan for what testing is going to be performed. In this case, there should be a statement in the informed consent about secondary uses of materials. Subjects should be asked if they would permit the use of their genetic material for future tests or if they allow researchers to contact them to obtain consent for secondary use of the sample(s). In many cases when genetic material is used for secondary research, all banked specimens will be stripped of patient identifiers (American College of Medical Genetics, 2005a, 2005b).

Recipient investigators of banked specimens should not have access to the identities of the donors. If they do have such access, they need to obtain an assurance of compliance and IRB review and approval of the research being proposed (Lahl, 2005).

The Office for Human Research Protections does not consider research involving coded information as human subject research if (Lahl, 2005)

- The specimen has no personal identifiers
- No interaction occurs between the investigator and the individual to whom the specimen belongs
- The key to the code is destroyed before the research begins
- The investigator has an agreement with the key holder that the key will not be released while the individual is alive
- IRB policies and procedures are in place to prevent the release of the key to coded information.

It is imperative that the specimens are protected and all regulations are followed. If any of these regulations are not adhered to, it is possible that the individual whose specimen is being studied may have his or her privacy compromised, thus allowing the potential for discrimination as discussed previously.

Resource Limitations

With the recent advances made in the completion of the human genome, a new area of medicine, that of genetic medicine, has become part of the public health agenda. Figure 33-5 lists some of the organizations that provide genetic resources for CTNs. Unfortunately, because of the speed at which the advances are being made, medicine has not yet been able to integrate all of these findings into practice. The availability of genetic healthcare services is neither uniform nor consistent. It is imperative that everyone has equal access to state-of-the-art genetic healthcare services.

According to the International Society of Nurses in Genetics (2003), three basic elements are needed to form the framework of genetic medicine in health care: establishment of an infrastructure that will provide the services, education of both healthcare providers and the general public about services that are available in genetic health, and equal access to genomic health care for individuals. This can occur only with adequate planning, funding, and allocation of resources, especially of specialty-trained individuals in this field. Although barriers to access exist, they can be overcome if the state and federal legislatures provide support to prevent insurance and employment discrimination and to promote education and access to quality health care for everyone.

Nursing Implications

The evolution of the field of genetics greatly affects the role of the nurse. It is imperative that the oncology nurse, the oncology APN, and the genetics APN are knowledgeable about the role that genetics plays in health care. Today, genetics is incorporated into nursing curricula. Numerous continuing education programs exist to update nurses in the advances that have occurred, as well as to reinforce oncology nurses' roles in genetic health care (Oncology Nursing Society, 2004).

Oncology nurses must be patient advocates from the bedside to the legislative level. They must

- Work diligently to educate patients about genetics in health care
- Advocate for an individual's right to choose whether to pursue genetic testing
- Lobby legislators at both the state and federal levels to pass bills that protect the privacy of the person undergoing genetic testing and to make any acts of discrimination related to genetic testing illegal.

The oncology nurse should refer patients to genetic specialists as a given situation dictates. The nurse also must incorporate genetic research findings into clinical practice.

As the field of genetics continues to grow, so will the role of the nurse in educating patients about new findings. The challenge of yesterday in science is here in health care today. The nurse, as a critical member of the healthcare team, must respond to the challenges that genetic health care poses to both individuals and to society as a whole. Figure 33-6 lists U.S. regulatory and advisory boards that provide genetic resources for nurses.

Summary

Genetic testing is a rapidly evolving component of health care that requires the balance of personal privacy

---

Figure 33-5. Organizations Providing Genetic Resources for Nurses

- American Nurses Association Center for Ethics and Human Rights
- International Society of Nurses in Genetics
- National Institute of Nursing Research, NIH—focuses on the development of core curriculum for nurses
- National Coalition for Health Professional Education in Genetics—a registry established by the American Medical Association, American Nurses Association, and National Human Genome Research Institute for information about various curricula and educational programs in genetic education
- Oncology Nursing Society

Figure 33-6. Key U.S. Regulatory and Advisory Boards

- Center for Biologics Evaluation and Research (CBER)
- Centers for Disease Control and Prevention (CDC)
- Food and Drug Administration (FDA)
- National Human Genome Research Institute (NHGRI)
- National Human Research Protections Advisory Committee (NHRPAC)
- National Institutes of Health (NIH)
- Office for Human Research Protections (OHRP)
- Office of Genomics and Disease Prevention (OGDP)
- President's Council for Bioethics
- Recombinant DNA Advisory Committee (RAC)
- Secretary's Advisory Committee on Genetic Testing (SACGT)

Note. Based on information from Janson-Smith, 2002.

---

concerns with public health needs. Genetic information presents unique bioethical and psychosocial issues to healthcare providers. The CTN plays an important role in many aspects of providing care for those undergoing genetic testing and in the management of genetic information. Maintaining an awareness of the complex issues and implications surrounding advancements in genetics can enhance the nurse's ability to advocate for others as an educator, clinician, consultant, and researcher (Bove, Fry, & MacDonald, 1997; Scanlon & Fibison, 1995).

References

Adams, A. (2003, December 24). *Genetic health. What is genetic counseling?* Retrieved October 4, 2005, from http://www.genetichealth.com/Resources_What_Is_Genetic_Counseling.shtml

American College of Medical Genetics. (1995a). ACMG statement. Statement on storage and use of genetic materials. American College of Medical Genetics Storage of Genetics Materials Committee. *American Journal of Human Genetics, 57,* 1499–1500.

American College of Medical Genetics. (1995b). Points to consider: Ethical, legal, and psychological implications of genetic testing in children and adolescents. *American Journal of Human Genetics, 57,* 1233–1241.

American Society of Human Genetics Board of Directors. (1996). Statement of informed consent for genetic research. *American Journal of Human Genetics, 59,* 471–474.

Bove, C.M., Fry, S.T., & MacDonald, D.J. (1997). Presymptomatic and predisposition genetic testing: Ethical and social considerations. *Seminars in Oncology Nursing, 13,* 135–140.

Clayton, E.W., Steinberg, K.K., Khoury, M.J., Thompson, E., Andrews, L., Kahn, M.J., et al. (1995). Informed consent for genetic research on stored tissue samples. *JAMA, 274,* 1786–1793.

Collins, F. (2003). *A brief primer on genetic testing.* Retrieved September 27, 2005, from http://www.genome.gov/page.cfm?pageID=10506784

International Society of Nurses in Genetics. (2003, September 19). *Access to genomic healthcare: The role of the nurse* [Position statement]. Retrieved October 31, 2007, from http://www.isong.org/about/ps_genomic.cfm

Janson-Smith, D. (2002, July 19). *Human genetics: Key US regulatory and advisory bodies.* Retrieved September 21, 2005, from http://genome.wellcome.ac.uk/doc_WTD021013.html

Koliopoulos, S. (2001). *Predictive genetic testing—Do you really want to know your future? The topic in-depth.* Retrieved October 1, 2005, from http://www.dnafiles.org/about/pgm4/topic.html

Lahl, L. (2005, April 22). *Biological specimens and personal data.* Retrieved October 1, 2005, from http://www.uh.edu/pharmacy/ohrp/ppt/Linda_lahl-biological_specimens_and_personal_data_Houston.ppt

Miller, P.S. (2005). *Analyzing genetic discrimination in the workplace.* Retrieved September 22, 2005, from http://www.eeoc.gov

National Human Genome Research Institute. (1998, September 19). *Genetic information and the workplace.* Retrieved September 22, 2005, from http://www.genome.gov/10001732

National Human Genome Research Institute. (2005a). *Ethical legal and social implications research program.* Retrieved September 22, 2005, from http://www.genome.gov/page.cfm?pageID=10002329

National Human Genome Research Institute. (2005b). *Genetic discrimination in health insurance.* Retrieved September 22, 2005, from http://www.genome.gov/page.cfm?pageID=10002328

National Human Genome Research Institute. (2005c). *An overview of the Human Genome Project.* Retrieved September 22, 2005, from http://www.genome.gov/12011238

National Human Genome Research Institute. (2005d). *Privacy and discrimination in genetics* Retrieved September 22, 2005, from http://www.genome.gov/10002077

Office for Protection from Research Risks. (1997, November 7). *Issues to consider in the research use of stored or data tissues.* Retrieved October 4, 2005, from http://www.hhs.gov/ohrp/humansubjects/guidance/reposit.htm

Oncology Nursing Society. (2004, October). *The role of the oncology nurse in cancer genetic counseling* [Position statement]. Retrieved September 22, 2005, from http://www.ons.org/publications/positions/CancerGeneticCounseling.shtml

Rice, W. (2005). *What is genetic testing?* (Lawrence Berkley Memorial Library). Retrieved October 9, 2005, from http://www.mydna.com/resources/tests/alltests/topics/tests/genetics/whatgt.html

Scanlon, C., & Fibison, W. (1995). *Managing genetic information: Implications for nursing practice.* Washington, DC: American Nurses Association.

University of California, San Diego, Human Research Protections Program. (1997). *Issues on DNA and informed consent.* Retrieved October 1, 2005, from http://irb.ucsd.edu

U.S. Department of Energy Office of Science. (2004a). *Frequently asked questions.* Retrieved September 21, 2005, from http://www.ornl.gov/sci/techresources/Human_Genome/faq/faqs1.shtml

U.S. Department of Energy Office of Science. (2004b). *Genetics privacy and legislation.* Retrieved September 21, 2005, from http://www.ornl.gov/sci/techresources/Human_Genome/elsi/legislat.shtml

CHAPTER 34
Pharmacoeconomic Studies

Patricia McLaughlin, RN, MSN, AOCN®

Introduction

The recent movement in health care to cut costs is strong. Many feel that as a result of this, quality is being compromised. This cost cutting and possible compromised quality particularly is experienced by the older adult population, which comprises 12.7% of the total population. The 65-and-older age group consumes more than one-third of total prescriptions. As the "baby boomers" (those born between 1946 and 1964) are aging (U.S. Census Bureau, 2005), the 65-and-older age group is increasing by 6,000 people every day (Zagaria, 2004).

In the current healthcare climate, cost cutting is going to continue. The goal of those who work in healthcare professions, however, is to cut costs without sacrificing quality. Evidence-based studies must be done, and these need to be based on scientific methodologies in the area of pharmacology and economics. This chapter will explore what pharmacoeconomics is, what methods are used to conduct studies, and the role the clinical trial nurse (CTN) plays in this process.

Pharmacoeconomic Principles

According to Zagaria (2004), pharmacoeconomics is "the discipline of placing a value on drug therapy and seeks to describe and analyze the costs of drug therapy to the healthcare system and society" (p. 34). In the past, pharmacoeconomics only dealt with costs and safety (Reeder, 1995). Today, outcomes such as the impact of drug therapy on society are a major consideration.

Reeder (1995) described the economic, clinical, and humanistic outcomes as a model for planning and conducting a pharmacoeconomic evaluation. A combination of these three factors is used to examine the value of a drug. *Clinical outcomes* relate to medical events that result from disease or treatment. *Economic outcomes* involve direct, indirect (e.g., cost of nursing time), and intangible costs, such as pain, suffering, and grief. Last, but equally important, are *humanistic outcomes.* These involve the consequences of treatment or disease on the functional status of the individual or quality-of-life issues such as psychosocial functioning, patient preferences, and patient satisfaction (Zagaria, 2004).

Pharmacoeconomic Methods

Zagaria (2004) defined pharmacoeconomic research as "the process of identifying, measuring, and comparing the costs, risks, and benefits of programs, services, or therapies, and determining which alternative produces the best health outcome for the resource invested" (p. 33). Pharmacoeconomic methods can be viewed from two perspectives, economic and humanistic. Five types of analyses can be performed. The four that are most widely used are cost-minimization analysis, cost-effective analysis, cost-utility analysis, and cost-benefit analysis (Beltz & Yee, 1998).

In *cost-minimization*, the basic assumption is that all outcomes are the same. Costs are studied as dollars. This is the simplest form of analysis and looks for the least expensive alternative. The problem with this method is that if the basic assumption is wrong, then the results are not accurate.

In *cost-effectiveness* analysis, costs are expressed "as the numerator in monetary units (e.g., dollars) and effectiveness is expressed in the denominator in some unit of effectiveness" (Beltz & Yee, 1998, p. 6). The units of effectiveness are the clinical outcomes like those used in clinical research or practice. An example of this is survival (i.e., life-years gained). A drawback of this method is that a number of ways exist to express effectiveness. The effec-

The author would like to acknowledge Maribeth Hohenstein, RN, BSN, OCN®, CCRC, for her contribution that remains unchanged from the first edition.

tiveness of a given treatment may vary based on different diseases (Beltz & Yee).

Cost-utility analysis takes into account the effectiveness of a particular treatment or drug measured in quality-adjusted life-years in analyzing cost-effectiveness. The major advantage to this model is that it looks at both mortality as well as morbidity. Cost-utility analysis is especially useful in evaluating new chemotherapeutic agents because some treatments do not extend life but may have fewer associated side effects. Although this type of analysis is very useful, it is not easy to do. Cost-utility data usually are not collected in clinical trials because of the additional costs associated with data collection and analysis (Beltz & Yee, 1998).

Cost-benefit analysis expresses costs and benefits in the same units (e.g., cost versus a decrease in the number of disability days). Although this model is simple to use, it is difficult to actually assign a measure to benefits (Beltz & Yee, 1998). Assumptions and biases are inherent in this type of analysis and therefore decrease its effectiveness.

In addition to the four methods listed previously, Zagaria (2004) described one additional economic method and three humanistic methods. A *cost-of-illness* evaluation involves the analysis of the cost of a particular disease on the patient population. From a humanistic perspective, health-related quality of life, patient preferences, and patient satisfaction are all taken into account.

Interpretation of Results of Pharmaco-economic Studies

According to Beltz and Yee (1998), "When an intervention is considered to be cost effective, it implies that the therapeutic benefit is worth the cost" (p. 7). Therefore, although the intervention may not necessarily be cost *saving*, it may be the most cost effective because of the benefit that is gained; hence, the humanistic outcomes are being considered. It is very important that the results of pharmacoeconomic studies be carefully scrutinized. The investigators, inaccurate assumptions, and sources of the data collected, for example, may influence the results of the studies. If the studies are conducted by pharmaceutical companies, as many are, they may be biased so that the outcomes look favorable. It is critical that those who have experience in and a clear understanding of pharmacoeconomics analyze the results. One tool that is used to test the "robustness of the results and conclusions" is *sensitivity analysis* (Coleman, Reddy, Quercia, & Gousse, 2003, p. 382). If the results do not change using a wide range of variables, then confidence in the results of the study is enhanced (Coleman et al.).

The Use of Clinical Research Trials in Conducting Pharmacoeconomic Evaluation

According to the International Society for Pharmacoeconomics and Outcomes Research (ISPOR) Health Science Strategy Ad Hoc Group (n.d.), neither purely pharmacoeconomic methods nor methods used in clinical trials are sufficient to answer the questions involving decisions about which drugs should be used for a given illness. According to ISPOR, the following four key issues need to be considered:

- When is it appropriate to use randomized clinical trials to be the primary basis of decisions regarding the question of value?
- What changes in the design of clinical trials would improve their usefulness in the pharmacoeconomic and health economics decision-making process?
- When is it appropriate to use observational trials as an assessment of value?
- What changes in the design of observational studies would make them more useful in decisions regarding economic value?

The Role of the Clinical Trial Nurse in Pharmacoeconomics

Because economic analysis may be included in a clinical trial, it is important that the CTN understand the role he or she plays in helping to carry out the study. In the past, clinical trials were predominately concerned with the safety and clinical efficacy of the treatment being tested. Now, policy makers also are concerned about analyzing the cost associated with the outcomes. A pharmacoeconomic study may be designed as a primary study or as a companion or secondary study that is incorporated into a treatment trial. Regardless of the type of pharmacoeconomic study, the regulations related to obtaining informed consent must be followed.

The following is an example of a statement that may be included in a consent document in which the economic analysis is a secondary objective of a phase III study.

> In addition, an analysis will be done to compare the potential economic benefits of Drug A to Drug B. This pharmacoeconomic analysis (an analysis of the economic value of a drug) requires that the investigator of this study or his/her designee obtain a copy of your billing records for the duration of the study. Your name will be coded on these records to keep your identity strictly confidential. You will receive no personal benefit from this economic analysis.

Researchers must obtain institutional review board approval for the pharmacoeconomic study being conducted. In addition, the objectives of the study must be fully disclosed to potential participants. The methods used to collect the information must be explained to the patient. This may involve analysis of medical bills, number of procedures and physician visits, and the cost associated with side effects resulting from the treatment.

The collection of billing information could potentially involve a great deal of time on the part of the research staff. When different offices and facilities (e.g., radiology, laboratory) need to be contacted in order to obtain information, the time required for this should be factored into the analysis as an indirect cost related to the study.

Summary

Clinical research is an exciting vocation for the CTN. With the pharmaceutical industry rapidly developing new drugs and new treatments for patients with cancer, there is no loss for alternate treatment options. As new therapies are developed, methods are needed to compare them against existing therapies. By including a pharmacoeconomic analysis, economic, therapeutic, and humanistic outcomes can be reviewed with side-by-side comparisons of the standard care versus the investigative agent. Pharmacoeconomic studies will help to improve the understanding of the costs and benefits of clinical therapies.

References

Beltz, S., & Yee, G. (1998). Pharmacoeconomics of cancer therapy. *Cancer Control: Journal of the Moffitt Cancer Center, 5*(5). Retrieved October 14, 2005, from http://www.moffitt.usf.edu/pubs/ccj/v5n5/article4.html

Coleman, C.I., Reddy, P., Quercia, R.A., & Gousse, G. (2003). Cost-benefit analysis of a pharmacy-managed medication assistance program for hospitalized indigent patients. *American Journal of Health-System Pharmacy, 60,* 378–382.

International Society for Pharmacoeconomics and Outcomes Research Health Science Strategy Ad Hoc Group. (n.d.). *Health science strategy.* Retrieved October 13, 2005, from http://www.ispor.org/workpaper/healthscience/report.asp

Reeder, C. (1995). Overview of pharmacoeconomics and pharmaceutical outcomes evaluations. *American Journal of Health-System Pharmacy, 52*(Suppl. 4), 5–8.

U.S. Census Bureau. (2005). *Data sets.* Retrieved September 21, 2005, from http://www.census.gov/main/www/cen2000.html

Zagaria, M. (2004). Pharmacoeconomics in senior care. *U.S. Pharmacist, 29*(6), 32–37.

CHAPTER 35
Nursing Companion Studies

Joyce M. Tokarsky, RN, MSN

Introduction

Survival rates for patients with cancer have increased dramatically over the past 35 years, which is attributed primarily to earlier diagnosis and treatment, as well as the development of more accurate diagnostic and therapeutic measures. As the number of patients surviving cancer far beyond the end of treatment increases, oncology health-care professionals will continue to monitor and care for an increasing number of patients living with cancer as a chronic illness. These individuals and their families will present unique physiologic and psychological situations that will challenge oncology nurses.

Because clinical advances for the treatment of cancer continue to outpace the development of new nursing theory, a clear set of research priorities is needed to focus nurse researchers' efforts to fill existing gaps in practice knowledge. All patients must be cared for with knowledge that is based on a solid scientific foundation, and the best knowledge available serves as the basis for nursing interventions (Haberman, 1997).

A study conducted by Bakker, Trottier, and McChesney (1997) demonstrated that oncology nurses in the United States value nursing research and perceive a role within the research arena for nurses. Those participating in this study identified the major barrier to conducting nursing research as poor administrative and collegial support. Topics for nursing research can be identified from the results of research priority surveys or from issues that arise as priorities within individual care settings. Another study conducted in Queensland, Australia, surveyed members of the Oncology Nurses Group of Queensland and was aimed at describing research experience, attitudes, opinions, priorities, and strategies for developing cancer nursing research. Similar to the U.S. nurses, they believed that nursing research should be a priority; however, very few nurses were actually involved in developing research protocols, participating in research, and publishing their findings (Yates et al., 2002).

Oncology nurses have participated in numerous research priority surveys conducted by the Oncology Nursing Society since 1981. Topics ranked by oncology nurses as research priorities can be found in Table 35-1. Because an increased number of patients and families are living with cancer as a chronic illness, a novel research area for nurses to explore includes the psychological impact on family and caregivers, which may include coping style, marital adjustment, and family functioning (Blanchard, Albrecht, & Ruckdeschel, 1997).

Nursing Companion Studies

Companion studies offer nurses the opportunity to conduct independent research within a supportive framework through collaboration with other investigators that will advance the specialty of oncology nursing. Nursing companion studies may be performed with a variety of disciplines but most often are associated with medical research. Two general types of companion studies exist: *collaborative* and *parallel*.

Collaborative Companion Studies

Collaborative companion studies are conducted in association with an ongoing medical study. These studies are initiated and implemented by a nurse researcher, although interdisciplinary effort by the nurse and physician investigator is imperative. In this situation, two or more studies are carried out jointly; subject accrual, day-to-day management, data collection, and analysis often overlap between the two. Collaborative studies are the most successful type of companion studies.

Parallel Companion Studies

A parallel companion study is one in which a nurse investigator implements a study as a result of a nursing concern that may have arisen from observations of patients enrolled in an ongoing medical study. Parallel studies usually address general nursing issues such as nausea, stomatitis, quality of life, fatigue, and pain (Ferrell & Cohen, 1991).

Table 35-1. Top 20 Research Priorities Ranked by Mean Importance Ratings for the Total Membership Sample, Adjusted for Doctorate Group Oversampling[a], With Comparisons to the 2000 Survey

Topic	Rank Order	X̄ Importance Rating[b] (SD)	2000 Survey Rank Order
Quality of life	1	1.52 (0.718)	2
Participation in decision making about treatment in advanced disease[c]	2	1.54 (0.701)	18
Patient/family education[c]	3	1.55 (0.742)	19
Participation in decision making about treatment[c]	4	1.58 (0.701)	43
Pain	5	1.59 (0.746)	1
Tobacco use and exposure[d]	6	1.60 (0.848)	–
Screening/early detection of cancer	7	1.60 (0.746)	3
Prevention of cancer/cancer risk reduction	8	1.61 (0.754)	4
Palliative care	9	1.62 (0.727)	17
Evidence-based practice	10	1.62 (0.810)	78
Nurses as advocates[d]	11	1.65 (0.773)	–
Fatigue/lack of energy	12	1.66 (0.773)	9
Cancer recurrence	13	1.67 (0.704)	20
Curative treatment/care[c]	14	1.67 (0.733)	37
Patient outcomes of cancer care[c]	15	1.67 (0.743)	8
Cognitive impairment/mental status changes[c]	16	1.67 (0.750)	70
Late effects of treatment[c]	17	1.68 (0.722)	24
Hospice/end of life	18	1.69 (0.790)	6
Initial cancer diagnosis[d]	19	1.69 (0.764)	–
Ethical issues	20	1.70 (0.752)	10

[a] Adjusted by weighting to correct for oversampling of doctorally prepared nurses
[b] Scores ranged from 1 (extremely important) to 5 (not at all important).
[c] Item wording was not identical to the 2000 survey.
[d] New question, not asked in the 2000 survey

Note. From "Oncology Nursing Society Year 2004 Research Priorities Survey," by A.M. Berger, D.L. Berry, K.A. Christopher, A.L. Greene, S. Maliski, K.K. Swenson, et al., 2005, *Oncology Nursing Forum, 32,* p. 285. Copyright 2005 by the Oncology Nursing Society. Reprinted with permission.

Barriers and Benefits of Companion Studies

Regardless of the type of study conducted, the success of companion studies depends a great deal on positive interdisciplinary collaboration. Lancaster (1985) first described the importance of teamwork in carrying out these types of studies by introducing the "six C's" of companion research. She defined these characteristics as contribution, compatibility, communication, consensus, commitment, and credit. For a companion study to be successful, all healthcare members involved in the research project must embrace these attributes, have the ability to work well together, possess mutual respect for each other's efforts, and be coauthors on any publication. A nurse researcher may initiate a companion study (as an investigator) or be a member of a multidisciplinary team designing a companion study.

Companion studies have many potential benefits, but barriers to conducting these studies exist, as well. Researchers must be aware of the potential challenges and benefits prior to embarking on this endeavor. Benefits of conducting companion studies include gaining access to a larger population of subjects than would be available to nurse researchers conducting an independent study. Through collaboration, access to subjects is enhanced, and opportunities for enrollment at multiple sites may be possible. Patient accrual, therefore, might be accomplished in a shorter period of time, or a larger and more diverse sample size may be made a reality.

Frequently, companion studies can be conducted at a lower cost because expenses can be shared between studies. Shared expenses might pertain to patient screening, accrual, and follow-up; data collection and management; and blood sampling.

Finally, another advantage to conducting companion research studies is the opportunity for interdisciplinary collaboration. These studies allow novice investigators to take an active role in the research process, affording them an opportunity they otherwise might not have had to evaluate patient outcomes. Companion studies also can provide a challenge to the experienced researcher because they may extend beyond the individual's scope of research.

Despite these advantages, companion studies also have potential drawbacks. Although medical studies and companion studies may be implemented at the same time, they are, in reality, two separate trials based on complete and separate protocols and must be capable of standing alone in terms of scientific merit and patient safety. Each study requires extensive, comprehensive planning before implementation, just as if each had been implemented independently. Each must meet the institution's Research and Human Rights Committee requirements and receive approval. A principal investigator who will assume accountability for the study must be identified for each study. When planning these studies, investigators must keep in mind that although some costs may be shared, each study requires a separate budget. Each also must have a time frame established before initiation and be monitored closely. Analysis of study results, ownership of the data, and plans for dissemination through publication or presentation must be negotiated in advance.

Often, other investigators may view companion studies as being less important than the medical study, but these studies are based on a complete and separate protocol with unique and valid study questions or hypotheses, objectives, framework, methodology, and outcomes. These are the studies that move nursing care forward and improve the care that patients receive.

Currently, only a handful of national and/or regional nursing companion studies are actively recruiting patients. These include protocols sponsored by the National Surgical Adjuvant Breast and Bowel Project, the Eastern Cooperative Oncology Group, the Southwest Oncology Group, the Radiation Therapy Oncology Group, the National Institute of Mental Health, the National Cancer Institute and many universities within the nursing program. Table 35-2 lists examples of active protocols in January 2007.

As evidenced by the paucity of available national and regional nursing companion studies, much room exists for growth. These types of studies must be conducted at both the local level within individual care settings and in conjunction with cooperative group clinical trials. All levels of nursing staff should be encouraged and mentored to accomplish meaningful research. Those institutions that participate in national or regional clinical trials must actively accrue patients to companion studies that will assist investigators in understanding how treatments affect patients' quality of life or the effectiveness of particular nursing interventions. Such studies promote the discipline of nursing.

Table 35-2. Examples of Regional/National Nursing Companion Studies, January 2007

Title	Sponsor
Quality of Life in Younger Breast Cancer Survivors (E2Z04)	ECOG
A Quality of Life Substudy of Subjects Enrolled in "A Clinical Trial of Adjuvant Therapy Comparing Six Cycles of 5-Fluorouracil, Epirubicin, and Cyclophosphamide (FEC) to Four Cycles of Adriamycin and Cyclophosphamide (AC), in Patients with Node-Negative Breast Cancer" (NSABP B-36)	NSABP
Study to Assess Compliance with Long Term Mercaptopurine Treatment in Young People with Acute Lymphoblastic Leukemia in Remission	COG
Musical Therapy or Book Discussion in Improving Quality of Life in Young Patients Undergoing Stem Cell Transplant	COG
Evaluating Quality of Life in Patients Enrolled in "A Phase III Randomized Open-Label Study Comparing Gemcitabine Plus Cetuximab (IMC-C225) Versus Gemcitabine as First-Line Therapy of Patients With Advanced Pancreatic Cancer" (SWOG S0205)	SWOG
Patient Reported Outcomes in Long Term Survivors with Colon and Rectal Cancer (LTS-01)	NSABP

ECOG—Eastern Cooperative Oncology Group; NSABP—National Surgical Adjuvant Breast and Bowel Project; SWOG—Southwest Oncology Group

Summary

Nursing companion studies have the potential to advance nursing research and ultimately nursing practice. Nurses in all settings should be encouraged to participate in the research process. More comprehensive information regarding cancer therapy and its potential toxicities can be gained through nursing companion studies that are based on solid research procedures.

References

Bakker, D.A., Trottier, T., & McChesney, C. (1997). Clinical oncology nurses' perceptions of research. *Canadian Oncology Nursing Journal, 7*, 150–161.

Blanchard, C.G., Albrecht, T.L., & Ruckdeschel, J.C. (1997). The crisis of cancer: Psychological impact on family caregivers. *Oncology, 11*, 189–194.

Ferrell, B.R., & Cohen, M.Z. (1991). Companion studies. *Seminars in Oncology Nursing, 7*, 252–259.

Haberman, M. (1997). Advancing cancer nursing through nursing research. In S.L. Groenwald, M.H. Frogge, M. Goodman, & C.H. Yarbro (Eds.), *Cancer nursing: Principles and practice* (4th ed., pp. 1678–1690). Sudbury, MA: Jones and Bartlett.

Lancaster, J. (1985). The perils and joys of collaborative research. *Nursing Outlook, 33*, 231–238.

Yates, P., Baker, D., Barrett, L., Christie, L., Dewar, A.M., Middleton, R., et al. (2002). Cancer nursing research in Queensland, Australia: Barriers, priorities, and strategies for progress. *Cancer Nursing, 25*, 167–180.

SECTION VIII.

Off-Treatment Follow-Up

CHAPTER 36
Off-Treatment Protocol Considerations

CHAPTER 37
Long-Term Follow-Up

CHAPTER 38
Off-Treatment Documentation

CHAPTER 36
Off-Treatment Protocol Considerations

Mary Ellen Haisfield-Wolfe, RN, MS, OCN®

Introduction

Study participants must abide by many post-treatment requirements. In most institutions, the research staff is responsible for coordinating effective patient follow-up. This chapter addresses study and institutional review board (IRB) considerations, data management considerations, and patient considerations during the off-treatment study phase. The terms *closed to accrual, off treatment, off study,* and *study termination* can be confusing because they are closely related. A definition of each term is provided in Figure 36-1, as an understanding of these terms can guide the clinical trial nurse (CTN) in decisions regarding follow-up, form submission, and regulatory requirements.

Study and Institutional Review Board Considerations

Regulatory issues involving IRBs, informed consent, toxicity reporting, maintenance of accurate records, and drug accountability logs continue when patients are off treatment but are still being followed for late effects or survival. The primary purpose of follow-up is to ensure continued medical surveillance and to collect accurate long-term data. These data ultimately will provide researchers with information upon which to base future treatment decisions.

According to the *Code of Federal Regulations* (CFR), 21 CFR Part 56, Institutional Review Boards, any clinical investigation that involves human subjects started after July 21, 1981, is required to follow the U.S. Food and Drug Administration (FDA) regulations for IRB requirements (FDA, 2007). An IRB review of research protocols must continue to follow FDA guidelines to protect the rights and welfare of human subjects.

Continuation reviews and reapprovals are required at various intervals appropriate to the degree of risk for the

protocol but not less frequently than once a year (FDA, 2007). The determination of the frequency and extent of the

---

Figure 36-1. Definitions of Terms

- **Closed to accrual:** No additional subjects will be enrolled in the study. Study activity is ongoing and may include interventions and interactions with the subject or continued use of the drug or device or follow-up (Johns Hopkins Medicine Institutional Review Boards, 2007).
- **Off treatment:** The individual study participant is no longer on the study treatment (medication or device), whether the treatment ended according to the protocol, the individual was taken off because of an adverse event, or the subject decided to withdraw from the treatment. The defining issue is that the subject has stopped the study treatment (Stone, 2006).
- **Off study:** The individual study participant no longer is on the study protocol, whether the patient completed the study per protocol, withdrew consent to continue the protocol, or was taken off the study for some other reason. The defining issue is that the subject will not have any additional study procedures or treatment. The participant has completed the study activities outlined in the protocol (M. Michaels, personal communication, May 16, 2006).
- **Study completion:** This term is essentially the same as off study. Study completion is sometimes referred to as study discontinuation. The term also is used when the individual study participant completes the study per protocol (M. Michaels, personal communication, May 16, 2006).
- **Study termination:** All the study participants have completed their final visit and follow-up at the study site. All data collection from all subjects is finalized. At this time, a final report (study termination report) usually is submitted to the sponsor or sponsor representative (Johns Hopkins Medicine Institutional Review Boards, 2007).
- **Study closure:** The study is open at the site until a study closure report is submitted and received by the institutional review board (Western Institutional Review Board, 2006). The sponsor or sponsor representative has concluded all study activities and has indicated that the study is closed at the site (Western Institutional Review Board). For studies conducted under federalwide assurance, all data analyses are completed at this time.

The author would like to acknowledge Maria Karigan, RN, MSN, CCRC, for her contribution that remains unchanged from the first edition.

continuation review must be sufficient to ensure continued protection of research participants until the study is terminated at the site. Consequently, continuation study review continues until the study is terminated at the site. IRB reporting requirements for continuing review are specific to each institution and may include the number of patients on study, participant withdrawals, adverse events, data safety monitoring reports, new protocol amendments, protocol violation reporting, and changes to the study (e.g., new personnel or forms) (Western Institutional Review Board, 2006). Chapter 13 includes more information about IRBs.

Continuation reviews serve many purposes. They help to ensure the continued protection of human participants and to evaluate the continued quality of a study. A copy of the approved protocol and any subsequent revisions must be provided to the treating physician(s), the pharmacy, and other healthcare personnel who use the protocol. The most current protocol outlines time frames and schedules for the study, off-treatment, and follow-up requirements.

Data Management Considerations

In addition to the protocol requirements for physical evaluations, data management requirements also must be followed. When protocol therapy is completed, patients are followed according to a protocol-specific calendar. Figure 36-2 provides a hypothetical example of a follow-up study calendar. Most protocols outline the form submission schedule required during follow-up. Off-study summaries, protocol-specific follow-up forms, flow sheets, and toxicity forms are examples of documents submitted to study groups and/or sponsors at specified intervals. Side effects, toxicities, and all treatment-related procedures must be completely documented as outlined in the protocol. In some cases, the effects of the intervention and/or the drug toxicities may last quite a while, even after the treatment has been discontinued. Often, the CTN or data manager is the first to be aware of physical changes, toxicities, protocol violations, or other events requiring further attention (Ocker & Pawlik Plank, 2000).

Long-term patient follow-up can be challenging. Some study groups require long-term patient follow-up data as long as the patient is alive, regardless of whether the patient received or completed treatment. In addition, institutions must remain committed to patient follow-up—even if funding or membership status within that group changes (Southwest Oncology Group [SWOG], 2007). These issues related to data collection can compete with the demanding workload and responsibilities of the CTN.

Awareness of follow-up schedules and off-study requirements, and careful completion of necessary forms, are crucial. Some patients are followed for survival status only. Other patients are considered off treatment, off study drugs, or off protocol therapy and are followed according to the specified protocol requirements. In addition to identifying treatment-related toxicities, study documentation summarizes a patient's status at any given point in time. If a patient dies while on study follow-up, a death summary is completed, and the institution's IRB is notified. If it is suspected that a patient's cause of death is protocol-related, an adverse event form and other appropriate forms also must be submitted to the study-coordinating center and the institution's IRB. Because long-term survival data are crucial, submission of this information is vital to accurate analysis of the therapy under study (Gordis, 1996).

Patient Issues

The patient's cooperation and compliance once off treatment are essential to overall study results. Research personnel must encourage and support the patient and family members to continue with study protocol requirements during this phase (Grant & De Pew, 1999).

During patient follow-up, the CTN serves as both a patient advocate and as a liaison between the physician's office and the patient. This ensures proper clinical trial conduct and adherence to follow-up schedules. Thus, providing a current protocol calendar to the primary physician and notifying him or her of any revisions or amendments specific to follow-up care are important. Sending friendly reminders regarding tests, evaluations, or other specific protocol requirements prior to patient appointments can help the physician to adhere to protocol specifications.

As outlined in all protocols, patients are required to return at specified intervals to provide follow-up data. The CTN must clearly explain to the patient the rationale for this follow-up compliance. Some institutions use protocol-specific guidelines or specially developed educational tools that outline off-treatment protocol requirements. Only the patient and the physician's office can use these. One excellent example of a study educational resource is the National Surgical Adjuvant Breast and Bowel Project's (1997) *Breast Cancer Prevention Trial Participant's Notebook*, which is designed to help patients to comply with the additional two years of follow-up required once study medication is completed.

Research staff use a wide variety of data retrieval methods to obtain and receive off-treatment information. Sources of data include, but are not limited to, patient telephone calls, e-mail communications, patient progress notes, medical records from outside facilities or outpatient clinics, tumor registries, state or central registries, direct contact with the patient and/or family members, protocol-specific questionnaires, primary care physicians, referring physicians, nursing home records, visiting nurses' associations, and death reports. In addition to these resources, information available via the Internet also can provide research personnel with pertinent patient information that otherwise would be difficult to obtain. One example of a useful, up-to-date Internet database is the U.S. Social Security Death Index at www.ancestry.com/ssdi/advanced.htm (SWOG, 2007).

Audits should be performed routinely to ensure study integrity and quality data. Types of audits are self-audit,

Data Points	Post Treatment						
Figure 36-2. Off-Treatment Follow-Up Study Calendar							
	Week 1 Follow-Up	Week 2 Follow-Up	Week 3 Follow-Up	3-Month Follow-Up	6-Month Follow-Up	Year 1 Follow-Up	Annual Follow-Up Year 2–Year 10
Clinical assessment							
Physical exam	X	X	X	X	X	X	X
ECOG/Zubrod performance status	X	X	X	X	X	X	X
Weight	X	X	X	X	X	X	X
Vital status and recurrence assessment					X	X	X
Radiology							
Chest x-ray			X		X		
CT scan						X	X
Sample collection							
Serum and plasma						X	
Safety assessments							
Adverse events	X	X	X	X	X	X	
Concomitant therapies and medications					X	X	

CT—computed tomography; ECOG—Eastern Cooperative Oncology Group

institutional audit, or an audit by an outside monitor. The need for continuous monitoring of quality control procedures cannot be overemphasized (see Chapter 47). All efforts must be made to ensure the accuracy and validity of the results (Hulley et al., 2001).

Summary

Continued long-term off-treatment follow-up data must be submitted in a timely manner. Regulatory compliance during all phases of the study will facilitate a successful trial, and accurate, complete data are crucial for final study analysis. Reports of unusual results, toxicities, or adverse reactions could lead to early protocol closure. In addition, survival data must be reported promptly. Components of successful clinical trial implementation include a consistent, dedicated research team, a prudent principal investigator, and a patient/family with adequate knowledge and support. Individuals who remain involved in the ongoing care of the patient can help to ensure that off-treatment, protocol-specific requirements will be followed accurately and consistently (Hulley et al., 2001).

References

Gordis, L. (1996). *Epidemiology.* Philadelphia: Saunders.

Grant, J.S., & De Pew, D.D. (1999). Recruiting and retaining research participants for a clinical intervention study. *Journal of Neuroscience Nursing, 31,* 357–362.

Hulley, S.B., Cummings, S.R., Browner, W.S., Grady, D., Hearst, D., & Newman, T.B. (2001). *Designing clinical research: An epidemiologic approach* (2nd ed.). Philadelphia: Lippincott Williams & Wilkins.

Johns Hopkins Medicine Institutional Review Boards. (2007). *Institutional review boards.* Retrieved March 21, 2007, from http://irb.jhmi.edu

National Surgical Adjuvant Breast and Bowel Project. (1997). *Breast cancer prevention trial participant's notebook: A guide for participants who have completed five years of study.* Pittsburgh, PA: Author.

Ocker, B.M., & Pawlik Plank, D. (2000). The research nurse in a clinic-based oncology research setting. *Cancer Nursing, 23,* 286–292.

Southwest Oncology Group. (2007). *Clinical research associate (CRA) manual.* Retrieved March 21, 2007, from https://gill.crab.org/txwb/CRAManual.aspx

Stone, J. (2006). *Conducting clinical research.* Cumberland, MD: Mountainside MD Press.

U.S. Food and Drug Administration. (2007). *Code of federal regulations (Title 21, Vol. 1, Part 56).* Retrieved March 21, 2007, from http://www.accessdata.fda.gov.scripts/cdrh/cfdocs/cfcfr/CFRSearch.cfm?fr=56.104

Western Institutional Review Board. (2006). *Study closure.* Retrieved April 28, 2006, from http://www.wirb.com/shell.php?content=content/quick_notify_wirb

CHAPTER 37
Long-Term Follow-Up

Tasha D. Hall, RN, MS, OCN®, CCRP

Introduction

An adverse event of a drug or device approved by the U.S. Food and Drug Administration can be identified after the drug or device has been on the market for many years. The need for long-term assessment of study participants for adverse events is reinforced by the identification of increased cardiovascular risk from COX-2 inhibitors (Bresalier et al., 2005; Solomon et al., 2006). Treatment studies typically include requirements for long-term follow-up of study participants to assess for late-occurring adverse events. The end points, or objectives section, of a research protocol determine what length of follow-up is required for the study. If a study has survival listed as an end point, the subjects will be followed until death. Examples of long-term follow-up end points are survival, time to recurrence, and determination of long-term toxicities. Phase I, II, III, and IV studies have the potential for long-term follow-up. Specific case report forms are used to capture the follow-up data. An example of a follow-up schedule is provided in Figure 37-1.

Methods of Contact

In the era of modern technology, several methods exist for contacting the patient to retrieve follow-up data. Telephone, fax, mail, or e-mail can be used to maintain communication with the patient. The clinical trial nurse (CTN) may contact the patient's physicians for follow-up information. When consenting a patient for a study with long-term follow-up requirements, recording the name and number of a family member or friend of the patient is important. The alternative contact person can be used if the nurse is unable to contact the patient. If the patient does not respond to mail, the information/requests can be sent by certified mail. This allows for tracking of the mail and serves as documentation that every attempt was made to contact the patient. If a patient does not respond to mail or the telephone and an alternative contact person is not available, then the CTN must become creative. Sug-

Figure 37-1. Example of a Follow-Up Schedule
Year 1—At 6, 9, and 12 months
Year 2—Every 3 months
Years 3, 4, and 5—Every 6 months
Year 6 and beyond*—Annually
*At progression/relapse; at death

gestions for addressing these situations include contacting the patient's physician to learn if medical records were transferred to another physician and checking community resources, such as the board of elections, city directories, or the bureau of traffic safety (MacLachlan, 1988). The ease of coordinating a patient's follow-up care is dependent on the patient's level of compliance.

To ensure compliance with the Health Insurance Portability and Accountability Act (HIPAA), information outlining the length of follow-up and how the CTN will be contacting the patient after active treatment on a study is completed should be described in detail in the patient consent form. A patient may withdraw from a study at any time. Under HIPAA, the subject must withdraw in writing to revoke authorization of the use of the patient's personal health information. Once a subject has revoked authorization, no new data can be collected or submitted to a sponsor on that subject (Woodin, 2004).

Compliance

Compliance has a variety of definitions and is defined here as following the instructions of the coordinator as indicated by the protocol. A woman who met the requirements for follow-up by having yearly mammograms, clinical breast examinations, and gynecologic examinations as required by most breast cancer protocols is an example of a compliant patient in a breast cancer study. When screening patients for participation in a study, compliance cannot be determined by examination of demographic data. Patients who have a history of missing physician appointments or failing to have prescriptions filled may not be compliant with study treatment or follow-up. The CTN should work closely with the participant before enrollment and during the trial to increase the patient's compliance with long-term follow-up (Woodin, 2004). Establishment of an open and honest relationship will assist with patient retention and compliance throughout the study.

Examples of Areas Related to the Follow-Up of the Patient's Compliance

Several follow-up activities are dependent on a patient's compliance. Patients need to continue to report adverse events as they occur during the follow-up portion of the study. Failure of a patient to report adverse events that occurred in the recent past or between physician appointments can greatly affect the collection of long-term toxicity information. The key is open communication between CTN and patient. Patients also need to be encouraged to report any physician visits other than those with members of their healthcare team. A physician other than the oncologist may order testing that is not required by the study. For many studies, such data need to be captured on follow-up forms. If an outside physician performs a study requirement, the CTN needs to know so that the test is not repeated unnecessarily. Sometimes outside testing reveals adverse events. For example, an unscheduled complete blood count may reveal anemia.

Patients need to be compliant with the study schedule by attending scheduled appointments and testing. The CTN assists patients in completing follow-up care and ensures that they do not "fall between the cracks."

Methods to Ensure Compliance

Barriers can be encountered when trying to ensure that follow-up requirements are completed and that data are retrieved. Several strategies can be used to ensure that study requirements are met. The most valuable action a CTN can take when initiating a patient on a study that requires follow-up is to educate the patient about the necessity of adherence to study requirements. By explaining the objectives of the study to the patient, the CTN increases the patient's active participation in reaching the goals of the study.

Patients are sometimes referred to large medical centers or large practices for participation in protocols. Some patients choose to be followed by their local physician after the completion of study therapy and not the oncologist associated with the study. In this situation, maintaining communication with the local physician throughout the course of protocol therapy is important. When protocol therapy begins, having the patient sign a consent form for release of information from the local physician to the institution where the study therapy is being performed is useful.

Providing the patient with a calendar that indicates when long-term follow-up requirements are scheduled helps with patient compliance. This calendar can be used as a reminder of appointments and for recording long-term toxicities. Mailing personal notes one month before the studies are required can serve as a personal reminder.

Ensuring that the requests for follow-up testing adhere to the guidelines of the individual's insurance carrier or method of payment also can increase compliance. Sometimes it does not adhere; pharmacy companies often will pay for extra tests not considered to be standard operating procedure if the costs are included in the study budget. Being aware of what tests are being covered by the study budget will assist in managing follow-up testing. The insurance carrier often specifies where tests can be performed. A referral may be needed for all appointments. Prescription plans also are very specific. The CTN needs to consider these issues in the follow-up plan.

Requesting that patients keep a diary of adverse events during active treatment is common. The diary should be maintained through the follow-up portion of the study. Frequently, six months to one year passes between contacts with the protocol team, and adverse events can occur during this long time period that the patient may forget during a brief physician appointment. Asking the patient to keep a record of all appointments with physicians other than the oncologist is another strategy that will assist in gathering data that may have an impact on the study outcome.

Strategies in Protocol Development

If the CTN is able to review a protocol in the developmental stage, he or she should be proactive when it comes to defining long-term follow-up requirements. Ensuring that the follow-up requirements are outlined clearly in the study is imperative so that the requirements may be interpreted correctly. A chart is the clearest way to show what is required at specific time points. This is especially true for ongoing studies because the CTN enrolling the patient in the study may not be the same one working with the patient for the entire follow-up. Comparing objectives of the study to follow-up requirements should be done to ensure that the appropriate follow-up requirements are present in the protocol to meet the objectives of the study. The CTN's responsibility related to follow-up spans from the beginning of the protocol to the end, when all the study questions are answered.

Summary

Many protocol objectives can be met only with detailed and accurate long-term follow-up, and the CTN has a critical role in this process. Long-term follow-up can be very time-consuming for the CTN. Creating and maintaining a system to track follow-up patients and documentation at the initiation of a protocol will help to ensure success.

References

Bresalier, R.S., Sandler, R.S., Quan, H., Bolognese, J.A., Oxenius, B., Horgan, K., et al. (2005). Cardiovascular events associated with rofecoxib in a colorectal adenoma chemoprevention trial. *New England Journal of Medicine, 352,* 1092–1102.

MacLachlan, M. (1988). *Never say lost! A practical guide for establishing and maintaining long-term follow-up on clinical trials patients* (3rd ed.). Pittsburgh, PA: National Surgical Adjuvant Breast and Bowel Project.

Solomon, S.D., Pfeffer, M.A., McMurray, J.V., Fowler, R., Finn, P., Levin, B., et al. (2006). Effect of celecoxib on cardiovascular events and blood pressure in two trials for the prevention of colorectal adenomas. *Circulation, 114,* 1028–1035.

Woodin, K.E. (2004). *The CRC's guide to coordinating clinical research.* Boston: Thomson CenterWatch.

CHAPTER 38
Off-Treatment Documentation

Mary Ellen Haisfield-Wolfe, RN, MS, OCN®

Introduction

Documentation is important during all phases of a study. Missed data points or inaccurate information can threaten the integrity and successful completion of a clinical trial. This chapter addresses documentation during the off-treatment phase of the study, regulatory requirements, and U.S. Food and Drug Administration (FDA) audits.

Clinical Trial Records

Two basic types of records are kept during a clinical investigation: (1) case history records and (2) the study protocol and related documentation. This chapter focuses on the documentation required for the off-treatment, follow-up phase. Chapter 40 provides information regarding documentation and form submission during the active treatment phase of a clinical trial. The off-treatment phase is a *continuation of the study* until the participant completes all activities as outlined in the protocol. When the participant completes these activities, he or she is off study. When all enrolled participants complete the off-treatment phase and all follow-up activities, the study is terminated at the site (Johns Hopkins Medicine Institutional Review Boards, 2007).

Off-Treatment Documentation

Study-specific case report forms (CRFs) and source reporting provides the documentation for the off-treatment phase. The off-treatment study phase requires follow-up visits, activities, and documentation as outlined in the protocol and study calendar. In this study phase, the purpose of the patient visits and data collection is to monitor the treatment effect. The protocol defines the length of the follow-up intervals and the data points to be followed.

Completing documentation during the off-treatment phase sometimes is difficult because of missed patient visits and perceptions that data collection is more important during active treatment. Failure to follow up affects the study through missing data, which can result in diminished credibility of findings, biased results, and diminished statistical power (Hulley et al., 2001). The study monitor and the clinical trial nurse should routinely examine reasons and trends for missed follow-up visits. One strategy for reducing missed follow-up visits is to coordinate required follow-up data collection to correspond with patient's clinical follow-up.

Off-Study Case History Records

Investigators are required to prepare and maintain adequate and accurate case histories for both the active treatment and follow-up phases that document all observations and other data pertinent to the study about each participant treated with the investigational agent or enrolled as a control. Investigators are required to maintain these records even though the research sponsor may have identical records. Complete and accurate case history records are critical to the scientific integrity of every study and are essential for a study audit.

Figure 38-1 presents the five basic elements of case history records. Case history records should be kept and maintained such that all information regarding each individual in a study is attributable to that individual. Case history records must include the source information obtained from tests and examinations; laboratory results; x-ray reports; treatments received; progress notes; consultations; correspondence; information and data on the subject's condition before, during, and after the clinical investigation; diagnostic test results; diagnoses made; concomitant or concurrent

The author would like to acknowledge Bertie A. Ford, RN, MS, AOCN®, for her contribution that remains unchanged from the first edition.

Figure 38-1. Elements of Case History Records

1. Basic subject identification information
2. Eligibility information showing that each subject meets the study selection criteria or justification for otherwise enrolling the subject
3. Treatment or agent under investigation and information of each subject's exposure to the test or control article, including the date (and time, if relevant) of each administration, the quantity administered, and any administration delays or modifications
4. Disease outcome/response determination information such as tumor measurement, protocol direct response criteria, sites of involvement, or failure to detect cancer progression
5. Toxicity information such as grade, type, and adverse event reporting

Note. From *Southwest Oncology Group Quality Assurance Audit Guidelines* (Appendix B1), by E. Armstrong, D. De Los Santos, L. Rowen, M. Hernandez, and C. Bonugli, 2007, San Antonio, TX: Southwest Oncology Group. Adapted with permission.

---

therapy; and factors that might alter the test article's effects (e.g., development of an intercurrent illness).

To substantiate that each participant meets the selection criteria, the investigator must maintain records of the subject's medical history before enrolling the patient into the study—even if these records exist in the investigator's own files or hospital files. In most cases, the investigator is not obligated to seek past medical history records from other physicians who may have treated the subject or referred the subject to the investigator. If the subject has had no previous contact with the investigator, an initial medical history and protocol-specific tests are used to demonstrate that the patient meets the study eligibility requirements.

Additionally, investigators should maintain correspondence sent to or received from the study sponsor and the monitor, including the protocol or investigational plan, materials to be used in obtaining informed consent, protocol modifications, and records of institutional review board approval and of other communications/actions pertaining to the study (see Chapter 13). Because much of the communication regarding the study is done through e-mail, copies of specific issue-related e-mail messages should be retained.

The investigator may maintain all of the off-study records or, in cases in which the patient is in a hospital or other facility, the records may be maintained as part of the patient's hospital or clinic records. Even if a hospital or clinic keeps the records, the investigator must ensure that the records are retained at least for the length of time required by federal and sponsor regulations.

An investigator may retain off-study records either in their original form or by means of microfilm, microfiche, photocopies, or other accurate reproductions of the original records. If copies are used, however, they must be legible, and the investigator is required to ensure that such reproductions are true and accurate copies of the original. When reproduction techniques (e.g., microfilming) are used, a reader and

photocopying equipment should be readily available. If written notes, erasure marks, or other changes are not apparent on the reproduction, a clear notation of this fact should be on the reproduction of the record, and the original record should be retained for the required length of time.

Data entered directly into a computer system are considered to be the original or true copy of the data, whether printed out as a hard copy or stored as computer files. An acceptable computerized data collection system would be one that allows data entry only by authorized individuals, controls the ability to delete or alter previously entered data, provides an audit trail for such data changes (e.g., modification file), protects the database against tampering, and ensures data preservation. If records are retained in a computer data system, suitable equipment should be readily available to produce a hard copy of any portion of the data.

U.S. Food and Drug Administration Requirements

The FDA and study-specific regulatory agencies assess compliance with the regulations governing clinical trials, review the progress and conduct of these studies, and, ultimately, evaluate the safety and effectiveness of the study article by reviewing a variety of documents. For these purposes, accurate and complete study documentation is required before, during, and after the study. Therefore, documentation of the off-treatment study phase, which is the follow-up phase, after active treatment in the study is important. The off-treatment phase should not be confused with off-study or study termination. *The participant is not off the study until all protocol-outlined activities are completed.*

Participant expectations concerning confidentiality will vary depending on the purpose of the study and the subject's relationship to the clinical investigator. Because FDA oversight responsibilities may compromise participant confidentiality, the agency requires informed consent documents noting that the FDA may inspect the records and a description of the extent to which the investigator must maintain confidentiality (FDA, 2007a). The participant must be informed if anyone other than authorized hospital or research personnel will have access to records containing their identities. Although FDA regulations neither require nor prohibit sponsor access to study records, participants must be made aware of the extent to which such access will be allowed.

When clinical investigators conduct a study for submission to the FDA, they agree to allow the FDA access to the study records. The investigator is responsible for making the participant's records available to the FDA for inspection and copying. The agency will inspect and copy records, regardless of whether the participant has agreed to such a review (FDA, 2007c).

U.S. Food and Drug Administration Audit

The FDA may audit any and all records that might support microfilm, microfiche, or other stored data. These records must be maintained just as paper CRFs must be maintained (see Chapter 47).

The FDA understands the need to protect the privacy of research participants. Study records need not identify subjects by name, but they do need to provide some type of identifier to permit cross-indexing of a subject's study record. Identifying information must be available to respond to queries that may arise, such as a claim that a subject's consent was not obtained or that the study records do not represent actual studies or do not present the actual results. When an individually identifiable medical record is copied and reviewed by the agency, the FDA safeguards the information and uses or disseminates the information only under conditions that protect the individual's privacy to the fullest possible extent consistent with laws related to public disclosure and the agency's law enforcement responsibilities.

The FDA assesses study results through a scientific evaluation of the data contained in case report tables summarizing the data in CRFs. The case report format and content will vary from investigation to investigation. CRFs are a critical part of the investigation records, but they cannot serve as the complete investigation record. The CRFs should contain all data required by the protocol but need not duplicate all of the investigator's records on the subjects' medical histories. Likewise, everything in the CRFs need not be duplicated in the medical records. The FDA does not require that special medical records be established to meet its requirements.

When the FDA needs to verify the validity and completeness of the case report data submitted to the agency, it may audit case history records in the possession of the investigator or the investigator's institution (FDA, 2007c).

FDA regulations require investigators to retain records for a specified time period. These time periods are different than those required for IRB records (see Chapter 13). For investigational new drug studies (and medical food and food-additive studies), records are to be maintained for *two years following the date of marketing application approval* for the drug for the indication for which it was being investigated. If no application is filed or if the application is not approved for the indication, the records are to be retained for two years after the investigation. For device studies, records are to be maintained for two years after the later of the following dates: the date on which the investigation is terminated or completed or the date that the records are no longer required to support a premarket approval application or a notice of completion of a product-development protocol (see Figure 38-2).

To comply with FDA record-retention requirements, clinical investigators should arrange with study sponsors to be kept informed of the status of the application for their respective studies. To illustrate, for an active study, FDA regulations require sponsors to notify each investigator if the FDA approves the new drug application (NDA) or product license application (PLA) or if the investigation

Figure 38-2. Investigator and Sponsor U.S. Food and Drug Administration (FDA) Responsibilities for Retention of Clinical Trial Records

FDA	Record Retained
Application for new drug	Two-year period following the date of a marketing application/drug approval for the drug indication studied in the clinical trials investigation
No application filed	Two years after the investigation is discontinued and FDA notified
Application is not approved for such indication of the drug	Two years after the investigation is discontinued and FDA notified
Note. Based on U.S. Food and Drug Administration, 2007d.	

is discontinued. Therefore, investigators should insist that their contract with a sponsor include a provision requiring the sponsor to notify the investigator of any action with regard to the test article (e.g., submission or approval of an NDA or PLA, withdrawal of an investigational new drug, placement of an investigational new drug on inactive status).

Retention of accurate and complete records is essential to establish the validity and completeness of a report on a clinical investigation that is submitted to the FDA in support of an application for a research or marketing permit. The investigator, not the sponsor, is responsible for the accuracy and completeness of his or her study records, and the investigator is responsible for any discrepancies found in these records during inspection.

Investigators must have some documentation of medical records because the CRF cannot be the patient's only medical record. In addition to the previously mentioned records, sponsors and investigators must prepare and maintain additional records at the end of a study. The sponsor must be able to document that all of the investigational material associated with the study is accounted for and that all of the information on adverse experience is included in appropriate reports.

Source Documents

Source documents are the documents in which information regarding a subject is first recorded. Investigator patient files or hospital records generally are the basis of source document information (FDA, 2007b). The monitor should discuss with the investigator and study staff the type of information expected to be contained in the source documents. The monitor must take into account the sponsor's procedures when establishing requirements for the source documents. If necessary, the monitor can provide a source document format or checklist to the sponsor's site (see Figure 38-3).

The information in the source documents is used to complete the CRFs. Having source documents signed or

---

Figure 38-3. Source Document Checklist

- Hospital chart
- Clinic chart
- X-rays or scans
- Lab reports
- Operative reports
- Pathology reports
- Radiotherapy records
- Chemotherapy records
- Informed consent form

Note. From *Southwest Oncology Group Quality Assurance Program Guidelines* (p. 10), by E. Armstrong and N. McCasland, 2004, San Antonio, TX: Southwest Oncology Group. Copyright 2004 by Southwest Oncology Group. Reprinted with permission.

---

initialed by the individual completing them is common industry practice. The subject's study identification number or code should appear on each page, and all corrections should be initialed and dated by the individual making the change. Hospital records serving as source documents generally do not have changes initialed and dated because a number of individuals make notations on these records, and they often are not involved with the study. The source documents should contain at least the following information (Stone, 2006; Weiss, Armstrong, Herrera, & McCasland, 1997).

- Any adverse experiences, illnesses, or problems reported by the patient during the course of the study
- Ancillary work sheets
- Current physical condition
- Current illnesses and injuries
- Current medications
- Current test results that establish study eligibility
- Dates of the participant's study-required visits
- Indication that study procedures (e.g., laboratory samples, x-rays, electrocardiograms) were completed, including dates and results
- Medications discontinued within the last month (or longer, if required by the protocol)
- Medical history, including relevant history for the disease being treated
- Missed visits and explanations
- Number of study treatments received by the patient
- Nurses' notes and charts
- Patient diaries and appointment books
- Statement that the informed consent form was signed by the subject
- Study medication administration

Any additional information relevant to the study should be included in the source documents (e.g., special dressings, treatments specific to the study protocol). In particular, any deviations from the study protocol or procedures should be recorded in the source documents. For example, if study-required procedures are not completed or are completed outside the time frame specified in the protocol, the reasons for the deviations should be explained in the source documents. The clinical trial nurse should submit the study-specific form related to this information, such as the development of a new diagnosis, or death forms, as required.

Summary

Documentation during the off-treatment phase is as important as documentation during the active phase of the study. Case history records, source documents, and CRFs are an integral, important part of any clinical study. The CRFs are the forms into which the data from source documents are transcribed so that the sponsor can analyze data from multiple sites. The design of CRFs and their completion by study personnel require special attention by the sponsor. Whether the clinical trial nurse completes the documentation personally or oversees the data collected by a clinical research associate, he or she must make sure that, even though the patient may be off treatment, required evaluations are still completed as required by the sponsoring body.

References

Johns Hopkins Medicine Institutional Review Boards. (2007). *Institutional review boards.* Retrieved March 21, 2007, from http://irb.jhmi.edu

Hulley, S.B., Cummings, S.R., Browner, W.S., Grady, D., Hearst, N., & Newman, T.B. (2001). *Designing clinical research: An epidemiologic approach* (2nd ed.). Baltimore: Lippincott Williams & Wilkins.

Stone, J. (2006). *Conducting clinical research.* Cumberland, MD: Mountainside MD Press.

U.S. Food and Drug Administration. (2007a). *Code of federal regulations (Title 21, Vol. 1, Part 50.25(a)[5]).* Retrieved March 21, 2007, from http://accessdata.fda.gov/scripts/cdrh/cfdocs/cfcfr/cfrsearch.cfm

U.S. Food and Drug Administration. (2007b). *Code of federal regulations (Title 21, Vol. 5, Part 312.57).* Retrieved March 21, 2007, from http://fda.gov/cder/about/small/CFR.htm

U.S. Food and Drug Administration. (2007c). *Code of federal regulations (Title 21, Vol. 5, Part 312.68).* Retrieved March 21, 2007, from http://fda.gov/cder/about/small/CFR.htm

U.S. Food and Drug Administration. (2007d). *Code of federal regulations (Title 21, Vol. 5, Part 312.62).* Retrieved March 20, 2007, from http://accessdata.fda.gov/scripts/cdrh/cfdocs/cfcfr/cfrsearch.cfm

Weiss, G.R., Armstrong, E., Herrera, C., & McCasland, N. (1999). *Southwest Oncology Group quality assurance program guidelines.* San Antonio, TX: Southwest Oncology Group.

SECTION IX.

Data Management and Reporting

CHAPTER 39
The Need for Data Management Tools

Betty Razvillas, RN, OCN®, CCRC

Introduction

Clinical trial outcomes depend upon study data being reported in an accurate and verifiable manner to ensure acceptance by regulatory agencies for review and decision-making purposes (PSC Clinical, 2007). Data must be treated with a scrupulousness that exceeds the care with which we treat most information in daily life (Whitbeck, 2006). Investigators must know what type of information should be captured and how that information can be communicated in the most scientifically appropriate manner (Green, Benedetti, & Crowley, 2003). This chapter will examine the need for data management tools to preserve the scientific integrity of the research protocol.

Background

The identification of data items necessary for answering the study objectives and the design of the tools that will be used to collect data should be determined while the protocol is being developed (McFadden, 1997). Specialized cancer clinical trial nurses (CTNs), because of their vital role in the research project, should be involved in the development of the protocol. Many of the tasks associated with the protocol, such as identifying potential study participants, submission and maintenance of regulatory documents, discussion of the study with potential subjects, and education of clinical staff are undertaken by CTNs (Eisenhauer, Twelves, & Buyse, 2006). The review of these functions by the CTN can lend valuable insights to the design of data collection tools prior to study initiation, thus avoiding the need to revise instruments during the course of the study. Spilker and Schoenfelder (1991) asserted that the use of a consistent tool throughout a protocol enables investigators to obtain data of higher quality.

During the course of the study, early data may be reported in abstracts presented at scientific meetings, especially data from large, multicenter phase III trials conducted by National Cancer Institute cooperative groups. Data may be analyzed at specified time points during the study. Investigators can ensure that accrual goals and study objectives are being met. Also, a Data Safety and Monitoring Committee can review safety information. At the conclusion of the study, all the data are analyzed and the findings submitted for publication (Green et al., 2003).

A variety of tools are used for capturing data. Use of the appropriate tools will facilitate data collection, data auditing, and data processing (Spilker & Schoenfelder, 1991). Tools range from hand-completed paper forms to more advanced computerized data collection methods. The tools may be preprinted forms provided by the sponsor of the trial or hand-developed tools created by a study coordinator or investigator. The most common method of data collection is the completion of a protocol-specific case report form (CRF).

Protocol-Specific Tools

Sponsors of trials usually provide protocol-specific CRFs as tools that are completed by the CTN at a participating site. The CRF ensures standardization and consistency of data across multiple sites (McFadden, 1997). Protocol-specific forms can be used to gather data at specified points as mandated by the protocol. The design of CRFs will vary with each sponsor. In addition, each sponsor may impose different parameters for recording the same information, such as adverse events and concomitant medications. One should be knowledgeable about the sponsor's expectations for completion of the CRFs before the first patient is en-

The author would like to acknowledge Susan Bakke, RN, Patricia Davis, RN, BS, OCN®, Valerie Dyer, RN, BSN, Donna Headlee, RN, BSN, Florentino Merced, RN, MSN, and Thelma Watson, RN, OCN®, for their contribution that remains unchanged from the first edition.

rolled in the study. This will reduce the number of queries or edits necessary when the forms are submitted to the sponsor for review (Woodin, 2004).

Standard Tools

When standard tools are developed, different members of the research team should provide input so that clarity and consistency can be maintained (Spilker & Schoenfelder, 1991). The language used in such tools should be clear and simple. Leading and ambiguous questions should be avoided, questions should be self-explanatory, and instructions should be kept brief and to the point (Spilker & Schoenfelder).

Standardized forms are appropriate for all types of protocols. Standardization allows the person who is completing numerous forms to do so more quickly and allows for clearer and easier data collection. Standardization also assists the trial auditor who reviews the forms. Standardized forms should be designed at the outset of the trial to ensure that all essential data are collected without capture of extraneous information and to take into account the data needed for the final manuscript. Forms should be designed to facilitate the creation of the study database (Eisenhauer et al., 2006). As CTNs become familiar with the forms, data entry will become more efficient, and errors will be minimized. Some types of standardized forms are those used for collecting demographic information about patients, history and physical assessment information, and information about previous treatments. Figure 39-1 shows an example of a standard form used to capture patient history information. The CTN or clinic nurse could complete this form with the patient during the initial visit. Although the form is lengthy, its use will ensure that collection of important information will not be inadvertently forgotten or missed. Figure 39-2 shows an example of a new form designed to condense a lengthy, cumbersome, previously used tool.

Supplemental Tools

Occasionally, additional tools will be needed for capturing data that may not be available in the source document. The use of these tools may help to fulfill regulatory requirements for source documentation. Tools such as diaries, calendars, questionnaires, phone logs, mail surveys, and computers assist patients in documenting adverse events and side effects as they are occurring and can be used to document patient compliance with self-administration of oral study medication. Questionnaires also can be used to capture quality-of-life measurements.

Tools for Use by Patients

Patients may use a variety of tools such as visual analog scales, open-ended questions, and checklists. Visual analog scales may be used to represent several dimensions of appetite, pain, fatigue, and other symptoms experienced during certain periods of the day. The most common visual analog scale is a 100 mm long horizontal line with right-angle vertical lines, or "stops," at each end of the line (Burns & Grove, 2007). The left stop may be represented by the number "0" and the right stop by the number "10," indicating a range of intensity from none, or "0," to the most intense, or "10." The subject indicates the degree of intensity of the symptom by placing a vertical line that intersects the horizontal line at the area the patient feels best represents the degree of the symptom he or she is experiencing. Results are obtained by measuring the number of millimeters from "0" to the mark placed by the patient (Waltz, Strickland, & Lenz, 2005). For a more exact measurement, scales may specify a range of 0 to 100 millimeters. The value, recorded in millimeters, can be entered onto a CRF or entered into a database.

Open-ended questions allow patients to list possible causes of their symptoms and to describe how they manage those specific symptoms (Wood & Ross-Kerr, 2006). Daily diaries and calendars have been shown to minimize problems related to recall and to result in more accurate documentation than that achieved by retrospective interviews. Ultimately, the use of forms or other tools is important for fostering patients' participation in their own care.

Study Drug Diaries

With the increasing availability of orally administered treatment agents, patient compliance becomes an important concern. A researcher cannot be present each time the participant self-administers drugs at home, but some method of verifying patient compliance is necessary. Patient cooperation can be promoted by delivering clear and well-written instructions and samples during the initial orientation (Richardson, 1994). Instructions about study drug administration and the use of the diary should be given to the research participant when each cycle of the study drug is dispensed. The completed diary and any unused drug should be collected and verified by study personnel at the end of the cycle. The diary should be signed and dated by study personnel and then placed in the subject's research file as source documentation and back-up for the drug administration CRF. A sample drug diary appears in Figure 39-3.

Symptom Diaries or Calendars

The focus of diaries or calendars should be on eliciting and providing comprehensive, patient-centered information. Diaries may be constructed as journals, in which all health events are entered daily on the same page, or as ledgers, in which separate pages are used for different entries, ranging from medications to symptoms (Richardson, 1994). The diary or calendar must elicit the specific information required by the protocol.

The diary or calendar should be easy to complete, usually within less than five minutes; otherwise, patients may perceive it as a nuisance or a burden, a perception that

---

Figure 39-1. History Form

MEDICAL AND SOCIAL HISTORY INFORMATION

PLEASE COMPLETE THE FOLLOWING:

Name:_____ Today's Date:_____

Address_____ Home Phone :_____

City: _____ State:_____ Zip Code _____ County_____

Sex: _____ Date of Birth: _____ *Race:_____ *Ethnicity: _____

Employment Status: ☐ Employed   Occupation:_____ Work Phone:_____

☐ Unemployed   (Reason_____)   Social Security # _____

PSYCHOSOCIAL INFORMATION

Marital Status (please check one):
☐ Married
☐ Divorced
☐ Single
☐ Separated
☐ Widow/widower

Do you live:
☐ With a spouse   Name: _____
☐ With a significant other   Name: _____
☐ Alone
☐ With family

Whom do you rely on most for support?_____
How many children do you have? _____
What are their ages? _____

Do you have an advance directive/living will? ☐ Yes ☐ No
Healthcare power of attorney?   ☐ Yes ☐ No

Highest level of education completed:
☐ High school
☐ College degree
☐ Graduate degree
☐ Some college but no degree
☐ Technical school

NURSE'S INTERVIEW INFORMATION

*Race: ☐ White   ☐ Black   ☐ Asian   ☐ Pacific Islander

*Ethnicity _____
(Based on place of birth or heritage according to NCI criteria)

What is your average family income/year?
☐ $10,000–$20,000
☐ $20,000–$30,000
☐ $30,000–$40,000
☐ $40,000–$50,000
☐ $50,000–$60,000
☐ $60,000–$70,000
☐ $70,000–$80,000
☐ $80,000–$100,000
☐ Above $100,000
☐ Do not care to respond
(We are asking for this information as a request of the Federal Government.)

Method of payment (mark primary method only):
☐ Private insurance
☐ Medicare
☐ Medicaid
☐ Medicare/Medicaid
☐ Medicare & private insurance
☐ Military/Veterans sponsored NOS
☐ Military sponsored (i.e., Champus)
☐ Veterans sponsored
☐ Self pay (no insurance)
☐ No means of payment
☐ Other _____

EMERGENCY CONTACT INFORMATION

Who should we call in case of an emergency?

Name _____ Relationship _____

Address _____

City/State _____ Zip Code _____

Phone No. (Home) _____ (Work) _____

(Continued on next page)

Figure 39-1. History Form *(Continued)*

Patient Name _____

ALLERGIES	**MENSTRUAL HISTORY** *(If applicable)*

ALLERGIES

Are you allergic to anything?   ☐ Yes ☐ No

If yes, please list all allergies:_____

_____

_____

_____

Describe the type of reaction you have (dizziness, rash, etc.):___

_____

_____

_____

MENSTRUAL HISTORY *(If applicable)*

Have you stopped having periods?   ☐ Yes ☐ No
If Yes, when? _____

Has your uterus been removed?   ☐ Yes ☐ No
If Yes, when? _____

Have your ovaries been removed?   ☐ Yes ☐ No
If Yes, when? _____
If yes, were both ovaries removed?   ☐ Yes ☐ No

Are you using birth control?   ☐ Yes ☐ No
If yes, what type? _____

YOUR FAMILY CANCER HISTORY

Relative	Type of Cancer	Date of Diagnosis

YOUR FAMILY MEDICAL HISTORY

Relative	Age (if living)	Present Health	If dead, give age at death and cause of death
Mother:			
Father:			
Spouse:			
Brothers: Number living _____ Number dead _____			
Sisters: Number living _____ Number dead _____			
Children: Number living _____ Number dead _____			

(Continued on next page)

Figure 39-1. History Form *(Continued)*

Patient Name _____

PATIENT MEDICAL HISTORY: *Have you ever had any of the following conditions? Place a check (√) in the box next to the appropriate condition. Check all that apply.*

<u>Previous Conditions</u>
☐ Angina (chest pains)
☐ Gastric problems (ulcer, irritable bowel)
☐ Heart attack
☐ Heart failure
☐ Heart murmur
☐ High blood pressure
　　If yes, is the high blood pressure currently controlled:
　　☐ Yes ☐ No
☐ Stroke
☐ Pulmonary embolism
☐ Blood Clots
☐ Transient ischemic attack (TIA)
☐ Superficial phlebitis

☐ Depression
☐ Nervous or emotional disorder (anxiety, mood swings)
☐ Psychiatric problems (schizophrenia, bi-polar disorder)
☐ Cataracts
☐ Glaucoma
☐ Macular degeneration
☐ Diabetes
　　If yes, is the diabetes currently controlled:
　　☐ Yes ☐ No
☐ Liver disease (yellow jaundice, hepatitis, cirrhosis)
☐ Thyroid trouble (overactive, underactive, goiter)
☐ Tuberculosis (TB)
☐ Other _____

<u>Previous surgeries (not related to cancer)</u>
Date of Surgery___/___/___ Reason for Surgery _____

Date of Surgery___/___/___ Reason for Surgery _____

Date of Surgery___/___/___ Reason for Surgery _____

Date of Surgery___/___/___ Reason for Surgery _____

List all medicines (including over-the-counter products, herbals, vitamins) you are now taking and the reason for taking them. *Use the back of the page if more room is needed.*

Medication and Dose	Reason for Taking	Date Started	Nurse's Interview Information

(Continued on next page)

Figure 39-1. History Form (Continued)

Patient Name _____

PREVIOUS RESEARCH TRIALS AND CANCER TREATMENT

Have you ever participated in any clinical trial?   ☐ Yes   ☐ No

If YES:
Name and/or purpose of trial: _____

Names of any drugs received during the trial: _____

What date did you start on the study? _____ What was the last day you were on the study? _____

Have you had any prior standard treatment for cancer?   ☐ Yes   ☐ No   *(Use back of page if needed)*
If yes, please check all that apply:

☐ Chemotherapy: Start date __/__/__ End date __/__/__ Drugs given_____
☐ Radiation Therapy: Start date __/__/__ End date __/__/__ Areas radiated _____
☐ Surgery: Surgery date __/__/__ Type of surgery _____
☐ Hormone Therapy: Start date __/__/__ End date __/__/__ Drugs given _____
☐ Biological Therapy: Start date __/__/__ End date __/__/__ Agents given _____
☐ Other Therapy: _____

CURRENT PHYSICAL CONDITION: *TO BE COMPLETED BY NURSE*

VITAL SIGNS   DATE TAKEN:_____

B/P _____
HEIGHT (measured) _____ Unit: ☐ Inches   ☐ cm
WEIGHT (measured)_____ Unit: ☐ lbs.   ☐ kg

REVIEW OF SYSTEMS

System	Normal	Abnormal	Abnormality

Integumentary System:
    Skin
    Hair
    Nails
	☐
	☐
	☐
		☐
		☐
		☐	

Head	☐	☐	
Eyes	☐	☐	
Ears	☐	☐	
Nose, nasopharynx, paranasal sinuses	☐	☐	
Mouth, oropharynx	☐	☐	
Neck	☐	☐	
Breasts	☐	☐	

Cardiovascular System
    Heart
    Peripheral vascular
	☐
	☐
		☐
		☐	

Respiratory System	☐	☐	
Gastrointestinal System	☐	☐	
Gynecologic System	☐	☐	
Urinary System	☐	☐	

(Continued on next page)

Figure 39-1. History Form *(Continued)*			
Musculoskeletal System	☐	☐	
Central Nervous System	☐	☐	
Endocrine System	☐	☐	
Constitutional	☐	☐	

Comments:_____
_____
_____
_____
_____
_____
_____
_____

This information has been reviewed by: _____ **Date Reviewed:** _____

Note. Developed by B. Razvillas, 2003, University of Texas Health Science Center at San Antonio.

may result in incomplete documentation and compliance. The healthcare team can ensure patients' optimal reporting by providing them with oral and written instructions about how to complete the diary or calendar. Ideally, such teaching should be performed individually or in a small-group setting and in a quiet environment. Healthcare professionals should ensure that each patient interprets the questions and criteria in the diary or calendar the same way the healthcare provider interprets them. Patients should be encouraged to report both medical and psychosocial issues; such reporting will empower them to document all aspects of their symptoms.

Healthcare professionals must review the diary or calendar individually with each patient so that symptoms and toxic effects can be properly documented and missing data can be obtained. When a diary or calendar must be recorded for a lengthy period, it may be best to allow the patient to compile the information every other day rather than daily.

Although one advantage of the diary or calendar is that it minimizes recall errors, one disadvantage of this type of data collection is poor rates of patient compliance and motivation. Initially, compliance rates may be as high as 84%; after time, however, compliance rates consistently decline (Sullivan et al., 1995). If the follow-up period is longer than six or eight weeks, data collection can be facilitated by having patients mail or fax diaries or calendars at set intervals. Unfortunately, the diary or calendar is not always an all-inclusive tool; therefore, data sometimes may be omitted (Richardson, 1994).

Nonetheless, the CTN should encourage patients to look to the dairy or calendar as their own data collection tool in which they can record pertinent information (Freer, 1980). As the CTN continues to work with patients on their diaries or calendars, it will become clear that requiring patients to provide daily information about their health status is effective in helping them to manage their medical care and symptoms. This realization may, in turn, encourage patients to become more involved in providing optimal documentation.

Usable Data Management Tools

Study coordinators may find that standard instruments do not exist that are adequate or appropriate for their needs. They may find it beneficial to create their own tools to assist them in performing their daily work (Waltz et al., 2005). The tools can serve a variety of functions, several of which are discussed in this section.

Data Tracking Forms

Study coordinators may find tracking logs useful for a complicated study with multiple time points for study evaluations and data submission. The tracking log will help the study coordinator to maintain timely submission of data and collection of specimens required by the study. An example of a study evaluation tracking log is presented in Figure 39-4.

Telephone Interviews or Logs

Telephone interviews often are conducted during a follow-up period after patients have been discharged from a healthcare facility or an outpatient setting. Healthcare professionals should document the information gathered by such interviews in the medical record for the purposes of accountability and for retrieval. Individual healthcare records, including inpatient hospital charts, outpatient ambulatory care charts, and immunization records, are designed to document the observations, treatments, and services of healthcare providers. Telephone logs can be easily created and can readily become part of the healthcare

Figure 39-2. Condensed On-Study Form

Pt Name: _____

Pt Initials: _____

Patient ID: _____-_____-_____-_____

Type: A = Antiretroviral, B = Biologic, C = Chemotherapy, F = Antifungal, G = Gene, H = Hormonotherapy, I = Immunotherapy, O = Other, R = Radiation, S = Surgery, T = Bone Marrow Transplant, X = Antibiotic

Prior Therapy ___ (check here) if no prior therapy

Type	Start Date	Stop Date	Agent	Schedule Site	Dose	Response

Prior Radiation ___ (check here) if no prior radiation

Type	1st Dose	End Date	Site	Schedule Total	Dose	Response

Prior Surgery ___ (check here) if no prior surgery

Date	Procedure	Findings	Extent of Disease

Note. Developed by T. Merced, 1998, National Institutes of Health, Bethesda, MD.

Figure 39-3. Drug Diary for a Patient to Complete

Protocol No.	Site Number	Patient Number	Patient Initials	Date					Course No.
	☐☐☐	☐☐☐☐	☐☐☐	☐☐	☐☐	☐☐			☐☐
				DD	M M	Y	Y		

PATIENT MEDICATION DIARY
INSTRUCTIONS

Please take the capsules as instructed on the bottle labels. Capsules should be taken with a glass of water BEFORE meals, preferably on an empty stomach (at least 10 minutes before meals) and at 12-hour intervals.

Please record below, the exact time you took the capsules (see example below).

3	30	Example = 3:30

hr:min

		DAY 1	DAY 2	DAY 3	DAY 4	DAY 5	DAY 6	DAY 7
WEEK 1	**am dose**	hr:min	hr:min	hr:min	hr:min	hr:min	hr:min	hr:min
DATE __/__/__	**pm dose**	hr:min	hr:min	hr:min	hr:min	hr:min	hr:min	hr:min

		DAY 1	DAY 2	DAY 3	DAY 4	DAY 5	DAY 6	DAY 7
WEEK 2	**am dose**	hr:min	hr:min	hr:min	hr:min	hr:min	hr:min	hr:min
DATE __/__/__	**pm dose**	hr:min	hr:min	hr:min	hr:min	hr:min	hr:min	hr:min

		DAY 1	DAY 2	DAY 3	DAY 4	DAY 5	DAY 6	DAY 7
WEEK 3	**am dose**	hr:min	hr:min	hr:min	hr:min	hr:min	hr:min	hr:min
DATE __/__/__	**pm dose**	hr:min	hr:min	hr:min	hr:min	hr:min	hr:min	hr:min

Date Diary Returned: _____   Signed: _____ RN

Number of Bottles Returned: _____   Number of Capsules Returned _____

THANK YOU FOR YOUR COOPERATION

Note. Developed by B. Razvillas, 2000, University of Texas Health Science Center at San Antonio.

Figure 39-4. Study Evaluations Form for Study Coordinators

DEPARTMENT OF MEDICINE, DIVISION OF HEMATOLOGY

Study Title_____

STUDY EVALUATIONS-Page 1

Patient Initials _____ Study #_____ SS# _____ Treatment Site _____

Pre-PBSC Mobilization Tests/Evaluations	Purpose	Performed	Date Performed
Bone marrow biopsy sample (Send to _____)	Research	☐ Yes ☐ No	___/___/___
20 cc heparinized blood (Spin & store)	Research	☐ Yes ☐ No	___/___/___
50 cc heparinized peripheral blood (Send to _____)	Research	☐ Yes ☐ No	___/___/___
40 cc (45 cc if WBC < 2000) heparinized venous blood (Send to____ _____) **Females only**	Research	☐ Yes ☐ No	___/___/___
1–2 cc heparinized marrow aspirate (Spin & store)	Research	☐ Yes ☐ No	___/___/___
Complete H&P w/ careful description of tx requirements & liver and spleen size **Submit completed H&P form**	Routine	☐ Yes ☐ No	___/___/___
Documentation of performance status using the Karnofsky scale	Routine	☐ Yes ☐ No PS=_____	___/___/___
Bone marrow aspirate and biopsy for routine morphologic studies **Submit report**	Routine	☐ Yes ☐ No	___/___/___
Cytogenetics exam **Submit report**	Routine	☐ Yes ☐ No	___/___/___
3 cc heparinized blood for CD34+ measurement **Submit report**	Routine	☐ Yes ☐ No CD 34+= _____	___/___/___
*CBC w/diff and platelet count **Submit lab spreadsheet for all labs** *Preferably drawn same day as CD 34+	Routine	☐ Yes ☐ No WBC=___ Hct=____ Plt=_____	___/___/___
Retic count **Submit report**	Routine	☐ Yes ☐ No	___/___/___
Coagulation profile (PT/PTT) **Submit report**	Routine	☐ Yes ☐ No	___/___/___
Chemistries: lytes, BUN, creatinine, LFTs (SGOT, SGPT, ALP, Bili, GGT), albumin, total protein, LDH **Submit report**	Routine	☐ Yes ☐ No	___/___/___
Chest x-ray	Routine	☐ Yes ☐ No	___/___/___
EKG	Routine	☐ Yes ☐ No	___/___/___
Pulmonary function tests	Routine	☐ Yes ☐ No	___/___/___
MUGA scan (as indicated) **Send report if abnormal**	Routine	☐ Yes ☐ No	___/___/___
Pregnancy test (if applicable)	Routine	☐ Yes ☐ No	___/___/___
CMV, HSV and HTLV1 serologies	Routine	☐ Yes ☐ No	___/___/___
HIV test	Routine	☐ Yes ☐ No	___/___/___
Urinalysis	Routine	☐ Yes ☐ No	___/___/___
Abdominal ultrasound to determine spleen and liver size **Submit report and measurements**	Routine	☐ Yes ☐ No	___/___/___

(Continued on next page)

Figure 39-4. Study Evaluations Form for Study Coordinators *(Continued)*

DEPARTMENT OF MEDICINE, DIVISION OF HEMATOLOGY

Study Title_____

STUDY EVALUATIONS-Page 2

Patient Initials _____ Study #_____ SS# _____ Treatment Site _____

During PBSC Collection			
50 cc heparinized peripheral blood-Collect on day 1 before pheresis (Send to lab)	Research	☐ Yes ☐ No	____/____/____
10 cc of each day's PBSC product (Spin & store)	Research	☐ Yes ☐ No	____/____/____
CD 34+/38– measurement of stem cell product	Research	☐ Yes ☐ No	____/____/____
PBSC product-(Send as much as possible to lab)	Research	☐ Yes ☐ No	____/____/____
5 cc of PBSC-**Females only** (Send to _____)	Research	☐ Yes ☐ No	____/____/____
Measurement of CD34+ content of PBSC product	Routine	☐ Yes ☐ No	____/____/____
Daily CBC	Routine	☐ Yes ☐ No	____/____/____
2 cc PBSC product for cytogenetics (if cytogenetic abnormality present at baseline)	Routine	☐ Yes ☐ No	____/____/____
1 Month After Transplant			
10 cc heparinized blood (Spin & store)	Research	☐ Yes ☐ No	____/____/____
30 cc (45 cc if WBC < 2000) heparinized venous blood-**Females only** (Send to _____)	Research	☐ Yes ☐ No	____/____/____
2 cc heparinized marrow (Spin & store)	Research	☐ Yes ☐ No	____/____/____
Bone marrow aspirate & biopsy (and cytogenetics if abnormal pretransplant **Submit reports**	Routine	☐ Yes ☐ No	____/____/____
CBC, Retic count, PEw/PS, hx of transfusions **Submit reports**	Routine	☐ Yes ☐ No	____/____/____
3 Months After Transplant			
10 cc heparinized blood (Spin & store)	Research	☐ Yes ☐ No	____/____/____
30 cc (45 cc if WBC < 2000) heparinized venous blood (Send to _____) **Females only**	Research	☐ Yes ☐ No	____/____/____
2 cc heparinized marrow (Spin & store)	Research	☐ Yes ☐ No	____/____/____
Bone marrow aspirate & biopsy (and cytogenetics if abnormal pretransplant) **Submit reports**	Routine	☐ Yes ☐ No	____/____/____
Abdominal ultrasound w/ liver & spleen measurements (if enlarged pretransplant) **Submit reports**	Routine	☐ Yes ☐ No	____/____/____
CBC, Retic count, PEw/PS, hx of transfusions **Submit reports**	Routine	☐ Yes ☐ No	____/____/____
12 Months After Transplant			
10 cc heparinized blood (Spin & store)	Research	☐ Yes ☐ No	____/____/____
2 cc heparinized marrow (Spin & store)	Research	☐ Yes ☐ No	____/____/____
Bone marrow aspirate & biopsy (and cytogenetics if abnormal pretransplant) **Submit reports**	Routine	☐ Yes ☐ No	____/____/____
CBC, Retic count, PEw/PS, hx of transfusions **Submit reports**	Routine	☐ Yes ☐ No	____/____/____

Note. Created by B. Razvillas, 2000, University of Texas Health Science Center at San Antonio.

record. These logs can provide clear documentation of symptoms and their management while patients are active in the study and can be made part of the medical record. The importance of healthcare records as sources of data for research cannot be overstated. However, wide variability exists in how the records are used (vonKoss Krowchuk, Moore, & Richardson, 1995).

Mail Surveys

Mail surveys are another common method of data collection. A mail survey is not subject to interviewer bias, and patients can answer the questionnaire at their leisure (De Leeuw, Hox, & Snijkers, 1995). This method of data collection is not costly, but compliance may be a problem. However, including a preaddressed, postage-paid reply envelope with the survey can improve compliance.

The disadvantages of this method include the inability to pursue questions in other areas, such as specific details of symptoms (i.e., frequency and severity) (De Leeuw et al., 1995). Another area of concern is whether the survey meets the patient's reading ability and comprehension level.

Information Technology

Clearly, computers are already a valuable tool for data collection and management (De Leeuw et al., 1995). A set of standardized or open-ended questions can be stored on the computer and can guide the interviewer and patient to specific end points (Spilker & Schoenfelder, 1991). One advantage of this method is that the interviewer does not have to be present; the patient may answer the questions directly on the computer, and the absence of an interviewer may encourage patients to respond more freely to the questions (Schmitt, 1994). Data collection tends to be more consistent with a prepared text and with direct entry of responses into the database (De Leeuw et al.). This method allows the database to be updated with greater ease and provides for quicker data retrieval. Some institutions provide portable computers for patient use, and voice-recognition computer software also has been developed. Of course, not every patient or institution will be able to have a computer because of the related cost, but for those that do, this equipment may provide an excellent opportunity for facilitating data collection. The expansion of computer technology has resulted in the availability of dozens of software programs for data management, as well as advances in scanning programs and Internet use (Waltz et al., 2005). New technology also has introduced new issues: Points to be considered include whether data will be entered online or off-line, the type of equipment that will be needed, the amount of training and type of personnel needed, and the amount of support from a technician that will be required.

Off-Line Data Entry

A less technical and straightforward method of data capture is off-line data entry. Many off-line programs will work with basic office software, and this compatibility results in lower technology costs and lower training costs. The start-up times are often faster because programming a CRF page requires only a few minutes, and the form can be used immediately. Files can be exported into spreadsheet programs such as Microsoft® Excel® or Microsoft® Access®. A disadvantage is the fact that access to the data is limited to people who are able to use the particular computer or computer drive on which the data were entered (Maes, 2005).

Scanning Technology

Important technologic changes have occurred during the past 10 years in the area of document scanning. Drastic improvements have been made in scan interpretation software, which has become a powerful tool in the field of data capture, as it enables complicated forms to be scanned into a computer. Portable scanners can be carried to a hospital or another site and can be used there to scan patient records into a file. When selecting scanning software, investigators should understand the different types of data recognition available: optical character recognition (OCR), intelligent character recognition (ICR), and optical marking recognition (OMR).

The most common type of scanning software uses OCR. This technology transforms paper documents into editable computerized files; the software also can recognize handwritten characters. ICR goes further, because it recognizes handwritten documents. Often, these two technologies can be used together for optimal results. The third type of technology available, OMR, allows recognition of marks such as bar codes, marks on answer sheets for multiple-choice questions, or CRFs that consist of check boxes. An important consideration in choosing any of these programs is the program's ability to allow the editing of scanned documents (Maes, 2005).

Online Data Entry

The use of online data entry has steadily increased over the past 10 years. This approach allows data to be entered into a centralized data bank and results in consistency in the quality of data entry and the paper flow processes. Some methods of online data entry are data entry via a site-to-site connection over a virtual private network (VPN), data entry via a Web application, and electronic data gathering at the source.

A VPN connection works via a direct link to the sponsor's server. The most commonly used VPN application is Oracle®, but setting up these entry screens requires some level of expertise. Online data entry via a Web application allows the entire data management process to be performed online, including the design of CRFs and the entry of data. Electronic data gathering allows the direct input of digitized data. An investigator or coordinator can enter data at the patient's bedside by using a personal digital assistant (commonly known as a PDA), a smart pen, or another device that is directly linked to a server.

Although the advances in technology have helped to streamline the data management process, they also usher in new sets of concerns. The greatest concerns relate to the security of data and protection of patients' confidentiality. Precautions such as the use of separate networks, secured lines, password protection, and dedicated computers can enhance security. Computers should be set up with appropriate firewalls and should be located in secure areas. The number of people with access to the computers should be limited, and the users should sign confidentiality agreements.

Another concern about electronic data entry is the need for adequate information technology support. Personnel should be available to assist with difficulties in data entry. In the case of a computer failure, or "crash," immediate action is necessary for preventing loss of data or for recapturing data if possible (Maes, 2005). Another method of preventing the loss of data is to perform daily back-ups. Data can be sent to a remote location for storage. The data should be tested before back-ups are performed so that investigators can ensure that the data are not contaminated (Good, 2002).

Summary

Data management tools and study protocols should be developed concurrently. Tools are essential for facilitating the collection, auditing, and processing of data. Several methods of collecting and retrieving data from clinical trials have been presented. The tools of data collection include diaries or calendars, questionnaires, phone interviews or logs, mailed surveys, and computers. Each method and tool has advantages and disadvantages, and the choice of tools usually is influenced by personal bias, availability of resources, and cost. The ultimate goal is to ensure that data are as reliable and as easily retrievable as possible.

References

Burns, N., & Grove, S.K. (2007). *Understanding nursing research: Building an evidence-based practice.* St. Louis, MO: Elsevier Saunders.

De Leeuw, E.D., Hox, J.J., & Snijkers, G. (1995). The effect of computer-assisted interviewing on data quality: A review. *Journal of the Market Research Society, 37,* 325–344.

Eisenhauer, E.A., Twelves, C.B., & Buyse, M. (2006). *Phase 1 cancer clinical trials: A practical guide.* New York: Oxford University Press.

Freer, C.B. (1980). Health diaries: A method of collecting health information. *Journal of the Royal College of General Practitioners, 20,* 279–282.

Good, P.I. (2002). *A manager's guide to the design and conduct of clinical trials.* Hoboken, NJ: Wiley-Liss.

Green, S., Benedetti, J., & Crowley, J. (2003). *Clinical trials in oncology* (2nd ed.). Boca Raton, FL: Chapman & Hall/CRC.

Maes, B. (2005). Data capture in the 21st century: A European perspective. *Monitor, 19*(3), 43–45.

McFadden, E. (1997). *Management of data in clinical trials.* New York: Wiley.

PSC Clinical. (2007). *Written procedures for clinical research.* Retrieved March 20, 2007, from http://pscclinical.com/index.php?option=com_content&task=view&id=1&Itemid=25

Richardson, A. (1994). The health diary: An examination of its use as a data collection method. *Journal of Advanced Nursing, 19,* 782–791.

Schmitt, N. (1994). Method bias: The importance of theory and measurement. *Journal of Organizational Behavior, 15,* 393–398.

Spilker, B., & Schoenfelder, J. (1991). *Data collection forms in clinical trials.* Baltimore: Lippincott Williams & Wilkins.

Sullivan, L., Dukes, K., Harris, L., Dittus, R., Greenfield, S., & Kaplan, S. (1995). A comparison of various methods of collecting self-reported health outcomes data among low-income and minority patients. *Medical Care, 33*(Suppl. 4), AS183–AS184.

vonKoss Krowchuk, H., Moore, M.L., & Richardson, L. (1995). Using health care records as sources of data for research. *Journal of Nursing Measurement, 3,* 3–12.

Waltz, C.F., Strickland, O.L., & Lenz, E.R. (2005). *Measurement in nursing and health research* (3rd ed.). New York: Springer.

Whitbeck, C. (2006, August 28). *The responsible collection, retention, sharing, and interpretation of data.* Retrieved July 1, 2007, from http://onlineethics.org/CMS/16371.aspx

Wood, M.J., & Ross-Kerr, J.C. (2006). *Basic steps in planning nursing research: From question to proposal* (6th ed.). Sudbury, MA: Jones and Bartlett.

Woodin, K.E. (2004). *The CRC's guide to coordinating clinical research.* Boston: Thomson CenterWatch.

CHAPTER 40
Documentation and Forms Submissions

Tasha D. Hall, RN, MS, OCN®, CCRP

Introduction

Data generated from a clinical trial are analyzed to determine the results of the trial. It is the responsibility of the investigator to "prepare and maintain adequate and accurate case histories that record all observations and other data pertinent to the investigation on each individual administered the investigational drug or employed as a control in the investigation" (21 CFR 312.62 [U.S. Food and Drug Administration, 2006]). Information from a study participant's clinical record is transcribed onto specific case report forms (CRFs) for the clinical trial. By transcribing the data onto CRFs, the clinical trial nurse (CTN) is preparing the data for evaluation. The CRFs and supporting data—for example, signed and dated consent forms, medical records, progress notes of the physician, the individual's hospital chart(s), and the nurses' notes—are included in the case histories. The nature of the study dictates the number and complexity of the forms required for submission. The basic rules of documentation, as well as the rules specific to research, apply when completing forms for a clinical trial. This chapter provides an overview of the basic rules for documentation, source documents, forms organization, and submission.

Basic Rules of Documentation

When documenting any client record, source document, or CRF, the CTN has to do so in a legal manner. Erasing or covering mistakes is prohibited. To cross out an item, one single horizontal line should be drawn through it. Then, the writer must initial and date the crossed-out information. Only site personnel may make corrections or modifications to a CRF. All documentation in client records and on clinical trial forms should be completed in ink, not pencil. Ensuring that all handwritten information is legible also is important. No abbreviations may be used on the forms for a clinical trial unless the specific protocol indicates that they are appropriate. Although standards for nursing and medical documentation have emerged,

best practices for research record keeping still are evolving (Schreier, Wilson, & Resnick, 2006).

Source Documents

The *source data* entered onto CRFs are obtained from source documents (see Figure 40-1). A *source document* is any document where data are first recorded (see Figure 40-2). Source documentation serves to substantiate the integrity of the trial data, confirm observations that are recorded, and confirm the existence of study participants (Woodin, 2004). A source document is needed to support any information documented on a form for a clinical trial. A CRF can become a source document if the original collection of data is done on the CRF. An example would be a rating scale or questionnaire completed by the patient.

Forms Preparation and Organization

Multiple methods exist for the preparation and organization of CRFs for submission. They can be organized by visit or type of data collected or a combination. If CRFs are organized and designed in a user-friendly manner, it will increase the probability that the data are collected in a comprehensive manner. Headlee (2004) suggested a variety of strategies to facilitate their use. For example, for handwritten forms, limit the handwriting needed, use a

---

Figure 40-1. Source Data

Source Data
All information in original records and certified copies of original records of clinical findings, observations, or other activities in a clinical trial necessary for the reconstruction and evaluation of the trial. Source data are contained in source documents (original records or certified copies).

Note. From *Guidance for Industry: E6 Good Clinical Practice: Consolidated Guidance* (p. 7), by U.S. Food and Drug Administration, 1996. Retrieved July 4, 2007, from http://www.fda.gov/cder/guidance/959fnl.pdf

---

Figure 40-2. Source Documents

Source Documents
Original documents and records including, but not limited to, hospital records, clinical and office charts, laboratory notes, memoranda, subjects' diaries or evaluation checklists, pharmacy dispensing records, recorded data from automated instruments, copies or transcriptions certified after verification as being accurate and complete, microfiches, photographic negatives, microfilm or magnetic media, x-rays, subject files, and records kept at the pharmacy, at the laboratories, and at medico-technical departments involved in the clinical trial.

Note. From *Guidance for Industry: E6 Good Clinical Practice: Consolidated Guidance* (p. 7), by U.S. Food and Drug Administration, 1996. Retrieved July 4, 2007, from http://www.fda.gov/cder/guidance/959fnl.pdf

---

consistent format for date and time, and avoid modifying the forms once a study is open. A clinical study may require several types of forms, including on-study forms, patient history forms, treatment forms, adverse event forms, patient diaries, and follow-up forms. The forms used by a study reflect what data the investigators are interested in capturing. For example, a study with an end point of quality of life (QOL) will have QOL questionnaires and submission forms as a part of the CRFs.

On-study, or entry, forms vary from study to study but usually include similar information. Documented information includes family history, concomitant medications, history of current cancer diagnosis, history of other medical problems, and review of current symptoms. Some studies have patient history forms specifically for historical information. Active treatment forms generally report the treatment given and adverse events experienced. Treatment forms frequently have spaces for the drug administered, route administered, date administered, and results of studies done prior to treatment (e.g., complete blood count, differential, platelets). Adverse event information may or may not be requested on a separate form. Adverse event information includes signs and symptoms of events experienced during and after treatment. All serious adverse events (e.g., hospitalization) need to be submitted within a narrow time frame from the occurrence of the event. Serious adverse event forms need to be submitted to a variety of groups (see Chapter 28 for more information on adverse event reporting).

As more patients are administering treatment to themselves in the home setting, patient diaries to document administration of study drugs and side effects are becoming a key component of study documentation. Patient diaries are subjective but provide a method of documenting adherence and nonadherence (see Chapter 30). Follow-up forms for many studies are completed over the lifetime of the patient. Survival information, long-term side effects of study medication, and diagnostic evaluations may be included on follow-up forms. The frequency of follow-up data collection will vary, depending on the nature of the study. The CTN retains a copy of all forms submitted. These records are maintained in a research chart to which the coordinator will refer during an audit. For easy reference, copies of key source documents should be maintained in the research chart along with copies of the forms submitted. The CTN who completes the form is responsible for all data listed or not listed on the forms. Errors of omission can occur and need to be monitored carefully, especially with multicenter studies. Data monitoring committees make decisions about multicenter studies based on the information submitted to them on the forms. If key data are omitted or reported incorrectly, erroneous conclusions may be made regarding study outcomes.

Forms Submission

The CRFs are forwarded to the study sponsor, and copies of the CRFs are kept on file at the trial site for possible audit and verification of source documentation. Many studies are utilizing electronic data capture (EDC) (see Chapter 41). EDC has multiple advantages, including that as data are entered, automated data edit checks alert the site to possible errors. This assists the site in avoiding costly errors early in the process.

Electronic records and electronic signatures are covered in 21 CFR 11 (FDA, 2003). Part 11 applies to records in electronic form that are created, modified, maintained, archived, or transmitted under any requirements set forth in FDA regulations. It addresses electronic CRFs, electronic patient diaries, electronic health records, software validation, and source documents. Parameters for both open and closed systems to ensure authenticity, integrity, and confidentiality of the electronic records are included in the regulation. Certification of all electronic signatures is required.

Summary

The CTN frequently is responsible for ensuring that CRFs are accurately completed. Although this can be viewed as a mundane task, it is vital to the success of a clinical trial. Data recorded on study forms are used, for example, to evaluate the efficacy of an investigational agent. All of the forms need to be completed accurately and in a timely manner to ensure the successful completion of the study. The quality of the study is directly affected by the quality of the study documentation.

References

Headlee, D. (2004, May). The paper trail: CRFs, source documents, and data collection tools. *SoCRA Source*, pp. 30–33.

Schreier, A., Wilson, K., & Resnick, D. (2006). Academic research record-keeping: Best practices for individuals, group leaders, and institutions. *Academic Medicine, 81*, 42–47.

Woodin, K.E. (2004). *The CRC's guide to coordinating clinical research.* Boston: Thomson CenterWatch.

U.S. Food and Drug Administration. (2003). *Guidance for industry: Part 11, electronic records; electronic signatures—scope and application.* Retrieved March 1, 2007, from http://www.fda.gov/cder/guidance/5667fnl.htm

CHAPTER 41
Electronic Data Capture in Clinical Trials

Joanne C. Ryan, RN, MS

Introduction

Ensuring the collection of high-quality data is critical to any clinical research study. The methods by which these data are collected have evolved from simple paper-based tools to more efficient remote data entry (RDE) approaches. As computers have come to play a greater role in daily life, it is anticipated that the speed and convenience that this technology provides could be applied to the clinical trial arena. This chapter will explore the evolution of data capture from paper-based to electronic and the requirements for utilizing RDE in the clinical research setting.

The Evolution of Data Collection Methods
Case Report Forms

Up until the 1980s, data for clinical trials were solely collected on paper. The information obtained at a subject's visit was initially recorded in the subject's chart or medical record and, thus, became the source document for the trial. The data were then transcribed onto a paper case report form (CRF), which was designed by the study sponsor (e.g., pharmaceutical company, cooperative group) to capture specific information appropriate to the clinical trial. These CRFs were monitored for their completeness and accuracy against the source documents (source document verification [SDV]) by a person designated by the sponsor in an effort to ensure the validity of the data. Following this, the CRF would be collected and sent to the sponsor for entry into its database. The data would be "cleaned," and the site would be required to respond to queries to provide missing information, clarify inconsistencies, or correct errors. This approach was cumbersome and resulted in long time intervals, perhaps months, between the subject's visit and the time at which the data were entered into the database. The delay contributed to the length of the clinical trial and ultimately the overall cost of the study.

In an effort to shorten the time frame from subject visit to database entry, changes were made in the 1990s to the process by which an investigational site could fax its unmonitored paper CRFs to the sponsor upon completion. The sponsor would scan these documents and enter the information into the database from the scanned image. Query generation would be performed after data entry, and the site could respond to the query before the monitor conducted a site visit and SDV. However, any changes to information on the CRF needed to be made on the original document. This modified CRF would need to be faxed back to the sponsor for scanning, so that the hard copy and scanned copies were identical at all times. A monitoring visit often resulted in additional changes, thus requiring more corrections, faxing, and scanning to take place. This overall approach did shorten the time from subject visit to data entry but added some additional steps to the process and still required the use of paper CRFs.

The next step in the evolutionary process came with the development of electronic CRFs (eCRFs) in the late 1990s. For the most part, these electronic documents are identical to the paper CRFs. In the initial phase of utilization of eCRFs, the sponsor often was required to provide the investigational site with a personal computer (PC), appropriate software, and telephone modem capabilities because most sites did not have the technical resources. Sponsors often developed their own software programs to manage the data collection. The site staff were required to complete a paper CRF from the data found in the source documents and then enter this data into an eCRF, resulting in double data entry. At predefined time intervals, the data were then sent either via modem or on diskette by regular mail to the sponsor for entry into the database. Thus, the process known as RDE emerged. While shortening the time to database entry, RDE also opened the door to additional transcription errors as the staff had to copy the data from the source document into the paper CRF and once again into the eCRF. The monitor was then required to compare all three sets of data for consistency.

The next phase of development involved utilizing the Internet for entering and transmitting clinical trial data. Web-based approaches to data collection became possible in the late 1990s, and the clinical trials industry moved from RDE to electronic data capture (EDC) technology (Marks, 2004). Although similar to RDE, the use of EDC provides for the immediate transfer of data and the ability to build more edit checks into the system so that some data entry errors can be identified and fixed up front. Monitors can conduct SDV directly with the data on the Web page, and reports can be generated easily. Trends in data entry errors can be easily and quickly identified and remedied.

A number of vendors have taken advantage of this new direction and have developed programs for Web-based data entry such as Datatrak EDC™ (Datatrak International) and InForm™ (Phase Forward). etrials® Worldwide has gone a step further and developed the eClinical Suite system. This system is intended to incorporate data from other sources in a clinical trial (e.g., central laboratories, randomization systems, supply management) and to integrate this with the data analysis programs, thereby allowing for a single, complete system to collect, manage, and analyze all data in a clinical trial.

Each method of data collection has advantages (see Figure 41-1). Factors that contribute to the decision to use either method include the length and complexity of the trial, available resources and capabilities of clinical investigative sites and the sponsor, and the subject population.

Figure 41-1. Advantages of Paper Versus Electronic Data Collection Methods

Advantages of Paper Data Collection
- Little training required
- Easy to transport
- No electronic malfunctions
- No modem/Internet access required
- Cost of development is less than for electronic system
- No equipment costs or maintenance requirements for handheld devices or Web-based programs

Advantages of Electronic Data Collection
- Shortened time from subject visit to data entry
- Incorporation of rules/edit checks up front, decreasing queries later on
- Rapid report generation
- Decreased overall length of the trial
- No need to decipher handwriting
- No transcription errors if data are entered directly
- No storage space required for case report forms with direct data entry
- Real-time data collection (diaries/tools)
- Rapid and timely data transmission from multiple sites simultaneously
- Can confirm subject compliance with diaries and instruments
- Manageable audit trail
- May be able to incorporate data from other sources (i.e., laboratory data)

Subject Diaries and Instruments

Clinical trials frequently require the use of subject diaries or validated scales with which to assess pain, quality of life, patient-reported outcomes, and other important measures. These outcomes often are the basis for nursing research and may include symptom management or survivorship. Paper versions of these tools have been used most often, and compliance with completion of these documents is well known to be a challenge (Bolger, Davis, & Rafaeli, 2003). Under most circumstances, it is critical to have the subject complete his or her documentation during the protocol-specified time frames. This provides the most accurate reflection of the subject's current state rather than relying on recall, which is quite limited and fraught with inaccuracies. Paper diaries and questionnaires are unsupervised and do not always reflect reality, as they may contain missed questions, delayed or incomplete entries, and recall bias (Lauritsen et al., 2004; Nyholm, Kowalski, & Aquilonius, 2004). Telephone and electronic versions of instruments recently have been created and implemented in clinical trials with the hope of increasing compliance and capturing data in "real time."

To compare reported and actual compliance with diary keeping, Stone, Shiffman, Schwartz, Broderick, and Hufford (2002) recruited 80 adults with chronic pain into a study that compared a paper diary versus an electronic diary. These 80 patients were evenly divided into two groups and assigned to complete either a paper or an electronic version of the diary. For the paper diary, the patient-reported compliance was 90%, but actual compliance was 11%. The actual compliance with the electronic diary was 94%. The researchers also assessed "hoarding" (when the diary binder was not opened but for which diary cards were completed), and 32% of the days contained no diary openings, yet the patients reported their compliance as 92%. Of the 40 patients using paper diaries, 75% had a minimum of one day of hoarding. Although the "auditory prompts" made by the handheld electronic device probably contributed to the greater compliance rate, this can be seen as an advantage to using this method of data collection.

The results of this study demonstrated the degree of noncompliance that occurs with paper instruments, yet in most clinical trials the compliance rate is unknown. Therefore, the data are assumed to be accurate, results are published, and clinical practice is potentially affected. Using a method of data collection that verifies compliance and increases the reliability of the data should be the goal regarding patient-reported outcomes and measures.

EDC seems to be a big step toward achieving this goal. In addition, many of the handheld devices utilize "touch screen" technology, making their use simple for those participants who have little or no computer experience. Whether via handheld or Web-based technology, some programs even allow for flexibility and targeting by which the subject's response to the current question determines the next question presented. For example, if asked about the presence or absence of a particular side effect of therapy, a positive response by the patient may generate a question related to the severity of that side effect, whereas a negative response may generate a question asking if a completely different side effect is present.

Considerations in Electronic Data Capture

While paper CRFs require very little in the way of physical resources, RDE and EDC have greater needs. A computer (laptop or PC) is required at the investigational site for data entry and, depending upon the goals of the trial, handheld devices for subject diaries or instruments may be necessary. High-speed Internet access (via broadband telephone or cable lines) is essential for EDC to have easy access to eCRFs and rapid turnover of data. Although many clinical trials are global in nature, instances have occurred where this service is not available; this then becomes a factor in determining whether a study uses only EDC, uses EDC in combination with paper CRFs, or simply uses paper alone.

Training of site staff is necessary whether using paper or electronic CRFs. As more practices are converting to electronic charting, healthcare practitioners are becoming more familiar with data entry procedures. However, the use of EDC may result in a greater learning curve depending upon the user's prior experience and comfort with the technology (Lopez-Carrero et al., 2005). As the use of electronic medical records becomes more widespread, clinical trial staff will become more comfortable with using electronic systems and will strengthen their data entry skills. Of course, the more user-friendly and efficient a system is, the more likely its users will accept this change. The same can be said for the ability and comfort of subjects/patients to enter their information into computerized systems (Mullen, Berry, & Zierler, 2004).

Summary

One of the greatest challenges facing the clinical research enterprise today is the ability to increase the efficiency of clinical trials while generating the highest-quality data and ensuring protection of participants. To accomplish this, the industry needs to develop and maintain an electronic system that will interface with all necessary sources of information. In addition, such a system would need to meet regulatory requirements (i.e., secure, valid, reliable, auditable), be cost effective and user friendly, enable rapid turnover of data without requiring additional steps, and demand a reasonable amount of training. To date, significant advances have been made in moving toward this goal; however, more investment is required.

Clinical research is critical to the development of new treatment options and to gaining a better understanding of the patient's experience. Because trials can be costly and labor intensive, improvements in speed and efficiency have become central to their success. It appears that embracing technology and moving to a more efficient electronic data collection approach would benefit sponsors, investigational site staff, and participants alike. The clinical trial nurse can be instrumental in helping to move this initiative forward, as the role of the research nurse is central to the successful conduct of clinical trials.

References

Bolger, N., Davis, A., & Rafaeli, E. (2003). Diary methods: Capturing life as it is lived. *Annual Review of Psychology, 54,* 579–616.

Lauritsen, K., Degl' Innocenti, A., Hendel, L., Praest, J., Lytje, M.F., Clem–memsen-Rotne, K., et al. (2004). Symptom recording in a randomized clinical trial: Paper diaries vs. electronic or telephone data capture. *Controlled Clinical Trials, 25,* 585–597.

Lopez-Carrero, C., Arriaza, E., Bolanos, E., Ciudad, M., Municio, J., & Hesen, W. (2005). Internet in clinical research based on a pilot experience. *Contemporary Clinical Trials, 26,* 234–243.

Marks, R.G. (2004). Validating electronic source data in clinical trials. *Controlled Clinical Trials, 25,* 437–446.

Mullen, K.H., Berry, D., & Zierler, B.K. (2004). Computerized symptom and quality-of-life assessment for patients with cancer, part II: Acceptability and usability. *Oncology Nursing Forum, 31,* 84–89.

Nyholm, D., Kowalski, J., & Aquilonius, S.M. (2004). Wireless real-time electronic data capture for self-assessment of motor function and quality of life in Parkinson's disease. *Movement Disorders, 19,* 446–451.

Stone, A.A., Shiffman, S., Schwartz, J.E., Broderick, J.E., & Hufford, M.R. (2002). Patient non-compliance with paper diaries. *BMJ, 324,* 1193–1194.

CHAPTER 42
Clinical Data Management Systems

Dianne M. Reeves, MSN

Introduction

Advancements in cancer detection, prevention, and treatment have a foundation in the data generated from clinical trials. This critical connection underscores the need to guarantee the quality of data gathered, managed, and shared. The data are arguably the most important outcome from the conduct of clinical trials. Thus, the need to institute systems and processes that yield high-quality data is paramount for any organization engaged in the conduct of clinical trials.

Clinical data management systems must be chosen, implemented, and maintained in accordance with policies that reflect the needs within an organization. Decisions of scope, scalability, interoperability, security, and the underlying structure of the system should be reached only after careful examination of local and future requirements.

This chapter addresses the *indicators* of clinical data management systems (e.g., scope, scalability, interoperability, security, standard operating procedure, semantic interoperability), and the *components* of a data management system (e.g., data entry, source documents, procedures, performance improvement, training/education, measures of success). A discussion of available resources also is provided for the reader.

Qualities of Clinical Data Management Systems

Today's world of clinical data management is characterized by the expanding scope and complexity of the research environment. There is a growing realization that a single solution for the management of data is not always possible; instead, the ability to make several systems interoperable is the key to transforming approaches. This means that a variety of approaches can be implemented to support data quality, system security, data aggregation, the integration of various data formats, workflow, and observance of subject compliance with regulatory guidelines.

The current literature usually discusses the realm of data management systems in research as overwhelming electronic in nature. Ambinder (2000) defined a clinical data management system as computer-based, with the ability to store and communicate data in a way that supports clinical decision making. In fact, the partnering of information technology (IT) with clinical research in the past two decades has accelerated the ability to provide innovative and successful approaches to data capture and management. The skills and focus of each community have produced multiple software systems that can be used to support clinical trials. This synergistic relationship allows the researcher to function more clearly in the role of domain or subject expert, identifying requirements for a data management system but not charged with finding a solution. Based on requirements from the research team, IT may decide to customize and/or use a commercially available software product (commercial off-the-shelf product) or to create a new one. The creation and maintenance of a data management approach must be a coordinated effort between IT and the research team, reflecting a balanced relationship between human and machine (Nemeth, Nunnally, O'Connor, Klock, & Cook, 2004).

Scope

Multi-institutional and multicenter research consortia trials are becoming commonplace. In settings where data are being collected and entered from disparate sites, the use of a common data management solution makes good business sense. Data management systems can operate from a single point of access (i.e., all data entry occurs at a single work station) or can provide a Web-based portal for all data entry. Systems that use *electronic data capture* (EDC) provide a level of convenience that is invaluable; a user logs into the system through a URL that uses password information to display customized forms and entry tools (see Chapter 41).

The merits of a remote entry system must be balanced with the increased security risks to data, the need to provide

Glossary of Terms

21 CFR Part 11— Title 21, Part 11 of the *Code of Federal Regulations,* which identifies criteria under which an organization considers electronic records and signatures to be essentially equivalent to handwritten records (Waters Laboratory Informatics, n.d.)

attribute—a property or characteristic of an object

audit trail—a chronologic record of computer activities used to reconstruct and examine a sequence and/or changes in events

case report form (CRF)—a primary data collection tool used in clinical research

clinical data management system—a computer-based system to capture, store, and/or share clinical data used for clinical decision making

commercial off-the-shelf (COTS) product—a software product that is commercially available to the public; the use of COTS can reduce software development costs and time.

common data element (CDE)—a fully described study variable or single data point. A CDE includes both the question being asked and a description of how responses will be captured.

configuration management—a process to ensure that only authorized changes will be made to a system

controlled vocabulary—a complete set of terms that has been identified; all terms in a controlled vocabulary should have unambiguous, nonredundant definitions.

cross-team training—education of personnel to facilitate coverage across a number of groups (teams) without a loss of efficiency or effectiveness

curation—the process of examining and preparing content to go into a database

data—information stored on the computer system; the actual results of a clinical trial or investigation

database—a structured repository to hold data, usually stored in a computer system

data collection instrument (DCI)—a form or set of forms used to collect information

data integrity—a state that exists when computerized data are the same as that in the source documents and have not been exposed to accidental or malicious alteration or destruction

data repository—a database acting as a storage facility

dataset—a collection of data or information that has a common theme

discrepancy—a difference between the data captured and the expected entry

electronic CRF (eCRF)—data collection forms that are implemented in computerized (electronic) form

electronic data capture (EDC)—alternative to the traditional paper-based recording of clinical trial data in which data are entered directly into an electronic computer system

enterprise (level)—a large-scale, organizationwide computer network

firewall—a security barrier that exists between a local private network and a public network, such as the Internet

information technology (IT)—forms of technology used to create, store, exchange, and utilize information in its various forms

International Electrotechnical Commission (IEC)—the international standards commission that prepares and publishes all standards for electrical, electronic, and related technologies

Internet—a network of computer networks that are publicly accessible and provide the basis for the World Wide Web (Web)

interoperability—ability of two or more computerized systems to exchange and then use the information that is shared

ISO 11179—International Organization for Standards 11179, an information standard for metadata registries

iterative process—series of updates and changes that evolve to a final and improved product

metadata—description of the data being collected or studied

metrics—measures used to indicate progress or achievement

network—a set of connected components for computers that enables communication and the sharing of data and software

protected health identifiers (PHI)—variables that can be used to uniquely identify a study subject that are protected by Health Insurance Portability and Accountability Act regulations

scalability—the ability of a software application or business approach to expand without significant loss of efficiency or effectiveness

security—the effort to create a secure computing platform, designed so that agents (users or programs) can only perform actions that have been allowed. This involves specifying and implementing a security policy.

semantics—the unique meaning given to a set of symbols in a language to differentiate it from all/any other symbols

semantic interoperability—the ability of computer systems to exchange information and then to meaningfully use the shared information

software system—computer program

source document—information in original records and certified copies of original records of clinical findings, observations, or other activities in a clinical trial necessary for the reconstruction and evaluation of a trial

stakeholder—an individual or group with an interest in the success of an organization

standard operating procedure (SOP)—document that defines a process for accomplishment of a specific task. SOPs are maintained by an organization through a formalized process of review and dissemination.

subject/domain matter expert (SME)—an individual with expertise in a specific domain or area of knowledge

terminology—standard set of symbols or words used to describe concepts and objects in a specified area of interest

URL—universal resource locator, the electronic address for a document on the Web access for various groups of users beyond traditional institutional firewall limits, and the challenges of data sharing and ownership (Geissbuhler, 1998; Marenco, Wang, Shepherd, Miller, & Nadkarni, 2004). Each institution or user group needs to conduct a thorough *assessment* of its own data management needs based on their scope, projected outcomes, and resource requirements.

Scalability

State-of-the-art clinical data management systems (sometimes referred to as CDMSs or CDMs) are electronic systems that are designed to permit growth as the programs that support them expand. *Scalability* is the ability of an application or business approach to grow without a significant loss of efficiency or effectiveness and must be considered from the inception of a project. Clinical data management systems that are easy to learn and use, require a reasonable amount of time to do various tasks, and produce output reliably and efficiently are good candidates for adoption by a large community of users.

Other areas that affect scalability can be the requirements for support systems (such as a "Help Desk" function to assist users) and the ability of these support mechanisms to create reusable resources to respond to questions and problems. In settings where performance actually improves with the addition of users, the system can be considered to be "scalable."

Interoperability

Interoperability is a critical attribute for successful data management systems. Electronic systems must be integrated or function together to create a robust set of data for the researcher. For example, data from laboratory systems or imaging systems represent a huge addition to a clinical data management system. Instead of manually reentering data from one application to another (which is time intensive as well as fraught with error), it is highly desirable to have the laboratory and imaging data electronically merge with the clinical data when they are needed. Data can be housed in a single repository or pulled from several sites in the form of a query or report when needed.

Quality data management systems use widely accepted external standards, such as the Logical Object Identifiers Names and Codes, or LOINC® (Regenstrief Institute, Inc.), terminologies. LOINC is one of the standards for use in U.S. federal government systems to exchange healthcare data, is supported by the National Library of Medicine, and was identified in 1999 as the preferred set of laboratory test names for use by healthcare facilities. LOINC provides a universal coding system for laboratory test data that facilitates the capture, storage, aggregation, and exchange of lab results from multiple sites (McDonald et al., 2003).

Interoperability is supported through activities that harmonize semantic differences in research questions, providing a data dictionary approach through the use of standards and controlled vocabularies (Marenco et al.,

2004). Instead of loosely defined data points that need to be redefined with each successive trial iteration, a comprehensive set of well-defined terms that can be reused and expanded over time is a much more efficient approach to the creation of a data management system.

Security

Confidentiality of patient data is a pivotal requirement for most healthcare organizations in the United States. The Health Insurance Portability and Accountability Act (HIPAA) of 1996 mandated the adoption of federal regulations for the protection of individually identifiable health information (HIPAA, 2000). Every healthcare provider who electronically transmits health information for certain transactions is covered by this act. Using electronic technology in itself does not meet the terms for consideration as a "covered entity." However, transactions such as healthcare claims benefit eligibility inquiries or referral authorization requests are covered by the HIPAA requirements. These requirements translate into the need to strip identifiable personal information from a subject's healthcare information and to use standard stipulated code sets in order to safeguard a subject's identity.

The HIPAA requirements for the protection of patient data provide a challenge for data management systems. The need to find more examples in the literature of the ability to maintain anonymity in real time in a database is paramount (Pace et al., 2003). The test of anonymity used in this citation was the ability of an expert to link events in a meaningful way that could be used to reconstruct an organization's or individual's identity.

In another example, physicians in an emergency department setting participated in a test of a Web-based, multisite system to collect real-time research data in compliance with HIPAA Privacy Act requirements (Kline, Johnson, Webb, & Runyon, 2004). Using extensive planning and analysis of requirements and data encryption, they linked nonprotected health identifiers or non–personal health information (PHI) data to PHI data (18 data elements identified with the HIPAA regulations as requiring anonymity) with appropriate password/login protection to access decrypted/reidentified data. Their measure of successful implementation was demonstrated by a 98.8% rate of data being reusable from all fields and was interpreted as no evidence of data intrusion or loss.

A more recent report described an algorithmic approach to clinical research database design that allowed analysis, distribution, and publication of clinical research without disclosing HIPAA PHI (Schell, 2006). Included in this report was notation that this algorithm did not include the cost or the design effort for the collection of clinical data.

Standard Operating Procedures

A broader and more fundamental requirement for all clinical data management systems is Title 21 of the *Code of*

Federal Regulations, Part 11 (21 CFR Part II). Approved in 1997, the law requires that people who use electronic systems to "create, modify, maintain, or transmit electronic records shall use procedures and controls designed to ensure the authenticity, and when appropriate, the confidentiality of electronic records" are required include (but are not limited to)

- Validation of systems to ensure they are accurate and reliable
- Protection of records to support ready and reliable retrieval
- Limiting system access to only authorized individuals
- Use of secure, computer-generated, time-stamped audit trails
- Clear linking of signatures to specific records
- Proper use of passwords and authority to use the system
- Proper training and preparation of all system users.

The use of standard operating procedures (SOPs), therefore, is integral to current enterprise-level data management systems. SOPs should offer guidance to a system's user that will guarantee the proper use and controls will be in effect. A set of SOPs should exist within each data management system organization, be accessible to system users, be reviewed and updated on a regular basis, and be subject to a configuration management strategy that will reliably handle versions and supporting documentation. SOPs also can support changes in workflow and social and organizational climate that will result from the introduction or change in data management systems. Institutions can apply existing guidelines for format, creation, and maintenance to the creation of data management SOPs.

Semantic Interoperability

Semantic interoperability is the ability of a data management system to clearly and unambiguously define the data that are being collected and then to share data in a way that retains their full meaning. When two separate collection systems define a data point exactly the same, the results can be aggregated or shared without an intermediate step to transform the data in some way. Semantic interoperability requires that data points be defined often through the use of controlled vocabularies and clearly defined variables. For example: A question on a case report form may ask for a subject's performance status. Institution A defines this as a self-reported score, whereas Institution B defines this as the result of using the Karnofsky Performance Status scale, which results in a set of clearly defined scores. If these two groups wish to combine their data for a larger analysis, the ability to aggregate "subject performance status" would not be possible. This variable is not defined nor captured using the same set of terms.

The clear definition of data points and questions creates "metadata," or descriptors that provide semantic uniqueness and clarity for a question. Creation of a set of common data elements (CDEs) is based on a collection of metadata profiles that can standardize the way in which data elements/questions can be asked, collected, stored, exchanged, and reported. The International Organization for Standardization (ISO, 2004) and the International Electrotechnical Commission, through ISO Standard 11179 (specification and standardization of data elements), support this approach to semantic interoperability.

The use of CDEs as a basis for data management systems is a good approach for biomedical inquiries, which change as the science evolves. Metadata can be easier to revise and reuse, as compared to the maintenance of multiple unsynchronized sets of study case report forms (CRFs) and data collection instruments (DCIs) that each implement a different version of a set of questions. Therefore, scalability is also supported through the metadata approach in data management systems (Brandt, Gadagkar, Rodriguez, & Nadkarni, 2004).

CDEs can support complex metadata relationships, but the creation and maintenance of these elements can be a challenge. Metadata holds the system's knowledge and thus must be created with great care. A *curation process* that involves subject/domain experts, iterative processes to confirm that the correct attributes are preserved, and a careful review are all necessary (Winget et al., 2003). Questions need to be defined precisely, with consensus reached among all members of the user community. The result will be a set of well-defined metadata that will reduce redundancy in data management efforts.

The metadata approach requires that a change-control strategy be used to create versions as questions change, with proper reference to the actual data collected. The regulation 21 CFR Part 11 requires the preservation of all versions of CRFs/DCIs used in a clinical study (Brandt et al., 2004). A well-documented approach to metadata and form versions must be part of every quality data management system.

One recent report described a group's committee-driven approach to create metadata to support prostate cancer studies (Patel et al., 2005). Their group developed 145 CDEs to annotate prostate tissue samples; these CDEs were used in multiple tissue sample requests and in dozens of tissue banking efforts. Their elements were ISO 11179 compliant and freely available for reuse. The outcome of this activity was an overall improvement in data collecting in terms of completeness and consistency across all questions.

Data content must be semantically defined and tagged with metadata descriptors to best support interoperability efforts (Covitz et al., 2003). Attributes, such as a complete definition, maximum permitted field length, and data type, must be fully documented. The true foundation of a CDE is the use of registered concepts or terminologies that can be referenced for review and reuse.

Fragoso, de Coronado, Haber, Hartel, and Wright (2004) described the National Cancer Institute's Thesaurus, a reference terminology holding more than 110,000 terms in more than 36,000 concepts used to create CDEs and other metadata. Each concept is a distinct unit of meaning complete with annotations and references to external authorities. Concepts also are defined by their relationships to other concepts in the thesaurus. Use of *registered concepts* facilitates interoperability across programs by mapping to commonly accepted terms, thus supporting data sharing. Initially labor intensive, the use of CDEs or metadata is conducive to supporting large research groups and multi-institutional cancer research efforts. Pooled data can be stored or warehoused or analyzed at later successive time points.

Components of a Clinical Data Management System

Elements of a clinical data management system are outlined in Figure 42-1. In its most simplistic form, it does not include features such as event scheduling, billing, and drug supply management, although it should be structured to support these other functions. The concept of modules that can be upgraded over time is important to consider. This approach allows organizations to customize a data management system to meet their own needs while retaining required functional components.

Data can be entered through a variety of means: entered manually, scanned into the system, fed into the system electronically through integrated sources of information (such as lab data), or even migrated in electronically from legacy electronic systems. The timeliness of entry from the time of an event should be addressed in SOPs, but should be as close temporally to an event as possible. An expert data manager who is comfortable with the system, educated in the handling of source documents, and equipped with good resources to resolve questions is an organization's most valuable asset in the establishment and maintenance of quality data management practices.

Data Entry

CRFs or DCIs remain the basic unit of data collection and entry in data management systems. Data of the same type or related in content are entered together. This permits the investigator and sponsor to sort through large datasets more efficiently. For example, batching all adverse event data together allows safety and monitoring groups to scan records more efficiently. It also permits the data manager to ascertain more quickly if key data points are missing from medical records or source documents.

Typically, CRFs are named to reflect the activities that occurred to support the primary activities of a clinical trial.

Figure 42-1. Elements of a Data Management System

- The software application itself
- Supporting standard operating procedures and documentation required to capture, edit, manage, and transmit data
- Training and support materials required for system users

If a trial is focused on the administration of a chemotherapeutic agent, CRFs would be expected to capture eligibility of the subject, pre-agent work-up and evaluation, study drug administration and associated events, follow-up activities including those conducted to assess response, and survival. A significant portion of the data collected may be expected to include labs, adverse events, and related procedures.

Electronic CRFs (eCRFs) should be envisioned as more than simply computerized paper CRFs (see Chapter 41). Data are entered directly into the computer instead of abstracting them first from some source documents onto a paper report form. The eCRFs often include additional and useful electronic features, such as data validation rules to entries, notation of mandatory fields that need to be completed, instructions on permissible values or formats, or calculations and support of complex data dependencies (such as "skip patterns" in questionnaires and surveys). Additional electronic support can be provided through interactive or real-time validation of entered values and context-sensitive help (Brandt et al., 2006). CRFs should use standard approaches and well-written user instructions to promote entry from multiple sites that typically use a variety of computer hardware configurations and personnel. The better the instructions to and education of personnel completing eCRFs, the higher the expected integrity and completeness of the data.

Data management systems that employ the CDE or metadata/data dictionary approach to questions on a CRF/DCI will use a significant number of items that have constrained or "choice list" entry fields. This is a move away from the collection of data in free text or comment fields on CRFs. Applications that use well-defined data questions can be programmed to look for deviations or "discrepancies" from an accepted list of permissible responses and then "flag" an entry to alert the data manager of a needed action. The use of constrained value sets needs to be supplemented on a case-by-case basis by the addition of text fields that capture verbatim descriptions of events or subject narratives.

The key to data integrity from the entry perspective is the principal investigator's agreement that the questions, data elements, CRFs, report templates, and reports all reflect the intent of the protocol document. Within the body of the protocol, all study specifications and specialized terminology (such as specialized rating scales for adverse events or lab data collection requirements) must be clearly delineated, with a plan for repeat measures of data points. This also is the logical spot to define study-specific terms, such as the length of a course of treatment, the end-of-treatment date, the follow-up period for a study registration, and study-specific requirements that need to be collected, stored, and reported.

Source Documents

Source documents, as defined by the *Guideline for Good Clinical Practice* (International Conference on Harmonisation [ICH], 1997), are original or primary documents, data, and records. Once CRFs are constructed, the source documents are reviewed and abstracted into the computerized entry screens. Personnel entering the data should be trained and supervised as needed to produce the type of quality outcomes mandated by an institution.

Although the use of original healthcare records as sources for research data purposes is critical, the user must remember that these records are intended to document observations, not specific information pertaining to research end points. Actual medical records may suffer from missing data and various types of errors (e.g., illegibility, incorrect entries, incorrect corrections of entries), and data management systems must be able to account for this type of data. The ability to note that data are missing, that a subject refused to answer a question, or that a critical value was not part of the source document are critical requirements of any quality data management system.

Procedures

All data management activity should be conducted under controlled conditions that support a quality outcome. Data entry procedures often are viewed as repetitive, tedious, and subject to error. Electronic clinical data management systems can be a source of error because of entry error, user inexperience, or system limitation. The generation and use of SOPs provides an indicator of an organization's ability to comply with the *Guideline for Good Clinical Practice* (ICH, 1997) and 21 CFR Part 11. SOPs should outline the content and scope of the tasks typically performed by the data management personnel, research nurses, and all other members of the research team. Activities such as the abstraction of data from source documents, the generation of reports and other forms of output, performance of quality assurance activities, and the review and resolution of data discrepancies all lend themselves to descriptive SOPs. These documents are used during internal and sponsor audits and during site visits as tools to assist an organization in the identification, correction, and reduction of errors in clinical data.

Quality Control Practices

Data management procedures are grounded in the need to incorporate robust quality assurance surveillance and monitoring activities into work procedures. Procedures to improve the product—the data—should be part of the daily work routine. Quality assurance exercises performed to document the institution's compliance with recognized levels or standards of excellence must be implemented within the context of creating an environment that values regular and critical reviews of the data. Emphasis must remain on review and correction of items and on improvement in processes employed in data handling.

Data cleaning activities are needed to identify and correct errors in an effort to minimize their effect upon trial results (Van den Broeck, Cunningham, Eeckels, & Herbst, 2005). This exercise reaffirms the value placed upon the data and does not transform or manipulate it in any way. Priority areas to begin with include those items that will have a major effect in areas of analysis and review and that can contaminate derived calculations of results, such as gender, critical dates, and primary study end point measures.

The Society for Clinical Data Management's *Good Clinical Data Management Practices*, version 4, published in May 2007, noted that regulations and guidelines do not delineate a minimum acceptable data quality level for clinical trials data. This is a standard that must be established *by each institution.* Data cleaning activities can lead to the identification of a number of common causes for erroneous data, such as writing or transcription errors, illegibility, out-of-range values, incorrect entries and/or changes to entries, data extraction or transformation errors, and sorting errors.

The application of quality control practices to collected data must be an integral part of a data management system. Random samples of entries may be reviewed on an ongoing basis; some organizations subject all of their data transmitted to sponsors to a routine review to ensure that it is validated and complete. Metrics should be maintained and shared with data entry personnel. Identified needs for improvement should be filtered back into the training program for users of the application.

Today's clinical data management systems can be configured to catch errors using a set of validation rules that will inform the data manager rapidly of the need to edit an entry or will at least attach a note to confirm that the data as entered are correct. Once data have reached the point that they are not going to be modified, they should have the capability to be locked. This gives perhaps only one person the ability to edit any portion of the dataset, and this person assumes responsibility for any further changes to the data.

Training and Education

The training and education of personnel who work with clinical research data is an investment in the future of the system and the organization. Data management staff, clinical trial nurses, study coordinators, and physicians accessing the system need to maintain a high level of awareness and expertise when working with electronic data. Certain concepts can be customized for each role.

The regulation 21 CFR Part 11 stipulates that people who work with clinical data management systems must have the education, training, and experience or any combination thereof necessary to perform their assigned tasks. Qualified individuals must perform training, and records of training must be maintained.

Data management personnel benefit from *cross-team training* for numerous reasons. Components of a skills inventory for these personnel may be as specific as institutional requirements demand. A standardized approach to procedures such as data entry, report generation, and the conduct of data audits should be reflected in data management SOPs and skills inventories. Such an approach incorporates a quality improvement philosophy into work processes. A number of professional organizations and societies have journals that can provide continuing education and updates on topics of interest to the clinical trial nurse (see Figure 42-2).

Measures of Success

Determination of a successful data management system can be based upon a number of criteria. Is the system able to accommodate data entry from all sources in a timely manner? Can input data from various sources be compiled in a logical way to be useful to the investigator? Are the data able to be reported to sponsors and monitoring agencies without a series of interim data transformation steps?

In their review of clinical information systems, Van der Meijden, Hange, Troost, and Hasman (2003) found that the stakeholders (people or groups who have a stake in the outcome of a project), the organization, and the objectives of the system determine success. They also discovered that definitions of success tend to change over time and are dependent upon the perspectives of the stakeholder performing the evaluation. One approach to gathering ongoing measures of success is to create an inventory of system requirements and desired outcomes at the inception or adoption of a data management system. Requirements should be concisely phrased with measurable outcomes. An example of an outcome may be that data entry formats will be standardized across individual studies, with reuse of the same CRFs in each study.

The ability to gather metrics concerning generation of data discrepancies and their resolution, completeness, and timeliness of data entry should be obtainable from a quality data management system. Program directors should make use of this valuable information to plan and budget resources for system support and to prescribe improvements in quality assurance and quality improvement programs. Practice issues should be analyzed and used to revise SOPs on a regular basis, improving an organization's quality improvement program expectations.

Summary

Clinical data management systems must be chosen, implemented, and maintained in accordance with policies that reflect the needs of an organization. Decisions of scope, scalability, interoperability, security, and the underlying structure of the system should be reached only after careful examination of local and future requirements. Difficult decisions can be guided through the construction of realistic-use cases that illustrate the breadth and complexity of biomedical research. The *Guideline for Good Clinical Practice* and adherence to regulatory guidelines must be reflected in the day-to-day functioning of the system.

Although the literature and case studies supply a number of indicators (see Figure 42-3) for the creation or choice of quality clinical data management systems, ultimately each organization is charged with making the best decisions based on its own requirements. Careful planning with ongoing analysis is necessary to ensure a thorough evaluation of active clinical data management systems.

Figure 42-3. Indicators of Quality Data Management Systems

- Electronic application
- Standardized, well-constructed electronic case report forms for data entry
- Support for scope of work
- Data security
- Scalability
- Interoperability
- Semantic definition of data points (data dictionary, common data elements, metadata registry)
- Standard operating procedures
- Training program for all users
- Support of standards and controlled vocabulary where appropriate
- Report capabilities
- User support systems—online help, help desk functions
- Quality improvement program with ongoing collection/analysis of metrics
- Quality assurance program with data validation activities
- Health Insurance Portability and Accountability Act compliance for covered entities
- 21 CFR Part 11 certification of implementation

Figure 42-2. Computer-Related Journals in Health Care

- *Artificial Intelligence in Medicine*
- *BMC (Biomed Central) Cancer*
- *British Journal of Healthcare Computing and Information Management*
- *Cancer Informatics*
- *Clinical Trials*
- *Computers in Biology and Medicine*
- *Computers in Nursing*
- *Contemporary Clinical Trials*
- *Health Informatics Europe*
- *Health Information Management*
- *Healthcare Computing and Communications*
- *Healthcare Informatics*
- *Informatics Review*
- *International Journal of Medical Informatics*
- *Journal of Biomedical Informatics*
- *Journal of Information Systems Management*
- *Journal of the American Medical Informatics Association*
- *Nursing Management*

References

Ambinder, E. (2000). Oncology and the information revolution. In D.W. Kufe, R.E. Pollock, R.R. Weichselbaum, R.C. Bast, Jr., T.S. Gansler, J.F. Holland, et al. (Eds.), *Cancer medicine* (5th ed., pp. 2454–2467). London: B.C. Decker.

Brandt, C.A., Argraves, S., Money, R., Ananth, G., Trocky, N.M., & Nadkarni, P. (2006). Informatics tools to improve clinical research study implementation. *Contemporary Clinical Trials, 27,* 112–122.

Brandt, C.A., Gadagkar, R., Rodriguez, C., & Nadkarni, P.M. (2004). Managing complex change in clinical study metadata. *Journal of the American Medical Informatics Association, 11*, 380–391.

Covitz, P.A., Hartel, F., Schaefer, C., De Coronado, S., Fragoso, G., Sahni, H., et al. (2003). caCORE: A common infrastructure for cancer informatics. *Bioinformatics, 19*, 2404–2412.

Fragoso, G., de Coronado, S., Haber, M., Hartel, F., & Wright, L. (2004). Overview and utilization of the NCI thesaurus. *Comparative and Functional Genomics, 5*, 648–654.

Geissbuhler, A. (1998). Clinical information systems—What is the bottom line? *Journal of the American Medical Informatics Association, 5*, 585–586.

Health Insurance Portability and Accountability Act. (2000). Standards for privacy of individually identifiable health information—Rules and regulations. *Federal Register, 65*, 250.

International Conference on Harmonisation. (1997). *Guideline for good clinical practice: ICH harmonized tripartite guideline.* Geneva, Switzerland: Author.

International Organization for Standardization. (2004). *Specification and standardization of data elements Part 3: Basic attributes of data elements.* Retrieved December 16, 2007, from http://www.iso.org

Kline, J.A., Johnson, C.L., Webb, W.B., & Runyon, M.S. (2004). Prospective study of clinician-entered research data in the Emergency Department using an Internet-based system after the HIPAA Privacy Rule. *BMC Medical Informatics and Decision Making, 4*, 17.

Marenco, L., Wang, T., Shepherd, G., Miller, P.L., & Nadkarni, P. (2004). QIS: A framework for biomedical database federation. *Journal of the American Medical Informatics Association, 11*, 523–534.

McDonald, C.J., Huff, S.M., Suico, J.G., Hill, G., Leavelle, D., Aller, R., et al. (2003). LOINC, a universal standard for identifying laboratory observations: A 5-year update. *Clinical Chemistry, 49*, 624–633.

Nemeth, C., Nunnally, M., O'Connor, M., Klock, P.A., & Cook, R. (2004). Getting to the point: Developing IT for the sharp end of healthcare. *Journal of Biomedical Informatics, 38*, 18–25.

Pace, W.D., Staton, E.W., Higgins, G.S., Main, D.S., West, D.R., & Harris, D.M. (2003). Database design to ensure anonymous study of medical errors: A report from the ASIPS Collaborative. *Journal of the American Medical Informatics Association, 10*, 531–540.

Patel, A.A., Kajdacsy-Balla, A., Berman, J.J., Bosland, M., Datta, M.W., Dhir, R., et al. (2005). The development of common data elements for a multi-institute prostate cancer tissue bank: The Cooperative Prostate Cancer Tissue Resource (CPCTR) experience. *BMC Cancer, 5*, 108.

Schell, S.R. (2006). Creation of clinical research databases in the 21st century: A practical algorithm for HIPAA compliance. *Surgical Infections, 7*, 37–44.

Society for Clinical Data Management. (2007, May). *Good clinical data management practices (GCDMP), version 4.* Milwaukee, WI: Author.

Van den Broeck, J., Cunningham, S.A., Eeckels, R., & Herbst, K. (2005). Data cleaning: Detecting, diagnosing, and editing data abnormalities. *PLoS Medicine, 2*, e267.

Van der Meijden, M.J., Hange, H.J., Troost, J., & Hasman, A. (2003). Determinants of success of inpatient clinical information systems: A literature review. *Journal of the American Medical Informatics Association, 10*, 235–243.

Waters Laboratory Informatics. (n.d.). *21CFRPart11.com.* Retrieved from http://www.21cfrpart11.com

Winget, M.D., Baron, J.A., Spitz, M.R., Brenner, D.E., Warzel, D., Kincaid, H., et al. (2003). Development of common data elements: The experience of and recommendations from the early detection research network. *International Journal of Medical Informatics, 70*, 41–48.

CHAPTER 43

Cancer Trials Support Unit: A Service of the National Cancer Institute

Mechelle Barrick, BSN, RN, OCN®, CCRP

Introduction

The Cancer Trials Support Unit (CTSU) is a pilot project of the National Cancer Institute (NCI) that provides clinicians across the United States and Canada with access to cancer clinical trials. CTSU programs and services include regulatory support, patient registration, clinical data management, help desk support, promotion, education and training, site performance evaluation, and site financial management.

Background

In 1996, NCI and its Board of Scientific Advisors convened the Clinical Trials Program Review Group to evaluate NCI-sponsored extramural clinical trial programs. Based on the review group's recommendations, NCI decided to create the CTSU, whose aim would be to increase access and accrual to phase III trials sponsored by NCI (Abrams et al., 2001). In 1999, NCI initiated plans to develop the CTSU. Initial funding grants for the project were awarded to three groups: Westat (prime contractor), Coalition of Cancer Cooperative Groups (CCCG) (subcontractor), and Oracle Corporation (subcontractor). Westat is an employee-owned research corporation founded in 1961 and based in Rockville, MD. It is a leading statistical survey research organization with expertise in multiple research areas, including clinical trials. Westat Clinical Trials oversees protocol management including protocol design, patient evaluation and enrollment, statistical data collection, management and analysis, adverse event submission, data queries, and interfacing with participating cooperative groups for assurance of accurate and timely data submission and compliance. The CCCG provides the leadership and direction for the CTSU and oversees education and training, financial and regulatory management, and site evaluation and audits.

Goals of the Cancer Trials Support Unit

One of the organizational goals of the CTSU is to provide a wide selection of NCI clinical trial options to as many investigators as possible, thereby involving more institutions in the clinical trial accrual process (Abrams, 2002). Through this effort, additional patients could be enrolled to cancer clinical trial protocols, and overall accrual numbers would increase. The CTSU aims to provide a streamlined approach to regulatory management, allowing for the central management of enrollment, data management, and safety monitoring. This process results in a more efficient means of managing patient information and allows smaller oncology practices to enroll patients with minimal internal staff resources.

Registration

By registering with the CTSU, physicians who are current members of a clinical trial cooperative group are able to enroll their patients in other cooperative group clinical trials without being a member of that specific cooperative group (see the CTSU Web site [www.ctsu.org] for a listing of clinical trials groups). Cooperative group members, including investigators and staff, must initially register using the Cancer Therapy Evaluation Program (CTEP) Accounts Management System (AMS), available at the CTSU Web site. CTEP enrollment provides the CTSU with the ability to centrally validate and maintain updated information on all staff participating in CTSU trials.

Physicians who are not members of any of the participating cooperative groups must initially apply to the CTSU to be considered as a CTSU Independent Clinical Research Site (CICRS). Online application forms are available. Once the application is submitted, the CTSU will review the individual and institutional site credentials. Upon approval, physicians then are granted support and access to all protocols. No mandatory accrual minimum is required for ongoing participation in this program. All clinical trials available through the CTSU have received Central Institutional Review Board (CIRB) approval. CIRB approval does not preclude local sites from obtaining the necessary local institutional approval as specified by each individual's institutional site. However, the CIRB provides a full review process that allows the site to download all CIRB approved protocol, consent, and supporting documents for a facilitated local review.

Active Participation

In an effort to streamline regulatory management, all sites submit regulatory documents to a central regulatory support system (RSS). This central repository manages the database containing all investigator credentials, site enrollment, and performance and institutional review board (IRB) requirements. Once active enrollment is established, protocols and supportive documents are available at the members' page on the CTSU Web site. Protocols of interest, including amendments, safety updates, case report forms, adverse event forms, and educational materials, can be downloaded from the site, and needed documents can be submitted to the site's local IRB for review. All required regulatory documents (CTSU IRB certification form, regulatory approval transmission sheet, IRB-approved consents, and any protocol-specific regulatory documents) then are submitted to the RSS after local IRB approval and prior to patient enrollment.

Patient Enrollment

Before patient enrollment to a specific trial can take place, all regulatory documentation must be submitted to and processed by the CTSU. The site and investigator must be registered CTSU members. Protocol eligibility, including protocol-specific patient consent, inclusion and exclusion criteria, and pretreatment evaluations, is verified by the site. Registration materials then are faxed to the CTSU using protocol-specific registration forms and the patient enrollment transmittal form. Within one hour of receiving the documents, the site will be notified of enrollment status, including the patient's treatment group assignment and protocol identification number.

Data Submission

Data submission guidelines are protocol-specific. For the majority of studies, data forms are submitted to the group leading the trial using the methods outlined in the CTSU Logistical Appendix of each protocol document. The CTSU also monitors sites for delinquency of data submissions, volume of queries, and response time. Quarterly reports are issued regarding data quality, and an improvement plan is needed by sites failing to meet current CTSU standards. Standard site audits are conducted as part of cooperative group audits.

The instructions for reporting an adverse event vary among cooperative groups. The adverse event reporting guidelines using toxicity assessment in accordance with the NCI Common Terminology Criteria with guidelines and additional information can be found on the CTSU member Web site.

Educational and Supportive Services

Educational materials and promotional documents are available on the CTSU member Web site and include the following: the CTSU operations manual, eCourse, protocol-specific physician fact sheets, protocol screening cards, and treatment evaluation/events sheets. PowerPoint presentations also are available to use for staff education and training. For an example of some of the resources that are publicly available, see Figure 43-1.

Outcome of the Cancer Trials Support Unit

Since its inception, the CTSU has registered approximately 12,000 patients to clinical research trials, with an average monthly accrual in 2005 of 600 patients (Riordan, 2005). A bimonthly online newsletter is sent to all members that includes updates regarding the status of clinical trials, including activations, terminations, and protocol amendments. Additionally, the CTSU is moving forward to pilot the use of remote data capture in several of its studies. This process would allow for a more timely collection of data and subsequent study events, thus decreasing time and costs for overall study management. With more than 10,000 registered users, the CTSU can assist in promoting protocols in numerous ways. Broad participation and rapid accrual have led to several important studies achieving results much faster than was possible before the advent of the CTSU (NCI, 2006).

Summary

The CTSU developed as NCI recognized the need to provide oncologists and patients with a means to access a variety of clinical research trials in a standardized and streamlined process (Donovan, 2001). Today, the CTSU provides practitioners with the ability to increase clinical trial opportunities for patients and to streamline the enrollment process. Each year, monthly enrollment increases and more physicians have signed on as members. With several new projects, including remote data capture and ongoing educational efforts, the

---

Figure 43-1. Publicly Available Cancer Trials Support Unit (CTSU) Educational and Supportive Materials*

- **eCourse:** This is an online educational program that introduces and explains the CTSU for those interested in learning more and/or becoming registered members.
- **CTEP-AMS fact sheet:** This fact sheet guides new investigators/noninvestigators on how to register with the CTSU by establishing an account with the Cancer Therapy Evaluation Program-Account Management System (CTEP-AMS).
- **RSS fact sheet:** This fact sheet defines the regulatory support system (RSS) and how it is utilized by the CTSU.
- **Study status list:** This list of studies provides all the protocols that are active on the CTSU menu.
- **CTSU process checklist:** This checklist provides a step-by-step tool that outlines protocol-specific site/patient enrollment registration. A separate checklist is available for Canadian participants.

* Available at www.ctsu.org

CTSU can only continue to be more successful in supporting clinical trial recruitment efforts. The clinical trial nurse can help to educate others about this valuable NCI resource, especially patient advocates and physicians who do not currently participate in cancer clinical trials.

References

Abrams, J.S. (2002). Clinical trials referral resource. Current clinical trials of the cancer trials support unit (CTSU), an NCI pilot program. *Oncology, 16,* 1074–1077, 1080.

Abrams, J.S., Gotting, V., Whitehouse, J., Riordan, S., Meadows, B., Chiausa, A., et al. (2001). Development of web-based systems to facilitate phase III clinical trials enrollment: Early results from the CTSU pilot project [Abstract No. 2619]. *Proceedings from the American Society of Clinical Oncology, 20.* Retrieved January 15, 2008, from http://www.asco.org

Donovan, C. (2001). CTSU provides tools that link research and practice. *ONS News, 16*(10), 14–15.

National Cancer Institute. (2006). CTSU increases patient and physician access to clinical trials. *NCI Cancer Bulletin, 3*(42), 1–8.

Riordan, S. (2005). Note from the CTSU project director. *CTSU Quarterly Newsletter, Issue 3,* pp. 1–2. Retrieved October 15, 2005, from https://members.ctsu.org

CHAPTER 44
Clinical Trial Registries

Nina M. Trocky, MSN, RN, CCRA, and Cynthia Brandt, MD, MPH

Introduction

A clinical trial registry is a repository of information about clinical trials that are open and enrolling patients as well as closed trials. The process by which a clinical trial is registered, such as posting descriptive information on a specific Web site, is in fact the beginning of a public declaration that the study exists. This chapter provides the clinical trial nurse (CTN) with an overview of clinical trial registries, their history, recent developments, and examples of registries that are currently active.

Clinical Trial Registries

Tonks (1999) stated that "registering a clinical trial of a new drug or intervention means putting on public record some basic information about the trial from its inception" (p. 1566). This is called *prospective registration*. She further explained that the aim of a registry is to provide reliable intelligence concerning the research process, while *in progress*, to various stakeholders, including the public, researchers, funding bodies, and healthcare providers. The World Health Organization (WHO, 2005a) defined a trial registry as a directory that lists key administrative and scientific information about planned, ongoing, and completed trials that is sufficient to identify that trial's existence. Registries also may be used for recruiting trial participants or for other purposes. Similarly, the Institute of Medicine (IOM) described a clinical trial registry as a vehicle that serves as a repository for various related information specific to ongoing clinical trials (IOM: Committee on Clinical Trial Registries, 2006).

When discussing clinical trial registries, the terms *results database* ("Fair Access to Clinical Trials Act," 2007; Fisher, 2006), *trial bank* (Sim & Detmer, 2005), and *results registers* (Rockhold et al., 2005) may be used, as these terms refer to separate yet complementary repositories of information. These databases can augment the registries as a vehicle to disseminate trial results, outcomes, or end products and to supplement information similar to that published in peer-reviewed journals. The separate or unconnected databases

may be linked through the use of a unique identifier to the clinical trial registries for a more seamless continuum of information. The results database also can serve to publish all trial results, regardless of the outcomes of the study.

Clinical trial registries aim to improve the accessibility of trial information for the purpose of aiding in more informed decision making and expanding access to interested and eligible patients. Although no single or comprehensive registry exists, multiple registries are available that serve the public and professionals who need to learn more about open and enrolling trials, thereby enhancing the decision-making process (McCray, 2000).

Additionally, both the conduct and the outcomes of clinical trials must be publicly known and easily accessible, as these data will lay the foundation of evidence-based medicine and ultimately transparency throughout the research continuum (Dickersin et al., 2004; Dickersin & Rennie, 2003; McCray, 2000; Sim & Detmer, 2005). Currently, there is significant movement toward consolidation, centralization, and standardization of the type and amount of information on both the clinical trial registry and the results database. Taken individually, clinical trial registries serve as a starting point from which patients and professionals may find and locate clinical trials.

Purpose of Clinical Trial Registries

Figure 44-1 outlines the basic purposes of a clinical trial registry: access to information, notification, education, choice, and communication. Registries serve as a vehicle to support enrollment of patients into clinical trials as well as to inform physicians of open trials to which they may refer potential study participants (Dickersin & Rennie, 2003; McCray, 2000; McCray & Ide, 2000; Rockhold et al., 2005). Registries are not considered recruitment tools because recruitment materials must be reviewed and approved by an organization's institutional review board (IRB). Fisher (2006) stated that a registry is a public record that serves two primary purposes: (a) to educate patients about the specific clinical trial requirements, el-

Figure 44-1. Purposes of a Clinical Trial Registry

- Offer access to open and enrolling clinical trials information.
- Facilitate public notification that a clinical trial exists.
- Promote subject recruitment into a clinical trial.
- Educate the public and professionals.
- Notify the public when the clinical trial has closed to enrollment.
- Serve to alert the public that trial results should be available.
- Support evidence-based medicine and scientific advances.

igibility criteria, and protocol summary to include study purpose and recruitment status, and (b) to establish an expectation that summary information and trial results would be publicly disseminated upon study completion.

In the 1980s, clinical trial registries focused on addressing special conditions or diseases. Targeted in their focus, registries initially were conceived to facilitate enrollment into specialty or disease-specific trials (e.g., AIDS, breast cancer). Patients and healthcare providers could access trial information, such as eligibility criteria, as they searched for treatments, thereby expanding their care options (Dickersin et al., 2004; McCray, 2000; McCray & Ide, 2000). For example, the AIDS Clinical Trials Information Service, AIDS Education Global Information System, and CancerNet were specialty registries that focused on AIDS and cancer clinical trials (McCray; McCray & Ide; Tonks, 1999).

The IOM and the National Academies (IOM: Committee on Clinical Trial Registries, 2006) noted consensus building among the International Committee of Medical Journal Editors (ICMJE), scientists from the National Institutes of Health (NIH) and the U.S. Food and Drug Administration (FDA), and representatives from the pharmaceutical and biotechnical industries as they identified the goals of a robust central clinical trial registry. Figure 44-2 describes the four goals of a central clinical trial registry.

Currently, several different registries exist that include similar study-specific information, yet each registry varies in content, types of trials included, format, and search properties. The lack of standardization among them may present

Figure 44-2. Four Goals of a Central Clinical Trial Registry

1. To provide patients and their healthcare providers with adequate and reliable information about clinical trials that may be enrolling patients.
2. To provide healthcare providers, patients, and others with the results of a clinical trial once the trial is completed and the product is available for prescription.
3. To link each clinical trial initiated with a reported outcome, thereby preventing selective or biased reporting of results.
4. To meet the first three goals in a way that protects proprietary research data, as necessary, and preserves innovation.

Note. From *Developing a National Registry of Pharmacologic and Biologic Clinical Trials: Workshop Report* (pp. 1–2), by Committee on Clinical Trial Registries, Institute of Medicine of the National Academies, 2006, Washington, DC: National Academies Press. Copyright 2006 by the National Academies Press. Reprinted with permission.

an added weight or complexity, beginning with the sheer volume of information, for even the most astute healthcare professional to navigate a focused and productive search.

Information Contained in a Clinical Trial Registry

Numerous registries exist today, the majority of which are Web accessible. The target of each registry varies in the degree of comprehensiveness (directory of trials versus phases of trials), spectrum of therapeutic areas (pharmaceutical, preventive, nonexploratory, behavioral, device), geographic areas (national or international), and sponsorship (FDA-sponsored, pharmaceutical-sponsored, investigator-initiated). Each registry is designed to disclose specific details of new studies at or before their inception and definitely prior to the beginning of the patient accrual process.

Interested individuals can review the information contained in a registry to identify clinical trials that would be most appropriate to their needs. An adequate description should be included so that people seeking information can quickly narrow their search to the most appropriate and meaningful trials. The IOM (IOM: Committee on Clinical Trial Registries, 2006) set forth several guiding principles that contribute to a robust and valid clinical trial registry, which are presented in Figure 44-3.

Figure 44-3. Desirable Guiding Principles and Goals for a Clinical Trial Registry

- Be global in perspective.
- Offer access to the public at no charge.
- Be located on a single website or linked via a single portal.
- Be open to all prospective registrants.
- Be managed by a not-for-profit organization or trusted governmental agency.
- Have the capacity for electronic searches.
- Provide a mechanism to ensure the validity of the registration data.
- Have a process to ensure adherence to the registry standards.
- Avoid reducing any incentives to conduct clinical research, whether public or privately funded.

Note. From *Developing a National Registry of Pharmacologic and Biologic Clinical Trials: Workshop Report* (p. 19), by Committee on Clinical Trial Registries, Institute of Medicine of the National Academies, 2006, Washington, DC: National Academies Press. Copyright 2006 by the National Academies Press. Reprinted with permission.

WHO is leading the effort to move beyond a national focus to a more inclusive international focus of standardization or harmonization. Building on earlier efforts and standards proposed by others, such as the ICMJE (DeAngelis et al., 2004, 2005a, 2005b), WHO (2005b) established minimum data set requirements for international trial registry listings (see Figure 44-4).

The purpose of a minimum data set is to identify a uniform group of elements that serve to organize and *standardize* specific information. This means that each clinical trial registry would contain the same information in the same

Figure 44-4. World Health Organization 20 Items Minimal Registration Data Set (Version 1.0)

1. Primary register and trial ID number
2. Date of registration in primary register
3. Secondary IDs
4. Source(s) of monetary or material support
5. Primary sponsor
6. Secondary sponsor(s)
7. Contact for public queries
8. Contact for scientific queries
9. Public title
10. Scientific title
11. Countries of recruitment
12. Health condition(s) or problems studies
13. Interventions
14. Key inclusion and exclusion criteria
15. Study type
16. Date for first enrollment
17. Target sample size
18. Recruitment status
19. Primary outcome(s)
20. Key secondary outcomes

Note. From *World Health Organization Trial Registration Data Set*, by World Health Organization, n.d. Retrieved April 6, 2007, from http://www.who.int/ictrp/data_set/en/print.html. Copyright 2006 by the National Academies Press. Reprinted with permission.

format. While the WHO directives are consensus driven, they serve primarily as the building blocks from which they will advance the consolidation and unification efforts. WHO, in addition to defining the minimum data set of 20 items, also has established a project titled the International Clinical Trials Registry Platform (ICTRP) (WHO, 2005c). The *platform,* as it is referred to, facilitates access to information about clinical trials and their results. The ICTRP's purpose is to lead the way in setting international standards and norms for both clinical trials registration and results reporting. The objectives of the platform are to

• Ensure that all clinical trials are registered.
• Attest that all clinical trials are publicly declared and uniquely identifiable.
• Ensure that a minimum set of data will be reported at trial completion.
• Ensure that trial results will be publicly reported and publicly available.

WHO's focus is on establishing a higher global standard for streamlining the clinical trial accrual process, increasing public trust by facilitating publication of all trial results, and establishing core data elements facilitating consistency and equity. Several clinical trial registries currently exist. Each varies in content, focus, and orientation. Before beginning a search, it is important to have a clear idea of what information is sought so that the search can be directed and focus-oriented to the specific need or area of interest.

Examples of Clinical Trial Registries

Healthcare providers, researchers, and patients currently have access to the following examples of Web-based clinical trial registries. It is important to note that not all clinical trial registries address only cancer-related trials; many include information about any disease site or treatment trials. Of the registries highlighted in the following section, none have a fee or associated charge for searching their databases.

Government-Sponsored Registries

Physician Data Query, commonly called PDQ®, is the National Cancer Institute's (NCI's) comprehensive cancer database. Launched in 1984, the original intent was to aid in the rapid dissemination of research findings, provide oncology professionals and patients with the most advanced information on cancer treatment, and facilitate recruitment to clinical trials. It comprises three main sections: PDQ Cancer Clinical Trials Registry, PDQ Cancer Information Summaries, and PDQ Directories of Health Professionals and Organizations Involved in Cancer Care. All sections can be accessed through www.cancer.gov/cancertopics/pdq/cancerdatabase.

The PDQ Cancer Clinical Trials Registry contains only oncology clinical trials. Considered an extensive resource, this registry includes two databases: one containing more than 4,000 *abstracts* of open cancer clinical trials and another including more than 15,000 abstracts of trials that are closed to accrual and completed. PDQ Cancer Clinical Trials Registry primarily includes NCI-sponsored trials, but, to a lesser degree, non-NCI–sponsored trials are incorporated (e.g., pharmaceutical-sponsored trials).

Performing a basic search is simple. A search field with a drop-down box allows the searcher to select from a variety of cancer types. Once the type of cancer is selected, the stages or subtypes of that cancer are identified in the field below the original selection. With the stage or subtype identified, the type of trial may be selected. Treatment, supportive care, screening, and genetics are a few of the trial types available. The final criterion is the geographic location of the research site. A basic search for supportive care trials for patients with follicular thyroid identified four trials within a 100-mile radius of Washington, DC.

Each search provides an abstract that includes basic trial information, trial description, summary, further trial information, eligibility criteria, and trial contact information. Each abstract may be viewed in lay or technical language.

The PDQ Cancer Clinical Trials Registry is periodically merged with an NIH database called ClinicalTrials.gov. The exchange of information between NCI's PDQ and NIH's ClinicalTrials.gov ensures harmony between the two registries with respect to cancer trials. Therefore, trials registered in the one registry will be registered in the other.

The two other sections, PDQ Cancer Information Summaries and PDQ Directories of Health Professionals and Organizations Involved in Cancer Care, offer summaries of peer-reviewed articles and treatment digests and contact information of health professionals and services, respectively.

In February 2000, the National Library of Medicine and the NIH launched ClinicalTrials.gov as a result of the FDA Modernization Act, Section 113. The act was passed into law in November 1997 (Center for Drug Evaluation and Research [CDER], 2002) and specifically requires that the U.S. Department of Health and Human Services (DHHS) establish a clinical trial registry program through the NIH. The result was an Internet-accessible databank, ClinicalTrials.gov, which contains

- Information about both federally and privately funded clinical trials for experimental treatments for patients who have serious or life-threatening disease and conditions
- A description of the experimental agent
- Eligibility criteria
- Locations of recruitment sites
- Contact information for patients seeking enrollment.

ClinicalTrials.gov contains approximately 29,500 efficacy clinical studies sponsored by the NIH, other federal agencies, and private industry. Studies listed in the database are conducted within the United States plus in more than 130 countries internationally. Entry of a condition and a location can generate a combination search. Selecting a specific trial will list the sites, geographic location, and contact information for that particular trial. ClinicalTrials.gov is open and accessible to both public and healthcare professionals and serves as a registry for researchers to post trials, as well as an open-access site for the general public. ClinicalTrials.gov focuses on serious and life-threatening illness and those trials that include well-controlled hypothesis testing and excludes exploratory and non-hypothesis–generating trials. Data from the AIDS Clinical Trials Information System and PDQ are included in ClinicalTrials.gov, and all may be accessed on http://clinicaltrials.gov.

Commercially Sponsored Registries

TrialCheck® is an oncology-focused clinical trial registry developed by the Coalition of National Cancer Cooperative Groups (2006). Located at www.trialcheck.org/services, TrialCheck is intended primarily for oncology professionals—physicians, oncologists, nurses, clinical research associates, and patient advocates—and is another example of a Web-based application. The uniqueness lies in its focus: cooperative group oncology trials. According to its Web site (Coalition of National Cancer Cooperative Groups), the TrialCheck database contains the active clinical trials of the Cancer and Leukemia Group B, Eastern Cooperative Oncology Group, North Central Cancer Treatment Group, National Surgical Adjuvant Breast and Bowel Project, Radiation Therapy Oncology Group, and Alpha Oncology. Trials conducted by other cooperative groups are highlighted under a section called intergroup studies.

The TrialCheck Web site offers initial screening options and serves as a preliminary vehicle for searching for oncology trials by protocol and eligibility criteria, location of physician researcher, or treating institution. Specifically, TrialCheck offers oncology professionals the

options of screening the registry for clinical trials appropriate for their patients, searching for specific cancer clinical trials using a unique protocol ID and/or title, searching for research facilities that are participating in the various trials, and searching for a physician from an online data roster or directory. TrialCheck also offers a brief tutorial of the registry's features and guides the user through a featured search. It has a comprehensive frequently asked questions section that explains how to navigate, enter data and updates, and perform other operational tasks necessary for users who are accessing and posting information to the site (Coalition of National Cancer Cooperative Groups, 2006).

Thomson CenterWatch Publishing Company hosts www.centerwatch.com, which lists more than 41,000 active industry- and government-sponsored clinical trials, including listings of new drug therapies in research and those recently approved by the FDA (Thomson CenterWatch, n.d.). The CenterWatch Web site lists patient-focused and industry-specific resources. A variety of clinical trials are posted, including dermatology, plastic surgery, oncology, trauma/emergency, and healthy patient trials. The search parameters used are medical condition and geographic location. A search for non-small cell carcinoma of the lung identified 485 total sites within the United States and internationally. Each site is listed separately, which may suggest that 485 different non-small cell carcinoma trials exist. Upon closer inspection, however, multiple sites are geographically dispersed but with the same identifier number. The CenterWatch registry is available to patients and professionals alike (Thomson CenterWatch).

TrialsCentral™ was launched in 2001 (www.trialscentral.org/aboutus.htm). According to its Web site, TrialsCentral's mission is to improve access to current and comprehensive clinical trials information to support informed healthcare decision making. Kay Dickersin, PhD, has been a proponent of prospective registration of clinical trials and in 1987 began the maintenance of the International Register of Clinical Trials Registers. Dr. Dickersin's goal in launching the TrialsCentral Web site is to make timely clinical trials information more available to a broader group of users via the Internet.

Openly available to both the public and healthcare providers, the TrialsCentral registry provides free and confidential access to listings of multiple clinical trials. Searches may be performed in one of two ways: by specific condition and geographic location of the research site or by sorting through the list of online registries. Searching by registry type identifies an expansive assortment of options. The format in which the search options are grouped facilitates a focused search. For example, approximately 193 different hospital and clinical research centers and approximately 122 nonprofit foundations and organizations are identified. This is a defining feature of this registry. National and international studies are included as well. Located under the resources tab are a variety of patient education materials with associated directed Web links. For the healthcare professional, references to publications, evidence-based practice guidelines, care practices, and search engines such as Medline (http://medlineplus.gov) link to other evidence-based healthcare sites.

Pharmaceutical Company–Sponsored Registries

Many pharmaceutical companies have clinical trial registries that solely focus on trials they sponsor. Similar to a disease-focused registry, the company-oriented registry offers a narrower set of options by virtue of the parameters or orientation of choices. For example, a specific pharmaceutical company may not be conducting prostate cancer prevention studies; therefore, that company's registry may be of less help to an individual who is performing a search for that type of study. Knowing how to focus and navigate a search may require some practice.

The following are examples of pharmaceutical company registries and serve only as examples; the list is not intended to be comprehensive. However, it is important to note that pharmaceutical registries are narrowly focused and limited to trials that research the company's products.

The GlaxoSmithKline (GSK) clinical trial registry provides an easily accessible repository of data from GSK-sponsored clinical trials, patient-oriented materials such as defining the phases of clinical trials, medical publications, updates from scientific meetings, and basic prescribing information. The trials listed in the registry are exclusively GSK-sponsored trials. Trial results are listed for those GSK-sponsored trials that have completed enrollment and data analysis. Patients and professionals may access information on this site (http://ctr.gsk.co.uk/welcome.asp) (GlaxoSmithKline, 2006).

Similarly, Eli Lilly hosts a clinical trial registry that lists initiated and ongoing clinical trials sponsored and conducted by Eli Lilly. Users can search by disease state or medical condition. Each trial is listed by a unique identifier, and once a condition is selected, such as osteoporosis, the protocol-specific information is displayed along with a comprehensive list of all recruitment sites, both in and outside the United States. Additionally, trial results are listed by therapeutic area and product. Patient education materials such as terminology and definitions and an explanation of the drug development process are included. Supplemental links to additional resources, for both patients and healthcare providers, also are included, such as ClinicalTrials.gov and the Center for Information and Study on Clinical Research Participation (Center for Information and Study on Clinical Research Participation, 2003; Eli Lilly & Company, 2006).

Several registries are available that offer information on trials conducted outside the United States. These internationally oriented and country-focused registries provide additional options and may complement a basic search.

International-Sponsored Registries

The publishing company BioMed Central established Current Controlled Trials, which is part of the Science Navigation Group of companies (www.sciencenavigation.com), based in London, England. Access to searches is free of charge; registration of trials is not. A search may be performed by one of two methods: by using the ISCRTN identifier or by using the metaRegister of Controlled Trials (referred to as mRCT) database. Because the company is based in the United Kingdom, trials sponsored by the National Health System (NHS) are included, many of which are conducted across the world. Currently, 11 different registries are listed from which searches can be performed. For example, Action Medical Research, Leukaemia Research Fund, NHS Trusts Clinical Trials Register, and ClinicalTrials.gov are listed. The key difference with the Current Controlled Trials registry is that it consolidates information from several registries so that a search may cross multiple databases. The registry offers a full range of open-access peer-reviewed journals published by its partner company, BioMed Central (Current Controlled Trials, 2006).

Countrywide Developed and Maintained Registries

Of note, several nations have initiated countrywide registries (Dickersin et al., 2004). For example, the Australian Clinical Trials Registry (ACTR) is a national, online registry of clinical trials conducted solely in Australia (see Chapter 54: Australia). The registry includes numerous clinical trials in varied therapeutic areas, including pharmaceuticals, surgical procedures, preventive measures, devices, treatment and rehabilitation strategies, and complementary therapies. The registry is limited to clinical trials involving Australian researchers or Australian participants (ACTR, 2006).

The National Research Registry (NRR) is an open-access Web site that locates clinical trials sponsored by the United Kingdom's NHS (see Chapter 64: United Kingdom). The NRR contains only descriptions of clinical trials. Trials are organized within four primary categories: national and regional trials, single-center trials, lead centers for multisite trials, and participating centers within multisite trials. More than 350 organizations referred to as *data providers* submit information to the NRR. The data providers, as opposed to individual researchers, submit information to the NRR because data providers receive funding from the NHS Trusts (Department of Health, 2006).

Locally Developed and Maintained Registries

Many clinical research centers, healthcare institutions, and academic centers maintain a locally developed clinical trial registry. The trials that are included on these Web sites are specific to that institution or facility. Even narrower in scope than the clinical trial registries mentioned previously, these registries serve to register and prospectively announce trials being conducted by researchers within that institution. Several of these hospital-based or institution-based Web sites may be found on the TrialsCentral Web site (TrialsCentral, 2004).

The lack of integration and the duplication of trial information on one or more registries may present an obstacle for both patients and CTNs. The fragmentation may be decreased through the joint and coordinated efforts of the ICMJE and WHO as well as through legislation by the federal government. Refinement, consolidation, standardization, and greater transparency linked with mandatory registration requirements could strengthen the ease of access, reliability, integrity of registry content, and, ultimately, decision-making processes for healthcare providers, patients, and the scientific community.

Current Trends

The WHO, as a global, neutral, and independent body, has defined and finalized the minimum registration data set, which, if adopted universally and made mandatory, should significantly decrease the variability among registration information. WHO continues to seek support while negotiating agreement from the various industries and health care, as well as the international community (Korn & Ehringhaus, 2006). By beginning to define universal registry characteristics and requiring international acceptance, WHO aids the movement toward global access, using a standard Internet-based system, free of undue constraints, fees, or barriers. Trial sponsors must

- Release and not mask details such as the description of the intervention, target sample size, and outcome including negative results.
- Fully disclose reports of early-phase (I and II) as well as later-phase (III and IV) studies.

The WHO is firm with these requirements, despite objections from pharmaceutical manufacturers. They argued that doing so would impinge on innovation and impose undue commercial risks to their company (Vanchieri, 2006b). Industry officials preferred masking specific data fields and keeping the data in a "lockbox" until the study was completed. Dr. Philip A. Pizzo, a committee chairman at the IOM meeting in May 2006, supports the goal to convey information that engenders public trust (Vanchieri, 2006a). He believes that conveying some, but not all, information to the public "doesn't cut it" (Vanchieri, 2006a, p. 415). Pizzo noted that providing a complete record of a drug trial once a drug was approved would guide "developers, insurers, and those who monitor quality of care in the United States" (Vanchieri, 2006a, p. 415).

International agreement on a minimum data set for all registries will force discussion about how best to ensure compliance. Although registering trials continues to be voluntary, at the time of publication of this manual, no mechanism exists to ensure compliance with either the prospective registration process or the updating of pertinent information, such as the addition of new research sites. The FDA is exploring ways to induce or facilitate registration compliance (Dickersin & Rennie, 2003). IRBs (see Chapter 13), which are responsible for ensuring the protection of human subjects, may find themselves involved in the process of establishing criteria for protocol submissions. These criteria may include prospective registration and confirmation of updates to information on the registry as part of the annual review process.

Legislative influence also will affect clinical trial registries. In draft legislation, Senate bill 467, titled the U.S. Fair Access to Clinical Trials Act (FACT) of 2007, amended the Public Health Service Act that originally directed DHHS through the NIH to create the ClinicalTrials.gov registry. It now mandates that the registry be maintained, organizing all ongoing trials for serious or life-threatening diseases and conditions. Furthermore, FACT directs the FDA to assist in the maintenance of the ClinicalTrials.gov site. FACT mandates that trial results from all publicly and privately funded trials be reported regardless of the outcome of the trial and that these results be made available to both patients and physicians. FACT legislation requires that all trials be registered in order to obtain IRB approval. Foreign trial sponsors that intend to submit data to the FDA or plan to advertise within the United States must register their trials at the time of submission. FACT also mandates that clinical trial registry information conform to the minimum data set requirements that have been defined by WHO and adopted by the ICMJE. Additionally, FACT seeks to establish a method or process of an enforcement mechanism as well as a process for performing periodic compliance auditing (U.S. Senate Committee on Finance Report, 2005).

In February 2007, senators Edward Kennedy, chair of the Committee on Health, Education, Labor, and Pensions (HELP), and Mike Enzi, HELP committee member, reintroduced the Enhancing Drug Safety and Innovation Act ("Kennedy, Enzi Reintroduce Vital Drug Safety Legislation," 2007). Initially introduced in August 2006, the legislation mandated the FDA and pharmaceutical companies to initiate stringent safety control and planning initiatives earlier in the drug development process and well before the drug enters the general market. Mitigating risk and improving public safety were the focus of the original legislation. The Kennedy-Enzi bill not only stressed the original elements of the drug safety legislation, but it also included other provisions. One provision was to establish a central clearinghouse trial database available to the general public that would guarantee public notification, information about trial enrollment, and results reporting. This new database, built upon clinicaltrial.gov, would require trial registration and include all phases of clinical trials. The emphasis continues to be on affording the public and healthcare professionals the most up-to-date information so that they have the best information to make healthcare decisions. Additionally, greater emphasis is placed on consumer safety. Providing greater transparency may help patients and healthcare providers to make safe, appropriate, effective, and informed healthcare decisions.

Finally, the Oncology Nursing Society (ONS) clearly stated its commitment concerning access to cancer research and clinical trial participation in its position "Cancer Research and Cancer Clinical Trials" (ONS, 2006). As stewards and agents of change, ONS members are integral in mitigating the barriers related to access and enrollment in clinical trials, including system barriers, healthcare provider barriers, and patient barriers. Additionally, the membership has the opportunity to support international efforts, which may streamline and standardize the registration process and ultimately the public reporting of trial results (ONS).

Summary

It is imperative that CTNs become knowledgeable about trends and influences that affect patients' ability to acquire information specific to clinical trials. Currently, no single point of access exists, thus resulting in a patchwork of informational sources, choices, and options. No all-inclusive directory of clinical trials is available, and trial registration remains a voluntary process. A variety of registries exist that can assist both CTNs and their patients in initiating a directed and ultimately productive search for open and enrolling clinical trials. Accessing information on the Internet can be daunting for patients and family members, who may be experiencing anxiety over their condition or may be novices to the World Wide Web. Assisting them in securing reliable, current, and appropriate information is critical.

References

Australian Clinical Trials Registry. (2006). *Australian clinical trials registry.* Retrieved July 2, 2006, from http://www.actr.org.au

Center for Drug Evaluation and Research. (2002, January 24). *Guidance for industry information program on clinical trials for serious or life-threatening diseases and conditions.* Retrieved June 30, 2006, from http://www.fda.gov/cder/guidance/4856fnl.htm

Center for Information and Study on Clinical Research Participation. (2003, June 30). *FAQs for patients and families: An introduction to clinical trials.* Retrieved June 30, 2006, from http://www.ciscrp.org/information/patients.asp

Coalition of National Cancer Cooperative Groups. (2006). *TrialCheck: A quick and easy way to check for cancer clinical trials.* Retrieved June 30, 2006, from http://www.trialcheck.org/services

Current Controlled Trials. (2006). *Welcome to current controlled trials.* Retrieved June 30, 2006, from http://www.controlled-trials.com

DeAngelis, C.D., Drazen, J.M., Frizelle, F.A., Haug, C., Hoey, J., Horton, R., et al. (2004). Clinical trial registration: A statement from the International Committee of Medical Journal Editors. *JAMA, 292,* 1363–1364.

DeAngelis, C.D., Drazen, J.M., Frizelle, F.A., Haug, C., Hoey, J., Horton, R., et al. (2005a). Clinical trial registration: A statement from the International Committee of Medical Journal Editors. *Archives of Otolaryngology—Head and Neck Surgery, 131,* 479–480.

DeAngelis, C.D., Drazen, J.M., Frizelle, F.A., Haug, C., Hoey, J., Horton, R., et al. (2005b). Is this clinical trial fully registered? A statement from the International Committee of Medical Journal Editors. *JAMA, 293,* 2927–2929.

Department of Health. (2006). *The national research register.* Retrieved June 30, 2006, from http://www.nrr.nhs.uk/default.htm

Dickersin, K., Davis, B.R., Dixon, D.O., George, S.L., Hawkins, B.S., Lachin, J., et al. (2004). The society for clinical trials supports United States legislation mandating trials registration. *Clinical Trials, 1,* 417–420.

Dickersin, K., & Rennie, D. (2003). Registering clinical trials. *JAMA, 290,* 516–523.

Eli Lilly & Company. (2006). *Initiated trials.* Retrieved June 30, 2006, from http://www.lillytrials.com/initiated/initiated.html

Fair Access to Clinical Trials Act of 2007, S. 467, 110th Cong. (2007). Retrieved April 3, 2007, from http://thomas.loc.gov/cgi-bin/query/F?c110:1:./temp/~c110sTLrCI:e0:

Fisher, C.B. (2006). Public health. Clinical trials results databases: Unanswered questions. *Science, 311,* 180–181.

GlaxoSmithKline. (2006). *GlaxoSmithKline clinical trial register.* Retrieved June 30, 2006, from http://ctr.gsk.co.uk/welcome.asp

Kennedy, Enzi reintroduce vital drug safety legislation. (2007, February 1). Retrieved April 3, 2007, from http://kennedy.senate.gov/newsroom/press_release.cfm?id=7c1a651c-d965-4283-ae99-ec5d19d0d9ab

Korn, D., & Ehringhaus, S. (2006). Principles for strengthening the integrity of clinical research. *PLoS Clinical Trials, 1*(1), e1.

Institute of Medicine: Committee on Clinical Trial Registries. (2006). *Developing a national registry of pharmacologic and biologic clinical trials: Workshop report.* Washington, DC: National Academies Press.

McCray, A.T. (2000). Better access to information about clinical trials. *Annals of Internal Medicine, 133,* 609–614.

McCray, A.T., & Ide, N.C. (2000). Design and implementation of a national clinical trials registry. *Journal of the American Medical Informatics Association, 7,* 313–323.

Oncology Nursing Society. (2006, October). *Cancer research and cancer clinical trials* [Position statement]. Retrieved June 30, 2006, from http://www.ons.org/publications/positions/CancerResearch.shtml

Rockhold, F., Freeman, A., Metz, C., Merchant, T., Fuell, D., Gallacher, T., et al. (2005). From study initiation to publication—the role of clinical trial registers. *Applied Clinical Trials, 14*(9), 38–46.

Sim, I., & Detmer, D.E. (2005). Beyond trial registration: A global trial bank for clinical trial reporting. *PLoS Medicine, 2,* e365.

Thomson CenterWatch. (n.d.). *Clinical trials listing service.* Retrieved June 30, 2006, from http://www.centerwatch.com

Tonks, A. (1999). Registering clinical trials. *BMJ, 319,* 1565–1568.

TrialsCentral. (2004, October 20). *Your source for online clinical trials information.* Retrieved June 30, 2006, from http://www.trialscentral.org/AllRegistersByType.aspx

U.S. Senate Committee on Finance. (2005, February 28). *Press release floor statement of Senator Chuck Grassley: Grassley co-sponsors clinical trial registry legislation.* Retrieved August 2, 2006, from http://finance.senate.gov/sitepages/grassley.htm

Vanchieri, C. (2006a). Championing transparency in clinical trials. *Community Oncology, 3,* 415–416.

Vanchieri, C. (2006b). The pressure is on for full disclosure in clinical trials reporting. *Community Oncology, 3,* 455–456.

World Health Organization. (2005a). *International clinical trials registry platform: Frequently asked questions.* Retrieved August 2, 2006, from http://www.who.int/ictrp/faq/en/index.html

World Health Organization. (2005b). *International clinical trials registry platform: Trial registration data set.* Retrieved June 26, 2006, from http://www.who.int/ictrp/data_set/en/index1.html

World Health Organization. (2005c). *International clinical trials registry platform: Welcome to the WHO international clinical trials registry platform.* Retrieved June 26, 2006, from http://www.who.int/ictrp

SECTION X.

Quality Management

CHAPTER 45
Good Clinical Practice

Patricia C. Woltz, RN, MS, CCRP

Introduction

At the core of good clinical practice (GCP) related to the conduct of clinical trials is a broad set of rules, standards, and recommendations with two overarching objectives: to protect study participants' rights, safety, and well-being and to ensure that trial data are credible. Compliance with GCP regulations and recommendations ensures that a standard for ethical and scientific quality in carrying out clinical trial research is achieved. Thus, an understanding of GCP is essential to all those involved in clinical trial research. Yet, confusion arises when the terminology *good clinical practice* is used in different contexts by various parties (Grimes et al., 2005; Lepay, 2001; Mackintosh, Molloy, & DeCherney, 2000). To clinicians who use this terminology to describe clinical practice, *good clinical practice* for the conduct of clinical research seems somewhat of a misnomer and might be more accurately called "good clinical *research* practice." In fact, three different GCP standards for clinical trial research currently exist: the International Conference on Harmonisation of Technical Requirements for Registration of Pharmaceuticals for Human Use (ICH) GCP guideline, the U.S. Food and Drug Administration (FDA) program, and evidence-based best practices (Duke Clinical Research Institute, 2003; Mackintosh et al., 2000). This chapter reviews the historical background of GCP to facilitate readers' understanding of how GCP is defined, its purpose, key aspects of the ICH guideline, and the emerging need for evidence-based best practices for issues pertaining to clinical trial conduct.

Definitions

It is widely accepted that clinical trials involving drugs and biologics should be conducted in accordance with the ICH *E6: Good Clinical Practice: Consolidated Guideline*. The ICH guideline defines GCP as "an international ethical and scientific quality standard for the design, conduct, performance, monitoring, auditing, recording, analyses, and reporting of clinical trials that provides assurance that the data and reported results are credible and accurate,

and that the rights, integrity, and confidentiality of trial subjects are protected" (ICH, 1996, p. 1). A standard may be defined as that which represents accepted or mandated obligations, behaviors, and ethical expectations for one's profession (Duke Clinical Research Institute, 2003). Standards in the conduct of clinical research have evolved and are viewed as necessary to (a) provide the public with assurance that trial participants are protected and, thus, the guidelines are fundamental to recruiting adequate numbers of participants into studies, and (b) assure the public and policymakers that credible and reliable evidence exists on which informed decisions can be made to affect medical practice and public health (Njie & Thomas, 2001; Ottevanger et al., 2003).

The terminology *good clinical practice* also has been coined by the FDA to collectively refer to its regulations, guidance documents, and information sheets designed to protect human participants in clinical research (Grimes et al., 2005; Holobaugh, 2005; Lepay, 1998). Regulations are mandatory, legally binding requirements, whereas guidance and guidelines assist in explaining how to comply with the requirements, and information sheets are guidance documents that offer detail and instructions (Duke Clinical Research Institute, 2003). Of the many GCP guidance documents for FDA-regulated clinical trials, the ICH GCP guideline is but one. The FDA maintains a Web site that references its GCP requirements and recommendations at www.fda.gov/oc/gcp, from which a selected listing is provided in Table 45-1. For convenience, this chapter refers to the compilation of FDA recommendations and requirements as *FDA GCP*. The differences between FDA and ICH GCP will be reviewed in more detail.

Background

The evolution of providing assurances for quality in human research has been guided by historical events of scientific misconduct and economic globalization (Lepay, 2001). Exploring the background of these forces provides insight into the proscriptive nature of the ICH GCP standard.

Table 45-1. Selected List of U.S. Food and Drug Administration (FDA) Regulations and Guidance Related to Good Clinical Practice in Clinical Trials

Document	Content
Regulations	
Part 11	Electronic Records; Electronic Signatures
Part 50	Protection of Human Subjects
Part 54	Financial Disclosure by Clinical Investigators
Part 56	Institutional Review Boards
Part 312	Investigational New Drug Application
Forms	
Form FDA 1571	Investigational New Drug Application
Form FDA 1572	Statement of Investigator
Guidances	
	FDA Information Sheet Guidances for Institutional Review Boards, Clinical Investigators, and Sponsors
	Financial Relationships and Interests in Research Involving Human Subjects: Guidance for Human Subject Protection
	Guidance for Industry: Acceptance of Foreign Clinical Trials
	Guidance for Industry: Computerized Systems Used in Clinical Investigations
	Guidance for Industry: Financial Disclosure by Clinical Investigators
	Guidance for Industry: Guideline for the Monitoring of Clinical Investigators
	Guidance for Industry: Information Program on Clinical Trials for Serious or Life-Threatening Diseases and Conditions
	Guidance for Industry: IRB Review of Stand-Alone HIPAA Authorizations Under FDA Regulations
	Guidance for Industry on Part 11—Electronic Records; Electronic Signatures—Scope and Application
	ICH E3: Guideline for Industry Structure and Content of Clinical Study Reports
	ICH E5: Ethnic Factors in the Acceptability of Foreign Clinical Data
	ICH E6: Good Clinical Practice: Consolidated Guidance
	ICH E10: Choice of Control Group and Related Issues in Clinical Trials

ICH—International Conference on Harmonisation of Technical Requirements for Registration of Pharmaceuticals for Human Use

Note. Based on information from U.S. Food and Drug Administration, n.d.; U.S. Food and Drug Administration Center for Devices and Radiological Health, 2006; U.S. Food and Drug Administration Center for Drug Evaluation and Research, 2002.

Although much of the following reflects U.S. history, similar developments have occurred in the European member states of the ICH (Otte, Maier-Lenz, & Dierckx, 2005).

GCP for the conduct of clinical research had its beginnings in the United States in the 1950s (Health and Human Services, 2000). Milestones in the evolution of GCP include the passage of the Kefauver-Harris amendments to the Food, Drug, and Cosmetic Act in 1962, which occurred in response to the discovery of a tragic link between fetal abnormalities and the use of thalidomide. The Kefauver-Harris amendments required that written informed consent be obtained to participate in an experimental therapy and, for the first time, required that drug manufacturers show drug efficacy prior to obtaining market approval (FDA, 1999). In 1978, work that later became known as the Belmont Report was published as an essential reference for institutional review boards (IRBs) reviewing federally funded, human subject research proposals and established boundaries between practice and research (Office for Human Research Protections [OHRP], 2005; Otte et al., 2005). In 1991, the U.S. Department of Health and Human Services (DHHS) Federal Policy for the Protection of Human Subjects (i.e., Subpart A of the *Code of Federal Regulations* Title 45, Part 46, also known as "The Common Rule") was formally adopted by the FDA and codified in Title 21, Parts 50 and 56. Indeed, human subject protections and investigational new drug procedures have been enforced and regularly updated over the years to build the FDA version of GCP that is in force today.

Unfortunately, despite the evolution of GCP, new cases of scientific research misconduct persist. Attention to the oversight of clinical research and the safety of research participants increased significantly following the deaths at leading academic institutions of a participant in a gene transfer study in 1999 and a healthy volunteer in a lung physiology study in 2001. Investigations into these sentinel events revealed extensive noncompliance with regulations and resulted in the HHS OHRP suspension of related, federally funded research until corrective action plans could be implemented (Baker, 2002; Rhoads, 2003). Such events cause negative publicity for the research community and erode public trust in the integrity and merit of research (Njie & Thomas, 2001), which are critical for funding of and recruitment into clinical trials and confidence in the treatments that result from the trials (American Society of Clinical Oncology [ASCO], 2003).

Coincident to sentinel events in research conduct, globalization also has had a major impact on the evolution of GCP and the current research landscape. Globalization has its roots in economic forces and good business practices and is defined as "the process of increasing the connectivity and interdependence of the world's markets and businesses" (InvestorWords, 2005). As costs associated with pharmaceutical research and development have risen (Sung et al., 2003), more industry-sponsored trials are being conducted overseas, where participants are more readily recruited and trials are less expensive to conduct (FDA, 2004; Shah, 2003).

With the availability of foreign clinical data, the need to generate similar data in another region might be obviated. Yet, in the United States, because of historically strict regulation, the FDA frequently rejected foreign study data that it considered inferior. Other countries interested in a share of the economic and intellectual drug development market have had to review their procedures to ensure trial quality. In 1990, following a long historical development, representative experts from regulatory bodies and the pharmaceutical industry in the European Union (EU), Japan, and the United States embarked on a process to develop a unified standard and harmonize the technical requirements for registration of pharmaceutical products in their collective countries. Using a process of expert working groups and consensus decision making, these experts gave rise to the International Conference on Harmonisation Tripartite Guidelines (ICH, n.d.). The ICH guidelines are organized into four topic categories: quality (Q), safety (S), efficacy (E), and multidisciplinary (M). The ICH documents are maintained on the ICH Web site at www.ich.org.

International Conference on Harmonisation Good Clinical Practice

One of the many ICH guidelines is the *E6: Good Clinical Practice: Consolidated Guideline* (ICH, 1996). With the overall aim of international standardization of the quality of clinical trials by standardizing trial conduct, the ICH GCP guideline was formulated with consideration of current practices in the EU, Japan, the United States, Australia, Canada, the Nordic countries, and the World Health Organization. Simply stated, ICH GCP represents what regulatory and pharmaceutical industry experts think constitutes a good drug trial for international purposes.

The ICH GCP guideline was approved by the ICH Steering Committee in 1996, and within the year, each of the three ICH regions had adopted similar, but not identical, versions of the guideline. The EU implemented the ICH GCP guideline as a legal directive in 1996 (ICH, n.d.); Japan translated the document and legally enacted its version in 1997 (Ono & Kodama, 2000); and the FDA adopted the ICH guideline as a guidance document in the *Federal Register*, May 9, 1997. Henceforth, ICH GCP became the new standard by which all international drug trials should be performed in order to achieve universal recognition. Despite differences among the versions of ICH GCP in the three regions, the regions agreed that (a) adherence to the GCP standard is nevertheless crucial to maintaining the harmonization reached, (b) the principles of ICH GCP (see Figure 45-1) are the same in all three regions, and (c) most of the differences among the three versions are without any real impact for the users (ICH, n.d.). Adherence to ICH GCP is required for all approved international submissions to regulatory agencies in the EU, Japan, the United States, and Canada ("International GCP Regulations: Implementation of ICH GCPs," 2005).

Highlights of the International Conference on Harmonisation Good Clinical Practice Guideline

ICH GCP is a consolidated guideline organized into eight sections. All those involved in clinical trials should

---

Figure 45-1. The Principles of International Conference on Harmonisation Good Clinical Practice (GCP)

1. Clinical trials should be conducted in accordance with the ethical principles that have their origin in the Declaration of Helsinki, and that are consistent with GCP and applicable regulatory requirement(s).
2. Before a trial is initiated, foreseeable risks and inconveniences should be weighed against the anticipated benefit for the individual trial subject and society. A trial should be initiated and continued only if the anticipated benefits justify the risks.
3. The rights, safety, and well-being of the trial subjects are the most important considerations and should prevail over interests of science and society.
4. The available nonclinical and clinical information on an investigational product should be adequate to support the proposed clinical trial.
5. Clinical trials should be scientifically sound, and described in a clear, detailed protocol.
6. A trial should be conducted in compliance with the protocol that has received prior institutional review board (IRB)/independent ethics committee (IEC) approval/favorable opinion.
7. The medical care given to, and medical decisions made on behalf of, subjects should always be the responsibility of a qualified physician or, when appropriate, of a qualified dentist.
8. Each individual involved in conducting a trial should be qualified by education, training, and experience to perform his or her respective task(s).
9. Freely given informed consent should be obtained from every subject prior to clinical trial participation.
10. All clinical trial information should be recorded, handled, and stored in a way that allows its accurate reporting, interpretation, and verification.
11. The confidentiality of records that could identify subjects should be protected, respecting the privacy and confidentiality rules in accordance with the applicable regulatory requirement(s).
12. Investigational products should be manufactured, handled, and stored in accordance with applicable good manufacturing practice (GMP). They should be used in accordance with the approved protocol.
13. Systems with procedures that assure the quality of every aspect of the trial should be implemented.

Note. From *Guidance for Industry: E6 Good Clinical Practice: Consolidated Guidance* (pp. 8–9), by the International Conference on Harmonisation of Technical Requirements for Registration of Pharmaceuticals for Human Use, 1996. Rockville, MD: U.S. Food and Drug Administration.

---

at a minimum be aware of the topics addressed and the purpose of the document. Clinical trial nurses also should be aware that some GCP topics have been more detailed in other ICH guidelines, such as *E2: Clinical Safety Data Management and Data Reporting* and *E8: General Considerations for Clinical Trials*. The following information from the ICH GCP document is reviewed in the order of its sections.

Glossary

The glossary provides definitions for terms frequently encountered in clinical trials. Some terms, such as *source data* and *source documents,* are defined more comprehensively in ICH GCP compared to that found in federal regulations.

Terms that provide a sampling of the glossary's usefulness are *adverse event, audit trail, case report form, compliance, legally acceptable representative, monitoring, quality assurance, quality control, subject identification code, unexpected adverse drug reaction,* and *vulnerable subjects.*

The Principles of Good Clinical Practice

The overriding principles for adherence to ICH GCP are paraphrased in Figure 45-1.

Institutional Review Board/Independent Ethics Committee

The responsibilities, function, composition, operations, and procedures are outlined, in addition to how these committees should maintain their records. The overriding function of the IRB/independent ethics committee (IEC) is to safeguard trial participants.

Investigator

Reviewing the role and responsibilities of the investigator, the guideline begins with qualifications and the availability of resources necessary to recruit adequate numbers of subjects and to carry out the trial. Expectations include communication with the IRB/IEC and compliance with the protocol. The investigator must obtain IRB/IEC approval before starting the trial and must obtain written informed consent before subjects take part. Protocol deviations, an often difficult metric to operationalize, are addressed. Specifically, anticipated deviations to eliminate an immediate hazard to trial participants should occur only after the sponsor and IRB/IEC agree that the deviation is necessary (GCP section 4.5.2); or, if a deviation occurs without prior approval, it should be to eliminate immediate hazards to subjects and then be submitted for review by others as soon as possible (section 4.5.4). Other topics include the accountability, use, and storage of the study product; randomization and unblinding procedures; and informed consent. Discussion of records, reports, and premature termination or suspension of a trial addresses the need for adequate communication between the investigator, sponsor, and IRB/IEC. Case report forms and documents that are considered essential to a drug trial are discussed in section 4.9 of the guideline.

Sponsor

An overview of quality assurance, quality control, and the agreements made between sponsors and institutions/investigators and those between sponsors and contract research organizations (CROs) is provided. Selection of investigators is largely based on training, experience, and adequate resources (section 5.6). The role of CROs in carrying out the sponsor's duties and functions depends on the written agreements between them (section 5.2). However, the sponsor remains ultimately responsible for the quality and integrity of trial data (section 5.2.1), for which the use of independent data monitoring committees is suggested (section 5.5.2). It is the sponsor's responsibility to notify the investigator/institution in writing when trial-related records no longer need to be retained, which is usually two years from the end of the trial (section 5.5.12). Sponsors are directed to indemnify the investigator/institution against trial claims, except for cases that arise from malpractice and/or negligence (section 5.8.1), and are directed not to release study drug to a site until all required documentation to conduct the trial is received (section 5.14.1).

To ensure safety, the sponsor is expected to implement a coding system that permits rapid identification of the product in a medical emergency but does not otherwise permit breaks in the blinding (section 5.13.4), delivers study drug to sites in a timely fashion (section 5.14.4), and treats adverse drug reactions that are both serious and unexpected in an expedited fashion (section 5.17). Sponsors require direct access to site records and should verify that each subject has signed consent (section 5.15). Monitoring to ensure GCP compliance and quality control functions requires that sponsor-appointed monitors have the scientific and/or clinical knowledge needed to monitor the trial adequately (section 5.18.2). The extent and nature of monitoring is largely based on the level of risk associated with the trial. Although not the norm, central monitoring may be appropriate if extensive training and written guidance has been provided (section 5.18.3). As part of quality assurance, audits in which the trial is evaluated for adherence to the protocol, defined standard operating procedures, GCP, and applicable regulations may be performed by auditors who are independent of the trial and its data collection systems (section 5.19). See Chapter 47 for more information on audits. The role of case report forms in multicenter trials is considered in section 5.23 of the guideline.

Clinical Trial Protocol and Protocol Amendments

This secion provides a template for a clinical trial protocol, as well as discussion of the incorporation of addenda into the protocol. The study should be supported by adequate nonclinical and clinical information and should be scientifically sound. The protocol should be clear and sufficiently detailed.

Investigator's Brochure

The investigator's brochure (IB) section delineates the minimum information that should be included in an IB and outlines the process for incorporation of addenda into the IB. The IB should facilitate understanding of the rationale for key features of the protocol and support the clinician's ability to best manage study participants during the course of the clinical trial. In some unique circumstances, an expanded background information section in the protocol may substitute for a dedicated IB.

A template for an IB is provided in the guideline. The current state of knowledge about nonclinical and human effects of the investigational product includes a review of toxicology, dose response, safety, efficacy, and any marketing or approval of the drug in other countries. The IB should provide a summary to give the investigator a clear understanding of the possible risks and adverse events and to provide guidance for recognition and treatment of overdose and adverse drug reactions based on previous experience(s). Applicable landmark publications should be referenced.

Essential Documents for the Conduct of a Clinical Trial

The ICH GCP guideline includes a minimal list of documents that individually and collectively are viewed as essential to permit evaluation of study conduct and the quality of the data produced. This section provides a convenient resource for clinical trial nurses (CTNs) who are regularly delegated responsibilities that relate to the management of collecting, organizing, and archiving documents that will serve to demonstrate compliance and provide an audit trail.

A summary of the key aspects of the ICH GCP guideline for investigative sites is as follows.

- The objectives, design, conduct, analysis, and reporting of a clinical trial should be defined in a written protocol before the study starts. After it is approved, the protocol should be strictly followed.
- Protection of subjects is the shared responsibility of the investigator, the sponsor, and the IRB/IEC.
- Select, train, and keep a log of study team members.
- Predict recruitment accurately, and keep an up-to-date subject enrollment log.
- Pay particular attention to the ethical considerations of vulnerable populations and informed consent, and scrupulously follow informed consent procedures.
- Report serious adverse events immediately to the sponsor.
- Precisely document product accountability.
- Diligently collect and record reliable study data.
- Keep all source documents, and maintain organized files and archives.
- Keep everyone fully informed.

U.S. Food and Drug Administration Good Clinical Practice

The FDA uses the terminology *GCP* to refer to its collection of regulations, guidance, and recommendations for clinical trials involving drugs and biologic products that are controlled under its auspices (see Table 45-1) The FDA adopted the ICH GCP document as a guide that represents its current thinking on GCP. Unlike Title 21 of the *Code of Federal Regulations,* which is legally binding and enforceable, implementation of the FDA's version of ICH GCP is not mandatory. The FDA chose to adopt the ICH GCP guideline without making it regulation under the assumption that everything in the guideline is already contained in the FDA's current regulations. However, they are not entirely equivalent. In general, ICH GCP is stricter than the federal regulations. A summary of noteworthy

differences between the ICH GCP guideline and FDA GCP is listed in Table 45-2.

The FDA recognizes that an alternative approach to the guidance may be used if such an approach satisfies local and state requirements. It is the FDA's view that "the principles established in the ICH GCP guideline should be applied to other investigations that involve therapeutic intervention in, or observation of, human subjects" (ICH, 1997, p. 25692).

Good Clinical Practice and Best Research Practices

Although the goals of GCP are appropriate, it is questionable whether the methods detailed in the ICH GCP guideline will achieve them. First, the scientific basis of the ICH GCP recommendations is unknown. The current standard for GCP evolved out of consensus decision making in which academia did not participate and for which no identified authors or cited references were given (Grimes et al., 2005; Sniderman, 1999). Furthermore, limited scientific studies have been conducted to determine whether established GCP methods affect outcome measures of trial quality. Second, existing GCP does not address many trial situations. Thus, it remains to be determined how GCP will be best applied to clinical trial processes and tasks that may vary widely from study to study (Bohaychuk & Ball, 1999; Mackintosh, Molloy, & Mathieu, 2005).

Finally, compliance with GCP guidelines is costly and resource intensive, and whether the added costs are justified or feasible is not yet known. New regulation and increased oversight may exceed the capacity of even the most dedicated institutions (ASCO, 2003; Sung et al., 2003). Much remains to be learned about the true costs of running a clinical trial (Evans, 2000). Pharmaceutical companies have adequate administrative support, but not all clinical trials are large and have the benefit of industry resources. Although the clinical research landscape in Japan is very different than that in the United States, implementation of ICH GCP has substantially increased costs to investigators, sponsors, and patients, but it also has increased the ethical and scientific quality of trials there (Ono, Kodama, Nagao, & Toyoshima, 2002). For now, it is unclear whether current GCP is impeding, facilitating, or improving clinical research.

Clinical research in oncology is complex in both the organization and management of the trials and in the ethical issues that surround them. Better understanding of the many variables that affect determination of best practices for trial conduct is needed. For example, best practices may have to overcome institutional and sponsor impediments and consider the type of research being conducted and the study phase (Roche et al., 2002). Related to randomized controlled trials, Knatterud (2002) outlined approaches to issues, such as study communication, trial complexity, subject stratification, and the degree of study risk, that are

Table 45-2. Some Notable Examples of Differences Between International Conference on Harmonisation (ICH) Good Clinical Practice (GCP) and the U.S. Food and Drug Administration (FDA) GCP

Topic	Comparison
Notification to primary care physician	ICH recommends that a clinical trial investigator inform a subject's primary physician, if the subject agrees, about the subject's study participation (section 4.3.3). FDA does not mention such a notice.
Institutional review board (IRB)	ICH requires that the clinical investigator provide the IRB with a copy of the investigator's brochure (4.4.2). FDA only requires that the pharmaceutical company sponsor provide it to the investigator; however, many clinical trial sponsors require documentation of receipt from the investigator's IRB (312.55a). ICH requires a statement from the IRB that it is organized and operated according to GCP (5.11.1b). FDA does not require clinical research sponsors to obtain such a statement.
Documentation of protocol deviations	ICH requires that the investigator document and explain any deviation from the study protocol (4.5.3). FDA does not address this issue.
Study medication	ICH requires that the clinical investigator maintain records that document adequately that the subjects were provided the doses specified by the protocol *and reconcile* all investigational products received from the sponsor. FDA requires only the return of unused supplies and does not specify who is responsible for reconciliation (312.62). ICH prohibits the pharmaceutical company sponsor (or the contract research organization if the responsibility was properly transferred) from providing study medication until all required documentation from the IRB has been obtained (5.14.2). FDA does not address this; however, most sponsors have internal procedures covering this.
Informed consent	The elements differ between ICH (4.8.10) and FDA (50.25a, 50.25b). ICH requires that the subject receive a *signed* and *dated* copy of the written informed consent (4.8.11). FDA requires that a copy be given to the subject but does not state that it must be a *signed* copy (50.27).
Financial records	ICH requires that the clinical investigator make *all* clinical trial–related records available for direct access by the clinical research associate, auditor, IRB, or regulatory agency (4.9.7) and that financial aspects of the trial be in the investigator's files (8.2.4). FDA currently does not require financial records, nor does it mandate "direct access" (312.62).
Signed protocols	ICH requires that the sponsor and clinical investigator sign the study protocol (5.6.3). FDA does not have this requirement; however, most sponsors require signatures.
Indemnification	ICH requires that the sponsor provide insurance or indemnify the investigator against claims arising from the trial (5.8.1). FDA does not have such a policy; however, most investigators request and obtain it from the pharmaceutical company or contract research organization.
Case report form (CRF) changes	ICH requires the monitor (clinical research associate) to ensure that changes/additions/deletions to the CRF are made, dated, explained (if necessary), and initialed *by the investigator* or an authorized member of the investigator's staff, such as the study coordinator. This authorization must be documented (5.18.4n). FDA does not require documentation of authorization to initial CRF changes.
Monitoring reports	ICH requires that a copy of the clinical research associate's study initiation monitoring report be stored in the investigator's files (8.2.20). FDA does not require this at this time.
Study documentation	ICH puts responsibility for ensuring that all study documents are on file at the investigational site on the clinical research associate and requires that the clinical research associate confirm that all necessary documents are at the site prior to closing the site (8). FDA holds the investigator responsible for the accuracy and completeness of the records related to the clinical trial. ICH requires curriculum vitae of both the principal investigator and any subinvestigators (8.2.10). FDA does not require curriculum vitae of subinvestigators, although this typically is a sponsor requirement. ICH requires a *signature sheet* to document signatures and initials of all people authorized to make entries and/or corrections on CRFs in both investigator and sponsor files (8.3.24). FDA does not require documentation of investigator/staff signatures; however, this typically is a sponsor requirement.

Note. From *A Comparison of FDA Versus ICH Regulations,* by S. Mayo, 2005. Retrieved October 20, 2005, from http://www.sendemissary .com/compass.nsf/key/ich.htm. Adapted with permission.

confronted when planning and executing multicenter clinical trials and suggested cost-sensitive solutions that adhere to GCP standards.

One of the goals of ASCO, the National Institutes of Health (NIH), and others is to enhance the efficiency and cost effectiveness of the clinical research oversight system. In a recent call by NIH for research proposals, applications are being solicited that will support activities for improvement in clinical designs, regulatory pathways, informed consent, and participant enrollment (NIH, 2005). Additionally, NIH is seeking activities that limit participant risk, enhance the capture of appropriate data, and determine the most efficient and effective ways to interact with trial participants. NIH also is seeking activities that possess design and analysis plans for studies of unique populations or very small numbers of subjects, and methods to address issues in diseases with limited treatment options.

Clinical Trial Nurses and Good Clinical Practice Best Practices

Practice standards are related to quality processes, and in clinical research, processes that include the application of GCP and the CTN role "address accountability of the research participants, maintenance of the integrity and credibility of the data, and protocol adherence" (Njie & Thomas, 2001, p. 234). CTNs are both research- and clinically trained. They function on the front line of clinical research where they *directly* contribute to protections afforded to research participants and the generation of source data. Yet, despite the central role of CTNs in managing oncology research trials, little more than anecdotal evidence of nursing-sensitive outcomes associated with GCP trial processes exist. In collaboration with other research team members, CTNs should contribute to the identification and validation of cost-effective best practices that will benefit study participants, benefit all patients with cancer, decrease costs associated with trials, and validate the vital functions of the CTN role in ensuring quality clinical trials. CTNs must ask what is the evidence that CTNs advocate for their clients enrolled in clinical trials? What level and type of training and education best serve nurses in ensuring trial quality? What are benefits and costs associated with nurses' good clinical research practices?

Summary

Clinical trials help to improve cancer care and define the standards for optimal clinical cancer treatment. CTNs play an instrumental role in ensuring research quality and integrity in clinical trials that lead to improved treatments for patients with cancer. Knowledge of GCP is essential for CTNs, as it is for all those involved in clinical trial research. ICH GCP is a widely accepted ethical and scientific standard that details the expectations of those who are responsible for the conduct of sponsored clinical research.

ICH GCP was founded on the premise that international standardization of trial conduct provides assurance that participants are properly protected and trial data are credible and facilitates submissions and approvals of new drugs and biologic products. Although they do not address all trial situations, ICH and FDA GCP guidelines provide a reference from which best practices may be formulated to apply to a wide variety of trial situations. CTNs should network with colleagues to share and validate best practices and should contribute to future research on issues of GCP while attempting to minimize unnecessary costs associated with clinical trial research.

References

American Society of Clinical Oncology. (2003). ASCO policy statement: Oversight of clinical research. *Journal of Clinical Oncology, 21,* 2377–2386.

Baker, D. (2002). *FDA letter of opportunity for hearing.* Retrieved October 16, 2005, from http://www.fda.gov/foi/nooh/Wilson.htm

Bohaychuk, W., & Ball, G. (1999). *Conducting GCP-compliant research.* Chichester, England: Wiley.

Duke Clinical Research Institute. (2003). *Keys to building a successful research site.* Retrieved September 15, 2005, from http://www.dcri.duke.edu/investigator/quickref.pdf

Evans, W.K. (2000). Cost-effectiveness analysis in oncology. *Schweizerische Rundschau für Medizin Praxis, 89,* 492–496.

Grimes, D.A., Hubacher, D., Nanda, K., Schulz, K.F., Moher, D., & Altman, D.G. (2005). The Good Clinical Practice guideline: A bronze standard for clinical research. *Lancet, 366,* 172–174.

Health and Human Services. (2000, May 23). *HHS fact sheet: Protecting human research subjects.* Washington, DC: U.S. Department of Health and Human Services.

Holobaugh, P. (2005). *Good clinical practices and FDA inspections* [Slide presentation]. Bethesda, MD: U.S. Food and Drug Administration. Retrieved September 19, 2007, from http://videocast.nih.gov/ppt/NIAID_gcp_041505.ppt

International Conference on Harmonisation of Technical Requirements for Registration of Pharmaceuticals for Human Use. (1996). *Guidance for industry: E6 good clinical practice: Consolidated guidance.* Retrieved August 15, 2005, from http://www.ich.org/cache/compo/276-254-1.html

International Conference on Harmonisation of Technical Requirements for Registration of Pharmaceuticals for Human Use. (1997, May 9). International Conference on Harmonisation; good clinical practice: Consolidated guideline; availability, notice. *Federal Register, 62,* 25692.

International Conference on Harmonisation of Technical Requirements for Registration of Pharmaceuticals for Human Use. (n.d.). *ICH guidelines.* Retrieved August 10, 2005, from http://www.ich.org/cache/compo/276-254-1.html

International GCP regulations: Implementation of ICH GCPs. (2005). Retrieved October 14, 2005, from http://www.peri.org/distance_tour/agcp/html/intgcpreg51.html

InvestorWords. (2005). *Globalization.* Retrieved July 14, 2005, from http://www.investorwords.com/2182/globalization.html

Knatterud, G.L. (2002). Management and conduct of randomized controlled trials. *Epidemiologic Reviews, 24,* 12–25.

Lepay, D. (1998). *GCP compliance: FDA expectations and recent findings.* Retrieved August 30, 2005, from http://www.fda.gov/cder/present/dia698/diafda2/sld001.htm

Lepay, D. (2001). *Emerging issues in FDA's oversight of clinical research.* Retrieved August 30, 2005, from http://www.fda.gov/ohrms/dockets/ac/01/slides/3799s1_12_Lepay/tsld001.htm

Mackintosh, D.R., Molloy, V.J., & DeCherney, G.S. (2000). GCP responsibilities of principal investigators revisited: Going far beyond the 1572. *Applied Clinical Trials, 9,* 59–64.

Mackintosh, D.R., Molloy, V.J., & Mathieu, M.P. (2005). *Good clinical practice: A question & answer reference guide.* Waltham, MA: Parexel International Corporation.

National Institutes of Health. (2005, October 12). *Fact sheet: NIH clinical and translational science awards (CTSA).* Bethesda, MD: National Center for Research Resources. Retrieved September 19, 2007, from http://www.nih.gov/news/pr/oct2005/FactSheetCTSAclearance.pdf

Njie, V.P., & Thomas, A.C. (2001). Quality issues in clinical research and the implications on health policy (QICRHP). *Journal of Professional Nursing, 17,* 233–242.

Office for Human Research Protections. (2005). *Belmont report.* Retrieved October 31, 2005, from http://www.hhs.gov/ohrp/belmontArchive.html#histReport

Ono, S., & Kodama, Y. (2000). Clinical trials and the new good clinical practice guideline in Japan. An economic perspective. *Pharmacoeconomics, 18,* 125–141.

Ono, S., Kodama, Y., Nagao, T., & Toyoshima, S. (2002). The quality of conduct in Japanese clinical trials: Deficiencies found in GCP inspections. *Controlled Clinical Trials, 23*(1), 29–41.

Otte, A., Maier-Lenz, H., & Dierckx, R.A. (2005). Good clinical practice: Historical background and key aspects. *Nuclear Medicine Communications, 26,* 563–574.

Ottevanger, P.B., Therasse, P., van de Velde, C., Bernier, J., van Krieken, H., Grol, R., et al. (2003). Quality assurance in clinical trials. *Critical Reviews in Oncology/Hematology, 47,* 213–235.

Rhoads, J.L. (2003, March 31). *FDA warning letter.* Retrieved September 19, 2007, from http://wlap.org/file-archive/cacr/CACR3WarningLetter.doc

Roche, K., Paul, N., Smuck, B., Whitehead, M., Zee, B., Pater, J., et al. (2002). Factors affecting workload of cancer clinical trials: Results of a multicenter study of the National Cancer Institute of Canada Clinical Trials Group. *Journal of Clinical Oncology, 20,* 545–556.

Shah, S. (2003). Globalization of clinical research by the pharmaceutical industry. *International Journal of Health Services, 33*(1), 29–46.

Sniderman, A.D. (1999). Clinical trials, consensus conferences, and clinical practice. *Lancet, 354,* 327–330.

Sung, N.S., Crowley, W.F., Jr., Genel, M., Salber, P., Sandy, L., Sherwood, L.M., et al. (2003). Central challenges facing the national clinical research enterprise. *JAMA, 289,* 1278–1287.

U.S. Food and Drug Administration. (1999, May 3). *Milestones in U.S. food and drug law history.* Retrieved October 30, 2005, from http://www.fda.gov/opacom/backgrounders/miles.html

U.S. Food and Drug Administration. (2004). *Innovation or stagnation: Challenge and opportunity on the critical path to new medical products.* Retrieved August 16, 2005, from http://www.fda.gov/oc/initiatives/criticalpath/whitepaper.html

U.S. Food and Drug Administration. (n.d.). *Guidances, information sheets, and important notices on good clinical practice in FDA-regulated clinical trials.* Retrieved October 29, 2007, from http:/www.fda.gov/oc/gcp/guidance.html#guidance

U.S. Food and Drug Administration Center for Devices and Radiological Health. (2006, April 1). *CFR title 21 database.* Retrieved October 29, 2007, from http://www.accessdata.fda.gov/scripts/cdrh/cfdocs/cfcfr/cfrsearch.cfm

U.S. Food and Drug Administration Center for Drug Evaluation and Research. (2002, July 17). *Drug applications.* Retrieved October 29, 2007, from http://www.fda.gov/cder/regulatory/applications/Forms.htm

CHAPTER 46
Standard Operating Procedures

Kelly J. Dustin, RN, MS, CCRC

Introduction

The International Conference on Harmonisation of Technical Requirements for Registration of Pharmaceuticals for Human Use (ICH) defined standard operating procedures (SOPs) as "detailed, written instructions to achieve uniformity of the performance of a specific function" (ICH, 1996, p. 8). SOPs are an integral part of clinical trial conduct at all levels to ensure good clinical practice in compliance with the *Code of Federal Regulations* (Titles 21 and 45) and ICH guidelines. Good clinical practices are key to conducting a quality clinical trial that can be reproduced and the results replicated. To accomplish this, clinical research site SOPs may include the following categories (Kolman, Meng, & Scott, 2000).

- Study planning
- Study team definition and responsibilities
- Study files policy
- Protocol review and validation
- Review of protocol amendments
- Case report form review and completion
- Investigator's brochure
- Estimation of projected patient enrollment numbers
- Ethics committee
- Indemnity, compensation, and insurance
- Laboratory
- Monitoring visits
- Patient recruitment
- Informed consent
- Randomization
- Blinding codes and code breaking
- Study drugs
- Adverse events and serious adverse event reporting
- Nursing procedures
- Clinical procedures
- Trial reporting
- Archiving
- Audits and inspections

SOPs should be customized according to the site's organizational specifics. Records throughout a clinical trial should show documentation that the patient meets eligibility criteria, informed consent is obtained, treatment is given according to protocol, response is assessed according to protocol, adverse events are reported promptly, and drug accountability records are correct. A paper or electronic trail of study events such as protocol approval, amendments, correspondence, protocol team meetings, and study reports helps to ensure the quality of the data from a clinical trial. The essential elements relevant to clinical trials nursing are discussed in greater detail.

Protocol Treatment Course: Eligibility

Integrating good patient care with good clinical practices is a challenge to all researchers. Many concerns exist related to the verifiability of eligibility of potential patients for a clinical research protocol, which begins with writing the protocol and ends when the final results of the study have been published.

All protocols must include a section about the eligibility criteria that determine the common factors that bring potential patients onto the research study. These eligibility criteria describe the patient population to be included in the research study and must be clear, concise, and unambiguous. Every patient enrolled in the study must meet the eligibility criteria to meet the specified objectives of a protocol. The similarity of the participants' backgrounds will contribute to the reproducibility of data. Enrollment of ineligible patients is a major concern and is not only wasteful of resources but also could lead to potential misinterpretation of results and compromised patient safety. See Chapter 22 for additional information on eligibility.

The principal investigator (PI) is the individual responsible for ensuring the quality of the protocol data, including that all patients entering a clinical trial meet the specified eligibility criteria. The clinical trial nurse (CTN) or data manager shares this responsibility with the PI to ensure that the patient is eligible for the protocol.

When the protocol is written, all of the participants in the project benefit from having clearly written eligibility checklists that serve not only as a reference to individuals working with potential protocol candidates but also as documentation of eligibility assessment criteria. The eligibility checklist should include general information such as protocol name and number and investigator. The list also should include patient identification and demographic information, as well as all data specifically needed to confirm eligibility (e.g., diagnosis, performance, status, prior therapy). Most items will be in a standard yes/no format, but some fields should include specific values (e.g., lab results and date). This checklist aids the individuals involved in the registration/randomization process in ensuring that patients have met all eligibility criteria, including a signed consent to participate, and helps them in their role as "gatekeeper" to verify the eligibility of all patients being registered for the protocol. Chapter 23 presents a computer tool to verify that eligibility requirements are met.

The office that conducts registrations should have written SOPs to ensure that all patients are eligible for the protocol prior to initiation of any research-related procedure. SOPs also must specify the process for dealing with patients who are not eligible for the study, as these patients, if enrolled in the study, could cause invalid results when the study is analyzed. Checklists can serve as validation of eligibility for the protocol to which patients are being entered and become a standard form for the research records.

Critical details to help to ensure the quality of the registration process include a list of individuals qualified to register patients and tracking systems to ensure that protocol-specified accrual ceilings are not exceeded and that accrual is proceeding according to projections. Communication patterns that involve all of the individuals/areas in the clinical research process (e.g., pharmacy, administration, CTNs, PIs), documentation of registrations, routine internal monitoring procedures that ensure the validity of the processes, and internal measures that ensure the security of the data, as well as a back-up system to protect the information that has been obtained, also should be included.

The critical elements for ensuring eligibility criteria and quality control of the process are clearly defined study objectives, concise eligibility criteria, SOPs, good patterns of communication, excellent documentation, routine monitoring processes, and security measures to protect the confidentiality of study participants.

Protocol Treatment Course: Treatment

During the treatment phase of a clinical trial, quality improvement measures are necessary to ensure compliance with the guidelines and procedures outlined in the protocol (Iber, Riley, & Murray, 1987). The protocol will delineate the specific requirements that must be met while the subject is undergoing treatment. The medical record should be monitored regularly to ensure that compliance with the protocol is documented accurately (National Cancer Institute Cancer

Therapy Evaluation Program [NCI CTEP], 2002). Security of all records should be maintained consistently, and back-ups should exist of all computerized data to prevent loss of critical information. In many cases, documentation in the medical record (or hospital chart) alone is impractical or inconvenient, and a second record, called a research chart, is established. The research chart usually is kept in the patient care area and should contain copies of all pertinent protocol materials and source documents. The research record may be obtained quickly and referred to when the permanent medical record is not readily available.

Several areas of compliance may be included during monitoring of the acute treatment phase. First, all pretherapy laboratory values and results of any pretherapy procedures should be documented. Second, clear documentation noting that the research therapy or medications were administered according to the protocol is essential. Medical records should confirm that the correct drugs, dosage, and schedule were given and that correct techniques of administration were followed (NCI CTEP, 2002). Nurses or other appropriate healthcare providers are responsible for documenting the administration of study medications. If a subject is to self-administer a study therapy or will receive treatment as an outpatient, a patient diary or other documentation tool should be used to record therapy administration. Documentation of written informed consent is essential. Consent documentation should note the volunteer's understanding of the informed consent and how that assessment of understanding was made.

Third, all adverse events or toxicities that occur during therapy must be documented, as well as any dose modifications or interventions mandated by the protocol (White-Hershey & Nevidjon, 1990). For example, if the protocol states that the dose of research drug X will be reduced and granulocyte–colony-stimulating factor (G-CSF) will be administered for grade 4 (severe) neutropenia, the medical records should indicate not only the abnormal laboratory value but also that the research drug dose was decreased and that G-CSF was administered in response to the neutropenia.

Fourth, any therapeutic or research-related interventions or procedures mandated by the protocol should be recorded. These interventions may include procedures such as phlebotomy, bone marrow biopsy, computed tomography scans, or pulmonary function studies. Documentation should include not only results but also data that confirm that procedures were performed according to protocol specifications. For instance, blood samples for pharmacokinetics often are drawn at critical, predetermined times, so the records should indicate that the correct specimens were obtained at the appropriate times.

Finally, clear and precise documentation of response to the investigational therapy should be kept (White-Hershey & Nevidjon, 1990). Guidelines for evaluation of response are determined by the written protocol. For instance, if the protocol states that a partial response is a reduction by greater than or equal to 50% of the size of all measurable lesions, then the medical record should include the appropriate tumor measurements confirming the response. In addition, if the protocol requires that a particular action be taken depending upon the response, then this should be documented, as well. For example, if progressive disease means the subject must be taken off the study, this should be recorded in the medical record with duplicate documentation placed in the research chart. Any contact with the study chair or PI regarding protocol questions and determination of response should be documented.

Protocol Treatment Course: Off Treatment

One of the issues that commonly arises during the research process is standardization of definitions and terminology in the protocol. For instance, what does *off treatment* mean in terms of the protocol? Does it mean that the treatment has been completed and the patient is "off study," or, although the treatment is completed, a specified period of follow-up will exist? Was the treatment stopped because of completion, toxicity, noncompliance, progressive disease, or other protocol-defined conditions? Therefore, a major component in the research process is standardization of terminology and the definitions to be used in the protocol so that all personnel involved in the study will understand what is meant when specific terms are used. The text of the protocol should be written to include clear definitions of terminology and the responsibilities of the investigators and others implementing the protocol (e.g., pharmacy, administration, CTNs). All of the partners in the research process must understand the definitions of terms such as *off study* and *off treatment*. The protocol should include specific criteria for determining when a patient has met the criteria for off study and ensuring that patients are not inappropriately taken off or left on a study. The patient records or database should clearly document a patient's on- or off-study status. This documentation should state why a patient was taken off study and that the patient was notified. Final study documentation is complete when it includes a plan for further treatment or follow-up as dictated by individual patient circumstances. The standards for ensuring off-study criteria are met and ensuring quality control of the process include clearly defined study objectives, standardization of terminology, excellent documentation, and a routine monitoring process.

Protocol Treatment Course: Adverse Events

Prompt and thorough reporting of adverse events is critical in clinical drug trials. An adverse event may be described as a decline from baseline conditions and may or may not be attributed to the study drug (ICH, 1996). Adverse events need to be documented and assessed before causality can be decided. For example, a patient fall may be an accident, but was the accident precipitated by neurocerebellar effects of the drug, hypotension, or sensory neuropathy associated with the study drug? Could additive effects of the study drug exist with concomitant medications or conditions? The medical chart and research record should document any concomitant medical conditions and nonstudy drugs. After weighing all of these factors and the temporal relationship of the event to the study drug, an attribution of toxicity can be made by a physician. If a reasonable possibility exists that the drug caused the experience, the toxicity would be recorded in the research record as an adverse event related to the study agent. If a patient had an allergic reaction to the study agent, this is commonly referred to as an adverse drug reaction.

Title 21, Part 312.32 of the *Code of Federal Regulations* (U.S. Food and Drug Administration [FDA], 2006) provides the safety reporting guidelines for investigational new drugs. Reporting guidelines define serious and unexpected adverse events. A written report of an adverse drug reaction must be submitted promptly to the FDA for serious, unexpected events. The institutional review board (IRB) also must be notified promptly. The sponsor is responsible for notifying the FDA by telephone of any unexpected fatal or life-threatening experiences.

Communication of adverse events must be made to other investigators, the pharmacy, the nursing staff, and the sponsor. The sponsor is responsible for notifying the FDA and investigators at other sites. Prompt reporting may alert the sponsor to close a trial early because of unacceptable toxicity. See Chapter 28 for a detailed discussion of adverse events.

Full documentation of the event in the medical record is the source documentation for the event. The research record would hold information on all of the adverse events for each patient, and the database would document specific events during the time the patient was on study. Adverse events may not be discerned in phase I and phase II trials because these trials accrue smaller numbers of research participants. In phase III trials, however, larger numbers of participants are exposed to the drugs, and new adverse events may be noted. All reports of adverse events must be recorded carefully in the research record.

Long-term follow-up is necessary to uncover late-onset adverse events as well as to determine resolution. When a study drug is stopped because of an adverse event, the medical record should document whether the study subject was rechallenged with the agent and if the toxicity reappeared. Again, this information should be recorded in the research record. It is important to remember that the medical record documents the medical care and condition of the patient, whereas the research record is a compilation of documents that show the patient's progress through the study. The research record can include copies of the registration form, lab flow sheets, patient diaries, study drug flow sheets, and toxicity forms.

Trials need to be monitored for the quality of documentation of adverse events. The monitoring can be performed by the sponsor, by a monitor hired by the sponsor, or by internal computerized checks. These events must be followed to resolution or until it is determined that toxicity will not resolve.

Protocol Treatment Course: Notification of Updated Information to Patients

New information that is discovered during a trial may necessitate a change in the informed consent or notification of patients who already are entered or who formerly participated in a clinical trial. If the information pertains to potential harm to the patient, immediate notification is necessary. This notification can be in the form of a telephone call from the investigator to the patient followed by a letter to the patient. Every effort should be made to locate former patients. Documentation in the medical chart and the research record should indicate when the patient was notified, the means by which he or she was notified, and that the patient actually received notification. Merely attempting to notify the patient is not sufficient. If the patient cannot be reached by telephone, then a certified letter may be sent. The patient's primary care/referring physician should be notified of updated information by telephone, fax, or letter, and a confirmation of receipt of this information should be documented.

For phase IV trials, in addition to physicians notifying individual patients, public announcements on radio, television, and newspapers can be used. The updated information may involve situations in which the study drug caused or may be thought to have caused serious side effects or delayed effects. An alternative treatment may be determined to be superior. If one arm of a treatment is found to be more effective than another arm, the study may be stopped early and the patient may be offered treatment with the effective therapy. In any of these cases, current or former patients should be notified.

Protocol Treatment Course: Continuing Informed Consent

Informed consent is an ongoing process that does not end when the patient signs the consent form. The study participant may withdraw his or her consent at any time, even during implementation of the protocol. If the patient is unsure about whether to continue on the protocol, the investigator could meet with him or her to clarify any information or offer to make an appointment with the bioethicist if the patient feels that he or she cannot drop out of the study.

When new information is known about the study drug or if treatment on the protocol has been changed, a new consent form must be written and submitted to the IRB and sponsor for approval. After approval, the consent form must be explained to the patient. The new signed consent form is kept on file along with the first consent under which the patient entered the study. New informa-

tion can include reports of unanticipated side effects, delayed toxicities, more severe toxicities, or the availability of new treatments.

All versions of approved consents must be kept on file with the protocol; they are not destroyed while the study is ongoing. Old and new signed consents must be kept in the research record. A copy of each version of consent signed by the patient also must be kept in the medical record. Original signed consents, both old and new, must be retained for documentation and quality assurance tracking. If the patient withdraws consent, it must be documented in the medical record. The patient's signature is not required, but the investigator should note in the record when the patient withdrew consent and the stated reason. The notation should be signed and dated by the investigator or a member of the research team and retained as a source document.

Protocol Treatment Course: Death on Study

Occasionally, research participants die during the course of a study. All events and abnormalities related to the death must be well documented in the medical record and research chart. The timing of a death and preexisting conditions may be of particular significance in determining whether the death was caused by the experimental therapy. The records should clearly show the temporal relationship between the therapy and the time of death. The existence of prior abnormalities and concomitant problems also should be clearly documented. For example, if a study participant received drug X on day one and died from an acute myocardial infarction (MI) on day seven, the records should include information that could help to determine whether the MI was a toxicity caused by drug X or by concomitant cardiac disease. Such information may include that the patient had a history of MI in the past, a long history of poorly controlled hypertension and angina, and perhaps a normal electrocardiogram prior to receiving drug X. When the relationship of death to protocol therapy is unclear, an autopsy can provide valuable information. If an autopsy is performed, the report should be included in the medical record and the research chart (Dunn & Chadwick, 1999).

Deaths on study and within a certain time period following experimental therapy (often 30 days) usually will require a report to the FDA, the study sponsor, and the IRB. Quality improvement should include monitoring records to determine that required reports were sent to the appropriate agencies in a timely manner (Lepay, 2001).

If deviations from the protocol are found when monitoring records for quality improvement, a process should be implemented to report and resolve the discrepancy. Deviations from the protocol should be evaluated to determine the source of discrepancies and to suggest solutions for identified problems (Iber et al., 1987).

Summary

Quality improvement is a vital part of the conduct of a clinical trial. From the time of protocol inception through the publication of final results, measures to ensure quality must be established and maintained. Compliance with the protocol should be monitored beginning with eligibility and continuing through treatment, adverse events, changes in protocol, going off study, and potentially death on study. Many methods are needed to ensure adherence, including eligibility checklists, tracking systems, good communication patterns, thorough documentation, and regular monitoring.

Establishing clear SOPs in advance will help to ensure a reliable process and quality outcomes. Adherence to the protocol and documentation of compliance with all criteria are necessary for successful results. Noncompliance with the standards of the protocol limits the reliability and reproducibility of the data and confounds any conclusions one may draw from the study.

References

Dunn, C.M., & Chadwick, G. (1999). *Protecting study volunteers in research: A manual for investigative sites.* Boston: CenterWatch.

Iber, F.L., Riley, W.A., & Murray, P.J. (1987). *Conducting clinical trials.* New York: Plenum Publishing.

International Conference on Harmonisation of Technical Requirements for Registration of Pharmaceuticals for Human Use. (1996, April). *Guidance for industry: E6 good clinical practice: Consolidated guidance.* Retrieved May 17, 2006, from http://www.fda.gov/cder/guidance/959fnl.pdf

Kolman, J., Meng, P., & Scott, G. (1998). Preparation, approval and review of SOPs. In J. Kolman, P. Meng, & G. Scott (Eds.), *Good clinical practice: Standard operating procedures for clinical researchers* (pp. 11–17). Chichester, England: Wiley.

Lepay, D.A. (2001). *GCP, quality assurance, and FDA.* Retrieved March 30, 2007, from http://www.fda.gov/oc/gcp/slideshows/lepay2001/SQAWeb.ppt

National Cancer Institute Cancer Therapy Evaluation Program. (2002). *The investigator's handbook: A manual for participants in clinical trials of investigational agents sponsored by DCTD, NCI.* Retrieved September 14, 2007, from http://ctep.cancer.gov/handbook

U.S. Food and Drug Administration. (2006). *Code of federal regulations (Title 21, Vol. 5, Part 312.32).* Washington, DC: U.S. Government Printing Office.

White-Hershey, D., & Nevidjon, B. (1990). Fundamentals for oncology nurse/data managers—preparing for a new role. *Oncology Nursing Forum, 17,* 371–377.

CHAPTER 47
Audit Preparation

Ellen A. Patricia, MS

Introduction

Cancer clinical trial practitioners have an obligation to protect the rights, safety, and welfare of the participants enrolled onto their trials, as well as to ensure that the data collected during the trial are credible and verifiable. Good clinical practice (GCP) must be followed, and data results must be properly documented. This chapter is devoted to audits, of which several types exist: federal audits (e.g., National Cancer Institute [NCI], U.S. Food and Drug Administration [FDA]), sponsor audits, cooperative group audits, and internal investigational site audits. When through reading this chapter, the reader will have a good understanding of what an audit is, the purpose of an audit, the types of audits, how to prepare for an audit, and how to conduct an audit.

What Is an Audit?

An audit is a mechanism for assessing the data quality and regulatory integrity of a clinical trial. It often is the final step employed by the FDA before it approves a drug or device for the market. Audits should not be feared but instead viewed as a quality improvement tool. Audit education targets everyone who participates in clinical trials and must be considered part of the process of long-term learning (Lepay, 2001).

What Is the Purpose of an Audit?

The purpose of an audit is to evaluate trial conduct and compliance with the protocol, internal standard operating procedures, GCP, and applicable regulatory requirements (federal, state, and local). Audits are necessary to assure the public, and in particular, the subject volunteers, that the data generated in cancer clinical trials are credible and that while the trial was being conducted, subjects' rights, welfare, and safety were upheld.

A clinical study site may be audited by one or all of the following entities: (a) the FDA, (b) the study sponsor,

such as a pharmaceutical company, (c) NCI, the National Institutes of Health, the Department of Defense, or a cooperative group (e.g., Southwest Oncology Group [SWOG], Eastern Cooperative Oncology Group [ECOG], Cancer and Leukemia Group B [CALGB]), or (d) an internal auditing group, such as a compliance office or quality assurance office. Regardless of the auditing body, the principles listed in Figure 47-1 apply to all audits of clinical research.

What Are the Types of Audits?
U.S. Food and Drug Administration Audits: Routine and "For Cause"

An FDA routine site audit typically occurs as a result of clinical data submitted in the form of a new drug application (NDA) and the need of the FDA to base important decisions on those data. Events that could trigger a "for-cause" audit may include a whistleblower report to the FDA, reports of fraud or unreported serious adverse events, or a complaint that an investigator is administering investigational drugs in an inappropriate manner. Because most FDA audits are routine audits, it is important to focus on these.

The FDA's Center for Drug Evaluation and Research (CDER) determines which clinical studies and study centers will be audited. Although CDER does not release explicit details of how it goes about selecting studies and sites for

---

Figure 47-1. Audit Purposes

- To determine that the rights, safety, and welfare of human participants enrolled in clinical trials are properly protected
- To ensure the integrity of scientific research and the reliability of the data generated by verifying that all data are obtained in compliance with good clinical practice
- To ensure that local, state, and federal regulatory requirements and procedures are adequately fulfilled
- To assist site personnel in the development of useful procedures to guide research endeavors
- To educate research staff and initiate follow-up mechanisms for problem resolution

audit, it is obvious that if a trial is an important trial in an NDA portfolio, it will be audited. CDER drug reviewers also consider the number of subjects enrolled at a particular site, the number of subjects who withdrew early, and those sites with very good response rates or, conversely, very poor response rates. In a March 2005 presentation, Joanne Rhodes, MD, director of CDER's Division of Scientific Investigations, noted that the agency

> may inspect from one to several clinical sites per pivotal multicenter trial. For crucial primary efficacy endpoints, FDA may check the accuracy of the sponsor's data listings versus source documents for a sample of up to 100 percent of the subjects. Other elements, for example, the integrity of the blinding, drug accountability and safety data such as the reporting of serious adverse events and adverse events to the sponsor and IRB [institutional review board], are checked for accuracy in a sample of the subject's records. (Mathieu, 2005, p. 181)

Also during her March 2005 presentation, Dr. Rhodes highlighted 11 determinations that an FDA inspector must make during a clinical investigator audit, as outlined below (Mathieu, 2005, p. 181).

- What was the source of the subjects?
- Did the subjects exist?
- Did they have the disease under study?
- Did they meet inclusion/exclusion criteria?
- Was consent obtained?
- Was IRB review obtained?
- Was the clinical protocol followed?
- Did the subjects receive the assigned study drug in the dose, route, and frequency specified by the protocol?
- Are the case report forms complete and in agreement with the source data (compare with NDA data listing)?
- Are adverse experiences reported to the sponsor and IRB?
- Are records adequate and complete?

Routine audits are scheduled in the following manner: (a) CDER chooses a clinical site for inspection, (b) the local FDA office nearest to the site is notified that a site audit must be scheduled, (c) the local investigator contacts the site principal investigator and requests an audit date, which typically is one to two weeks from the contact date, and (d) the local inspector arrives at the mutually agreed-upon date, presents his or her FDA credentials, and issues FDA Form 482, Notice of Inspection. At the conclusion of the audit, typically FDA Form 483, Inspectional Observations, will be issued. The 483 is the FDA inspector's report to the site of those things that, in the opinion of the inspector, may include violations. Receiving a 483 is not the end of the world and does not represent the FDA's final position on the inspection. When it is reviewed internally at the FDA, the 483 may be overturned completely. The 483 is used to develop an inspectional report, which will include a more detailed description of the violations uncovered during

the site inspection. This report is then reviewed at CDER, and they, in turn, will classify the inspection results in one of three ways:

- NAI (no action indicated)
- VAI (voluntary action indicated)
- OAI (official action indicated).

Both NAI and VAI classifications result in "untitled letters." An OAI classification typically results in a warning letter being issued. A warning letter is an advisory to a clinical investigator communicating the FDA's position on violations of regulatory significance (Mathieu, 2005). The FDA will ask the investigator to respond to the warning letter with a remedial action plan to address the compliance problems. In extreme cases of severe noncompliance, the FDA can disqualify investigators from ever using investigational products again.

Sponsor Audits

In preparation for an FDA audit, oftentimes the drug manufacturer/pharmaceutical sponsor will send an audit team to the investigational site to conduct a pre-audit. The auditors assist the investigational site in preparing for the inspection. The team will ensure that source documentation is complete and well organized and may conduct further source document verification to identify potential problems. Note: No data changes should be made after study closure. The audit team also will address site concerns and questions about the pending audit and may offer tips and suggestions on how the staff should conduct itself while the audit is taking place. An audit report typically is generated as a result of this type of audit, but the report itself is exempt from FDA review. The investigational site should not make this report available to the FDA inspector.

National Cancer Institute–Directed Monitoring and Auditing

The Division of Cancer Treatment and Diagnosis (DCTD) of NCI has developed policies governing the therapeutic development of new agents. Within the DCTD exists the Cancer Therapy Evaluation Program (CTEP), a division responsible for the design and implementation of development plans for new agents.

Protocol compliance and data accuracy form the major focus of the DCTD-sponsored quality assurance effort (NCI CTEP, 2002). Cooperative groups, such as SWOG, CALGB, and ECOG, monitor trial compliance in several ways: central pathology reviews, quality control in radiotherapy, protocol chair review of case report forms, and statistical office review of eligibility and response. The majority of cancer centers have procedures in place to assess central protocol compliance. CTEP has an on-site audit program that evaluates cancer center protocol compliance as part of its monitoring visits. These visits involve administrative review for central data management, protocol development, and data collection. Protocol compliance is assessed by the Clinical Trials Monitoring Service (CTMS). Phase I and phase II/III investigational sites submit raw data to CTMS on an ongoing basis, and then CTMS reviews the data carefully for compliance with the protocol. Reports of these evaluations are provided to the investigator and to CTEP.

Data accuracy is verified during on-site audits. The research record (case report form) is compared to the primary patient medical records. Treatment responses are verified by reviewing the patient's disease assessments for adherence to protocol-mandated methods of measurement. Procedural activities also are checked at an on-site audit and include the following.

- The informed consent process: Auditors must verify the existence of an IRB-approved consent form signed by the trial participant prior to the initiation of study-specific procedures.
- IRB approvals must be verified to have been obtained before the start of the trial, and at least annually thereafter, for each NCI-sponsored trial.
- Drug accountability procedures and records are verified.
- Adverse event reporting is monitored, as well.

On-site audits are conducted, on average, once every three years. Cooperative groups perform their own program of on-site audits, and these are conducted by a combination of central staff and group members with direct oversight by the Clinical Trials Monitoring Branch. Paid contractors (e.g., Theradex) perform on-site visits to each phase I contractor three times per year. Cancer centers are audited on-site by NCI or NCI-contracted auditors once every three years.

CTEP and cooperative groups have many action options when dealing with problems identified during on-site audits. In most cases, the measures are intended to be constructive and educational. The action options employed by CTEP and the cooperative groups can include probation status, letter of warning, suspension of patient-enrollment privileges, repeat audit, removal of access to investigational agents, or termination of grant or contract.

Internal Audits at the Investigational Site

Large investigational sites often have an office completely dedicated to internal protocol compliance. These offices are set up as a safeguard for the institution. Community hospitals and private practices generally are affiliated with a Community Clinical Oncology Program, a community-based auditing program, or they hire independent auditors to review compliance. Because a clinical study site may be audited by one or all of the following entities—the FDA, the study sponsor, a cooperative group—it makes sense to have an office devoted to assisting with the numerous outside audits that take place every year and to perform internal audits of those trials that do not undergo routine auditing (i.e., investigator-initiated trials). The focus of such a protocol compliance office would be to educate site faculty and staff of the local, state, and federal regulations governing their clinical research. This office would serve as the central contact center when compliance questions arise, as well. Oversight of this office would be performed by hospital administration or by a clinical trials office medical director.

All of the investigational site's therapeutic groups are subject to an annual internal audit conducted by an office of protocol compliance. A protocol is chosen for audit, and then a representative number of patient cases are reviewed (at least 10% of all enrolled subjects) (author's internal SOP). All associated regulatory documents also are audited. At the conclusion of the audit, an audit report is generated and distributed to study personnel and to the protocol principal investigator. A point-by-point response to the audit report must be submitted to the office and a general corrective action plan employed to ensure that further mistakes are not repeated (author's internal SOP). Education is the key to these internal audits. Focusing on the positive aspects of the study conduct is essential, and correcting problems before they become routine is critical.

How to Prepare for an Audit

Auditors prepare for an audit by reviewing the protocol, the site's internal SOPs, applicable regulations, sponsor guidelines, and internal protocol-specific files (e.g., scientific review committee files, disease team protocol reviews). These preparations are enacted to ensure an educated and efficient use of time and resources and also to ensure an audit result that increases staff education and compliance. In turn, the research team must properly prepare for an audit to facilitate the audit process and ideally to arrive at a positive audit outcome. Once the research team has received notification of a pending audit, the steps outlined below should be followed.

- Notify all parties of the audit date(s) (i.e., the investigational pharmacy, the IRB, all members of the research protocol team).
- Obtain pertinent audit information such as the number of auditors who will conduct the audit, the approximate times the auditors will work each day, whether an exit interview will take place at the conclusion of the audit, and if so, who will be required to be present at this meeting.
- Schedule a quiet room with enough space to comfortably accommodate the audit team. The room should be located near a copier, fax machine, and phone. A computer also should be made available for the auditors to view online medical records, x-ray and scan results, and online versions of the protocol.
- Order all patient medical records, including inpatient, outpatient, and those housed in the physician's office.
- If required, flag the medical records with color-coded sticky notes for easier record review. See Figure 47-2 for a suggested color-coded flag system.
- Pre-review the regulatory records and charts for any missing source documentation.
- Perform an internal data review with assistance from the research team, if time allows, before the audit date.

**Figure 47-2. Sample Flag Color Code Guide
(Taken From Author's Standard Operating Procedure)**

Prestudy requirements: Red
Pathology: Green
Lab results: White
Radiology results and tumor measurements: Blue
Drug administration records: Yellow
History and physical records: Orange
Toxicities: Purple

What Will Be Reviewed During the Audit?

Regulatory Files

The regulatory files will be reviewed to provide evidence that regulatory compliance regarding study conduct and records has been properly maintained throughout the study. To facilitate review of these documents, they should be well organized into sections. The files should contain a section where all versions of the protocol and consent are housed, including a copy of the initial protocol. The file should contain an IRB correspondence section (correspondence to and from the IRB) and an approvals section (including initial protocol and consent approvals, amendment approvals, and annual continuing review approvals, along with the IRB roster and meeting minutes as applicable). A special section should be devoted to adverse event (AE) reporting. This section must include evidence that AEs were properly reported to the IRB and to the sponsor. Also contained in this file will be a sponsor correspondence section (to and from the sponsor).

Informed Consents

All IRB-approved consent versions will be reviewed to verify that they contain all required elements of informed consent as mandated by 21 CFR 50.25 (FDA, 2006). The auditors also will review the consent versions to ensure that they reflect the appropriate risks, tests, and procedures for each version time period. Auditors attempt to uncover the methods employed by the research team during the consenting process, such as: Were patients introduced to the concept of clinical trials and then presented all of their potential treatment options? Was consent obtained for every subject enrolled onto the trial? Was it obtained prior to the initiation of any protocol-mandated procedures? Was a copy of the consent given to the patient to take home? Was the entire consent process well documented in the medical record? Was a new consent signed when new information became available that might affect the subject's participation in the trial? Was the correct version of the consent used for the appropriate time frame?

Drug Accountability

Accountability records for investigational agents, as well as for any other drug supplied by the sponsor for the trial, will be subject to audit. As was mentioned earlier, always inform the investigational pharmacist of any pending audit, as most certainly the pharmacy will be a stop on the audit trail.

Drug accountability records are compared to shipment records to ensure that the agents were properly received and logged in at the site. If products were transferred from one office to another or were shipped back to the sponsor, those records will be compared to ensure that all products are accounted for. A patient registration log should correlate with the drug dispensing records. The auditor must ensure that all enrolled subjects were dispensed the proper drug and dosage per protocol and, conversely, that no patient other than those registered to the trial received study-supplied products. The auditor also must check to see that commercial supplies versus investigational supplies were appropriately used and not interchanged.

The auditor will visit the pharmacy to ensure that the location is secure and that access to the area is restricted to pharmacy personnel only. If investigational products are present in the pharmacy at the time of the audit, the auditor will actually count the remaining drug to confirm the amount indicated on the inventory records.

Subject Records

The auditor will compare the case report forms or sponsor-supplied data print-outs against the patient's medical records (both inpatient and outpatient) to verify reporting accuracy and to ensure that no omissions were made in the reported data. This document review allows the auditor to assess how well the research staff followed the protocol requirements: Were the proper tests ordered and obtained? Were AEs reported and in a timely fashion? Specifically, the following will be reviewed in detail.

- Subject enrollment procedures—was the first subject enrolled after IRB approval was granted?
- Subject selection—were the subjects eligible for the trial?
- Informed consent—is there an original signed informed consent available for every audited subject? Additionally, the auditor will verify that the correct version of the consent document was signed, that it was signed before any protocol-specific procedures were performed, and that the entire consent process was well documented in the medical record.
- Subject data—the following will be reviewed for each subject chosen for audit.
  - Inclusion/exclusion criteria to ensure that only appropriate patients were enrolled onto the trial
  - Protocol treatment administration records: Were treatments held or modified correctly, as mandated by the protocol?
  - Tumor response: Was response documented at the appropriate time points and by the methods outlined in the protocol?
  - Toxicities and AEs: Were they reported to the appropriate entities (i.e., the sponsor, IRB, NCI) as required by the protocol? Were the AE source documents signed by the principal investigator, treating physician, or RN?

- Laboratory results
- Reasons for subject withdrawal
- Follow-up data

What Happens at the Close-Out Meeting?

A close-out meeting is typically held with the research team, including the protocol's principal investigator, the regulatory coordinator, the study coordinator, and the data manager. The positive audit findings should be highlighted at this meeting, and then the deficiencies reviewed. The auditor may suggest corrective actions at this time. Otherwise, the research team can wait until an audit report is generated and take time to formulate a thoughtful and meaningful response to the report.

Summary

Audits ensure that the data generated during a clinical trial are credible, that the federal regulations governing clinical trials are followed, and that participants' rights, safety, and welfare are upheld. Audits are educational tools employed to instruct research teams in the correct way to run a clinical trial. It is critical that when subjects volunteer to participate in a clinical trial, their participation counts for something and is meaningful. That should be the ultimate goal of clinical trial research, along with, of course, finding treatments that eventually will enhance the lives of patients with cancer and those who are at high risk for cancer.

References

Lepay, D.A. (2001). *GCP, quality assurance, and FDA* [Slide show]. Retrieved October 29, 2007, from http://www.fda.gov/oc/gcp/slideshows/lepay2001/SQAWeb.ppt

Mathieu, M.P. (Ed.). (2005). *Good clinical practice: A question and answer reference guide.* Waltham, MA: PAREXEL International Corporation.

National Cancer Institute Cancer Therapy Evaluation Program. (2002). *The investigator's handbook: A manual for participants in clinical trials of investigational agents sponsored by DCTD, NCI.* Bethesda, MD: National Cancer Institute.

U.S. Food and Drug Administration. (2006, April 1). *Code of federal regulations (Title 21, Vol. 1, Part 50.25).* Retrieved October 29, 2007, from http://www.accessdata.fda.gov/scripts/cdrh/cfdocs/cfCFR/CFRSearch.crm?FR=50.25

CHAPTER 48
Community-Based Clinical Trials

June Iesue-Queen, RN, MSN

Introduction

Over the past 20 years, progressive, dynamic development has occurred in outpatient, community-based cancer care treatment programs and services. As part of this evolution, patients who utilize cancer care services within their community may discover themselves invited to participate in a clinical trial. For patients with cancer, major advantages of community-based clinical trials include the benefit of receiving state-of-the-art cancer treatment, prevention, or symptom management strategies as well as the ability to receive these therapies close to home without having to travel to a distant academic cancer treatment setting (National Cancer Institute [NCI], n.d.).

In 1983, NCI implemented an innovative program called the Community Clinical Oncology Program (CCOP). In 1989, NCI also approved the Minority-Based CCOP to increase the involvement of racial and ethnic minority patients in research (NCI, n.d.). According to NCI (n.d.), this program was "established to provide a mechanism for community physicians to bring the benefits of clinical research to their patients."

The CCOP is a network for conducting cancer prevention and treatment clinical trials by community physicians and is funded by a peer-reviewed cooperative grant agreement. This network connects academic centers—NCI-designated cancer centers or cooperative groups who design and conduct the trials—with community physicians (NCI, n.d.).

In 2003, NCI celebrated the 20th anniversary of the CCOP and reported on the program's success, effectiveness, and impact on community-based cancer care. The analysis included the finding that "CCOPs accrue one-third of patients who participate in NCI-sponsored cancer treatment trials" (Moulton, 2003, p. 1824). The report further noted that since the program's inception, "CCOP participation has resulted in more than 98,000 patients on treatment trials and more than 77,000 people at risk for cancer on prevention trials" (Moulton, p. 1824).

Definition of Community-Based Clinical Trials

Cancer clinical trials that are referred to as *community-based* are research studies typically coordinated and administered in a nonacademic hospital or medical center or a freestanding cancer care facility located within a particular community (NCI, n.d.). The ability of the patient to remain close to home is regarded as an important, primary element included in this definition.

The American College of Surgeons Commission on Cancer (ACoS CoC) establishes standards to ensure comprehensive cancer care delivery in healthcare settings. These settings include community-based cancer programs. The ACoS CoC formally recognizes programs that commit to offering a full scope of cancer services with the inclusion of clinical trials.

Standard 5.1 of the ACoS CoC (2006) *Cancer Program Standards* states that "information about the availability of cancer-related clinical trials is provided to patients through a formal mechanism" (p. 63). To achieve formal CoC program approval, comprehensive community-based cancer programs that demonstrate 650 or more new annual cancer cases (as evidenced by hospital cancer registry database information) are mandated to fulfill the clinical trial provision standards. For community hospital cancer programs that register between 100 and 649 annual cancer cases, although not mandated, CoC approval remains strongly recommended for facilities that participate in clinical research (ACoS CoC).

To provide cancer clinical trials to patients, the community hospital or cancer treatment facility may choose to become affiliated with a specific research organization that will serve as "research central," such as a contracted research organization, to provide data management and other related services, or the facility may choose to join a CCOP.

As part of a CCOP membership agreement, the hospital (affiliate site) agrees to pay an annual membership fee for services and also agrees to provide necessary clinical research personnel, resources, and overhead. The CCOP may offer specific research operations services such as protocol review and approval per clinical research committee, regulatory and institution review board (IRB) services, pharmacy services (i.e., study drug ordering, storage, and dispensing), data quality assurance and improvement, data management, and clinical research protocol guidance and expertise. This example is modeled after one of the first CCOP programs, the Columbus CCOP in Columbus, Ohio, which was established in 1983.

The benefits of community-based clinical trials include
- Increased patient accrual and a more diverse patient population to minimize bias (Spilker, 1991)
- Opportunity for community-based physicians to participate in clinical trials, which may lead to career enhancement, increased opportunities for coauthorship, or access to grant monies
- Access to state-of-the-art cancer therapy for patients without requiring extensive travel to distant cancer treatment sites.

Challenges of Community-Based Clinical Trials

Clinical trials administered in the community setting pose a number of unique considerations and challenges. In the following section, this chapter will present four major challenges that clinical trial nurses (CTNs) have reported as being often encountered in the clinical trial patient care arena. These include clinical trial challenges related to community reaction and participation, protocol compliance and oversight, education of the cancer care team, and long-term follow up.

Community Reaction and Participation

Initially, patients diagnosed with cancer may be surprised to learn that clinical trials are available through their community hospital or local cancer treatment center. Patients tend to expect clinical trials to be offered and conducted in a large academic cancer care setting. They may be hesitant and fearful to participate in a clinical research study that will be administered by their "hometown" hospital. See Chapter 19 for additional information on psychosocial considerations.

The overall goal of the American Society of Clinical Oncology's (2003) policy statement on oversight of clinical research is to "enhance public trust in the cancer clinical trial process" (p. 2377). The first element of this policy states, "Ensure safety precautions for clinical trial participants and their fully informed consent" (p. 2377).

The oncologist is responsible for initiation of the informed consent process and may consult the CTN—this position also may be titled as oncology research nurse or protocol nurse—to meet with the patient and family members to provide additional details about the protocol requirements and treatment plan.

It can be reassuring for the patient and family to understand that the patient will be closely monitored and assessed throughout his or her clinical trial experience by the oncologist, the CTN, and other members of the cancer care treatment team. See Chapter 14 for detailed discussion of the informed consent process.

Protocol Compliance and Oversight

The cancer care team of the affiliate member hospital site, with additional oversight by the central research office, must maintain careful and diligent adherence to the protocol treatment plan and study calendar. This begins at the time of protocol screening, continues during the course of cancer treatment, and may extend throughout patient survivorship. The central research office may monitor major aspects of the clinical trial to ensure that the affiliate site follows regulatory processes, enrolls only eligible patients, follows all protocol requirements, and practices ongoing due diligence related to all aspects of the protocol.

As previously mentioned, the CTN is a key member of the cancer care team. The CTN, an experienced oncology nurse clinician, functions in a unique and independent role while orchestrating a variety of responsibilities, which may include protocol treatment oversight and also data management. The CTN serves as the patient care coordinator and liaison and remains in close and ongoing communication with the oncologist(s), affiliate site cancer treatment team, and research central office.

The CTN closely monitors the patient for adverse events, alerts the oncologist to required protocol dose modifications and other requirements, and reports serious adverse events immediately and as mandated per protocol guidelines to a designated IRB. The CTN also may be directed to formally notify the protocol sponsor or protocol safety contact in addition to completing required case report forms: serious adverse event case report form (known as an SAE CRF), Adverse Event Expedited Reporting System (AdEERS), MedWatch, and additional adverse event case report forms as directed by the protocol.

Education of the Cancer Care Team

Education of the cancer care team, often an additional responsibility of the CTN, also can pose significant challenges. In addition to the CTN, the cancer care team includes, but is not limited to, oncology physician specialists (i.e., medical, radiation, and surgical), pathologists, radiologists, lab technicians, chemotherapy nurses, pharmacists and pharmacy technicians, radiation therapists, and medical office personnel. It is important that the cancer care team understands their specific roles and responsibilities in order to correctly and safely implement the protocol treatment plan.

Investigational and new U.S. Food and Drug Administration–approved chemotherapy drug treatment regimens and dosing schedules as well as required protocol testing and clinical assessment methods may vary from the standard of care.

Also, the protocol may require additional treatment planning and clinical monitoring and documentation. The cancer care team may perceive these protocol requirements as complex as well as labor and time intensive, which can lead to resistance or reluctance from care team members required to alter their busy patient schedule and treatment routine.

The CTN can provide assistance by initiating educational opportunities to facilitate clinical trial implementation. This is an important measure in fostering a collaborative, cooperative relationship between the CTN and the cancer care team.

Creative education and communication strategies can be designed and incorporated, tailored to the specific protocol design. Educational in-services provide opportunity for clarification, questions, and feedback. Protocol-specific information sheets with frequently asked questions and copies of specific protocol sections placed in the patient treatment chart can provide a quick and convenient reference for the cancer care team as the patient progresses through the protocol course of treatment.

Long-Term Follow-Up

Another major challenge is in regard to long-term patient follow-up and data collection. As the patient/cancer survivor proceeds along the course of the cancer care journey and reaches completion of his or her cancer therapy course, the oncologist and CTN will continue to see the patient in follow-up at protocol-specified time points to assess and address long-term follow-up care and concerns. Often, it is the CTN's responsibility to keep both the physician and patient abreast of protocol-required follow-up visit intervals and testing requirements.

In many instances, patients who have participated in a cancer clinical treatment trial are followed over the course of their lifetime to allow close assessment of the development of late effects and adverse events possibly related to treatment. The patient also is followed to eventually determine important study end points such as disease-free survival and long-term survival.

Patients should be reminded of the importance of close and regular follow-up care and health monitoring and should be instructed to notify the oncology office of changes in contact information and health status to prevent lost-to-follow-up occurrences. This also is important so that the research team can continue to keep the patient abreast of clinical updates that may affect the individual's health as a result of his or her previous clinical trial participation.

Efforts to obtain health status and survival information may become a challenge if, over time, the patient becomes "lost to follow-up." Common examples include that the CTN eventually may discover that the patient has changed his or her name, relocated, or died. Securing information may become more difficult if the patient's chart has been archived or if the patient has been treated at a different healthcare facility. Information may be obtained by contacting one or more of the following sources, while making every attempt to obtain patient consent for release of information and maintain compliance with Health Insurance Portability and Accountability Act regulations:

- Community hospital cancer registry
- Oncology physician practice offices
- Community hospital medical records department
- Referring physician(s) offices.

Patients who demonstrate noncompliance with follow-up visit requirements but agree to provide periodic health information updates may be willing to complete a brief health history questionnaire. A well-designed questionnaire may be administered via telephone interview or mailed to the patient. This can provide important, ongoing health information and allow continuation of the long-term follow-up process.

Summary

Although challenges exist in the delivery of community-based clinical trials, patients may greatly benefit from receiving cutting-edge cancer control and treatment therapies. Patients with cancer, as well as their family members and support people, can experience the convenience of receiving treatment close to home within their own community. Working cooperatively, the cancer care team has the ability to provide patients with excellence in community-based cancer clinical trial care and treatment.

References

American College of Surgeons Commission on Cancer. (2006). *Cancer program standards 2004 revised edition*. Chicago: Author. Retrieved August 1, 2006, from http://www.facs.org/cancer/coc/cocprogramstandards.pdf

American Society of Clinical Oncology. (2003). American Society of Clinical Oncology policy statement: Oversight of clinical research. *Journal of Clinical Oncology, 21*, 2377–2386. Retrieved August 1, 2006, from http://jco.ascopubs.org/cgi/content/abstract/21/12/2377

Moulton, G. (2003). Community clinical oncology program celebrates 20 years of trials and a few tribulations. *Journal of the National Cancer Institute, 95*, 1822–1824. Retrieved March 3, 2007, from http://jnci.oxfordjournals.org/cgi/content/full/95/24/1822

National Cancer Institute. (2003, December 31). *Clinical community oncology program: Questions and answers.* Retrieved March 22, 2007, from http://www.cancer.gov/cancertopics/factsheet/NCI/CCOP

National Cancer Institute. (n.d.). *About the community clinical oncology program.* Retrieved August 1, 2006, from http://prevention.cancer.gov/programs-resources/programs/ccop/about

Spilker, B. (1991). *Guide to clinical trials.* New York: Raven Press.

CHAPTER 49
Drug Accountability

Siu-Fun Wong, PharmD, FASHP, FCSHP

Introduction

The U.S. Food and Drug Administration (FDA) has been conducting audits of the work of clinical investigators since 1962. These inspections had been conducted on an irregular and limited basis (Lisook, 1990). In 1977, the FDA established the Bioresearch Monitoring Program. This program consists of the development of compliance programs involving inspections of clinical investigators, sponsors, biopharmaceutical laboratories, institutional review boards (IRBs), and toxicology laboratories (Lisook). The purpose of the Bioresearch Monitoring Program is to ensure the quality and validity of studies in support of new drug applications or product license applications and to ensure the safety of participants in clinical studies. The intent of an FDA inspection is to verify the data submitted in support of a new drug claim (Lisook).

From June 1977 to February 1990, the FDA conducted 2,308 evaluable investigations in the drug areas, with the leading deficiencies found in the handling of consent forms (54%), followed by protocol nonadherence (26%) and inadequate drug accountability (25%) (Lisook, 1990). Unfortunately, the investigators have not made significant improvements in the area of drug handling. Inadequate drug accountability continues to be a major problem in subsequent audits. The purpose of this chapter is to provide easy-to-follow, stepwise instructions on proper handling of research study drugs according to the policy and procedures set forth by the National Cancer Institute's Cancer Therapy Evaluation Program (NCI CTEP, 2002b) and the FDA Good Clinical Practice guidelines (FDA, n.d.).

Receiving Research Study Drugs

Upon receiving study drugs at the study institution, the clinical trial nurse (CTN) or investigational pharmacist should review the shipment document (receipt) and identify the drug with the appropriate protocol. The correct and appropriate shipping condition also should be verified at this time. If the shipment is incorrect or damaged, the CTN should contact the supplier by phone and arrange for more shipment as necessary. The drug shipment form (receipt) with information noting that the correct drug was received and the date always should be filed so that it is readily accessible for future site audits. In some studies, the drug supplier will require that a copy of the shipment receipt be returned by fax or mail to the supplier to indicate acknowledgment of receipt. The CTN should refer to the protocol for appropriate handling (NCI CTEP, 2002a).

The CTN then should record the drug shipment received in the NCI Drug Accountability Record (DAR) (see Figure 49-1) or an equivalent form provided by the study sponsor. Separate drug accountability forms must be used for each protocol and research drug. If more than one strength or dosage form of the drug is being used for the same protocol, separate DARs must be used for optimal record keeping (NCI CTEP, 2002a).

When performing documentation of research study drugs, the CTN should use a pen with black ink to enter information. Furthermore, if an entry error is made, correction fluid should not be used to correct the error. Rather, the CTN should draw a line across the error, write in the correction, and initial the entry. When entering duplicate information on different rows of the form, a "ditto mark" should not be used to indicate repeated information. All information entered must be written in complete entry format.

To start a new DAR, the CTN should enter the following information in the upper portion of the form.

1. Page number (Record the page number consecutively on the forms for each drug used on the protocol.)
2. Control record (Place a check mark if the form is being used at the centralized pharmacy where the drug is stored.)
3. Satellite record (Place a check mark if the form is being used at the satellite pharmacy and not at the primary site. Please refer to Chapter 25 for the definition of a satellite pharmacy.)

Figure 49-1. Drug Accountability Form

Form approved:
OMB No. 0925-0240
Expires: 11/30/2007

National Institutes of Health
National Cancer Institute

Division of Cancer Treatment and Diagnosis
Cancer Therapy Evaluation Program

PAGE NO.

CONTROL RECORD ☐

SATELLITE RECORD ☐

Investigational Agent Accountability Record

Name of Institution:

NCI Protocol No.:

Agent Name:

Dose Form and Strength:

Protocol Title:

Dispensing Area:

Investigator Name:

NCI Investigator No.:

Line No.	Date	Patient's Initials	Patient's ID No.	Dose	Quantity Dispensed or Received	Balance Forward / Balance	Manufacturer and Lot No.	Recorder's Initials
1.								
2.								
3.								
4.								
5.								
6.								
7.								
8.								
9.								
10.								
11.								
12.								
13.								
14.								
15.								
16.								
17.								
18.								
19.								
20.								
21.								
22.								
23.								
24.								

NIH-2564
11/2004

4. Institution (Indicate the name of the institution/pharmacy to which the drug is shipped from NCI.)
5. Protocol number (NCI) (The institutional protocol number may be added, if necessary.)
6. Drug name, dose form, and strength
7. Protocol title (Abbreviations may be used if necessary.)
8. Dispensing area (Identify the location where the drug is dispensed [e.g., infusion center pharmacy]).
9. Investigator (Identify the name of the investigator in whose name the drug is ordered from NCI.)
10. Balance forward (Enter zero if the current page is the first page, or enter the balance total from the previous page.)

To make an entry in an existing DAR upon receiving a drug shipment, enter the following information in the DAR.

1. Date (Enter the date the drug is received.)
2. Patient's initials and study ID number (Enter "Received from [name of the distributor].")
3. Dose (Enter the strength and dosage form of the drug received.)
4. Quantity dispensed or received (Enter the quantity received preceded by a "plus" sign.)
5. Balance (Enter the balance total.)
6. Manufacturer and lot number (If the drug shipment contains more than one of the drug lot number, a separate entry should be made for each lot for optimal record keeping.)
7. Recorder's initials

After documentation, the CTN should label the drug storage bag or bin with the drug name, dosage form, and protocol number. The study drugs should be placed in the appropriate storage area to ensure proper storage conditions (e.g., temperature, lighting condition). The CTN should inspect all of the drugs on hand for lot number, expiration date, and balance total and verify the information on the DAR. Drugs for the same study but with different lot numbers should be stored separately.

Dispensing Research Study Drugs
Institution or Control Pharmacy

When dispensing study drugs at a control pharmacy, the CTN should enter the following information in the DAR (NCI CTEP, 2002c).

1. Date (Enter the date of dispensing and/or preparation.)
2. Patient's initials (Use the same patient initials as for the protocol registration.)
3. Patient's ID number (Enter the patient's study number or medical record number.)
4. Dose (Enter the actual dose to be administered.)
5. Quantity dispensed or received (Enter the quantity dispensed preceded by a "minus" sign.)
6. Balance (The balance total should equal the quantity on hand.)

7. Manufacturer and lot number (Enter the lot number[s] of the drug; if more than one lot number is being used, make separate entries for optimal record keeping.)
8. Recorder's initials

All drugs dispensed must be labeled per federal law requirements. Federal law requires that "investigational drugs" be indicated as such on the medication label.

If the drug is to be prepared at the satellite/affiliated facility, the drug should be handled as a transfer to the satellite/affiliated facility (NCI CTEP, 2002c). The CTN should enter the following information in the DAR of the control pharmacy.

1. Date (Enter the date of transfer.)
2. Patient's initials and ID number (Enter "Transfer to [name of satellite location].")
3. Dose (Enter the strength and dosage form of the drug transferred.)
4. Quantity dispensed or received (Enter the quantity transferred preceded by a "minus" sign; provide sufficient supply for at least one treatment.)
5. Balance (The balance total should equal the quantity on hand.)
6. Manufacturer and lot number (Indicate the lot number[s] of the drug; if more than one lot number is being used, make separate entries for optimal record keeping.)
7. Recorder's initials

The CTN should label the transport package with the drug name, protocol number, patient's name (optional), and storage condition.

Satellite/Affiliated Facility

Institutions that are separated geographically by significant distance (e.g., different cities or states) but share professional staff or have joint appointments are not considered to be satellites. They often are referred to as *affiliates*. The drug supplier should ship investigational agents directly to these sites.

For facilities that are located on the same campus or near the control pharmacy service so that an institution employee can transport drugs using appropriate temperature controls and hazardous/infectious transportation procedures when necessary, transferring the research study drugs is permitted. Agents supplied by NCI's Division of Cancer Treatment and Diagnosis (DCTD) must not be repackaged and forwarded by mail or overnight delivery services to another institution or site. The facility must be affiliated with the central pharmacy institution, and the professional staff should be shared or have joint appointments. The principal investigators of the facility also must have a current registration on file with the Pharmaceutical Management Branch (PMB).

Upon receiving the drugs, the satellite/affiliated facility should enter the following information in the DAR.

1. Date (Enter the date of receipt from the control pharmacy.)

2. Patient's initials and ID number (Enter "Received from control pharmacy.")
3. Dose (Enter the strength and dosage form of the drug received.)
4. Quantity dispensed and received (Enter the quantity received preceded by a "plus" sign.)
5. Balance (Enter the balance total.)
6. Manufacturer and lot number (Indicate the lot number[s] of the drugs; if more than one lot number is being used, make separate entries for optimal record keeping.)
7. Recorder's initials

The satellite/affiliated facility should follow the same procedures for drug preparation and dispensing, as well as the documentation required for the institution or control pharmacy.

For protocols that require accountability of returned drugs by patients (especially for oral medications that require compliance checks), in addition to the case report form, the CTN should enter the information of the returned drugs in the DAR for optimal record keeping.

Returning and Transferring Research Study Drugs

Return

For NCI-approved research study drugs, investigators are required to return drugs if

1. The study is completed or discontinued and the agent cannot be transferred to another DCTD-sponsored trial.
2. The drug is outdated (i.e., drugs with a firm expiration date or if a written notification from PMB is received).
3. Obvious excess in the inventory exists. (The investigator should make the best attempt to transfer drugs to another DCTD-sponsored trial.)
4. The drug is damaged or unfit to use (e.g., loss of refrigeration). (The investigator should contact the PMB to confirm stability concerns prior to returning the drugs.)

To return drugs to NCI, the CTN should complete the Return Drug List form (see Appendix 11) and make an entry in the DAR to reflect the balance on hand (NCI CTEP, 2002d). If the study is completed, the balance total should be brought to zero. *Do not* return opened or partially used vials or bottles unless specifically requested in the protocol. A copy of the Return Drug List form should be kept on file with the DAR for future audit. The drugs and the original Return Drug List form should be sent to NCI's Clinical Drug Repository at the address indicated on the Return Drug List form. This should be done using traceable mail, with the drugs packaged securely to prevent breakage. All drugs can be returned to NCI at room temperature because they will be disposed of thereafter. The investigator is responsible for the cost of shipment. "Collect" or "cash on delivery" shipments will not be accepted.

To return drugs from the satellite or affiliated facilities, the drugs must be returned to the control pharmacy first, before being returned to the sponsor. Documentation must be completed at both the satellite/affiliated facility and the control pharmacies.

In certain protocols in which drugs are obtained from suppliers other than NCI, the CTN should refer to the specific protocol or protocol coordinator for directions to return or dispose of the drugs. He or she should document the disposal or return on the DAR. Other documentation, such as a Return Drug List form, may be required. In general, if the research drug is cytotoxic, the method of disposal should follow the recommended guidelines provided by the Occupational Safety and Health Administration (1995) and American Society of Health-System Pharmacists (1996). A copy of the DAR and the Return Drug List form should be kept on file.

Upon receiving notification of drug recalls or expiration, the control pharmacy is responsible for notifying the satellite pharmacy or pharmacies as well as the affiliates and affiliated facilities.

Transfer

Institutions are now "legally" able to transfer DCTD-supplied research study drugs within an institution from one active protocol to another DCTD-approved protocol. Transfer of NCI-supplied agents only should be made between registered active NCI investigators. The transferring investigator must be the investigator who originally ordered the agent or the investigator to whom the agent was previously transferred (i.e., double transfer). The receiving investigator must be a participant on the trial to which the agent is being transferred.

Drug transfer should be restricted to the following situations.

1. The protocol is closed, and another protocol at the institution uses the same agent and formulation. However, transferring DCTD-supplied agents to non-DCTD approved protocols is not permitted under DCTD, NCI, or FDA policies and regulations.
2. Excessive inventory exists for a protocol, and the transfer will minimize drugs being wasted because they are outdated.
3. The study drug has short dating.
4. A medical emergency is imminent (e.g., an urgent approval of a protocol and a very sick patient who needs to begin therapy immediately).
5. A drug ordered for an individual patient on a special exception (compassionate) protocol is no longer required for the patient, and a DCTD-approved protocol is being conducted at the institution using the same study drug.

Drug transfer should never occur under the following circumstances.

1. Transfer of NCI-supplied agents for commercial use. This is both prohibited and illegal.
2. Replacement of NCI-supplied agents with commercial agents. This also is prohibited and illegal.

3. Agents for blinded studies. (Exception: Agents for blinded studies may be transferred between investigators with *prior* PMB approval.)

4. Borrowing of a study drug. Study drugs should not be ordered for one protocol to replace what was "borrowed" from another protocol. The transfer procedures should be used and followed in those circumstances.

5. Transferring agents between two institutions. Agents can only be transferred intra-institutionally at the control pharmacy.

Transferring DCTD-supplied study drugs from an active protocol requires prior PMB approval by phone at 301-496-5725 or fax at 301-402-0429. PMB should be notified by phone within the next working day if emergent transfers are required during weekends or holidays or after hours. An NCI Transfer Investigational Agent form (see Appendix 12) must be completed and submitted by fax (301-402-4612) to the PMB for each agent transferred. Transfer forms should be submitted within 72 hours of the actual transfer. A copy must be retained at the institution for accountability records and future audit. Do not return drugs to NCI if the drugs can be transferred. This will minimize waste.

Storing Research Study Drugs

In accordance with the guidelines by the American Society of Health-System Pharmacists (1991), whenever possible, the pharmacy department should be responsible for drug receipt, storage, accountability, and preparation.

All DCTD investigational agents should be stored and accounted for separately by protocols. If an agent is used for more than one protocol, separate physical storage and accountability should be available for each protocol. PMB provides and accounts for agents on an individual protocol basis.

All research study drugs should be stored in a locked, secure cabinet or in an area with limited access. The drugs should be stored separately from the commercially available drugs, preferably in a separate cabinet, area, or location. The drugs should be placed in separate containers according to protocol and dosage form. The containers should be labeled with the drug name, strength, and protocol number.

To maintain quality assurance of drug storage, the CTN should keep a daily temperature log for the refrigerator and freezer used for storing research drugs. This log should be readily available for audit inspection. Room temperature storage control also should be maintained at all times to avoid excessive heating of the drugs. Light-sensitive products should be kept in the original container before administration, or an amber light-protection bag should be used to provide the protection required.

Compassionate Use, Special Exemptions, or Emergency Use of Investigational Drugs

In some cases, patients may enroll in nonresearch (compassionate) use of investigational agents under three mechanisms: special exception, group C, and treatment referral center protocols. To be eligible, a patient must be refractory to standard measures, not be eligible for an ongoing research protocol, or have a cancer diagnosis for which an investigational drug has demonstrated activity and when standard therapies have been exhausted.

To begin the enrollment process, the physician or designee of the physician is required to contact the sponsor (contact NCI by phone at 301-496-5725 or by fax at 301-402-4870, or contact the manufacturer of the drug) to obtain approval to use the drug in a patient. The sponsor will require the following information.

- Patient's diagnosis and date of diagnosis
- Justification for requesting the study drug
- Previous cancer therapy
- Current clinical status
- Intended dose and schedule of the requested drug
- Any proposed concomitant cancer drugs or other therapies
- Patient's name or identification number, age, sex, height, and weight
- Basic laboratory values (e.g., complete blood count, comprehensive metabolic panel)
- Express delivery courier number and account number

Upon approval, the sponsor will provide verbal or written instructions on other information needed to complete the application. The IRB chair of the treating facility must provide written or verbal approval before the treatment is initiated. The initial shipment of the drug will be mailed upon approval of the application. Reordering of the drug will be handled as with other NCI- or pharmaceutical company–sponsored studies.

The handling and documentation of these agents should follow the same policy and procedures as other NCI-sponsored study drugs. Compassionate-use drugs can be transferred to other NCI-sponsored studies when the protocol for that drug is no longer active at the institution. If the agent is transferred, the site must follow the procedures listed in the "Drug Transfer" section.

Summary

Sponsoring agencies have recognized that research drug accountability continues to be a major problem observed through audits. With NCI's leadership, the major research cooperative groups are dedicated to educating their members on the proper handling and documentation of research study drugs. Various educational tools are being used to achieve this goal.

References

American Society of Health-System Pharmacists. (1991). ASHP guidelines for the use of investigational drugs in organized health-care settings. *American Journal of Hospital Pharmacy, 48,* 315–319.

American Society of Health-System Pharmacists. (1996). *ASHP guidelines on handling cytotoxic and hazardous drugs* (pp. 136–152). American Society of Health-System Pharmacists bulletins. Bethesda, MD: Author.

Lisook, A. (1990). FDA audits of clinical studies: Policy and procedures. *Journal of Clinical Pharmacology, 30,* 296–302.

National Cancer Institute Cancer Therapy Evaluation Program. (2002a). *Investigational drug accountability. Forms and instructions.* Bethesda, MD: Author.

National Cancer Institute Cancer Therapy Evaluation Program. (2002b). *The investigator's handbook: A manual for participants in clinical trials of investigational agents sponsored by DCTD, NCI.* Retrieved October 29, 2007, from http://ctep.cancer.gov/handbook/index.html

National Cancer Institute Cancer Therapy Evaluation Program. (2002c). *Policy and guidelines for investigational agent distribution.* Bethesda, MD: Author.

National Cancer Institute Cancer Therapy Evaluation Program. (2002d). *Policy and guidelines for the transfer of DCTDC supplied investigational agents.* Bethesda, MD: Author.

Occupational Safety and Health Administration. (1995). *OSHA instruction TED 1.15. Directorate of technical support: Controlling occupational exposure to hazardous drugs.* Washington, DC: Author.

U.S. Food and Drug Administration. (n.d.). *FDA regulations relating to good clinical practice and clinical trials.* Retrieved October 2, 2007, from http://www.fda.gov/oc/gcp/regulations.html

CHAPTER 50
Interdisciplinary Team Review

Carol Anne Bales, RN, MSN, CCRP, AOCN®, and Denise Dearing, RN, BSN, OCN®

Introduction

This chapter focuses on the function and operation of the hospital research steering committee. The process of interdisciplinary review for quality improvement is the primary responsibility of this committee. The distinguishing characteristics and purposes of such a committee are discussed. Benefits to the organization, committee membership composition and responsibilities, and committee operations are presented. Examples of forms used for submissions and budget worksheets are included in the chapter, as well.

Interdisciplinary Review Committees: Types and Purposes

Quality improvement is enhanced by the systematic and ongoing interdisciplinary review of clinical trials. This is accomplished through the services of several committees: the institutional review board (IRB), the hospital research steering committee, a medical/nursing executive council, and a pharmacy and therapeutics committee, among others. The latter three types of committees are distinguished from the institutional review committee by composition of membership, purpose, and function. For the purposes of this chapter, the term *research steering committee* describes a model system for interdisciplinary team review.

An IRB is composed of professional members of multiple disciplines as well as lay members who represent the perspective of participants in clinical trials. Each member should have adequate knowledge of the U.S. Food and Drug Administration's (FDA's) *Good Clinical Practice Guidelines* (2007) and the International Conference on Harmonisation of Technical Requirements for Registration of Pharmaceuticals for Human Use (ICH) *Good Clinical Practice: Consolidated Guidance* (1996) in addition to expertise in reviewing study documents to determine compliance with these regulations (see Chapter 13 for more information on IRBs). The other three types of committees include only representatives of specific health disciplines and ancillary support staff who are not necessarily familiar with FDA regulations but who can determine the acceptability and appropriateness of clinical trials for the patient population they serve. The purposes of the IRB are to protect the rights of the research participants, ensure that the benefits outweigh the risks of participating in a study, and ensure that trials are conducted in congruence with FDA regulations (FDA). The purposes of the other three types of committees differ widely depending on the specific healthcare institution in which they exist, but they should not overlap with the purposes of the IRB. The committees' charters describe their membership, goals, scope, and function. The hospital research steering committee is the committee that most commonly is charged with providing interdisciplinary review of clinical trials. However, the medical executive committee also may be charged with that responsibility. Clinical trial nurses (CTNs) frequently serve on steering committees and contribute to the quality improvement process.

Benefits to the Organization and Principal Investigators

Interdisciplinary review of clinical research trials benefits the institution or organization, the principal investigator (PI), and the study team. The review process helps study sponsors by screening out studies that are unlikely to be successfully conducted at their institution. Improved collaboration is achieved by including representatives from these areas during the initial study review and discussion. This helps the clinical trial team to prevent logistics and feasibility issues from jeopardizing the success of the trial once it is under way. Interdepartmental and interdisciplinary collaboration produces a sense of cohesiveness, enthusiasm, and momentum that otherwise might be lacking if members of the steering committee did not have a forum in which to interact and discuss their projects. The advantage of steering committee meetings is that the members can share their individual expertise and experience with

345

the group, thus providing many different professional perspectives from which to review and plan the conduct of a clinical trial. Institutions require PIs to present prospective research as a prerequisite for conducting clinical research trials at their site. During the meetings, the members may question the PI and the study coordinator for each clinical trial under review, and vice versa. Such interactive dialogue serves as a foundation of understanding upon which to build a successful relationship between the clinical trial team and the PI.

Additional benefits of a steering committee to the organization are the provision of a forum in which to discuss the development of new organizational research initiatives; the existence of a team devoted to developing the necessary human, financial, and material resources needed to ensure the success of each study approved by the committee; and the provision of a committee that can develop and review organizational policies and procedures that address clinical research.

Committee Composition

Composition of research steering committees will vary among hospitals and from the hospital setting to the outpatient setting. Membership should reflect and represent the departments, groups, and individuals that compose the clinical trial team. With the exclusion of parties external to the institution or organization conducting the study, the members of the steering committee are all stakeholders in the process and outcomes of the organization's research activities. The institution that is sponsoring the research appoints a chair and committee members. These individuals usually are employees of the institution, the chair usually being a medical or pharmacy administrator. Care should be taken to limit the number of committee members to ensure the efficiency of the review process; however, enough members should be included to represent each discipline involved in the research activities at every meeting. The committee size may be small if the organization is an outpatient center or large if it is a hospital network comprising several facilities. A senior member of the organization's administration should be appointed to the committee to provide a direct link to the governing bodies of the organization. A sample membership list for a typical research steering committee is provided in Figure 50-1. This type of system works equally as well in many types of institutions, from community healthcare networks or hospitals to government or academic healthcare facilities.

The medical and nursing staff should have representatives from each department that participates in clinical trials, such as surgery and recovery, intensive care, and nursing care units (e.g., cardiology, oncology, surgical postoperative units).

Responsibilities of Committee Members

Committee responsibilities should include but not be limited to a systematic review of all research projects—

Figure 50-1. Sample Membership Composition of a Steering Committee

- Chair (the person who is responsible for the organization's clinical trial program)
- Secretary (a member of the committee who volunteers for the position or an employee of the organization assigned to the job)
- Vice president of medical affairs or medical director of the organization
- Vice president of operations or nursing director of the organization
- Vice president of legal affairs or director of legal affairs
- Representatives of the following departments:
  - Ethics committee/pastoral care
  - Risk management
  - Finance
  - Clinical trial program
  - Planning and marketing
  - Medical staff (if organization has multiple sites, one from each site)
  - Nursing staff (if organization has multiple sites, one from each site)
  - Laboratory staff
  - Radiology staff (nuclear medicine, if involved in clinical trials) and other departments deemed appropriate by the committee

including clinical trials—before, during, and after each project's duration. Administrative support for research program direction, initiatives, and policy also is a responsibility of the committee. Quality improvement is included during systematic research project review. If the investigational product or treatment regimen under study has no potential to improve patient care (either directly or indirectly), the committee should ask the PI about the appropriateness and benefit to the organization of conducting the study. Specific roles of committee members will vary depending on their professional roles within the organization and pertinence to the clinical trial team. All members are responsible for reviewing all submissions specifically pertinent to their discipline and purview, attending committee meetings, and voting to approve or disapprove the conduct of each clinical trial. Each member serves as a liaison to the department that he or she represents and provides opinion and feedback about the feasibility and willingness of his or her department's participation in the conduct of the study.

Enforcement of institutional requirements for review by such a committee is provided by an inherent checks-and-balances system. Because institutions prohibit PIs from conducting research without first obtaining approval of the committee, the PIs' vested interest in their research projects serves as an impetus for committee members to provide the review and approval service. On the institution's side, many hospital accreditation and certification requirements include an institution's inclusion of clinical research as part of its healthcare services to the community.

The chair is responsible for appointing and replacing committee members, orienting new members to their roles and responsibilities, conducting meetings, providing direction to the secretary, and directing meeting follow-up activities and communications. The chair serves as the key contact person within the organization to whom all clinical research inquiries, submissions, compliments, and complaints are directed. The chair also serves as the committee's liaison to the IRB and the committee's resource on FDA and ICH regulations. The steering committee secretary is responsible for providing information about how to format a submission packet to the committee and for providing a copy of any forms that the committee uses to supplement study documents for review. The secretary receives, copies, and distributes study submissions before meetings, allowing enough time for members to thoroughly review the protocols, consent forms, investigator brochures, and study budgets. The secretary also is responsible for committee correspondence, filing of documentation, scheduling, arrangements, and communications for meetings, as well as recording meeting minutes. Appointing one member as parliamentarian ensures that meetings are conducted according to agreed-upon rules of order. If time-consuming projects result from conducting the business of the committee, the chair has the authority to appoint specific members to form a temporary subcommittee to complete such projects.

Committee Structure and Operation

Steering committees set their meeting schedule as frequently as needed to provide timely review of clinical trial submissions, adequate time in which to review submissions thoroughly, and a convenient meeting time for most of the committee members. Depending on the volume of clinical trials conducted within the organization, the committee may meet every other month, monthly, or more often as needed. A meeting lasting one-and-a-half hours allows adequate time to review four to six submissions, unless the nature of some of those submissions is complex, problematic, or controversial. The meeting place must afford privacy to the committee and guests, include a waiting area for study presenters, and have adequate acoustics so that all comments can be heard by everyone present. Provision of food and beverages adds to the comfort of the meeting. A committee quorum must be present at each meeting, representing a third or more of the committee membership. Members who are unable to attend the meeting should provide their individual comments and questions about each study to the committee chair in writing either before or on the day of the meeting. The committee secretary or appointed scribe should advise presenters that each study submission will be reviewed individually in the privacy of the committee, and a specific presentation time should be given to them before the meeting. They must understand that the privacy necessary to protect confidentiality of each study is afforded to each presenter and that they may need to wait or adjust their scheduled time, depending on the meeting proceedings. Research presentations take approximately 10–30 minutes.

Therefore, the PI does not need to attend the entire clinical research committee meeting.

The meetings should be conducted according to a procedure agreed upon by the members, with the chair presiding over the meeting and appointing one committee member to attend to greeting and directing the presenters appropriately. An agenda should be distributed to guide the presentation schedule and the conduct of committee business, and a formal procedure should govern the presentation, discussion, and voting regarding each specific submission. *Robert's Rules of Order* (Robert, Evans, Honemann, & Balch, 2000) contains standard parliamentary procedures that can be adopted by the committee. Other business of the committee should follow a more informal style, allowing committee members the opportunity to brainstorm, troubleshoot, problem solve, and freely discuss the organization's research initiatives, projects, business, and concerns.

Review Documents and Considerations

During the submission review process, different aspects of each project are addressed, including the appropriateness of the project for the institution and the population it serves; the feasibility of conducting the study in terms of human, material, and financial resources; and the benefits, both tangible and intangible, to the study participants, the institution, the PI, and the population served by the organization. These aspects must meet institutional criteria. Using forms that list frequently asked questions about the criteria will help to organize the review process (see Figure 50-2).

The submission review should begin with an introduction of the presenter (either the PI or study coordinator), followed by a study presentation that includes a summary of the clinical protocol, a discussion of the study logistics and procedures, and a review of the informed consent process. The committee chair should direct committee members and the presenter about when to ask questions or make comments at the appropriate time during the presentation, which should take approximately 10–30 minutes, depending on the complexity of the study and the length of the discussion. The chair also should tell the presenter when to expect notice of the committee's decision, thank him or her, and excuse the presenter after the presentation.

All study submission presentations should be completed consecutively, followed by a private voting session by the committee. As each study is voted upon, the committee should privately discuss internal concerns, objections, and suggestions. The committee then will approve or disapprove the protocol, consent form, and any advertisements or public relations summaries to be used to publicize the study or recruit participants. This review is made from the business, clinical, and legal perspective of the institution, which is different from the IRB's perspective of the rights and welfare of research participants. If the committee is voting on the study before approval by the IRB, the research steering committee's decision is contingent upon

Figure 50-2. Sample Steering Committee Study Submission Form

Date Submitted to Seton Network Research Office: _____   Submitting for: _____
                                                                                        Meeting date

The following must be submitted with this form:

❏ IRB Approval Letter   ❏ 16 Copies of Consent/Assent   ❏ Other relevant materials

❏ 16 Copies of Protocol   ❏ Investigator or product brochure   ❏ Steering submission fee paid (HOLD)

Please answer the following questions which must be completed prior to submission:

Principal Investigator: **Contact Phone #:**	
Sub-Investigators:	
Study Coordinators: **Contact Phone #:**	
Sponsor:	
IRB/s of record: **Approval date/s:** If any study personnel are affiliated with UTMB, then the study must also be approved by the UTMB IRB.	
Study Site/s:	
Estimated initiation date:	
Estimated length of site participation **(from initiation to close out)**	_____Months _____Years
Anticipated enrollment:	# of Patients_____
Estimated length of **study patient participation:**	_____Months _____Years
Is this a compassionate use study? (i.e. a one-time use of the protocol for treatment of a patient in a life-threatening situation for which no other treatment provides as good a chance of a satisfactory outcome)	**Check one:** ❏ Yes ❏ No
How many hospital days will be incurred solely for the purposes of this study?	
What patient care areas will be involved? You are responsible for ensuring that the manager of the department is notified and has agreed to have their area participate in this study.	Check all that apply: ❏ Preadmission testing ❏ Surgery ❏ ICU_____ ❏ Inpatient unit_____ ❏ Outpatient clinic_____ ❏ Emergency Dept ❏ Imaging unit_____ ❏ Radiation center_____ ❏ Other_____

(Continued on next page)

Figure 50-2. Sample Steering Committee Study Submission Form *(Continued)*	
What non-patient care areas will be involved? You are responsible for ensuring that the manager of the department is notified and has agreed to have their area participate in this study.	Check all that apply: ❏ Admissions ❏ Medical records ❏ Billing ❏ Educators ❏ Legal affairs ❏ Risk management ❏ Infection control ❏ Data analysts ❏ Nursing administration ❏ Other_____
What staff requires educational in-services?	Check all that apply: ❏ Physician ❏ Nursing ❏ Medical/Clinical Assistants ❏ Pharmacy ❏ Lab ❏ Imaging ❏ Radiation ❏ Other_____
Who will provide the in-services?	Check all that apply: ❏ Seton Research staff ❏ Study Sponsor ❏ Other_____

I attest that the above is true _____   _____
                                     Signature of PI or designee   ***Date***

*Please note: Completed submission packets must be received in the Seton Network Research Office at Brackenridge Hospital no later than 3 weeks prior to the meeting in which you wish to have it reviewed. Please call [the IRB Coordinator] at 512-xxx-xxxx for any questions.

Note. Figure courtesy of Seton HealthCare Network, Austin, TX. Used with permission.

IRB approval. If individual members of the committee are to receive any sort of compensation, whether financial, material, or intangible, they should abstain from voting for that study to avoid creating a conflict of interest (see Chapter 16 for information about conflicts of interest). The entire submission and review procedure can be carried out through correspondence, although the committee should meet at least quarterly to provide a forum in which general clinical research topics can be addressed in person.

Meeting Follow-Up and Ongoing Committee Business

The business tasks related to the committee are the responsibility of the institution's research department employees. A staff consisting of a research director, two to three study coordinators, and a department administrative assistant can handle a workload of approximately 75–100 active research studies per year.

Follow-up for each meeting should include notifying PIs verbally and in writing of the outcome of the study review, preparing the minutes, filing documentation, and shredding study documents that are no longer needed by committee members. Letters advising the PI of study approvals should clearly state the reporting expectations of the organization (e.g., renewal, interim, closure reports). Conversely, letters advising the PI of study disapproval should state the reasons why the study was unacceptable to the organization (e.g., recruitment competing with another ongoing study, lack of resources necessary to conduct the study, inadequate consent form, unanswered questions or concerns). Meeting minutes should be typed and filed chronologically for future use. The chair should ask committee members to pursue resolution of logistical barriers that caused studies to be rejected at the meeting and to help study coordinators to revise inadequate consent forms to render them acceptable to the committee. Providing such assistance to the PI and study coordinators strengthens the relationship between the organization and the study teams, ensuring a continual collaborative relationship between the two. The committee chair, in the role of liaison to the organization's IRB, sends the results of the study reviews to the IRB chair. Finally, the committee's secretary should file all documentation pertinent to the meeting for future reference. Ongoing business of the committee should include provision of assistance to those who wish to develop or conduct research projects and periodic literature review of articles related to clinical trials. Due diligence is necessary to keep abreast of international, federal, state, and local clinical research regulations.

Summary

The overall goal of the clinical research steering committee is to improve healthcare quality by ensuring that scientific inquiry conducted within the organization is congruent with its goals, mission, and values, as well as with all pertinent regulations. If the studies that the committee approves are both appropriate and feasible and all PIs are required to submit their studies for review and approval, then the research program will result in quality improvement.

Evidence-based practice is a term applied to healthcare practice improvements based upon the analysis and appropriate and judicious application of compiled results of peer-reviewed reports of clinical research studies. Interdisciplinary review accomplished by a clinical research steering committee helps to produce valid and useful research results, which are the foundation of evidence-based practice. Regular internal audits of committee proceedings, meetings, and documentation will provide the quality assurance necessary to continually improve the clinical research program of any organization. Such audits include a systematic review of the documentation, policy and procedure, and membership of the committee by a team composed of the organization's risk manager, a representative of legal affairs, medical staff familiar with clinical trials, and nursing staff familiar with the conduct of research studies.

Every organization in which clinical research is conducted should consider developing a forum, such as an interdisciplinary review committee, and tailor its composition, goals, policy, procedures, and operations to meet its needs. This chapter has provided a review of the possible composition, structure, function, operations, and responsibilities of such committees. CTNs serving on these committees provide their input on the feasibility, appropriateness, and logistics of implementing new research projects. These nurses represent key areas in which the research is conducted. Their participation benefits the institution by allowing investigators and hospital staff to troubleshoot potential problems before they occur and work out the practical details of conducting the studies before they are initiated. Through nursing involvement in clinical research, especially in interdisciplinary review committees, nursing practice is improved and expanded. Evidence-based practice, quality improvement, shared governance, and leadership development are benefits and goals of nursing research participation. Personal and professional growth, job satisfaction, and career advancement are benefits of serving on an institutional interdisciplinary review committee (Daughters of Charity Health Services of Austin, 1998).

References

Daughters of Charity Health Services of Austin. (1998). *Nursing News, 3*(9), 3.

International Conference on Harmonisation of Technical Requirements for Registration of Pharmaceuticals for Human Use. (1996, April). *Good clinical practice: Consolidated guidance.* Retrieved October 3, 2007, from http://www.fda.gov/cder/guidance/959fnl.pdf

Robert, H.H., Evans, W.J., Honemann, D.H., & Balch, T.J. (Eds.). (2000). *Robert's rules of order* (10th ed.). Reading, MA: Perseus Press.

U.S. Food and Drug Administration. (2007). *Good clinical practice program.* Retrieved October 3, 2007, from http://www.fda.gov/oc/gcp/regulations.html

SECTION XI.

Professional Development

CHAPTER 51
Specialization in Clinical Trials Nursing

CHAPTER 52
Mentorship

CHAPTER 53
Professional Continuing Education

CHAPTER 51
Specialization in Clinical Trials Nursing

Heidi E. Deininger, PhD, RN, AOCN®

Introduction

Oncology nursing has long been at the forefront of advancing patient care. As a well-established and recognizable nursing specialty, it has, over time, provided the foundation for the emergence of yet another specialty, clinical research nursing or clinical trials nursing. While oncology nursing has its origins rooted in pursuit of the magic bullet, clinical trials nursing also is grounded in the pursuit of inquiry.

A better understanding of the evolving role and responsibilities of these individuals can be instrumental in promoting the contributions and legitimacy of nursing to the successful conduct of clinical research. Efforts by nurse researchers to develop this knowledge base are emerging (Mueller & Mamo, 2000, 2002). Within oncology, Ehrenberger and Lillington (2004) have described a measure to delineate the clinical trials nursing role and have provided a cornerstone for this emerging specialty.

Historical Perspective
Clinical Trials Nursing: The Early Years

The first roles for oncology nurses in the United States were those associated with cancer research in the 1960s, during the very early clinical trials of chemotherapy. Nurses needed to develop new skills and new knowledge and assume a new, collaborative role with physicians in the care of patients enrolled in clinical trials (Hubbard & DeVita, 1976; Moore, 1978; Suppers, Yarbro, & Mayer-Scogna, 1979). In the 1980s, the integral role of the research nurse in the cancer research setting in relationship to other nursing roles was fully described (Gross, 1986; Henke, 1980; Hubbard, 1982; Hubbard & Donehower, 1980). The responsibilities of the research nurse were made explicit and were described as they relate to the development of a new cancer chemotherapeutic agent. Other nursing specialties also began to describe this emerging role (Mullin, 1984).

The early 1990s saw further descriptions of the oncology research nurse role and activities (Cassidy & Macfarlane, 1991; Engelking, 1991, 1992; Hazelton, 1991; McEvoy, Cannon, & MacDermott, 1991; Melink & Whitacre, 1991). Wheeler (1991) described the process of preparing nursing staff for successful implementation of a protocol, whereas other authors focused on the oncology nurse's emerging role in data management (Cassidy, 1993; White-Hershey & Nevidjon, 1990). Subsequent articles identified and acknowledged research nurse involvement in the informed consent process (Berry, Dodd, Hinds, & Ferrell, 1996; Rosse & Krebs, 1999). Others began to investigate the research nurse role, responsibilities, and contributions to clinical research (Freedman, 1998; Xanthos, Carp, & Geromanos, 1998). Although the amount of literature surrounding the research nurse role increased during the 1990s, it remained primarily anecdotal.

Clinical Trials Nursing: The Later Years

In early 2000, a shift was evident as more critical and substantive literature began to emerge surrounding the role of the research nurse. Ocker and Pawlik-Plank (2000) used a case study to explain how the research nurse role was systematically developed and integrated into a clinic-based oncology research setting. During the development phase, they identified several research nurse roles that incorporated the nursing process: educator, patient advocate, and protocol manager. Final implementation and integration of the research nurse in their setting led to increased job satisfaction for both research nurses and oncology nurse clinicians. In another study, Burnett et al. (2001) surveyed nurses' attitudes and beliefs toward cancer clinical trials at a comprehensive cancer center. Furthermore, the Clinical Trial Nurses (CTN) Special Interest Group of the Oncology Nursing Society provided a major contribution to the literature by publishing the *Manual for Clinical Trials Nursing* (Klimaszewski et al., 2000). This was the first comprehensive nursing work that included CTNs from across the globe. The manual was designed to address the needs of the novice CTN while also appealing to the sensibilities of the expert CTN.

Internationally, research nurses have made substantial gains in developing their role. The international section of this book details the CTN's role in 10 countries and the European Union countries. The adoption of the International Conference on Harmonisation of Technical Requirements for Registration of Pharmaceuticals for Human Use (1996) Good Clinical Practice guideline has added to both the importance and credibility of clinical trial research internationally. As in the United States, the CTN must support and monitor the integrity of the study and the safety of patients.

Today, the most common role for the general oncology nurse in clinical trials is the research nurse role (Groer, Krebs, & Elson, 1998; Sadler, Lantz, Fullerton, & Dault, 1999) (see Figure 51-1), although the literature reports the need for an advanced body of knowledge with the emergence of new opportunities (Zimmerman, 2000), such as nurse practitioners serving as the principal investigator for clinical studies (Saunders & Turner, 2000; Sellers, Shenkin, & Lavin-Tompkins, 1997) and doctoral-prepared nurses functioning as principal investigators for pharmaceutical trials (Rosenzweig, Bender, & Brufsky, 2005).

Although the literature related to the clinical research nursing role spans nearly 50 years, it has been primarily anecdotal in nature with a paucity of data-based articles. Key themes emerging from this review are identified (see Figure 51-2) and help to guide future efforts in the field.

Implications for Nursing

Indeed, while the clinical trials nursing role continues to undergo examination, it is up to nurses to "empirically demonstrate" that a CTN would provide an advantage as compared to non-nursing individuals in this field (Mueller, 2001).

Next steps include the establishment of the scope and standards of nursing practice for clinical research nursing at either the generalist or advanced practice level. Additionally, formally defined curriculum content for a nursing specialty of clinical research nursing will undoubtedly be forthcoming as the cadre of nursing educators in this area expands. The concurrent emergence of master's degree programs in clinical trials nursing or clinical research management within schools of nursing is noteworthy. Indeed, "the clinical research nurse management program(s) will provide advanced preparation, opportunity, and recognition to the many nurses who are now the invisible quotient in medical clinical research studies" (L. Ford, personal communication, December 2, 2006).

Nursing Specialty Certification

Most valid specialty areas now have a certification program administered through examination. Certification is based on education and recognition of knowledge, skills, and abilities or competence developed through experience in a specialty area of practice. Certification is a type of credential that affords title protection and recognition of accomplishment but does not include a legal scope of practice. Many state boards of nursing use such professional certification as a requirement toward granting authority for advanced practice registered nurses.

Approximately 30 organizations exist that grant certifications for nurses with training beyond the entry-to-practice

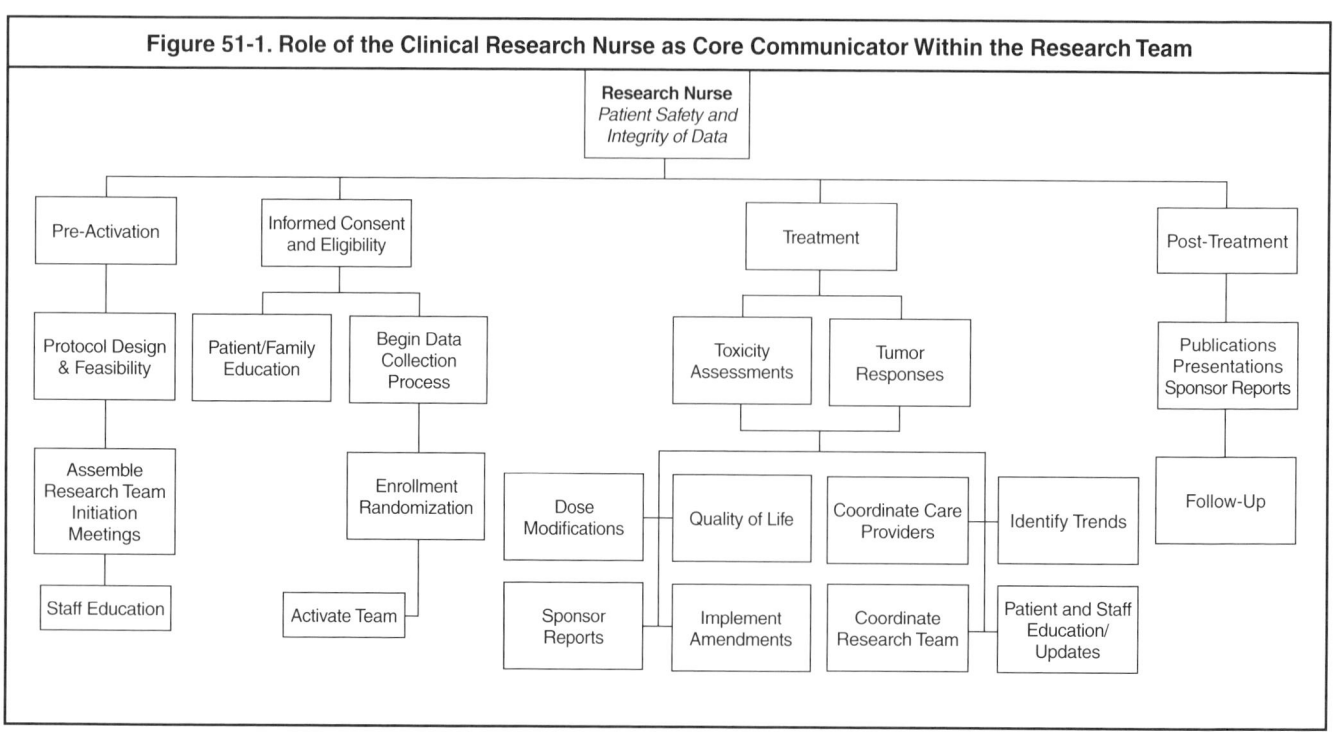

Figure 51-1. Role of the Clinical Research Nurse as Core Communicator Within the Research Team

Figure 51-2. Key Themes

- Absence of clear role definitions and lack of clarity of roles
- Variability in title
- Variability in educational requirements for research nurses
- Conflicting role expectations between different facets of the healthcare system
- Untapped potential of the role of the clinical research nurse within the research enterprise
- Emerging influence of clinical research nurses in community-based care
- Role adoption by non-nurses
- Absence of a cohesive model of professional development of the clinical research nurse in the United States

level. For example, the American Nurses Credentialing Center administers more than 37 specialty and advanced practice certification examinations each year. In addition, certifying bodies are now developing new subspecialty programs.

The author anticipates a nationally recognized specialty certification in clinical research nursing to be made available within the next five years. In the interim, certifications from non-nursing professional organizations, such the Association of Clinical Research Professionals (www.acrpnet.org) and the Society of Clinical Research Associates (www.socra.org), are available to CTNs.

Summary

The future remains bright for this cadre of highly specialized nursing professionals. Long the invisible quotient of the biomedical enterprise, advancement in autonomy is forthcoming for clinical trials nursing. Similar to the experiences of pioneer nurse practitioners in establishing advanced practice roles, CTNs, too, must progress through several stages (Brown & Draye, 2003). We are called to break free, mold the clay, encounter obstacles, survive the proving ground, stay committed, and build the eldership. Our future and that of our patients depend on it.

References

Berry, D., Dodd, M., Hinds, P., & Ferrell, B. (1996). Informed consent: Process and clinical issues. *Oncology Nursing Forum, 23*, 507–512.

Brown, M.A., & Draye, M.A. (2003). Experience of pioneer nurse practitioners in establishing advanced practice roles. *Journal of Nursing Scholarship, 35*, 391–397.

Burnett, C., Koczwara, B., Pixley, L., Blumenson, L., Hwang, Y., & Meropol, N. (2001). Nurses' attitudes toward clinical trials at a comprehensive cancer center. *Oncology Nursing Forum, 28*, 1187–1192.

Cassidy, J. (1993). The role of the data manager in clinical cancer research: An opportunity for nurses. *Cancer Nursing, 16*, 131–138.

Cassidy, J., & Macfarlane, D.K. (1991). The role of the nurse in clinical cancer research. *Cancer Nursing, 14*, 124–131.

Ehrenberger, H.E., & Lillington, L. (2004). The development of a measure to delineate the clinical trials nursing role. *Oncology Nursing Forum, 31*, 64–68.

Engelking, C. (1991). Facilitating clinical trials: The expanding role of the nurse. *Cancer, 67*, 1793–1797.

Engelking, C. (1992). Clinical trials: Impact evaluation and implementation considerations. *Seminars in Oncology Nursing, 8*, 148–155.

Freedman, T. (1998). The breast cancer prevention trial: Nurses' observations. *Cancer Nursing, 21*, 178–186.

Groer, M., Krebs, D., & Elson, G. (1998). A new path: Looking ahead. *American Journal of Nursing, 98*, 16B–16D.

Gross, J. (1986). Clinical research in cancer chemotherapy. *Oncology Nursing Forum, 13*(1), 59–65.

Hazelton, J. (1991). The role of the nurse in phase I clinical trials. *Journal of Pediatric Oncology Nursing, 8*, 43–45.

Henke, C. (1980). Emerging roles of the nurse in oncology. *Seminars in Oncology, 7*, 4–8.

Hubbard, S.M. (1982). Cancer treatment research: The role of the nurse in clinical trials of cancer therapy. *Nursing Clinics of North America, 17*, 763–783.

Hubbard, S.M., & DeVita, V. (1976). Chemotherapy research nurse. *American Journal of Nursing, 76*, 560–566.

Hubbard, S.M., & Donehower, M. (1980). The nurse in the cancer research setting. *Seminars in Oncology, 7*, 9–17.

International Conference on Harmonisation of Technical Requirements for Registration of Pharmaceuticals for Human Use. (1996, April). *Guidance for industry: E6 good clinical practice: Consolidated guidance.* Retrieved May 18, 2007, from http://www.fda.gov/cder/guidance/index.htm

Klimaszewski, A.D., Aikin, J.L., Bacon, M.A., DiStasio, S.A., Ehrenberger, H.E., & Ford, B.A. (Eds.). (2000). *Manual for clinical trials nursing.* Pittsburgh, PA: Oncology Nursing Society.

McEvoy, M., Cannon, L., & MacDermott, M. (1991). The professional role for nurses in clinical trials. *Seminars in Oncology Nursing, 7*, 268–274.

Melink, T., & Whitacre, M. (1991). Planning and implementing clinical trials. *Seminars in Oncology Nursing, 7*, 243–251.

Moore, P. (1978). Beyond the protocol. *Oncology Nursing Forum, 5*(3), 12–14.

Mueller, M. (2001). From delegation to specialization: Nurses and clinical trial co-ordination. *Nursing Inquiry, 8*, 182–190.

Mueller, M., & Mamo, L. (2000). Changes in medicine, changes in nursing: Career contingencies and the movement of nurses into clinical trial coordination. *Sociological Perspectives, 43*, S43–S57.

Mueller, M., & Mamo, L. (2002). The nurse clinical trial coordinator: Benefits and drawbacks of the role. *Research and Theory for Nursing Practice, 16*, 33–42.

Mullin, S.M. (1984). An acute intervention trial: The research nurse coordinator's role. *Controlled Clinical Trials, 5*, 141–156.

Ocker, B., & Pawlik-Plank, D. (2000). The research nurse role in a clinic-based oncology research center. *Cancer Nursing, 23*, 286–292.

Rosenzweig, M., Bender, C., & Brufsky, A. (2005). The nurse as principal investigator in a pharmaceutically sponsored drug trial: Considerations and challenges. *Oncology Nursing Forum, 32*, 293–299.

Rosse, P., & Krebs, L. (1999). The nurse's role in the informed consent process. *Seminars in Oncology Nursing, 15*, 116–123.

Sadler, R., Lantz, J., Fullerton, J., & Dault, Y. (1999). Nurses' unique roles in randomized clinical trials. *Journal of Professional Nursing, 15*, 106–115.

Saunders, C., & Turner, B. (2000). The role of nurse practitioners as principal investigators for clinical studies. *Research Practitioner, 1*, 129–133.

Sellers, M.A., Shenkin, D.J., & Lavin-Tompkins, J. (1997). Nurse practitioners coordinate clinical trials. *Nurse Practitioner, 22*, 151–152.

Suppers, V., Yarbro, C.H., & Mayer-Scogna, D. (1979). Nursing intervention in clinical research—a model program of nursing contributions to a cooperative study group. *Oncology Nursing Forum, 6*(4), 26–27.

Wheeler, V.S. (1991). Preparing nurses for clinical trials: The cancer center approach. *Seminars in Oncology Nursing, 7*, 275–279.

White-Hershey, D., & Nevidjon, B. (1990). Fundamentals for oncology nurse/data managers: Preparing for a new role. *Oncology Nursing Forum, 17*, 371–377.

Xanthos, G.J., Carp, D., & Geromanos, K.L. (1998). Recognizing nurses' contributions to the clinical research process. *Journal of the Association of Nurses in AIDS Care, 9*, 39–48.

Zimmerman, J.F. (2000). Clinical trial nurses must have an advanced body of knowledge and skills [Letter to the editor]. *ONS News, 15*, 3.

Additional Resources

Arrigo, C., Gall, H., Delogne, A., & Molin, C. (1994). The involvement of nurses in clinical trials: Results of the EORTC oncology nurses study group survey. *Cancer Nursing, 17*, 429–433.

Bowen, K., & Rice, L. (1998). Who is a clinical research nurse? Establishing guidelines and standards of practice for a growing profession. *Research Nurse, 4*, 1–4.

Carlson, C., Reilly, M., & Hitchens, A. (2005). An innovative approach to the care of patients on phase I and phase II clinical trials: The role of the experimental therapeutics nurse. *Journal of Pediatric Oncology Nursing, 22*, 353–364.

Cheng, A., Lai, Y., & Yu, Y. (1998). Research nurses for clinical trials of anti-cancer drugs: Developing a new subspecialty in Taiwan. *Drug Information Journal, 32*, 1279–1281.

Coulson, S., & Phelan, L. (2000). Clinical research in paediatric oncology and the role of the research nurse in the UK. *European Journal of Oncology Nursing, 4*, 154–161.

Di Guilio, P., Arrigo, C., Gall, H., Molin, C., Nieweg, R., & Strohbucker, B. (1996). Expanding the role of the nurse in clinical trials: The nursing summaries. *Cancer Nursing, 19*, 343–347.

Fishwick, K., Berridge, J., Coffey, M., Colussi, A., Di Giulio, P., Marinus, A., et al. (2002). The EORTC clinical research coordinators group. *European Journal of Cancer, 38*(Suppl.), 54–59.

Girault, V. (2003). [Clinical research nurses, the cornerstones of well-conducted clinical trials]. *Soins: La Revue de Référence Infirmière, 680*, 25–27.

Gwede, C., Johnsson, D., Roberts, C., & Cantor, A. (2005). Burnout in clinical research coordinators in the United States. *Oncology Nursing Forum, 32*, 1123–1330.

Joshi, T., & Ehrenberger, H.E. (2001). Cancer clinical trials in the new millennium: Novel challenges and opportunities for oncology nursing. *Clinical Journal of Oncology Nursing, 5*, 147–152.

Raja-Jones, H. (2002). Role boundaries—research nurse or clinical nurse specialist? A literature review. *Journal of Clinical Nursing, 11*, 415–420.

Rico-Villademoros, F., Hernando, T., Sanz, J., Lopez-Alonso, A., Salamanca, O., Camps, C., et al. (2004). The role of the clinical research coordinator—data manager—in oncology clinical trials. *BioMed Central Medical Research Methodology, 4*, 6. Retrieved June 11, 2007, from http://www.biomedcentral.com/1471-2288/4/6

Skrutkowska, M., & Weijer, C. (1997). Do patients with breast cancer participating in clinical trials receive better nursing care? *Oncology Nursing Forum, 24*, 1411–1416.

Stephens-Lloyd, A. (2004). The extended role of the clinical research nurse: Building an evidence base for practice. *NT Research, 9*, 18–27.

Stoeter, M. (2003). [Growing need for specialists in clinical research. Research assistants, "study nurses"]. *KrankenPflege Journal, 41*, 116–117.

Thompson, A., Pickler, R., & Reyna, B. (2005). Clinical coordination of research. *Applied Nursing Research, 18*, 102–105.

CHAPTER 52
Mentorship

Rose Ermete, RN, BSN, CCRP, OCN®

Introduction

The oncology nurse entering the arena of clinical trials assumes a variety of roles and responsibilities. These functions are dependent on many variables, such as the type and size of practice, patient population, and expectations of management and of the principal investigator. Clinical trial nurses (CTNs) may be responsible for the clinical aspects of managing a clinical trial patient, but in many settings, this is not their only role. The CTN also may be involved in data management, regulatory requirements, and budgeting (Joshi & Ehrenberger, 2001). This chapter will present mentorship and a program for mentorship of CTNs as a valuable process to orient nurses and other health professionals to clinical trial research.

Background

Clinical trials nursing is different from staff nursing and other areas of practice within oncology. New CTNs learn to quickly adapt to an environment of unfamiliar rules and regulations. Nurses evolve from being part of a team to coordinating the team (see Figure 52-1). Staff nursing tends to be task-oriented; however, in research, it often is the CTN providing directions and coordinating the plan of care. To function effectively, the CTN needs to be a team leader with a thorough knowledge of oncology and the science and regulations behind the research. The novice CTN needs to widen his or her focus from technical skills or issues surrounding a patient's condition to the meaning and impact this patient may have on the study and on the future standard of care for this disease (Lemery, 2002). This broader focus will provide the CTN with an understanding that encompasses clinical trials.

The novice CTN may experience significant role confusion in attempting to navigate a course toward professional growth. Role confusion is a result of the varying roles and responsibilities that surround the CTN profession. Coupled with increasingly complex studies and stringent regulations, the novice CTN may feel completely overwhelmed. Hurst and Koplin-Baucum (2003) observed that nurses who were unable to assimilate socially and clinically within 12 months of work would seek other employment. New CTNs need support from senior administration and CTN leaders who are willing to invest time and resources in them by providing mentoring and guidance to overcome these challenges. Without this needed support, nurses may explore other areas and abandon the profession (Wieck, Prydun, & Walsh, 2002).

Unfortunately, today's nursing shortage will affect the subspecialty of clinical trials nursing. The population of people older than age 65 will double by 2030 (Wieck et al., 2002). As nursing faculty retire, fewer nurses are entering

Figure 52-1. The Research Nurse's Central Role in the Coordination of Clinical Trial Activities

Clinical Trial Office
Physician
Treatment Staff
Sponsor
CTN
Patient
Clinical Research Associate
Ancillary Staff*

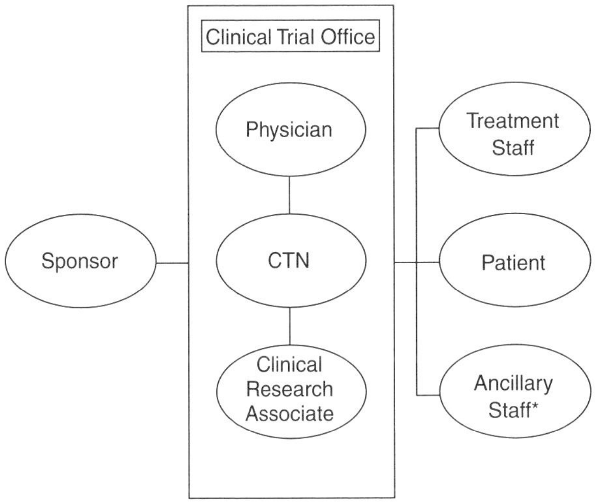

*Ancillary staff: Research Pharmacist, Social Worker, Dietician, Laboratory personnel and other assistive personnel.

CTN—clinical trial nurse
Note. From *CTN Mentorship Handbook*, by R.B. Ermete, 2003. Used with permission.

doctoral programs. Present trends indicate that the current nursing workforce will age without a great influx of new nurses (McKinley, 2004; Wieck et al.). It is important that experienced nurses pass their knowledge on to the next generation. In today's hurried workplace more time frequently is spent on developing processes and less time on developing people. When nurses retire, they will take with them their knowledge and expertise (Lemery, 2002). Experienced CTNs can create a legacy by passing their current knowledge to the next generation of CTNs. Through positive interaction with a more experienced CTN, novices will better assimilate into their new role while strengthening the subspecialty of oncology clinical trials nursing.

Mentorship Defined

The term *mentor* dates back to Greek mythology. When Odysseus left to fight in the Trojan War, he left his son, Telemachus, in the care of a trusted and wise friend, Mentor. Mentor not only raised Telemachus but also provided him with knowledge and guidance to prepare him for future responsibilities (Homer, trans. 1993).

A mentor has come to be known as a wise person who provides guidance and insight from experience. It is not the same thing as a coach or preceptor. Coaching generally is a top-down process that involves training toward predetermined goals that tend to revolve around the objectives of a team or organization. Precepting involves skills training that focuses on assisting a novice to function at a certain proficiency level as determined by the organization (Carroll, 2004; McKinley, 2004; Mitchell & Sawatzky-Girling, 2003). In contrast, mentorship has a broader focus. It fosters a supportive environment that nurtures advancement toward self-development and professional growth. The focus is on the developmental needs and goals of the novice. The mentor's role is to offer guidance and insight and to open doors to understanding so that the novice can see beyond what was originally thought to be possible (Carroll).

The Mentorship Process

To understand the mentorship process, it is essential to establish a theoretical framework for mentoring. Mentoring involves guiding or assisting others along a path to increased knowledge and professional growth. Several relevant learning theories exist that support this endeavor. McKinley (2004) discussed Kolb's theory on experiential learning and Malcolm Knowles' adult learning principles. Both theories, juxtaposed, support the goals of a mentorship program.

Knowles' (1990) theory of adult learning focuses on the needs of the adult learner. These needs are described using the Andragogical Model (see Table 52-1). Adults need to know why they need to know something and how it will apply to their life situations. They also must be ready to learn. Learning occurs more easily if it coincides with the developmental tasks of the adult. Adult learners bring with them differences in past experiences that will affect their

Table 52-1. The Andragogical Model	
Concept	**Description**
1. The need to know	Why do I need to know this?
2. The learners' self-concept	I am capable of self-direction.
3. The role of the learners' experience	I have many different types of experiences.
4. Readiness to learn	How does this relate to my developmental stage?
5. Orientation to learning	How will this help me to deal with problems I may confront?
6. Motivation	How will this help me to achieve self-esteem and quality of life?
Note. Based on information from Knowles, 1990; McKinley, 2004.	

interpretation and internalization of what is taught. Adults also are self-directed and are motivated to learn more by internal desires than by external stimuli (Knowles). This means that they will resist learning if it is perceived as enforcing the will or needs of others. These concepts need to be considered while mentoring a novice CTN. Employing the Andragogical Model in mentorship allows the mentor to guide novices to channel their energy toward their own professional growth and development.

Kolb's experiential learning theory focuses on the experiences of the person and how they relate to the learning milieu. McKinley (2004) and Smith (2001) reviewed the four steps in Kolb's theory. The first is the experience itself, followed by self-reflection to understand the outcome, or meaning of the experience. In the next step, generalization, the person begins to form concepts or create generalized principles that may be utilized in similar circumstances. The last step is to apply the new knowledge in future situations.

Carroll (2004) presented Rosemarie R. Parse's *Human Becoming Theory* as a model for mentorship. This model does not utilize stages of learning as in the previous theories. Here, the nurse is allowed to explore and draw on his or her own value system and creativity. Through this process, the novice envisions the nurse he or she wishes to become. The mentor then guides the nurse along the path toward the individual's professional goal.

The theories previously discussed help mentors to guide the learning of the novice CTN. This allows the mentorship process to be focused on the novice's needs rather than on an external entity. By allowing the novice to explore and problem solve, with guidance and insight from the mentor, the novice is able to build self-confidence and develop as a professional nurse.

The Mentoring Relationship

The success of mentoring depends on the individuals involved in the relationship. Triple Creek Associates (2005) has identified three vital ingredients to a mentoring relationship: respect, responsiveness, and accountability. Each person in the relationship must show appreciation for the other. Appreciation translates into mutual respect. Responsiveness means being sensitive and responsive to another person's needs. Accountability is living up to agreed-upon expectations and is vital to the development of trust.

Each person in a mentoring relationship has certain responsibilities (see Figure 52-2). Everyone has unique qualities that he or she brings to the relationship. For a successful mentoring relationship, the mentor and novice need to understand what their responsibilities are (Triple Creek Associates, 2004b). A lack of awareness of one's role can lead to misunderstandings and generate defective communication. Without communication, the relationship is stifled, and learning and growth cannot occur.

An essential ingredient in the mentoring relationship is the mentor. Whether a seasoned CTN is deciding to become a mentor or a novice is selecting a mentor, both need to be aware of the characteristics that a proficient mentor should possess. Lemery (2002), McKinley (2004), and Triple Creek Associates (2005) have identified several qualities of a successful mentor (see Figure 52-3). When choosing a mentor, the novice should look for a CTN who has achieved benchmarks that the novice wishes to achieve, such as skills, credibility, credentials, and leadership positions. The mentor should demonstrate a passion for clinical trials nursing. This means that the individual considers his or her work to be a career, not just a job. The mentor should be proficient in written and oral communication, utilize good problem-solving skills, and demonstrate objectivity when confronted with conflict. The mentor should be viewed as a role model, an approachable person, and one who views others positively. The mentor cannot be an intimidator, but instead is a person who continually encourages and promotes new thoughts and ideas. An ideal mentor also should possess

---

Figure 52-3. Qualities of a Mentor

- Has achieved benchmarks that the novice wishes to achieve
- Has a strong professional network
- Demonstrates the ability to think outside the box
- Thinks clearly through situations
- Demonstrates good oral and written communication skills
- Demonstrates good listening skills
- Maintains a positive attitude in difficult situations
- Demonstrates a high degree of motivation and commitment to the profession
- Is viewed as a role model by others
- Is approachable
- Empowers others

Note. Based on information from Lemery, 2002; McKinley, 2004; Triple Creek Associates, 2005.

---

the ability to empower others. Mentors should not solve problems for the novice. By providing insight and utilizing active listening, the mentor is able to assist the novice in developing successful problem-solving skills (McKinley).

Communication

Good communication is vital to the success of any relationship. Two elements are considered basic to good communication: dialogue and listening. These two elements together provide a foundation for interpretation of the thoughts being conveyed. It is the mentor's role to actively listen. Guidance begins with actively listening to what the novice has to say without interjecting opinions or judgments. A mentor should never assume that he or she knows more about a stated problem than the novice does. Paraphrasing, clarifying, summarizing, and empathy are all components of active listening (McKinley, 2004). Open-ended questions are an effective tool for clarifying a novice's experiences. These are questions in which the novice is forced to give an explanation and cannot simply answer yes or no. An open-ended question could be, "How did that make you feel?" as opposed to, "Did that make you angry when Dr. Smith disagreed with the patient's ineligibility?" Open-ended questions allow the novice to explore his or her feelings and thoughts on situations. Closed-ended questions, conversely, transfer the interpretation to the mentor, which prevents the novice from developing good problem-solving skills. The mentor should avoid providing answers to the novice. Instead, mentors need to encourage novices to utilize their own strengths and knowledge to work through situations and find answers (McKinley).

Providing feedback is an important skill in fostering professional growth. Without feedback, the novice might not realize where he or she needs to improve. Maintaining a supportive atmosphere that promotes growth is important when giving feedback. The novice should feel accepted, respected, and empowered. These feelings promote communication, and the novice will be more

---

Figure 52-2. Mentor Responsibilities

Mentees
- Initiate and drive the relationship.
- Identify initial learning goals.
- Seek feedback.
- Take an active role in their own learning.
- Initiate periodic update meetings.
- Allocate time and energy.
- Follow through on commitments or renegotiate appropriately.

Mentors
- Have reasonable expectations of the mentee.
- Be a resource.
- Provide feedback.
- Allocate time and energy.
- Help the mentee to develop an appropriate learning plan.
- Follow through on commitments or renegotiate appropriately.

Note. From "Role Clarity," by Triple Creek Associates, May 2004, *Newsletter: Masterful Mentoring*, pp. 2–3. Copyright 2004 by Triple Creek Associates, Inc. Adapted with permission.

likely to explore his or her thoughts and feelings without fear of ridicule.

Triple Creek Associates (2005) reviewed six components to providing effective feedback. First, the purpose of the feedback must be stated clearly. Both parties should understand why the feedback is taking place. Second, the information conveyed needs to be specific. The problem should be well described so that the novice understands what changes need to occur. The third component is relevance. The feedback given should be applicable to the situation or to the development of the novice. Fourth, the feedback should facilitate the novice to take action and initiate a change. Fifth, feedback should occur in a nonthreatening environment within a reasonable time period of the situation. Last, feedback should incorporate active listening. The novice should have the opportunity to provide a response. The mentor needs to incorporate good active-listening skills so that the response is understood. These steps provide a solid framework for positive change to occur.

During the mentoring experience, conflicts can arise. The mentor must understand how to address conflict in order to maintain positive, effective interaction. Conflict, handled inappropriately, can produce negative behavior. Negative behavior consumes energy that is necessary for constructive problem solving. The mentor must keep an open mind and avoid personal judgment. When addressing problems, opinions must not be confused with facts. The novice must have the opportunity to state his or her rationale without the mentor creating assumptions about what may have occurred. The conversation should be focused on what should have transpired, not just on what was done wrong. When confronting negative behavior, ample use of *I* statements should be used in place of *you* statements. For example: The statement "*I* am concerned that the case report forms were submitted without verifying them against the medical record" is preferable to the statement "*You* did not review all the source documents prior to completing the case report forms." *I* statements acknowledge the thoughts and feelings behind the mentor's comments. *You* statements put the novice on the defensive (Triple Creek Associates, 2005). When a person is defensive, attention is diverted away from the real issues. The mentor must keep the conversation focused on the present situation. Similar past situations have no relevance to the situation at hand. By correctly addressing conflict, the mentor assists the novice in acquiring the skills necessary to manage future problems and grow professionally.

Mentoring Programs

Mentoring can take place under a variety of different circumstances. It can occur through a formal program or through an informal arrangement with a colleague. A myth about mentoring is that it takes a great deal of time and involves long meetings and discussions between the mentor and the novice (Triple Creek Associates, 2004a). In today's hectic workplace, it is unrealistic to expect individuals to have time for this sort of mentoring. *E-mentoring,* a mentoring relationship that is conducted via the Internet, has begun to emerge as a reasonable alternative in today's fast-paced work environment (Griffiths & Miller, 2005).

The Southwest Oncology Group (SWOG) Nurse Oncologist Committee and the Clinical Trial Nurses Special Interest Group (CTN SIG) both have mentorship programs that are based on e-mentoring. SWOG's program utilizes a central contact person (the nurse mentorship chair) to collect information on potential mentors. New nurses then are matched with one who is more experienced. The matches are made based on the needs of the novice and the expertise of the mentor. Contact information is given to the mentor and the novice. The mentor contacts the novice by phone or e-mail to explore the nurse's needs. Subsequent contacts are on an as-needed basis. The response to this program has been positive (Ermete, 2004).

The CTN SIG utilizes e-mentoring through Triple Creek Associates. This program is in collaboration with the Oncology Nursing Society. CTNs log on to the Web site with a code from the CTN SIG Virtual Community page. They can either request a mentor or register as a mentor. Nurses looking for mentors enter information on what type of mentor they are seeking. The Web site matches the nurse with up to three potential mentors. The nurse then can review a profile on each of the mentors and choose the mentor that seems to best fit his or her needs. If the match is not suitable, the nurse can contact the other mentors. The Web site also offers a newsletter and handbooks on mentoring. This is a new program for the CTN SIG and is being evaluated for effectiveness.

Griffiths and Miller (2005) and Mitchell and Sawatzky-Girling (2003) discussed several benefits to e-mentoring. E-mentoring provides contacts far beyond one's local resources. Through this process, a new CTN has access to mentors that he or she normally would not encounter. E-mentoring also allows for flexibility with heavy schedules. Mentors and mentees can respond within their own time constraints. This delay in immediate response allows time for reflection. Another advantage is the elimination of possible feelings of intimidation or discomfort that can sometimes occur in a one-on-one relationship.

E-mentoring, however, presents some challenges. An efficient mechanism of electronic communication is required, but a personal touch needs to remain (Byrne & Keefe, 2002). Both parties must possess the ability to express themselves through the written word (Griffiths & Miller, 2005). With the loss of nonverbal clues, meanings may be misinterpreted. Differences between the individual's motivation and personal characteristics can hinder continuous effective interaction. If possible, there should be an opportunity to meet face to face. This could be accomplished by arranging to meet at a conference or research meeting. If meeting in person is not possible, follow-up phone calls should be employed.

E-mentoring programs should incorporate a mechanism that continually assesses the program's value. Changes should be made if the program is found to be ineffective.

Various other mentoring programs are available to CTNs. Some of these programs are listed in the mentorship resources at the end of this chapter.

Mentorship and the Future

Mentoring benefits the mentor, the mentee, and the profession. The mentee gains valuable experience while progressing toward and attaining professional goals. Through mentoring, the mentor creates a personal legacy that positively contributes to the profession. Mentorship is important to the future of the nursing profession. CTNs must continue to nurture and encourage new CTNs. Experienced nurses need to provide support and guidance for new ideas. New ideas lead to change. Without change, CTNs cannot move forward. If CTNs do not move forward, no growth can occur. Without growth, the CTN role and—the nursing profession—will not survive.

Summary

CTNs work in a variety of settings and assume various roles. Responsibilities differ greatly from that of the traditional staff nurse. These unique responsibilities create a need for mentoring. Through mentorship, a novice CTN can assimilate into the role and grow professionally. Many opportunities for mentoring exist both locally and through various organizations. The novice nurse should choose mentors who have good communication skills, have time for mentoring, demonstrate professionalism, and encourage professional growth and development. More experienced CTNs should consider becoming a mentor, not only to help guide the novice but also to sustain the continued growth of the profession.

References

Byrne, M.W., & Keefe, M.R. (2002). Building research competence in nursing through mentoring. *Journal of Nursing Scholarship, 34,* 391–396.

Carroll, K. (2004). Mentoring: A human becoming perspective. *Nursing Science Quarterly, 17,* 318–322.

Ermete, R.B. (2003). *CTN mentorship handbook.* Unpublished manuscript.

Ermete, R.B. (2004). Southwest Oncology Group's Clinical Trial Nurse Mentorship Program is open to SIG members. *Clinical Trial Nurses Special Interest Group Newsletter, 15*(3). Retrieved September 9, 2004, from http://onsopcontent.ons.org/Publications/SIGNewsletters/ctn/ctn15.3.html

Griffiths, M., & Miller, H. (2005). E-mentoring: Does it have a place in medicine? *Postgraduate Medical Journal, 81,* 389–390.

Homer. (1993). *The odyssey* (A. Cook, Trans.). New York: W.W. Norton Co.

Hurst, S., & Koplin-Baucum, S. (2003). Role acquisition, socialization, and retention: Unique aspects of a mentoring program. *Journal for Nurses in Staff Development, 19,* 176–180.

Joshi, T.G., & Ehrenberger, H.E. (2001). Cancer clinical trials in the new millennium: Novel challenges and opportunities for oncology nursing. *Clinical Journal of Oncology Nursing, 5,* 147–152.

Knowles, M. (1990). *The adult learner: A neglected species* (4th ed.). Houston, TX: Gulf Publishing.

Lemery, L.D. (2002). On mentoring. *Clinical Leadership and Management Review: The Journal of CLMA, 16,* 63–69.

McKinley, M.G. (2004). Mentoring matters: Creating, connecting, empowering. *AACN, 15,* 205–214.

Mitchell, C., & Sawatzky-Girling, B. (2003). Going provincial: Preceptoring and mentoring revisited in the health sciences. *Healthcare Management Forum, 16*(1), 37–39.

Smith, M.K. (2001). David A. Kolb on experiential learning. In *The encyclopedia of informal education.* Retrieved October 14, 2005, from http://www.infed.org/biblio/b-explrn.htm

Triple Creek Associates. (2004a, March). Mentoring myths. *Masterful Mentoring.* Retrieved September 3, 2005, from http://www.3creekmentoring.com/ONS

Triple Creek Associates. (2004b, April). Role clarity. *Masterful Mentoring.* Retrieved September 3, 2005, from http://www.3creekmentoring.com/ONS

Triple Creek Associates. (2005). *Web-based open mentoring, mentor guide: Self-paced workbook* (3rd ed.). Retrieved October 14, 2005, from http://www.3creekmentoring.com/ONS

Wieck, K.L., Prydun, M., & Walsh, T. (2002). What the emerging workforce wants in its leaders. *Journal of Nursing Scholarship, 34,* 283–288.

Additional Resources

Association for Women in Science, *Mentoring:* http://awis.org/careers/mentoring.html

International Mentoring Association: www.mentoring-association.org

The Mentoring Group: www.mentoringgroup.com/index.html

MentorNet®: www.mentornet.net

National Surgical Adjuvant Breast and Bowel Project (NSABP) Mentoring Program: https://members.nsabp.pitt.edu/Treatment_Mentor_Program.asp (Note: A password is needed to access this site. Nurses who use the NSABP will have a password.)

Oncology Nursing Society, *Clinical Journal of Oncology Nursing (CJON)* Mentor/Fellow Writing Program: www.ons.org/membership/mentoring/writing.shtml

Oncology Nursing Society, *ONS Mentoring Programs:* www.ons.org/membership/mentoring/index.shtml

Triple Creek Associates: www.3creekmentoring.com/ONS

Sigma Theta Tau International Chiron Mentoring Program: www.nursingsociety.org/LeadershipInstitute/chiron/pages/chiron.aspx

CHAPTER 53
Professional Continuing Education

Elizabeth Ness, RN, MS

Introduction

Nurses have a professional obligation to be lifelong learners, actively involved in their personal continuing education and professional development. The American Nurses Association (ANA) defined *nursing professional development* as "the lifelong process of active participation by nurses in learning activities that assist in developing and maintaining their continuing competence, enhancing their professional practice, and supporting achievement of their career goals" (ANA, 2000, p. 4). *Continuing education* is defined by ANA as "systematic professional learning experiences designed to augment the knowledge, skills, and attitudes of nurses and therefore enrich the nurses' contributions to quality health care and their pursuit of professional career goals" (ANA, p. 5). This chapter will review the characteristics of adult learners, explore different learning styles, and identify a variety of professional development activities for the clinical trial nurse (CTN).

Adult Learners

The field of adult learning was pioneered by Malcolm Knowles (1990). He identified the adult learner as *autonomous, self-directed, practical,* and *goal-oriented.* Adult learners have accumulated a foundation of *life experiences* and *knowledge* that may include work-related activities, family responsibilities, and previous education. Adult learners bring a variety of experiences, both personal and professional, including mistakes, to a learning situation. They are most interested in learning about subjects that have immediate relevance to their job or personal life, *and they need to be involved in the selection, planning, and evaluation of a learning activity.* The emphasis on adult learning in both general education and in nursing began during the 1990s.

In general, adult learning can be divided into three categories: formal education, informal education, and nonformal education. Formal education is education provided in a school, college, university, or other academic setting. Informal education is the learning that is experienced through normal activities of daily living or spontaneous day-to-day learning. Nonformal education is an organized educational activity that does not clearly fall within the formal education setting. Nonformal learning is deliberate, intentional, and has specific goals. The goals are the reason why the learning is undertaken, and the adult learner intends to retain and use what has been learned (Gopee, 2001). Many of the continuing education activities in which nurses participate today fall into the nonformal category.

Learning Styles

Learning styles classify the different ways people learn and how they approach, perceive, process, organize, and present information. The manner in which a learning style is conceptualized varies widely. Several models are available, many with several instruments from which to choose when assessing one's own learning style. For the purposes of this chapter, the sensory model, which is the most widely recognized, will be used (Avillion, 2004). Most people will have a dominant learning modality and a supporting learning modality.

One type of learner identified by the sensory model is auditory learners. These people learn predominately by hearing (e.g., lectures, discussions, audiotapes) and will tend to listen to a lecture and then take notes afterward or rely on printed notes. Often, information written down will have little meaning until it has been heard. Many auditory learners will read written information out loud. They will not benefit from written handouts or visuals, nor will they do as well with distance-learning activities such as computer-based learning. Educational strategies that best fit the auditory learner include interactive lectures and discussion, debates, audio/teleconferences, and audiotapes (Avillion, 2004).

Another type of learner, the visual learner, relates most effectively to written information, notes, diagrams, and pictures. The visual learner absorbs information best by taking very detailed notes, making lists to read later, reading information to be learned, and seeing a demonstration. Typically, they will be unhappy with a presentation where they are unable to take detailed notes. Some will even take notes despite having the printed materials in front of them (Avillion, 2004). Educational strategies that best fit the visual learner include lectures that utilize handouts, graphics and other printed/visual materials, including videotapes and books, and distance learning with a computer or other media (Avillion).

The third type is the tactile/kinesthetic learner. This type learns more effectively through touch, movement, and space and learns skills by imitation and direct hands-on involvement. The tactile/kinesthetic learner may use a pencil or highlighter pen to mark passages he or she finds meaningful. Taking notes and transferring information to book margins, a personal journal, or a computer also are examples of how tactile/kinesthetic learners learn. They are uncomfortable in classrooms that do not offer opportunities for hands-on experience. Tactile/kinesthetic learners need to be active, tend to take frequent breaks, and communicate by touching or gesturing. Educational strategies that best fit the tactile/kinesthetic learner include hands-on experiences, such as simulations, and activities with frequent breaks (Avillion, 2004).

Understanding one's own preferred learning style (both dominant and secondary) permits an individual to more effectively select appropriate professional development activities. This insight can lead to successful completion of a chosen activity, will maximize financial resources, and will build professional confidence.

Self-Development Activities for Professional Continuing Education

Whereas *lifelong learning* is a more global term, the concept of professional development includes a more structured approach and planned sequencing for learning. Professional self-development activities involve the following: assessing one's skills, abilities, and knowledge; identifying deficiencies or gaps; planning educational experiences to meet the deficiencies or gaps; and evaluating outcomes and the extent of completion of the identified learning program and goals. Through self-assessment and personal reflection, one can develop and maintain a professional portfolio. This allows the individual to monitor and track his or her professional development as well as supporting other activities, such as enrollment applications for formal education, applications for professional specialty certification, and promotion or workplace advancements (Beason, 2005).

The oncology CTN is a unique position because this individual is required to incorporate two distinct areas of subject matter when selecting professional development activities: oncology and clinical research practices. The CTN needs to stay current with both oncology practice and clinical research processes, for example, the latest treatment for cancer therapies, survivorship concerns, new federal regulations and guidelines (e.g., the Office for Human Research Protections' [2007] *Guidance on Reviewing and Reporting Unanticipated Problems Involving Risks to Subjects or Others and Adverse Events*, the U.S. Food and Drug Administration's [2006] *Establishment and Operation of Clinical Trial Data Monitoring Committees*), and trends in trial design for new noncytotoxic agents. Various formal and nonformal learning activities are available. They can be as simple as reading professional journals or more complex, such as preparing a manuscript for publication or completing a certificate or master's program in clinical trial management or regulatory compliance. Examples of professional self-development activities for the CTN include staying current with practice and research trends by reading the literature; attending conferences, seminars, and workshops; preparing written materials and presentations; seeking out mentorship experiences; and completing e-learning activities. Reading professional journals is important to staying current with practice and research trends. For the oncology CTN, journals of interest include, but are not limited to, the *Clinical Journal of Oncology Nursing, Journal of Clinical Oncology, Journal of Nursing Scholarship, Oncology Nursing Forum, Research Practitioner, SoCRA® Source,* and *The Monitor.* Each provides the reader with varying topics related to oncology and clinical research. Maintaining an awareness of the regulatory climate also is important for the CTN. Subscribing to various electronic mailing lists and visiting the Web sites of the U.S. Food and Drug Administration or the Office of Human Subjects Research to stay current with regulatory or guidance information can be beneficial. Numerous agencies have developed electronic mailing lists that will bring the CTN real-time updates to federal regulations and guidelines (see Figure 53-1).

Certification

Certification is the formal recognition based on specific criteria with established parameters that reflect assessment of educational preparation and knowledge, skills, and abilities or competence developed through experience in a specialty area of practice. The oncology CTN has opportunities to receive certification through at least three professional organizations: OCN® or CPON® from the Oncology Nursing

---

Figure 53-1. Electronic Mailing Lists

- Center for Biologics Evaluation and Research: www.fda.gov/cber/pubinfo/elists.htm
- Center for Device and Radiological Health: www.fda.gov/cdrh/subscribe.html
- Center for Drug Evaluation and Research: www.fda.gov/cder/cdernew/listserv.html
- Health and Human Services Office of the Inspector General: http://oig.hhs.gov/mailinglist.html
- Office for Human Research Protections: www.hhs.gov/ohrp/news/distributionlist.html
- U.S. Food and Drug Administration: www.fda.gov/emaillist.html

Society (ONS), CCRA or CCRC from the Association for Clinical Research Professionals, or CCRP from the Society of Clinical Research Associates (see Chapter 51 for more information on certification).

Conferences, Seminars, and Workshops

Numerous opportunities exist for the oncology CTN to attend a variety of conferences, seminars, or workshops, either at the local, regional, or national level. The professional associations noted previously offer annual meetings with a wide variety of learning activities that cover a broad range of topics, in addition to regional workshops. The oncology CTN is encouraged to attend the annual meeting of the American Society of Clinical Oncology, where data from current clinical trials and pivotal trials are presented. See Appendix 13 for additional professional associations of interest to the CTN.

E-Learning

Simply stated, *e-learning* is the delivery of an educational activity by electronic means. E-learning involves the use of a computer or other electronic device to provide training or educational materials. Many organizations develop training CD-ROMs and DVDs, which generally are disease-focused. Many professional organizations have e-learning activities for their members, such as virtual seminars, webcasts, audioconferences, and computer-based training activities.

Preparation of Written Materials and Presentations

According to a Latin proverb, "By learning you will teach; by teaching you will learn" (The Quotations Page, n.d.). Preparing for any type of presentation, whether at a local or national level, or publication, whether an abstract or manuscript, can be a daunting yet professionally fulfilling task. Important criteria include identifying the audience, understanding various learning styles, reviewing the literature, and planning revisions. The CTN is in a position to contribute his or her knowledge of both oncology and clinical research.

Mentorship Experience

ONS (n.d.) offers the following definition of mentoring:

> A personal enhancement strategy through which one person facilitates the development of another by sharing known resources, expertise, values, skills, perspectives, attitudes and proficiencies. It allows the learner to build skills and knowledge while attaining goals for career development. Conversely, it provides the opportunity for the experienced individual to further enhance his/her skill and knowledge areas by continuously reassessing and building upon those areas.

ONS offers a variety of mentoring programs that allow an individual to gain or provide peer support and guidance. In the spring of 2005, the CTN Special Interest Group began a mentorship program for CTNs. See Chapter 52 to learn more about mentoring and ONS's mentoring programs.

Institutional Activities for Professional Continuing Education

Many of the previously identified activities can be accomplished by an individual or coordinated by another organization. Identifying activities that can be coordinated by an individual or group within an institution is not as difficult as it may seem. Some examples are journal clubs, grand rounds, and brown bag lunches. These activities can be easily accomplished if at least one individual is motivated to take the first step, if that individual has the support of colleagues and administration, and if some basic steps are followed.

Journal Club

With improved methods for literature searching via the Internet and evidence-based nursing, a nursing journal club is an excellent educational strategy. The overall purpose of any journal club is to disseminate knowledge. In general, the three main goals of a journal club are to keep current with scientific and/or specialty knowledge, learn critical appraisal skills, and improve clinical practice (Forsen, Hartman, & Neely, 2003; Goodfellow, 2004). For the oncology CTN, the use of a journal club as a continuing education activity can focus on a variety of topics, such as oncology nursing practice, cancer clinical trials, new drug development, federal regulations governing clinical research, and research integrity. To initiate a journal club within an organization, the CTN will need to follow four basic steps: (a) develop the infrastructure of the journal club sessions (e.g., discussion leader, participants, session logistics), (b) select the design of the sessions (e.g., goals/objectives, type of literature to review, format of session), (c) determine how literature will be selected (e.g., chosen by the discussion leader or small working group, determined by a new regulation or pivotal trial results), and (d) evaluate the sessions (e.g., whether goals were met, participant satisfaction).

Grand Rounds

Nursing grand rounds have been cited in the literature since the 1960s with common purposes including providing nurses with opportunities to learn from experienced peers, acknowledging nursing expertise, decreasing nursing staff isolation, and promoting professional development (Lannon, 2005). For the oncology CTN, grand rounds provide a forum to strengthen nursing research and integrate nursing research into oncology nursing practice using an evidence-based practice framework. Because this proposed focus is broader than the clinical research domain, initiating grand rounds within an institution will require collaboration with nursing leadership. However, the basic steps are similar to those for initiating a journal club: (a) develop the infrastructure (e.g., committee or small working group, frequency of meetings and grand rounds sessions), (b) select the format (e.g., goals/objectives, topics to be presented), and (c) determine how to evaluate the sessions (e.g., whether goals were met, participant satisfaction).

Brown Bag Lunches

The concept of brown bag lunches is common among nursing staff development specialists, although little literature is found to support their use, benefit, or processes. Brown bag lunch sessions can provide an informal, supportive environment that allows staff to discuss clinically focused topics, the research process, and best practices or can even serve as a preview of presentations for professional meetings (King & Ness, 2007). Developing brown bag lunch sessions will follow similar steps as with journal clubs and grand rounds, and participants may include both CTNs and other oncology nurses.

Summary

The need for professional continuing education continues to increase as the pace of new knowledge escalates (Griscti & Jacono, 2006). Becoming a lifelong learner is no longer a choice but a necessity for oncology CTNs. Identifying one's learning style will assist the oncology CTN in selecting appropriate educational offerings for both oncology and clinical research management.

References

American Nurses Association. (2000). *Scope and standards of practice for nursing professional development.* Silver Spring, MD: Nursesbooks.org.

Avillion, A.E. (2004). *A practical guide to staff development: Tools and techniques for effective education.* Marblehead, MA: HCPor, Inc.

Beason, C.G. (2005). A new role in accreditation activities offers expanded horizons for registered nurses. *Journal of Professional Nursing, 21,* 191–196.

Forsen, J.W., Hartman, J.M., & Neely, J.G. (2003). Tutorials in clinical research, Part VIII: Creating a journal club. *Laryngoscope, 113,* 475–483.

Goodfellow, L.M. (2004). Can a journal club bridge the gap between research and practice? *Nurse Educator, 29,* 107–110.

Gopee, N. (2001). Lifelong learning in nursing: Perceptions and realities. *Nurse Education Today, 21,* 607–615.

Griscti, O., & Jacono, J. (2006). Effectiveness of continuing education programmes in nursing: Literature review. *Journal of Advanced Nursing, 55,* 449–456.

King, L., & Ness, E. (2007). The Center for Cancer Research Brown Bag Lunch sessions: The first year. *Journal for Nurses in Staff Development, 23,* 31–35.

Knowles, M. (1990). *The adult learner: A neglected species* (4th ed.). Houston, TX: Gulf Publishing.

Lannon, S. (2005). Nursing grand rounds: Promoting excellence in nursing. *Journal for Nurses in Staff Development, 21,* 221–226.

Office for Human Research Protections. (2007). *Guidance on reviewing and reporting unanticipated problems involving risks to subjects or others and adverse events.* Retrieved March 26, 2007, from http://www.hhs.gov/ohrp/policy/AdvEvntGuid.htm

Oncology Nursing Society. (n.d.). *How mentoring works at ONS.* Retrieved April 31, 2006, from http://www.3creekmentoring.com/ONS

The Quotations Page. (n.d.). *Latin proverb.* Retrieved March 26, 2007, from http://www.quotationspage.com/quotes/Latin_Proverb

U.S. Food and Drug Administration. (2006). *Guidance for clinical trial sponsors: Establishment and operation of clinical trial data monitoring committees.* Retrieved March 26, 2007, from http://www.fda.gov/cber/gdlns/clintrialdmc.pdf

SECTION XII.

International Considerations

CHAPTER 54
Australia

Catherine Johnson, RN, BSc, and Kathleen Scott, BSc(Hons), PhD

Introduction

Cancer clinical research has an established foundation in Australia through the work of national and state-based organizations, local hospital networks, and collaborations with international partners. Clinical trials conducted on the international stage increasingly share similar features with research nurses and site coordinators faced with common issues and problems in ensuring trials are conducted to recognized standards of good clinical practice (GCP). This chapter highlights some of the key features of conducting trials in the Australian research environment.

History and Background
Clinical Oncological Society of Australia

The Clinical Oncological Society of Australia (COSA) is the peak multidisciplinary society for health professionals working in cancer research or the treatment, rehabilitation, or palliation of patients with cancer. Formed in 1971, COSA conducts an annual scientific meeting, as well as seminars and educational activities related to current cancer issues (COSA, n.d.-c).

Groups Within COSA

COSA is composed of a number of groups that are either therapeutic-focused or dedicated to specialty areas in the field of cancer. Ten national cancer cooperative groups are affiliated with COSA, which cover a broad range of solid tumor types and hematologic cancers. In addition, two groups exist within COSA that specifically address clinical research as a discipline and the conduct of cancer clinical trials: the Cancer Research Group (CRG) and the Clinical Research Professionals Group (CRPG) (COSA, n.d.-b, n.d.-d).

The CRG, one of the first groups established within COSA, was originally envisioned as bridging the gap between basic, laboratory-based cancer research and applied research in a clinical setting (COSA, n.d.-b). The CRG is

exploring new means to fill this role, specifically facilitating COSA collaboration with relevant research-based societies, scientific networks, and research conferences.

A key goal is to ensure that barriers that limit the provision of optimal and improved cancer care are visible to the research community. Furthermore, the opportunity exists to ensure appropriate application of new knowledge concerning cancer biology, particularly that which is identified at the molecular level. Collaborations among COSA, the cancer collaborative groups, and the Australasian Biospecimens Network (ABN), a network of scientists who have initiated a number of tissue banks around Australia, are indicative of developments in this area. Alongside international collaborations, the coordination of biologic studies facilitates the collection of both tissue and blood samples within the context of clinical trial protocols. This permits the identification of prognostic factors (which will assist clinicians in determining cancer diagnoses and patient outcomes) as well as predictive markers to tailor individual patient treatment (ABN, n.d.).

Clinical Research Professionals Group

The COSA CRPG, formerly known as the Data Managers Group, represents cancer clinical researchers involved in the collection and management of data, including clinical trial coordinators, research nurses, clinical research managers, data managers, clinical research associates, and health information managers. The CRPG is committed to achieving and promoting excellence in cancer clinical research with the professional contribution of data managers through education, information, leadership, networking, and professionalism (COSA, n.d.-d).

The term *cancer research* now is widely recognized to be applicable to a broad range of activities, extending from epidemiology to clinical trials and including, for example, health services research. The CRG operates to accommodate all such activities, particularly within the annual scientific meetings of COSA. Clinical trials have helped to improve the survival of patients with cancer. They contribute to a reduction in the incidence of premature death and disability, improvement in the evidence behind cancer care, and creation of a health system that both is cost effective and guides best practice (*NSW Cancer Plan 2007–2010*, 2006).

Through the national cancer cooperative groups, a record of conducting research to a high standard has been established (COSA, n.d.-c). Both COSA and its close partner, the Cancer Council Australia (CCA), Australia's peak nongovernmental cancer control organization, have long advocated for infrastructure support for these groups and for improved participation in clinical trials. CCA's eight state and territory member organizations work together to undertake and fund cancer research and to prevent and control cancer, as well as to provide support and information for people affected by cancer (COSA, 2001; CCA, n.d.).

Infrastructure Support and Funding

COSA is committed to supporting cancer cooperative trials research. In 2001, COSA was the lead group in developing the Oceania Report on Cooperative Trials Research, which was pivotal in lobbying the government for additional infrastructure support for cooperative cancer trials research. In July 2005, COSA and the Australasian Cancer Cooperative Trials Groups were awarded a National Health and Medical Research Council (NHMRC) enabling grant. The investigators will receive $1.8 million over five years (COSA, n.d.-a).

The aim of the program is to enhance the capacity of all member cooperative trial groups of COSA to conduct high-quality clinical cancer research by developing and providing fundamental resources in three areas:

- Protocol development from concept outline to externally approved protocol
- Web-based randomization and data collection
- An independent, comprehensive quality assurance program (including standard operating procedures [SOPs]).

The CRPG of COSA is backing recent initiatives, such as providing support to clinical trial sites, through the purchase of SOPs from the United States, adapted for use in Australia. SOPs are available at a low price to sites to assist in the coordination of clinical trials in accordance with good clinical practice and regulatory requirements. The continued training of site staff, however, is an issue that requires further work, as is evaluating the uptake and updating of SOPs and assessing compliance at sites (COSA, n.d.-d).

Cancer Nurses Society of Australia

The Cancer Nurses Society of Australia (CNSA), established in 1998, is the national professional organization for cancer nurses and is affiliated with COSA. The CNSA is committed to achieving and promoting excellence in cancer care through the professional contribution of nurses. CNSA offers a research grant program to support the development

of cancer nursing. The purpose of the program is to provide financial assistance to facilitate research in the area of cancer nursing, which will contribute to improvements in the care of people with cancer (CNSA, 2006).

Australasian Health and Research Data Managers Association

The Australasian Health and Research Data Managers Association (n.d.) is an association of health researchers, research nurses, and data managers that was established in 1990. Its primary aim is to facilitate communication between staff working across a variety of disciplines in health-related research. Education and training also is a focus, with an annual scientific meeting in addition to the provision of professional development grants and scholarships to its members.

Government Initiatives in Cancer Research

Cancer Australia, an initiative of the Australian federal government, allocated $21.7 million over four years from 2005 to support Australia's capacity to undertake clinical trials for patients with cancer. This funding provides infrastructure support to cooperative groups to support group development and the initiation of clinical trials (Australian Government Department of Health and Ageing, 2005).

The state government of New South Wales (NSW) initiated Cancer Institute NSW, with key objectives including the increased participation of sites and enrollment of patients in cancer clinical trials. Funding is available to successful investigators and cooperative groups on application to initiate and run trials. New programs, such as establishing clinical trial research partnerships in tumor types that have a smaller research base in Australia, are more apt to receive funding.

Legal and Regulatory Issues

The Therapeutic Goods Administration (TGA), the national regulatory authority, regulates clinical trials in Australia under one of the two following schemes:
- The Clinical Trial Notification (CTN) scheme
- The Clinical Trial Exemption (CTX) scheme

The most common scheme used is the CTN scheme, which requires all study material related to the trial, including the protocol, scientific and background information regarding study drug(s), and information provided to study participants, to be submitted to the local Human Research Ethics Committee (HREC) for review. Once approval has been granted by the HREC, the completed CTN form, which is signed by (a) the study sponsor, (b) a representative for the HREC (usually the chair), (c) a legal representative for the institution (usually the hospital manager), and (d) the site investigator, is submitted to the TGA with an acknowledgment issued that the trial can commence. Phase III trials usually are conducted under the CTN scheme. The research nurse is responsible for ensuring that the CTN form is completed correctly and returned to the sponsor. If the site is acting as sponsor, it may submit the form directly to the TGA.

Under the therapeutic goods legislation, the HREC is responsible for monitoring the study at each associated institution. Serious unexpected protocol therapy–related serious adverse events (SAEs) that occur in Australian patients are required to be reported to the HREC and TGA. However, all other SAEs that occur, including safety letters or updates from sponsors regarding events that have occurred outside Australia, must be reported to the HREC only.

The CTX scheme is used less frequently and usually is only followed when a sponsor requests regulatory evaluation of an agent early in its clinical development (usually phase I/II) or for newer technologies such as gene therapy.

Whether conducted under the CTN or CTX scheme, all trials must be conducted in accordance with the protocol, associated documents, and the International Conference on Harmonisation of Technical Requirements for Registration of Pharmaceuticals for Human Use (ICH) *Note for Guidance on Good Clinical Practice (CPMP/ICH/135/95)* (ICH, 1996), which has been adopted by the TGA and legislated under Access to Unapproved Therapeutic Goods in 2001 (Australian Government Department of Health and Ageing, 2004).

Ethical Review

TGA legislation also covers the ethical review of clinical trials in Australia. HRECs generally are institutionally based and are governed by the Australian Health Ethics Committee (AHEC). The responsibilities of HRECs are outlined in the NHMRC's (2007) *National Statement on Ethical Conduct in Human Research 2007*, which also was adopted in TGA legislation.

Recently, the regulatory and ethics system in Australia has undergone extensive review, initiated on behalf of the TGA, to evaluate existing regulatory systems in both Australia and New Zealand in comparison to systems in Canada, the United States, and the United Kingdom (Banscott Health Consulting Pty Ltd., 2005). The establishment of a trans-Tasman joint regulatory agency between Australia and New Zealand has been proposed for the regulation of therapeutic products and currently is undergoing development. Concurrently, a number of initiatives are under way to move institutional-based HREC review to a multicenter HREC review system to reduce duplication and streamline the ethics review process.

Sponsoring Agencies

Australian regulations (the Therapeutic Goods Act of 1989 and subsequent amendments) require that a national sponsor (either a person, body, organization, or institution) is identified to take overall responsibility for the conduct of the clinical trial. The sponsor usually initiates, organizes, and supports the clinical trial and carries the medico-legal responsibilities with the conduct of the trial. For pharmaceutical-sponsored trials, the company affiliate will take on the role of sponsor, or it could be delegated to a contract research organization.

For investigator-initiated trials, the regulations permit an individual investigator or local institution to take on this sponsor role. In the case of multicenter trials, the collaborative or coordinating group often acts as a sponsor on behalf of many sites, whether initiated nationally or by international groups.

Defining sponsorship is a very complex aspect of trial setup, particularly when multiple parties are involved in a clinical trial contractually. Typically, pharmaceutical companies, who may be providing the study drug(s) in investigator-initiated trials, do not accept the role of trial sponsorship. Careful consideration of the responsibilities of each party is required, particularly which party will carry clinical trial indemnity, a factor that usually determines the trial sponsor.

Intergroup Trials

Collaborations among groups mainly exist between an Australian-based group, or a joint Australian and New Zealand group (Australasian), and overseas groups. Collaborations exist between many of the main tumor-specific cooperative groups in Australia (e.g., Australasian Gastro-Intestinal Trials Group) and established overseas groups (e.g., National Surgical Adjuvant Breast and Bowel Project [United States], National Cancer Institute of Canada Clinical Trials Group [Canada], European Organisation for Research and Treatment of Cancer [Belgium], Medical Research Council [United Kingdom]). International collaboration is the lifeblood of clinical trials, permitting the generation of data that are generalizable, as well as greater acceptance of the data for both publication and changes in clinical practice (COSA, n.d.-b).

Elements of a Protocol

In investigator-initiated trials, protocol development may occur at the site level, with the intention of running the trial as either a single-institution study or extended to multiple sites. The investigators usually write protocols; however, they may engage a number of team members to contribute in their area of expertise (e.g., statistician, research nurse, data manager, pharmacist). Completed protocols then undergo a peer review process to elicit any constructive criticism and further development. Locally generated case report forms (CRFs), which enable consistent data to be collected, also are developed.

For multicenter trials initiated under the umbrella of a collaborative group, a coordinating center is designated. This center is where the protocol is developed by an operations team, usually a clinical trial manager in consultation with the principal investigator, key coinvestigators, and the study statistician. The format of a protocol follows the elements outlined in the ICH Good Clinical Practice (GCP) guidelines (ICH, 1996), with relevant SOPs followed.

Studies initiated by international groups often permit Australian input through an international steering committee to review the protocol prior to finalization. This consultation reduces the number of protocols being initiated that, for whatever reason, are considered not feasible for participation, particularly because of differences in clinical practice or treatment protocols between countries. For both locally initiated and international studies, each collaborative group will scrutinize the protocol through scientific advisory committees to assess the scientific merit and feasibility of the protocol and to provide feedback and comments on the protocol design.

Protocol Considerations

Studies are considered by a site using set criteria, regardless of whether the study is investigator-initiated or run by a cooperative group or pharmaceutical company. The site first reviews the protocol to assess suitability for participation. Its review focuses on scientific rigor, patient population, eligibility criteria, and the individual capabilities of the site to conduct and adhere to the specifics of the individual protocol.

Once the site has agreed to participate, the protocol is prepared for submission to the local HREC. HREC applications vary from site to site and generally are prepared by site staff, including localized participant information and consent forms. Under a multicenter HREC system, standardization of application forms will become commonplace. The NHMRC cosponsored the development of a Web-based National Ethics Application Form (NEAF), which was released for use in 2006. The advantages for researchers are the completion of one form for submission to multiple HRECs, although only some HRECs have adopted the NEAF at the time of publication (National Commonwealth of Australia, n.d.).

On approval of the study by the HREC, sites prepare regulatory documents appropriate for the sponsor or investigator. After the required regulatory documentation is completed and collected, the study may commence. The sponsor or investigator and research nurse conduct a site initiation at the site. The site initiation includes communication to and education of the relevant staff, including ward and outpatient chemotherapy nurses, pharmacy, radiation, laboratory, and imaging staff.

The research nurse is responsible for ensuring that the trial is conducted according to protocol. Information aids may be adapted from material provided by the sponsor or developed by the research nurse specific to the needs of the site. As the complexity of clinical trials has increased over time, a corresponding increased need to provide accurate and detailed instructions to site staff has become necessary to ensure adherence to the protocol. Both site staff and protocol authors must pay specific attention to the effect of the study on the local indigenous (Aboriginal) population.

Determining Study Budgets

Site staff prepare a study budget based on estimated costs to conduct the study at the site. Generally, the budget provides an estimate of the accrual numbers anticipated during the life of the study and considers the complexity of study procedures and screening as outlined in Figure 54-1.

The site must have sufficient funding and resources available to conduct and complete the study. Reimbursement of costs via per-patient payments made by the sponsor is the usual method by which costs are recovered. Funding levels for clinical trials still vary greatly from study to study. Pharmaceutical-supported trials generally receive sufficient funding to cover the conduct of the study at each site. However, cooperative group and investigator-initiated studies may be funded to a lesser degree. Associated costs are covered through "in kind" use of resources to ensure that these clinical trials are conducted and patients gain access to a greater number of clinical trial options.

Studies run by cooperative groups usually require significantly greater funds to support the costs of the study at the central coordinating center. This ensures that study requirements are met and that the trial is run in accordance with GCP and local regulations. A budget is prepared based on projected costs of key trial activities, such as the resources and staff involved in project management, site management, data management, statistical analysis, and trial administration.

Following the development of a budget proposal, a number of factors will be considered as to where funding will be sought. For trials in which an international group or pharmaceutical company is involved, a per capita payment often is paid based on the recruitment of patients. Pharmaceutical companies frequently will provide an educational grant to support the study conduct, as well as the provision of study treatment, depending on the marketing status of the drug.

For a trial that has no direct involvement or relationship with external sponsors, funding usually is sought through grant-funding bodies such as the NHMRC, the lead government-funded research body, or from charitable organizations. However, funding is allocated on a competitive basis against other applicants from a wide range of disciplines, including basic science research.

Cofunding often can be sought from funding bodies to supplement income from sponsors or groups. CCA provides

---

Figure 54-1. Considerations for a Clinical Trial Budget

- The actual cost of all procedures and tests
- Investigator and study coordinator time
- Collection and preparation of specimens for shipment to the central laboratory
- Other requirements as and when necessary
- The administration costs of the study, including overheads, which are payable to the hospital institution

local infrastructure support for successful applications to employ site data managers/coordinators or research nurses. These studies have less central funding, with the aim of improving uptake to clinical trial research in general, including trials considered for the "public good" and not just commercially funded trials (CCA, n.d.).

Informed consent and patient recruitment specialist physicians inform patients of clinical trials available to them. However, patients increasingly are becoming aware of clinical trials through the media and the Internet and are seeking out treatment at sites based on participation in clinical trials. State and national bodies, such as the state-based cancer councils, also provide information about what a clinical trial is and the benefits of participation. Once the physician introduces a trial to a patient, information and education about the study are given both verbally and in writing. Although the format varies from site to site, all written participant information and consent forms are approved by the HREC and are in accordance with elements outlined in ICH GCP guidelines. All information provided to the patient discusses the study treatment and other options that may be available. Patients are advised of study results as they become available during the study period and after the conclusion of the study.

The research nurse plays a pivotal role throughout the consent process by acting as the primary contact for the patient and communicating the study's requirements. Patients then are given time to consider participation, commensurate with the imperative to commence treatment in a timely manner as appropriate to both the patient's condition and the study protocol timelines. The consent process is ongoing from the initial visit until the study is concluded; however, patients are formally reconsented if adverse reactions, changes to the protocol, or interim results indicate that this is necessary. This reconsent process is conducted verbally by the physician and in writing through an HREC-approved amended information and consent form.

Patient and Family Education

Although the role of the research nurse varies among sites, the research nurse generally fulfills the following two major functions.

- As a *specialist nurse* available to discuss problems and side effects with the patient, caregiver, and other team members
- As a *support nurse* for the patient, caregivers, and other team members, ensuring that the appropriate resources (physical, emotional, psychological, informational and educational) are available throughout the duration of the study. This role also extends to that of a *telephone clinic* where patients are encouraged to consult the nurse between visits.

Patient Selection and Eligibility

Eligibility criteria are clearly defined within each protocol, and the research nurse is responsible for patient assessment and ensuring adherence to eligibility criteria. Eligibility criteria may dictate the need for specific assessments and the time frames in which they are to be conducted. The research nurse, in consultation with the patient and the physician, coordinates these as required.

The research nurse assesses the patient's personal capacity to manage and adhere to the often-rigorous responsibilities that are associated with study participation, such as self-administration of treatments and the use of technologies (e.g., PDAs, infusional devices).

The research team and the patient must consider the ability of the site and the patient to meet the assessments, particularly in a geographically diverse country such as Australia. The patient may be required to travel great distances to receive specialist cancer treatments. Additional travel as a consequence of participation in a clinical study may place an undue or unnecessary burden on the patient and his or her caregivers. This is an important consideration for a patient being assessed for participation in a study who is faced with multiple visits for pharmacokinetics or prolonged periods of treatment. A number of centers or regional clinics now exist with clinical trial physicians and research nurses either on site or visiting from main centers, which permits greater patient access to new medicines or therapies and ensures adequate monitoring and follow-up.

Careful planning and good communication by the research nurse and physician with patients, site staff, and sponsors are required to ensure that eligibility criteria are met and that diagnostic assessments are conducted within the limits specified in the protocol. Time differences and public holidays may prove to be awkward when coordinating eligibility and randomization; thus, particular care needs to be taken to overcome these obstacles.

Administration of Protocol Agents

The research nurse, in consultation with the physician, is responsible for ensuring that the patient continues to be eligible to receive study treatment as dictated by the protocol. Any change in disease status or physical and psychosocial well-being of the patient should be considered within the context of the protocol, treatment modifications or delays specified, or criteria outlined on withdrawal from treatment. Psychosocial issues increasingly are being assessed by a variety of self-reporting tools that assess a range of physical and psychosocial issues. The research nurse and other health professionals work together with the patient, using a variety of methods and assessments to ensure that both the physical and psychosocial needs of the patient are met (National Breast Cancer Centre and National Cancer Control Initiative, 2003).

The hospital pharmacist generally is responsible for the correct preparation of cytotoxic treatment and any placebos that may be used during the study. The pharmacist also is responsible for correct documentation of the treatment in the study pharmacy manual. The administering nurse, who in some instances may be the research nurse, is responsible for the correct administration of the treatment according to the protocol, including appropriate monitoring of the patient before, during, and after the treatment as specified in the protocol.

Adverse Events

Adverse events or toxicities of the treatment are assessed at intervals prescribed in the protocol; however, more frequent assessment may be warranted if the patient experiences significant toxicities or if an SAE occurs. Cancer protocols usually follow the National Cancer Institute's Common Terminology Criteria for Adverse Events (version 3.0) for the evaluation and grading of toxicities (National Cancer Institute Cancer Therapy Evaluation Program, 2003). Appropriate baseline documentation of disease signs and symptoms is important, along with the documentation of any ongoing toxicities or side effects from any prior treatments, to be able to clearly differentiate between new and old toxicities or side effects. Continuing education of the patient and his or her caregivers is important so that they understand the importance of reporting new events and timely reporting so that the appropriate management of toxicities can be implemented.

SAEs *must* be reported to the sponsor and the HREC (per local requirements) within 24 hours of the site becoming aware of the event. It is the responsibility of the research nurse to ensure that the appropriate documentation is prepared and forwarded to the sponsor or local HREC.

Long-Term Follow-Up

The protocol usually specifies the follow-up intervals and duration. Treatment of cancer is becoming more successful with diagnoses occurring earlier, and, as such, the period of follow-up is increasing in duration. Monitoring patients over long periods of time is complex, and the research nurse has an important role in ensuring that contact is maintained with the patient at specified intervals and that the patient does not become *lost to follow-up*. Deteriorating levels of health and the remoteness of parts of Australia add additional challenges to maintaining contact with the patient during this follow-up period.

During follow-up, ensuring the patient's ongoing consent to participate is important. Toxicities and side effects that occurred during treatment continue to be monitored and treated, as well as any other issues identified during the treatment period. SAEs continue to be reported to the HREC and sponsor if they occur, usually until 30 days after the last dose of the study drug is given.

Ancillary Studies

Companion protocols (ancillary studies) increasingly are being included as components of clinical studies. Many clinical studies include a method of evaluating a patient's quality of life during treatment. Normally, the patient completes a questionnaire at regular intervals during and after the trial.

However, quality-of-life components are becoming more complex, sometimes involving frequent measurements recorded by patients using devices such as a PDA that transmits data electronically from the patient's home to the site. Other companion protocols may be included as an *optional extra* in which patients may elect to participate. These may include pharmacogenomic, pharmacokinetic, or pharmacoeconomic protocols involving

- The collection of additional blood and tissue samples
- The collection of data regarding the use of health-related resources, such as visits to a general practitioner or home health care.

Research nurses provide patients with additional education and information to ensure that they understand the nature of the questions and can answer appropriately.

Data Management

Historically, the research nurse recorded data on *paper* CRFs. More frequently, however, *computer-* or *Internet-based* CRFs are being used as a means of recording and transmitting data in a timely and efficient fashion to the sponsor.

The research nurse is responsible for the accurate documentation of data in the CRF as acquired from source documentation. It is important that source documentation is comprehensive and accurately reflects the experiences of the patient while the individual is participating in the study. The research nurse plays a vital role in ensuring that all team members understand what information is required for the study and that it is collected and documented as specified in the protocol. The research nurse is responsible for accurately assessing, screening, monitoring, and reporting patient data throughout a trial.

Historical means of communicating information regarding the study, including site activation, randomization, patient treatment, patient discontinuation, and so on, with the study sponsor via phone or post has largely been replaced by electronic-based methods, such as Interactive Voice Randomisation System, e-mail, and the Internet.

Clinical Trial Registries

The Australian Clinical Trial Registry (ACTR) was established in 2005 to assist both patients and health practitioners with access to information about trials, covering the full range of therapeutic areas, including cancer (ACTR, n.d.).

Prior registration with an authorized clinical trial registry is now a condition of publishing trials results. As of July 2005, the International Committee of Medical Journal Editors (which includes editors of the *Medical Journal of Australia, Lancet,* and the *New England Journal of Medicine*) will not publish in their journals the results of any clinical trial not already included in an authorized register at the inception of the trial (ACTR, n.d.). This is an important development that will assist cancer research nurses in providing patients with accurate information on clinical trials that are ongoing and planned.

Professional Development

Research is a rapidly evolving field of cancer care inclusive of advancing treatment technologies and increasing legal and ethical considerations. These developments place an imperative on the research nurse to keep abreast of changes that are integral to successful implementation of clinical studies.

Opportunities for professional development are important to the development of research nurses and their roles in cancer care today. The array of available professional development opportunities necessitates that research nurses carefully select the most advantageous experience to advance and maintain their knowledge base.

CNSA and COSA provide annual meetings that address aspects that are important to the continuing education and development of research nurses in cancer care in Australia. Many other opportunities exist through tertiary courses, international avenues such as the Oncology Nursing Society, the Canadian Association of Nurses in Oncology, and the International Society of Nurses in Cancer Care, and sponsor-driven events specific to clinical studies. Recently created in Australia, the NSW Cancer Institute provides support, information, funding, and seminars relevant to the role of the research nurse in cancer care in the state of New South Wales.

Research nurses are ideally placed to share and disseminate relevant information with the wider cancer care team at their institutions, thereby ensuring that optimal conditions exist to provide the best possible outcomes for patients participating in clinical studies and for the sponsor alike.

Summary

Cancer clinical trials are evolving in Australia. Research nurses work closely with physicians to ensure that patient safety, consent, and treatment maintain the integrity of the protocols and meet all regulatory requirements.

The authors would like to thank Margaret McJannett, Haryana Dhillon, Professor Bernard Stewart of COSA, Kate Cameron of CNSA, Burcu Cakir, and Rhana Pike of the NHMRC Clinical Trials Centre for their review and comments.

References

Australasian Biospecimens Network. (n.d.). *ABN—maximising valuable tissue resources for researchers.* Retrieved February 26, 2006, from http://www.abrn.net

Australasian Health and Research Data Managers Association. (n.d.). *Welcome to AHRDMA.* Retrieved February 26, 2006, from http://www.ahrdma.com.au

Australian Clinical Trials Registry. (n.d.). *Australian clinical trials registry.* Retrieved June 26, 2006, from http://www.actr.org.au

Australian Government Department of Health and Ageing. (2004, October). *Therapeutic Goods Administration (TGA): Access to unapproved therapeutic goods-clinical trials in Australia.* Retrieved February 26, 2006, from http://www.tga.gov.au/docs/pdf/unapproved/clintrials.pdf

Australian Government Department of Health and Ageing. (2005, May 10). *Investing in Australia's health: Strengthening cancer care.* Retrieved February 16, 2006, from http://www.health.gov.au/internet/budget/publishing.nsf/Content/health-budget2005-hbudget-hfact1.htm

Banscott Health Consulting Pty Ltd. (2005, February 22). *Report of the review of access to unapproved therapeutic goods.* Canberra, Australia: Therapeutic Goods Administration.

Cancer Council Australia. (n.d.). *Welcome to the Cancer Council Australia.* Retrieved February 26, 2006, from http://www.cancer.org.au

Cancer Nurses Society of Australia. (2006). *Grants and scholarships.* Retrieved October 24, 2007, from http://www.cnsa.org.au/grants_scholarship_research_travel.htm

Clinical Oncological Society of Australia. (2001, March). *Cancer in the bush: Optimising clinical services: Report and recommendations.* Retrieved January 18, 2006, from http://www.cosa.org.au/documents/Cancer%20in%20the%20Bush.pdf

Clinical Oncological Society of Australia. (n.d.-a). *Cancer Cooperative Groups.* Retrieved October 24, 2007, from http://www.cosa.org.au/content.cfm?randid=115351

Clinical Oncological Society of Australia. (n.d.-b). *Cancer Research Group.* Retrieved January 18, 2006, from http://www.cosa.org.au/content.cfm?randid=437586

Clinical Oncological Society of Australia. (n.d.-c). *Clinical Oncological Society of Australia: Welcome.* Retrieved January 18, 2006, from http://www.cosa.org.au/default.cfm

Clinical Oncological Society of Australia. (n.d.-d). *Clinical Research Professionals Group.* Retrieved January 18, 2006, from http://www.cosa.org.au/content.cfm?randid=743764

International Conference on Harmonisation of Technical Requirements for Registration of Pharmaceuticals for Human Use. (1996). *ICH: E6 (R1) note for guidance on good clinical practice (CPMP/ICH/135/95).* Retrieved October 24, 2007, from http://www.ich.org/cache/compo/276-254-1.html

National Breast Cancer Centre and National Cancer Control Initiative. (2003). *Clinical practice guidelines for the psychosocial care of adults with cancer.* Camperdown, NSW, Australia: National Breast Cancer Centre.

National Cancer Institute Cancer Therapy Evaluation Program. (2003). *Common terminology criteria for adverse events* (version 3.0). Bethesda, MD: National Cancer Institute.

National Commonwealth of Australia. (n.d.). *National ethics application form for submitting research proposals to human research ethics committees.* Retrieved February 13, 2007, from https://www.neaf.gov.au

National Health and Medical Research Council. (2007). *National statement on ethical conduct in human research 2007.* Canberra, Australia: Commonwealth Government of Australia.

NSW Cancer Plan 2007–2010. (2006). Sydney, Australia: Cancer Institute NSW.

About the Authors

Catherine Johnson, RN, BSc, is a research nurse based at the Calvary Mater Newcastle (CMN), New South Wales, Australia, managing a variety of medical oncology clinical trials. She has been working with clinical trials for 10 years and in nursing for 16 years. The CMN is very active in the conduct of clinical trials, in particular the Department of Medical Oncology, which has an established trials program and has been involved in the conduct of clinical research since 1985. Ms. Johnson currently is the deputy chairperson of the Cancer Nurses Society of Australia.

Kathleen Scott, BSc(Hons), PhD, is the head of site management at the National Health and Medical Research

Council Clinical Trials Centre (NHMRC CTC), University of Sydney, working predominantly in the management of oncology clinical trials programs. The NHMRC CTC is an academic center of clinical research excellence and the national coordinating and data center for cancer collaborative groups, including the Australasian Gastro-Intestinal Trials Group, the Australia and New Zealand Gynaecological Oncology Group, and the Germ Cell Trials Group.

CHAPTER 55
New Zealand

Belinda Egan, RN, PG Cert

Introduction

As stated on the Ministry of Health Web site (n.d.), "Cancer is a major health issue for all New Zealanders. One in three will have some experience of cancer, either personally or through a relative or friend." Although many achievements have been made in reducing mortality rates, many challenges still remain. This chapter describes important developments made and features of clinical trial research in New Zealand (NZ), its corresponding contribution in improving public health outcomes, and the pivotal role that the research nurse plays in achieving these goals.

History and Background

In NZ, six regional oncology centers provide medical oncology, radiation oncology, and hematology services. Radiation treatment is offered at all six centers; however, some chemotherapy and surgical services are offered in most other hospitals throughout the country.

The regional oncology centers are in Auckland, Hamilton, Palmerston North, Wellington, Christchurch, and Dunedin. Each of these centers has its own research unit. Before 1990, these research units were small, with only limited numbers of phase III trials being carried out. Over time, with the development of newer drugs and more innovative treatments, the research units have expanded, and they now are running phase I, II, and III studies. These primarily are pharmaceutical-company–sponsored studies and collaborative group studies.

The Health Research Council (HRC) of NZ is the main governing body that oversees research in NZ. Set up under the Health Research Council Act of 1990, the Council's functions include advising the minister of health on health research; administering funds in relation to the national health research policy; fostering the recruitment, education, training, and retention of those engaged in health research in NZ; and initiating and supporting health research (HRC, 2002). The HRC administers a number of committees, some of which are listed in Figure 55-1.

Figure 55-1. Health Research Council Committees

- Gene Technology Advisory Committee
- Standing Committee on Therapeutic Trials
- Independent Safety Monitoring Board
- Data Safety Monitoring Board

As NZ's population is only four million, the majority of oncology trials being conducted are initiated in other countries. The main collaborative groups, the Australia and New Zealand Gynaecological Oncology Group (ANZGOG), Australasian Gastro-Intestinal Trials Group (AGITG), Trans-Tasman Radiation Oncology Group (TROG), and Australia and New Zealand Breast Cancer Trials Group (ANZBCTG), are based in Australia, but a number of oncologists and research nurses from NZ play an active role within each of these groups.

In 2003, Cancer Trials New Zealand (CTNZ) was established. This is a collaborative group whose main goal is to support investigator-driven research in phase I and II trials in NZ. It assists with concept development, protocol writing, trial development, and central coordination where necessary. CTNZ also is investigating establishing links among and uses for rare tumor registries, national clinical databases, and pathology repositories.

Legal and Regulatory Issues

Before a patient can be registered into a study, the clinical site must have obtained approval for the current protocol, the local information, and the consent form from the relevant ethics committee. Each committee consists of 12 members, half of whom are laypersons. The committee must contain at least two members who have a recognized awareness of *te reo* Māori (the Māori language) and an understanding of *tikanga* Māori (the Māori culture) (HRC, 2002).

Approval is sought in one of two ways. If a study is to be conducted at a single center, an ethics submission is sent to one of the six Regional Ethics Committees. If a study is to be conducted at more than one center, a multiregion application must be completed and sent to the Multiregion Ethics Committee (MEC). The nominated lead center will complete the application and NZ-specific patient information and consent form on behalf of all the centers. This lead center then is responsible for communication between the MECs and the other participating sites.

Along with each ethics submission, the application must contain a signed document from the general manager of each district health board stating that the study has the hospital's approval to be conducted on site and that, as an institution, they have the necessary skills and resources to complete their study obligations (NZ Health and Disability Ethics Committees, 2005).

Before any study has final ethics approval in NZ, the researcher must have received approval from his or her local Maori committee. Each ethics application is sent to the local Maori research advisory committee, which ensures that the study is conducted according to the principles set out in the Treaty of Waitangi, signed February 6, 1840. These principles include the protection, participation, and partnership of Maori. The HRC guidelines (2002) state the following:

> Practices and beliefs of an ethnic and/or religious nature must be fully respected. Research must be undertaken in a culturally sensitive and appropriate manner, in full discussion and partnership with the research participants whatever their ethnicity or religious affiliation. (p. 21)

If an application is made for research involving the clinical trial of a preregistration drug, an application for Standing Committee on Therapeutic Trials (SCOTT) approval is required. This committee provides recommendations to the director-general of health on the scientific validity of applications for clinical trials of new medicines.

Section 30 of the Medicines Act (1981) empowers the director-general of health to allow the use of medicines that have yet to receive approval for registration in NZ in clinical trials for the purpose of obtaining clinical and scientific information. Trials involving postregistration medicines do not require the approval of SCOTT but still undergo the ethics committee review process (NZ Regulatory Guidelines for Medicines, 1998).

Once a study is open, the research nurse must forward any amendment or change to the patient information sheet or protocol to the ethics committee for reapproval before it can be used. Ethics committees require annual progress reports of each study until study completion. The research nurse and principal investigator who are responsible for each particular study compile these.

Protocol Considerations

The processes involved in the decision to take on a new clinical trial vary across centers, but the principles remain the same. New clinical trials are considered when a col-

laborative group or pharmaceutical company approaches oncology centers or investigators. Once a synopsis is received and reviewed, an external feasibility assessment is completed and returned to the group or company. If the study is considered suitable, it is discussed at a clinical trials meeting, which includes oncologists, research staff, pharmacists, radiation therapy staff, and oncology nurses. An internal feasibility assessment then is conducted to look specifically at the scientific question, potential patient numbers, allocation of resources, and research staff time required.

Once a site has received ethics approval, the research nurse must ensure that the regulatory documentation is completed prior to commencing patient recruitment. This includes liaising with the legal department from the relevant district health boards to ensure that the trial is being carried out in accordance with NZ law, including the appropriate indemnity. If the ethics committee decides that the study is not being done for the benefit of a drug manufacturer, the trial's indemnity will be covered under the accident compensation laws of NZ.

The accident compensation scheme provides coverage for injuries and accidents for all NZ citizens, residents, and temporary visitors, no matter who is at fault. This includes participants in a trial. In return, people do not have the right to sue for personal injury, other than for exemplary damages. It is funded by all New Zealanders paying premiums and by the government and is administered by the Accident Compensation Corporation (ACC). This is unique to NZ (ACC, 2005).

A study start-up meeting is organized by the sponsoring organization or company either in person or by teleconference. At the meeting, study-specific procedures are discussed with all relevant staff. This ensures that the trial conforms to the NZ guidelines for good clinical research practice (GCRP).

The NZ GCRP Guidelines are based upon the European Union, United Kingdom, Nordic, Australian, World Health Organization, and Committee for Proprietary Medicinal Products guidelines and codes for GCRP. GCRP guidelines ensure that clinical studies involving human participants are designed and conducted to the highest scientific and ethical standards. The first edition was legislated in September 1996, and the second, current edition was legislated in August 1998.

The research nurse will prepare study documentation, study diaries, and patient information folders and will ensure that all staff members are educated about the specific treatment as outlined in the protocol.

Patient Recruitment

Patients are made aware of current clinical trials through a variety of means, including direct contact with a specialist, information provided by the New Zealand Cancer Society, and Internet resources.

Participants are screened for recruitment in several ways, including the research nurse reviewing all new patient referrals and analyzing the database of the existing patient population. A study then will be offered to potential participants when treatment options are discussed in the clinic setting. The fact that only six main centers exist can present a barrier to recruitment to studies in NZ. This means that patients who live far from these centers, which are based in the six major cities, must agree to travel for all protocol-related procedures and treatment.

All patients with cancer in NZ are, however, equally assured of having health care available should they decline participation in a study.

Eligibility and Informed Consent

Eligibility criteria for each study are clearly stated in the protocol. The research nurse and the principal investigator for each specific study carry out assessment of participant eligibility. Factors assessed include the histologic diagnosis, the medical history, previous treatments, a patient's performance status, and ability to comply with all study requirements. Various tests such as computed tomography scans and blood tests are performed to confirm eligibility. Throughout this process, careful planning and coordination are required to ensure compliance with timeframes stated in the protocol.

Once the eligibility criteria have been met, the study is discussed with the participant, and she or he is given written information to take and discuss with family/*whanau*. (*Whanau* is the Māori word describing the close family links a person has with not just the immediate family but also the extended family of aunts, uncles, grandparents, and so on.) Informed consent is accepted as an ongoing process from the initial visit until completion of the trial. If the patient agrees to take part in the study, the patient and investigator sign a consent form. Special emphasis is placed on the collection of human tissue in NZ, as many Maori believe that their tissue is part of their extended family and they, therefore, do not have the right to consent to it being sent away. Consent forms must contain a choice as to whether patients agree to their tissue being used for research purposes (HRC, 2002; Sporle & Koea, 2004).

Separate guidelines and consents for children exist, and children are required to give their assent to participate where possible. When obtaining consent from older adults, special consideration is given to their comorbidities. Further explanation and time may be required to ensure their full understanding. All participants are encouraged to have a support person with them. Prisoners are treated no differently than the general population (HRC, 2002).

The research nurse performs baseline assessments as per the protocol, as no study-specific tests may be performed before the signing of consent. Education then is given to the patient and his or her family and friends about side effects of concurrent medication, chemotherapy, and treatment. They also are advised of whom to contact in an emergency. At the initial clinic visit and each clinic visit after that, patients are questioned by the investigator

and research nurse on their support network, how they are coping with the treatment, and whether they need help in any areas. Referrals to other disciplines, such as dietitians, social workers, and the palliative care team, are made as required.

Administration of Protocol Agents and Assessments

Drugs are prepared in the hospital pharmacy, with a research oncology pharmacist taking responsibility for the preparation, storage, handling, and distribution of the drug according to study protocols (Occupational Safety and Health Service, 1997).

Once a patient is randomized, he or she is scheduled for treatment, which usually is given in an outpatient setting. Cytotoxic-credentialed nurses administer chemotherapy. If required, the research nurse will take pharmacokinetic and study blood samples, electrocardiograms, and other prespecified tests during treatment.

Before each administration of the study drug, the investigator and oncology research nurse will see the patient in an outpatient clinic. Study-specific requirements will be carried out, blood results reviewed, and toxicities assessed and documented. A decision based on these assessments then will be made regarding continuing, dose modifying, or delaying treatment.

Side effects of treatment are assessed using the United States' National Cancer Institute Cancer Therapy Evaluation Program's (NCI CTEP) Common Terminology Criteria for Adverse Events (NCI CTEP, 2006). Tumor assessments are carried out according to protocol timelines and are reviewed using the Response Evaluation Criteria in Solid Tumors (RECIST). All of this information is recorded in source documentation, which then is used to correctly complete case report forms (CRFs). The District Health Boards and Nursing Council of NZ have strict guidelines on documentation requirements, which must be followed to the detail.

Often a patient will attend his or her first clinic visit armed with the latest information on treatments and care that the individual has found on the Internet. The research nurse is responsible for providing study-specific information that includes education about chemotherapy and its side effects. Written instructions are provided on what to do should the patient become unwell.

Printed booklets, developed in conjunction with the Cancer Society, are given to the patient. These cover a number of areas from general information about chemotherapy to diet and sexuality. The patient also has access to videos on radiation and its side effects. Additionally, the mental and emotional well-being of the patient and the patient's family are addressed by providing information on wig consultants, the "Look Good . . . Feel Better" self-esteem course, accommodations, transportation, and appropriate support groups. For some patients, a referral to a genetic service is made.

Long-Term Follow-Up

Follow-up for a study is determined by the protocol, stating the data to be collected at each visit. All toxicities are followed post-treatment, and if a serious adverse event should occur within 30 days after treatment, it must be reported to the company or sponsoring group. Toxicities considered to be drug related are followed until resolution. Follow-up visits usually take place in the oncology outpatient clinic; however, if a patient is from out of town, visits may take place in a satellite clinic held in smaller cities and towns in NZ.

Any new data or updates on long-term side effects must be provided to the patient at the individual's next follow-up visit. If necessary, the patient will be reconsented, ensuring that he or she has received the information in full. The patient is asked to explain back to the clinical trial nurse what his or her understanding is regarding any new information received.

Ancillary Studies

Increasingly, studies have ancillary components that are part of the main protocol. These may include quality of life, resource use, and optimism questionnaires, many of which are internationally validated tools, such as the European Organisation for Research and Treatment of Cancer quality-of-life questionnaire, the EORTC QLQ-C30. Ethnicity data also are collected on most studies, which then are used to target the future delivery of services.

Data Management Systems

One of the research nurse's main responsibilities is the entry of accurate documentation onto CRFs. The use of electronic CRFs is being studied with some new protocols; however, the majority of studies still use paper CRFs. Because of budget and time constraints, many CRFs are now being sent via e-mail or are downloaded directly from company Web sites. Sponsoring company monitors visit on a regular basis to check that data recorded on CRFs are accurate and of high quality.

Randomization of patients is accomplished either by faxing directly to the sponsor (company or group) or by using a telephone interactive voice recognition system.

Other tools used to assist in the smooth running of clinical trials are newsletters, CRF completion guidelines, data management manuals, patient study diaries, PowerPoint® presentations, and prompt cards for inclusion/exclusion criteria.

Professional Development

The NZ Nurses Organization has a long-established cancer nurses' group and a research nurses' group, both of which hold annual conferences. Both groups provide their members with regular newsletters, online discussion groups and online resources, articles of interest, and access to resources.

The majority of research conferences, study meetings, and ongoing education are held in Australia or elsewhere. However, in 1999, the NZ Haematology/Oncology Research Coordinators held its first meeting, and in 2004, the NZ Association of Clinical Research held its inaugural conference. Both of these meetings are now annual events.

NZ has a small population (4,238,879) (Statistics New Zealand, n.d.) and, as yet, has no postgraduate courses targeted specifically to clinical research. A number of options for continuing education are available to oncology nurses, including postgraduate diplomas in oncology and hematology nursing, courses in cytotoxic credentialing, and local in-service education. Further opportunities are expected to become available to research nurses and coordinators as cancer clinical trial research continues to expand in coming years.

Summary

Although NZ is a small country, its goals in relation to cancer research are the same as those worldwide: to improve the quality of care for those with cancer and to reduce the incidence and impact of cancer. With the development of better communication systems and worldwide research, people in NZ can have access to the same treatment as those overseas.

The role of a research nurse is both fulfilling and rewarding for the author. It is fulfilling in that no two days are the same, whether it is giving education, completing electronic CRFs, or designing patient information sheets; it is rewarding in being able to actively contribute to improving a patient's care and treatment.

The author would like to acknowledge and thank the following contributors: Anne Smith, RN, BA, Melanie Roberts, BN, Liz Thompson, RN, and Wendy Bourke, RN.

References

Accident Compensation Corporation. (2005). *About ACC.* Wellington, NZ: Health Research Council of New Zealand. Retrieved March 1, 2006, from http://www.acc.co.nz/about-acc/index.htm

Health Research Council of New Zealand. (2002). *Guidelines on ethics in health research.* Wellington, NZ: Author. Retrieved March 1, 2006, from http://www.hrc.govt.nz/assets/pdfs/ethgdlns.pdf

Ministry of Health. (n.d.). *Cancer control in New Zealand.* Retrieved May 12, 2005, from http://www.moh.govt.nz/cancercontrol

National Cancer Institute Cancer Therapy Evaluation Program. (2006). *Common terminology criteria for adverse events* (version 3.0). Bethesda, MD: National Cancer Institute. Retrieved May 27, 2005, from http://www.ctep.cancer.gov/reporting/ctc_v30.html

New Zealand Health and Disability Ethics Committees. (n.d.). *Application forms and guidelines.* Retrieved May 12, 2005, from http://www.newhealth.govt.nz/ethicscommittees/application.htm#Māori

New Zealand Regulatory Guidelines for Medicines. (1998). *Interim good clinical research practice guideline* (Vol. 3). Retrieved March 15, 2006, from http://www.medsafe.govt.nz/regulatory/guideline/medicines.asp

Occupational Safety and Health Service. (1997). *Guidelines for the safe handling of cytotoxic drugs and related waste.* Wellington, NZ: Department of Labour. Retrieved March 15, 2006, from http://www.osh.govt.nz/order/catalogue/pdf/cytodrug.pdf

Sporle, A., & Koea, J. (2004). Maori responsiveness in health and medical research: Key issues for researchers. *New Zealand Medical Journal, 117*, 1199.

Statistics New Zealand. (n.d.). *Population.* Retrieved October 17, 2007, from http://www.stats.govt.nz/people/population/default .htm

About the Author

Belinda Egan, RN, is an oncology research nurse at Christchurch Hospital in New Zealand. Her background includes 10 years working in a pediatric oncology ward, two years as a district palliative care nurse, four years working in the oncology outpatient department at Christchurch Hospital, and more recently, three-and-a-half years as an oncology research nurse specialist. She has completed a number of oncology and palliative care nursing courses and recently completed a University of Sydney postgraduate diploma in clinical data management. She is married with two children.

CHAPTER 56
Canada

Monica Bacon, RN

Background

The National Cancer Institute of Canada (NCIC) was founded in 1947 to conduct cancer research programs on behalf of the Canadian Cancer Society (CCS) and to provide funding for the majority of Canadian cancer research. Clinical trials supported by the NCIC began in the early 1970s, and an independent Clinical Trials Group (CTG) was created in 1977. The NCIC conducts site reviews (e.g., operations, data management, statistics) every five years at the CTG operations and statistics headquarters at Queen's University in Kingston, Ontario. The CTG conducts phase I and II investigational new drug (IND) and phase III adult cancer clinical trials in hematologic and solid tumors.

Quality of life (QOL), symptom control, economics, biologic markers, nursing, and methodology have joined standard end points (i.e., toxicity, response, and survival) in CTG phase III studies. These trials are managed with centralized trial teams composed of clinical trial assistants (CTAs), research associates (RAs), study coordinators (SCs), physician coordinators (PCs), and biostatisticians (Koski, 1998a), who are responsible for study conduct from protocol development through publication of results (NCIC, 1993, 1995, 1997).

As a private foundation, the NCIC is funded by charitable donations (primarily the CCS) and is not governed by political forces. The CTG grant is renewed per NCIC audits. Canadian centers participating in CTG studies are funded to offset costs (e.g., data management) on a per-eligible-case basis.

National centralization of medical care ensures basic health care and insurance for all Canadians, whereas the care delivery policies (e.g., drug formulary) are determined by the individual provinces and local communities. As well as *equal access* to health care, Canada is officially a bilingual country, operating in French and English. *Ethnic background* information is collected unless prohibited by local or regional regulations.

Although the CTG has not provided nursing summaries for protocols, trial teams provide trial-specific data management guidebooks, pocket reference cards, and current newsletters. The CTG has included nursing research questions as companions to large, randomized clinical trials (Bacon et al., 1996). The NCIC CTG has been extremely supportive in the founding and ongoing development of its Clinical Trial Nurses Special Interest Group (SIG).

Protocol Development

Ideas for new cancer clinical trials come from many varied sources (e.g., existing, pilot, or IND study results; intergroup or industry proposals). CTG disease-site committees are responsible for assessing the scientific merit and feasibility of proposals. Central office trial team members interact with the site committee in concept evaluation and study design and often survey centers for interest. If the site committee recommends proceeding, the concept then is considered by the Clinical Trials Committee (CTG executive committee), which ranks all proposals and approves only those that are of defined scientific merit and are able to be supported through available resources.

The study chair writes protocols and is assisted by the trial writing committee and the CTG trial team (Paul, 1992). In industry-sponsored studies and intergroup trials, input is received from representatives. The starting point is the CTG generic protocol (Koski, 1998a), which reflects the most current policies and procedures and provides a comprehensive blueprint to ensure complete content and consistent format. The protocol is the master reference document, which serves as a manual for the conduct of the study. It provides all information needed to enroll, treat, follow, and record the clinical course of trial participants (see www.ctg.queensu.ca for more information).

Concurrently, case report forms (CRFs) are developed to meet the data requirements of a given trial while using CTG generic models for consistency (Koski, 1997; Wainman, 1994). The same CTG generic module system is applied to the creation of the sample informed consent for each trial, thus ensuring that all required elements are included and explained at a common reading level (see www.ctg.queensu.ca).

The CTG generic protocol and forms module have allowed for a standardized Oracle® database dictionary (Pho & Koski, 1998), SAS® (Statistical Analysis System) variable names, data-checking programs (Day, 1997), and analysis across trials.

During protocol development, the senior biostatistician develops the statistical section and, with other trial team members, determines the appropriate randomization procedure based on stratification factors, sample size, and whether the study is blinded.

Trial-specific policies regarding *publication and authorship* are determined and included in the protocol. Generally, the CTG considers scientific input (from the study chair and writing committee) and activity (from the trial team and participants' accrual) in the criteria.

Although recognizing that honest errors can occur, the CTG has internal and external monitoring programs to safeguard, as much as possible, against fraud. This will be discussed further in the Quality Assurance section of this chapter.

Preparation

NCIC CTG trials are subject to regulations from various groups, including

- Therapeutic Products Directorate (TPD) of Health and Welfare Canada
- U.S. Food and Drug Administration
- U.S. Office for Human Research Protections (OHRP)
- National Cancer Institute (NCI) Cancer Therapy Evaluation Program (CTEP).

The agency involved depends on the nature of the study (e.g., the TPD if investigational agents are used; OHRP and CTEP if the United States is involved).

CTG trials are centrally activated (i.e., protocol and required documents are sent to centers) once the appropriate regulatory body approves the final protocol. All NCIC CTG member centers have local ethics committees and research ethics boards (REBs) established according to national guidelines. Evidence of local REB approval (protocol and consent), a participants list (including delegation of responsibilities and signatures), and other trial-specific administrative documents must be received, reviewed, and approved at the central office prior to *local activation* (accrual initiation) of a member center. Some centers require double ethics approval (e.g., affiliated university and local cancer center), and others submit to various local committees (e.g., nursing, pharmacy) for resource impact evaluation.

Industry-sponsored studies add extra regulatory concerns such as contracts, defined roles and responsibilities, additional serious adverse event (SAE) reporting classifications, extra monitoring, varied per-case funding, specific processes for drug availability, and increased data collection.

International intergroup studies have their own added complexities. For example, in trials affected by U.S. legis-

lation, Canadian centers must have cooperative project assurance and federalwide assurance numbers (issued by the OHRP) in order to participate. They also must have an REB constituted per U.S. guidelines. For trials led by the European Organisation for Research and Treatment of Cancer (EORTC), Canadian centers must submit ethics documentation to be issued an EORTC identification number and meet other requirements of the lead group (e.g., radiation therapy, quality assurance).

When the CTG is involved in intergroup studies (lead/coordinating or participant), every effort is made during protocol development to incorporate attention and allowances for national differences. These include variations in time zones, lab measurements, weights and measures, ethnic influences, adverse event reporting/adverse drug reactions, SAE reporting, language barriers, and accepted standards of treatment.

Because requirements vary among national health systems, consideration should be given to matters of insurance coverage, indemnification, confidentiality, and funding of participating centers. Matters concerning shipment of drugs, documents, x-rays, and body samples become complex issues when international borders and customs inspections are involved.

When Canadian centers participate in an intergroup study, the CTG central office is the conduit to and from the lead/coordinating group for registrations, questions, form flow, queries, and reminders. Although the lead/coordinating group may have differing policies, CTG centers also must abide by CTG policies.

The local REB is responsible for initial review and approval of all protocol and consent forms (Paul, 1997). During the course of the trial, revisions (i.e., administrative clarifications or modifications) and amendments must be brought to the attention of the REB, as well as all involved regulatory bodies and sponsors. Canadian centers are sent amended pages for insertion into the protocol. All centers are expected to submit proof of REB review for amendments as well as annual overall reapproval for CTG studies that are open to accrual. Once closed, REB approvals may be reviewed during local site audits. Local and trial-specific SAEs are summarized and also are reported to local REBs.

The compassionate release of drugs by pharmaceutical company sponsors is required less often in Canada than in the United States because of the country's national health coverage, but differences in regional formulary approvals do lead to some requests. Canadian rules for pharmacy management in receiving, storing, preparing, disposing of, and accounting for investigational drugs (including placebos and blinding) are equal to those of the United States.

Canadian centers evaluate the impact on resources before locally activating a study. Included in the assessments are staff (e.g., clinical research associates [CRAs], nurses, pathologists, pharmacists, radiologists), education (e.g., new skills/knowledge, policies and procedures), equipment, and hospital inpatients versus outpatients. Of particular concern are the effects on the resources of the system if the protocol requires more than the standard number or type of medications, lab tests, or other investigations and assessment visits for the study population. These factors can become obstacles to implementation.

Sometimes, the CTG will have start-up meetings for principal investigators (PIs) and CRAs, during which the basics of the study are taught. Otherwise, education related to study activity may be provided by a Web-based slide set. Trial workshops are presented, and opportunities for education abound at all site committee sessions where studies are addressed. The central office team and the local participating investigators and CRAs must address not only the skills and knowledge base related toward studies but also the attitudes of staff, patients, and families to research and components of the studies. The CTG provides educational materials and tools to the centers to facilitate local efforts (Paul et al., 1994). Increasingly, the education must extend to community bases as treatment and follow-up become geographically more suitable to patients.

Despite the national healthcare system in Canada, which covers all basic medical expenses, Canadian patients who participate in clinical trials are affected financially by loss of work, transportation needs, ancillary drug costs, and hidden costs such as unexpected child care/babysitting needs.

Promotion/Recruitment

NCIC CTG studies usually are distributed to all Canadian member centers (approximately 80 exist) for consideration unless restricted by protocol (e.g., IND), sponsor, or intergroup criteria. The local center representative and contact CRA receive these initial circulations for review and discussion with the appropriate investigators and other resources (e.g., pharmacy). The discussions often will extend to regional referring specialists (e.g., urologists, general practitioners), satellite treatment centers, and community clinics to assess interest and capabilities of the entire interdisciplinary team. Because Canadian cancer centers are connected under the CTG umbrella, potential future patient movement may be facilitated through another participating center.

Public and client education efforts in Canada are comparable to those in the United States. Because of the differences in healthcare systems, Canadian strategies for promotion and recruitment to clinical trials are focused more toward the medical community than the public. The public increasingly is using the Internet and disease-specific advocacy groups as resources in searching for information on the most up-to-date therapy.

The Canadian healthcare system provides equal access to basic health care for all Canadians. It is possible that the geography of the country would hinder access for outlying populations (especially northern residents), but referrals to cancer treatment centers capture those populations. Most importantly, all Canadian patients with cancer are equally assured of having health care available should they refuse the offer of clinical trial participation.

Eligibility

All CTG protocols clearly state the eligibility criteria for the study. Informed consent (as approved by the REB) must be obtained from each patient. Laboratory, x-ray, and other baseline tests must be obtained within the protocol-dictated time frames and within specified acceptable limits. Although the healthcare system guarantees coverage of the basic testing, patients' private insurance might be accessed for coverage for particular drugs, equipment, or other trial-specific extras.

Overall competence, health history, performance status, and geographic availability are evaluated, and diagnostic requirements are verified (e.g., pathology, stage, baseline symptoms). QOL assessment, if it is a component of the protocol, generally is mandatory unless the patient is truly incapable of providing the information (e.g., is illiterate in French or English). Canadian law requires that all patient materials be available in French and English (e.g., consent, questionnaires, diaries). NCIC CTG attempts to enforce a policy of allowing no exceptions to the eligibility criteria. Should there be a concrete, valid explanation for a request for an individual exception, the trial-specific SC and the PC review it at the central office prior to granting a waiver, which rarely is done (Koski, 1998b).

The trial-specific CTA (via the electronic NCIC CTG registration/randomization system called MANGO) completely verifies the eligibility checklist for every request for registration/randomization. This interactive process allows for clarifications, questions, and corrections; SCs and PCs are available if needed. The checklist verifies REB approval dates, eligibility criteria, and body surface area (BSA)/dose calculations and assignments. A study by CTAs (Sears et al., 1998) proved the benefit of the process in preventing ineligible accrual and providing education to both randomizing centers and central office trial teams. Although full checking may not be the policy of other groups, Canadian centers must participate in this interactive procedure for all registrations and randomizations requested through the CTG.

Baseline CRFs must be received within protocol-specified time frames and accompanied by copies of patients' signed consents, QOL questionnaires, and supporting documentation (e.g., lab and x-ray reports). The review of these documents and handling of central review materials (e.g., pathology, radiotherapy) are described in the Quality Assurance section of this chapter.

Active Treatment

Investigational agents for the NCIC CTG trials are procured either from the U.S. NCI or from a sponsoring pharmaceutical company. These may be shipped via CTG or directly to the centers. When a drug is supplied, centers identify a local or designated pharmacist on the trial-specific participant's lists. The pharmacist accepts responsibility with the CTG for receipt, storage, preparation, handling, disposal, and accountability according to agent-specific criteria.

Treatment is *blinded* by using an inactive compound (placebo) with the same appearance and management as the investigational agent when knowledge of treatment assignment might influence reported outcomes.

The CTG has an active pharmacy network committee with representation from all provinces. This network provides representatives to all disease-site committees and the Quality Assurance Committee and thus is involved in study proposal discussions and review of protocols. The representatives often create trial-specific information materials for use by pharmacists at participating centers. The network developed a pharmacists' clinical trials manual (Nakashima, Lin, & McBride, 1996) that gives clear explanations and descriptions of required criteria for locally involved pharmacists.

The protocol, including revisions and amendments, serves as the ultimate guide for proper study conduct. In CTG studies, the BSA is calculated at randomization (based on the DuBois method) using actual, not ideal, weight in kg unless the protocol states otherwise. Dose adjustments resulting from variations in the BSA throughout the patient's course are not required but are allowed. Blood values and other parameters (e.g., response) must be checked at each cycle prior to treatment and may require conversion to compare with protocol units/measures.

The protocol-dictated supplemental treatment (e.g., premedications, hydration, electrolytes) may be substituted with equivalents (with CTG permission) because of local nonavailability. The actual protocol agents under study may not be substituted, and dose modifications and treatment delays/discontinuations are as per protocol. The treating physicians and nurses confirm accurate dosing, timing, and route.

During treatment, patients are assessed for reactions, and expert oncology nurses provide emergency interventions if needed (Koski, Hale, & Bacon, 1994). Throughout the treatment phase of the study, SAEs are reported by telephone, and CTG SAE report forms are sent to the central office, local REB, and any other regulatory agencies as per protocol. Although 24-hour notifications may be impossible when events occur at a geographical distance and information is delayed from arriving at the participating center, reports are expected as quickly as possible.

For studies activated prior to March 1998, SAEs, toxicity symptoms, and hypersensitivity reactions were assessed according to the NCIC CTG Expanded Common Toxicity Criteria (Eisenhauer, Muldal, & Wainman, 1994), which provides detailed symptom identification categories and grading descriptions. The local investigator is responsible for reporting the relationship of all these side effects.

In 1997 and 2002, delegates from the NCIC CTG joined others from a multitude of American and international cooperative groups to participate in U.S. NCI-led initiatives to develop International Common Toxicity Criteria (NCI CTEP, 2003). Because all of the NCIC CTG Expanded CTC toxicities and grades were incorporated into the new collection with the expectation that they would vastly improve collaborative studies (and facilitate meta-analyses), the NCIC CTG began to implement the International Common Toxicity Criteria (version 2.0) in March 1998, which was renamed and implemented as the Common Terminology Criteria for Adverse Events (version 3.0) in 2003 (NCI CTEP, 1998, 2003).

Performance status is reported according to the scale identified in the protocol. Exact details of the treatment administered are collected from the CRFs and patients' diaries. Response assessments are performed at required intervals using specified measurement methods (e.g., computed tomography scan). All sites reported at baseline are reevaluated by the same technique throughout the study. Occasionally, the protocol imposes assessment definitions (e.g., Response Evaluation Criteria in Solid Tumors [known as RECIST] criteria), and those specified in the protocol must be followed.

Throughout the study (both on treatment and during follow-up), symptoms must continue to be reported and managed. Some of the physical side effects of systemic chemotherapy are long-term and irreversible. Similarly, toxicities from radiation therapy include acute and late reactions. Symptoms resulting from surgery, bone marrow transplant, biologic response modifiers, hormones, immunotherapy, gene therapy, and various modality combinations are known as acute but long-term effects and need to be documented and studied. Whether the symptoms result from the treatment or from the cancer must be clarified. The NCIC CTG shares this toxicity information with the U.S. NCI and other groups to ensure that united surveillance of emerging new and unexpected toxicity data may be complete.

Psychosocial side effects (e.g., fertility, sexuality, financial, employment) and interdisciplinary interventions (e.g., support strategies) are comparable to those in the United States and are assessed at each clinic visit by the nurse, social worker, or investigator. The approaches to patient/family education about treatment, side effects, and management strategies are also addressed.

Every CTG protocol includes a table outlining the schedule of expected CRF submissions (including accompaniments) and tables outlining expected tests and intervals. The documentation in the patient's medical record should provide all required information for the CTG CRFs. All members of the local interdisciplinary team must provide complete documentation in the patient's medical record (Paul et al., 1994).

Ancillary Studies

The NCIC CTG is committed to include a QOL component to all phase III studies unless the QOL committee deems this to be inappropriate (e.g., trial-specific). The QOL requirements are included in the eligibility criteria, and patients are excused only if they are incapable of completing the questionnaire (e.g., if they are illiterate in French or English). The QOL hypothesis is fully described in the protocol along with the schedule and specific instrument, usually EORTC QLQ 30 (plus site-specific modules). The consent form also contains QOL information. QOL compliance among Canadian patients has proved to be very good, with the local nursing staff recognized as bearing a large part of the responsibility and burden for facilitating proper data collection.

Nursing studies have been companioned to large NCIC CTG clinical trials. This collaboration has proved to be an excellent teaming of scientific and practical resources (e.g., data collection and entry, databases, analyses). A large ovarian cancer trial provided the opportunity for clinical trial nurses to gather gynecologic history data from the patients in a search for influences to toxicity outcomes that may guide preventive nursing management (Bacon et al., 1996). Economic, pharmacology, molecular biology, sexual health, and other companion studies have successfully teamed resources to examine interrelated questions. Admittedly, additional research questions add to the workload—particularly the length and breadth of CRFs and questionnaires. However, nurses have responded positively in their willingness to assist in the search for these interconnected answers (Bacon, 1994).

Off-Treatment Follow-Up

The CTG protocol clearly outlines the plan for follow-up, including the flow of forms. The patient's signed informed consent continues to be in effect, and important safety/toxicity discoveries during the trial are updated in the consent and patient notification. In Canada, all participating centers must submit proof of REB annual reapproval to the CTG as long as a trial is accruing patients. Thereafter, annual REB approvals, as long as data are being submitted, may be reviewed at the time of local site audits. If a non-Canadian group leads the study, the rules of the lead group regarding ongoing REB approval must be followed.

Increased feasibility of compliance to the follow-up schedule and requirements is possible through case transfers to other activated CTG member centers in instances of patient relocation. Centers are expected to make every effort to fulfill the follow-up reporting required to complete the (survival) analyses. Psychosocial issues, especially survivorship, do not differ from those in the United States.

Quality Assurance

To participate in NCIC CTG clinical trials, Canadian cancer centers must meet certain terms outlined in the "center agreement," or contract. CTG business is relayed through each center's representative and contact CRA; trial-specific business is relayed through the local PI and principal CRA. All PIs' curricula vitae must be approved by the CTG executive director and kept on file at the central office. For certain

studies, investigator agreements and proof of local lab and other accreditations are required.

Once a CTG trial has been centrally activated, the protocol is distributed to centers for consideration. Local activation occurs when a center has provided to the central office proof of REB approval of protocol and consent, the local participants list, curricula vitae, and other trial-specific documents that the trial SC has reviewed and approved. The local consent is compared with the protocol sample to ensure that all mandatory elements are present; centers are asked to amend any deficiencies.

Once locally activated, centers may request registrations and randomizations through the CTG central office. This is an interactive process, with the CTA verifying the eligibility via the MANGO system, including REB date, BSA and dose calculations, and treatment assignment. The center receives e-mail confirmation of allocation.

The SC and RA review baseline forms and supporting documents, including a copy of the signed consent, to confirm patient eligibility and authorize per-case funding. This review includes accompanying companion forms such as QOL questionnaires. If inconsistencies exist in the initial checklist, the centers are queried for clarification. The results may be recorded as deviations, stratification errors, or even retroactive ineligibility resulting from honest mistakes at the time of randomization. The SC also oversees and ensures any required central reviews (e.g., designated local reference pathologist review, central pathology review, surgical review, centralized real-time and final radiotherapy review, specimen collections).

Internal monitoring continues throughout the study, with SCs and RAs reviewing all CRFs and supporting documentation for proof of protocol compliance and questioning any inconsistencies or missing information. CTAs enter the data, and hard-copy print-outs are verified. Data submission is assessed for accuracy and timeliness. PCs may be consulted to resolve problems, and data-checking programs are run regularly to pinpoint inaccuracies.

The centers receive reminders for late CRFs and ethics documents. A Centre Performance Index, which monitors ineligibility, accrual, timeliness of data submission, and SAE reporting, is run and circulated to centers every six months and published in the CTG meeting book annually by the Audit/Monitoring Group. If minimum standards (i.e., eligibility ≥ 90% overall and ≥ 75% per trial; ≥ 75% of forms within time frames) are not met, centers receive a notification, warnings, and sometimes a suspension of trial privileges.

The CTG Audit/Monitoring Group office operates the external on-site monitoring program (Koski, 1996). An audit team visits all CTG centers at least every three years. The objectives of the audit team are to verify ethics, regulatory documents, and the informed consent process, examine study drug storage and accountability, ensure that current protocols are in use, and compare reported data with the medical record. A sampling of cases is reviewed for consent, eligibility, treatment, investigations, and response (using original radiology films), to confirm completeness, accuracy, and verifiability of data. Audit reports are sent to the center and regulatory bodies. Any audit findings for individual cases that will affect a trial database are forwarded to the lead/coordinating group. Standard CTG on-site audits focus on monitoring the center (as opposed to the sponsor's monitoring of all trial-specific cases).

Centers are expected to archive study patients' files, although the length of time required varies with the use of an investigational agent, the pharmaceutical company sponsor's policy, and routine. CTG studies that are sponsored by pharmaceutical companies or other cooperative groups often include frequent on-site monitoring visits by the industry/group representative(s).

Occasionally, CTG studies will include a final central radiology review of responders (Eisenhauer, Bacon, et al., 1994). This requires the centers to forward copies of all response assessment investigations (e.g., computed tomography films) performed throughout the study and can be a complicated extra workload for the related departments.

The Data Safety Monitoring Committee (DSMC) is composed of physicians, biostatisticians, ethicists, survivors (none can be members of the CTG), and liaison members (e.g., CTEP) for intergroup representation. The committee meets twice a year to review trial reports and conducts interim analyses when scheduled. The DSMC advises the CTG on matters related to ethics and safety of enrolled patients, including issues such as toxicities, recommended changes to protocols, and early termination considerations.

Environmental Safety

Although the agencies governing the handling of cytotoxic agents or bodily specimens are Canadian, the basic rules for safety mirror those of the United States. All handlers involved in the shipping, storage, administration, and disposal of these potentially hazardous materials observe universal precautions. The Canadian Guidelines for Handling and Disposal of Cytotoxic Drugs (which are the same as the Occupational Safety and Health Administration guidelines) govern the preparation and transport of these agents. Extra consideration must be given to labeling, packaging, timeliness, and expense when these agents or specimens are destined to cross international borders. Similarly, protection of staff and patients against radiation exposure is a priority. The key to a safe environment exists in the education of staff, patients, and families to eliminate risks and mythical fears.

Ethics

Canadian ethical standards have their historical origins in the Nuremberg Code (Trials of War Criminals, 1949) and the Declaration of Helsinki (World Medical Association, 1964). Of particular importance is the informed consent process. Although centers' REBs may modify the CTG pro-

tocol's sample consent to satisfy local regulations, certain mandatory elements required by national authorities must remain unchanged. Some clauses may not seem pertinent but still must remain. For example, issues of compensation, which are mandatory in the United States, are less relevant for Canadian participants but are required in the context of United States–CTG intergroup studies. In Canada, consent forms must be available in French and English and must use language that is comprehensible to the layperson. If further interpretation is necessary, this must be documented on the consent form and in the medical record. Local and regional regulations always supplement the protocol in issues such as the age of consent (e.g., age 14 in Quebec) and competence. Children are not required to sign a written assent; their parents' consent is required. Issues regarding older adults and prisoners are handled the same as in the United States.

Authorship and ownership issues are determined prior to trial activation and are described in the CTG protocol. Papers reporting CTG research results are evaluated for ethical standards before they are submitted to peer-reviewed journals for publication. The CTG's ability to carry out clinical trials (including IND, pharmaceutical company–sponsored, and intergroup studies) is dependent upon being assured that data from individual participants will not be reported or published separately. In a multicenter, multidisciplinary study, the validity of the results depends upon the maintenance of the integrity of the entire database.

To participate in collaborative clinical research, Canadian oncology nurses must be aware of the relevant ethical rules and safeguard their collegial responsibilities, especially in their role as patient and family advocates.

Data Management Tools and Systems

Accurate and timely data collection and management are crucial to the successful completion of cancer clinical trials (Paul et al., 1994). The CTG protocol, as the principal document, includes clear guidelines for the content and timing of data collection. CTG CRFs historically were provided on layered no-carbon-required paper from the central office to all participating Canadian centers, which guaranteed exact duplication. With the upsurge in automated data management options, recent CTG studies have begun to use direct data entry, remote data entry, datafax, and other methods. These tools increasingly are being used in Canada, and on-site training and development is popular among clinical trial nurses.

At the time of local activation, CTG centers receive patient-logging materials, eligibility-screening forms, QOL questionnaires, patient diaries and/or calendars, Common Terminology Criteria for Adverse Events (version 3.0) booklets, and any other trial-specific instruments (e.g., pocket reference cards). Certain complicated studies also are accompanied by data management guidebooks. Trial-specific newsletters are sent out periodically to update participants on items of interest.

More often, these materials are being provided on trial-specific Web sites. Many CTG studies involve a start-up education session that includes particular instructions related to data management. The annual NCIC CTG meeting always includes data management sessions and workshops. The standard resource for clinical trial nurses and CRAs is the CTG *Data Management Manual* (Paul et al., 1994), which is provided to all participating centers.

The NCIC CTG has a very active CRA committee, as illustrated in its *Goals and Objectives* publication (NCIC Data Management Committee, 1998). This committee's steering group oversees subcommittees involved with education and management, Ethics/Regulatory Affairs, Audit/Monitoring Group, manual updating, representation on all CTG site (e.g., breast) and modality committees, liaisons with clinical trial nurses and pharmacists, reviews of protocols and forms, and representation on the Clinical Trials Committee (the CTG Executive Board), as well as annual meetings and educational sessions for all CRAs. Thus, data management issues have multiple opportunities to be systematically addressed. Canadian clinical trial nurses are integral members of this group.

Information Systems and Resources

Similar to the American cooperative groups, NCIC CTG has established a Web site (www.ctg.queensu.ca) that includes information about the group and its research activities. Some Canadian cancer research centers also have developed Web sites to disseminate information via the Internet to prospective partner participants. More and more networking and communication among the CTG and both Canadian members and international colleagues are occurring via the Internet and e-mail. In general, the explosion in the use of electronic information systems and resources in Canada mirrors the experience in the United States. A national trial registry for Canadian patients is not necessary, as all Canadian trials are included in NCI's Physician Data Query database (known as PDQ®).

Professional Development

An increasing number of Canadian centers are recognizing the need for educational opportunities for nurses who are involved in research. These include not only cancer-center staff but also community and outpost nurses to ensure continuity of care. Clinical trial nurses often are educators and supporters to an ever-widening breadth of nurses working with patients and families who are involved in cancer clinical trials.

Canadian clinical trial nurses frequently perform a dual role as nurse and data manager/CRA. Thus, responsibilities extend to include accrual issues, documentation, form flow, patient scheduling, compliance management, and administrative duties. If not functioning as a CRA, the clinical trial nurse needs to develop team approaches with the CRA to best serve his or her particular locale and clientele. In the current Canadian climate of economic restraint and health-care restructuring, Canadian clinical trial nurses' activities toward role justification are in the forefront.

Commonly, clinical trial nurses are members of the Canadian Association of Nurses in Oncology (CANO) and actively contribute to its *Canadian Oncology Nursing Journal (CONJ)*. The Canadian Clinical Trial Nurses SIG was founded in 1993 and had 240 members as of 2006. Annual meetings and educational sessions are held in conjunction with and are supported by the NCIC CTG.

Some Canadian clinical trial nurses belong to American professional organizations, such as the Oncology Nursing Society (ONS) and its Clinical Trial Nurses SIG, the Society of Gynecologic Nurse Oncologists, and nursing committees of groups (e.g., Pediatric Oncology Group, National Surgical Adjuvant Breast and Bowel Project). Professional opportunities for Canadian nurses also include Canadian chapters of the Society of Clinical Research Associates and the Association of Clinical Research Professionals.

Opportunities for educational development for Canadian clinical trial nurses are available through the NCIC CTG, CANO (e.g., certification), hospital-based seminars, community college programs, and cooperative group meetings. In recent years, Canadian university nursing schools have evolved to include oncology-specific programs with increased emphasis on research (e.g., McMaster University in Hamilton, Ontario).

Summary

Clinical trial nurses share significantly in the clinical trial process in Canada. They assume multiple roles in ensuring the integrity of clinical trials and the safety of patients in those trials. Clinical trial nurses have presented and published widely both at home (e.g., *CONJ*, CANO conferences) and abroad (e.g., international cancer nursing conferences, ONS, American Society of Clinical Oncology, European Cancer Conference, Multinational Association of Supportive Care in Cancer, European ONS, Society for Clinical Trials). Clinical trial nurses are ever-vigilant in promoting the understanding and worthiness of multiple facets of their evolving roles.

The author would like to acknowledge Carrie Goudreau for typing and technical support, as well as Belinda Vandersluis, NCIC CTG Operations, and Bev Koski, NCIC CTG Quality Assurance, for their insightful reviews.

References

Bacon, M. (1994). Impact and opportunities of clinical trials for cancer nursing. In *Proceedings of the 8th International Conference on Cancer Nursing* (p. 8). Toronto, ON, Canada: Canadian Association of Nurses in Oncology.

Bacon, M., Myles, J., Fiander, W., Green, D., Craig, C., Papakonstationou, C., et al. (1996). Do pre-existing biologic characteristics influence chemotoxicities and, thus, nursing interventions? In *Proceedings of the 9th International Conference on Cancer Nursing* (p. 120). London: Royal College of Nursing.

Day, A. (1997). *SAS data checking system.* Kingston, ON, Canada: National Cancer Institute of Canada Clinical Trials Group.

Eisenhauer, E., Bacon, M., Atri, M., Lemort, M., Nolan, R., Petroons, P., et al. (1994). Radiologic review of response in ovarian cancer. *Proceedings of the American Society of Clinical Oncology, 13,* 257.

Eisenhauer, E., Muldal, A., & Wainman, N. (1994). *Expanded common toxicity criteria.* Kingston, ON, Canada: National Cancer Institute of Canada Clinical Trials Group.

Koski, B. (1996). *Guidelines for monitoring a QA document.* Kingston, ON, Canada: National Cancer Institute of Canada Clinical Trials Group.

Koski, B. (1997). *Generic forms module.* Kingston, ON, Canada: National Cancer Institute of Canada Clinical Trials Group.

Koski, B. (1998a). *Generic protocol module.* Kingston, ON, Canada: National Cancer Institute of Canada Clinical Trials Group.

Koski, B. (1998b). *Standard operating procedures.* Kingston, ON, Canada: National Cancer Institute of Canada Clinical Trials Group.

Koski, T., Hale, B., & Bacon, M. (1994). The evolving role of the clinical trials specialty nurse. In *Proceedings of the 8th International Conference on Cancer Nursing* (p. 38). Toronto, ON, Canada: Canadian Association of Nurses in Oncology.

Nakashima, L., Lin, J., & McBride, J. (1996). *Pharmacists network manual.* Kingston, ON, Canada: National Cancer Institute of Canada Clinical Trials Group.

National Cancer Institute Cancer Therapy Evaluation Program. (1998). *Common toxicity criteria* (version 2.0). Bethesda, MD: National Cancer Institute.

National Cancer Institute Cancer Therapy Evaluation Program. (2003). *Common terminology criteria for adverse events* (version 3.0). Bethesda, MD: National Cancer Institute.

National Cancer Institute of Canada. (1993). *Study coordinators manual.* Kingston, ON, Canada: National Cancer Institute of Canada Clinical Trials Group.

National Cancer Institute of Canada. (1995). *Clinical trials assistant manual.* Kingston, ON, Canada: National Cancer Institute of Canada Clinical Trials Group.

National Cancer Institute of Canada. (1997). *Computing team manual.* Kingston, ON, Canada: National Cancer Institute of Canada Clinical Trials Group.

National Cancer Institute of Canada Data Management Committee. (1998). *Goals and objectives.* Kingston, ON, Canada: National Cancer Institute of Canada Clinical Trials Group.

Paul, N. (1992). *Participants manual.* Kingston, ON, Canada: National Cancer Institute of Canada Clinical Trials Group.

Paul, N. (1997). *Requirements for local REB approval of studies.* Kingston, ON, Canada: National Cancer Institute of Canada Clinical Trials Group.

Paul, N., Smuck, B., Roche, K., Dionne, J., Bettello, P., Muldal, A., et al. (1994). *Data management manual.* Kingston, ON, Canada: National Cancer Institute of Canada Clinical Trials Group.

Pho, L., & Koski, B. (1998). *Oracle database dictionary (ODD).* Kingston, ON, Canada: National Cancer Institute of Canada Clinical Trials Group.

Sears, C., Mak, M., Bacon, M., Soroka, D., Dickson, M., Clark, A., et al. (1998). What is the utility of eligibility checklist screening [Abstract]? *Controlled Clinical Trials, 19*(Suppl. 3), S96.

Trials of war criminals before the Nuremberg military tribunals under control council law No. 10 (Vol. 2, pp. 181–182). (1949). Washington, DC: U.S. Government Printing Office. Retrieved May 16, 2007, from http://www.hhs.gov/ohrp/references/nurcode.htm

Wainman, N. (1994). *Data managers guide to IND standard forms.* Kingston, Canada: National Cancer Institute of Canada Clinical Trials Group.

World Medical Association. (1964). *The Declaration of Helsinki: Ethical principles for medical research involving human subjects.* Retrieved May 16, 2007, from http://www.wma.net/e/policy/b3.htm

About the Author

Monica Bacon, RN, graduated from the Royal Victoria Hospital School of Nursing in Montreal in 1969. Oncology nursing positions held by Ms. Bacon over the following 20 years in Montreal, Canada, and Vermont, United States, included various sites (e.g., breast, gynaecology), modalities (e.g., screening, treatment), and roles/responsibilities (e.g., beside, clinic, unit management, education). Since 1991, she has been employed as a study coordinator (gynaecology) at the NCIC CTG and is currently the International (non-U.S.) Intergroup Affairs Coordinator with that Group. Professional memberships include ONS (and its Clinical Trial Nurses SIG), CANO, Society of Gynecologic Nurse Oncologists, NCIC CTG Clinical Trials Nurses SIG (founder and coordinator), Royal Victoria Hospital Alumnae, American Society of Clinical Oncology, and others.

CHAPTER 57

Japan

Eriko Aotani, RN, MSN, CCRP, and Yuko Saito, MS, RN, CCRP

History and Background

Many cancer clinical trial groups have been established since the late 1970s in Japan. Some of them are nationwide, and others are provincial. The Japan Clinical Oncology Group (JCOG) was established as a multimodality cooperative group sponsored by the Ministry of Health, Labour and Welfare (MHLW) and has been conducting multi-institutional clinical trials since 1978. JCOG is the first and only cooperative study group that has been fully supported by the Japanese government's research funds. As of 2006, it consists of 13 disease-oriented trial groups, some administrative and operational committees, and a data center. JCOG has greatly contributed to establishing standard therapies against cancer and also has served as a model for other study groups in Japan (especially for the clinical trial infrastructure and operations) (Fujimoto & Saijo, 2003; Tamura, 2003).

Throughout the 1980s and 1990s, other nationwide cooperative groups, such as the Japanese Gynecologic Oncology Group (JGOG), the West Japan Thoracic Oncology Group, the Japan Adult Leukemia Study Group, and the Comprehensive Support Program for Oncology Research (CSPOR) were established. Figure 57-1 lists the national oncology cooperative groups in Japan. They established their own statistical data centers and conducted phase II and III clinical trials. These groups are nonprofit organizations or foundations supported mostly by charitable donations from pharmaceutical companies and individuals. They have conducted important clinical trials and made great contributions to the improvement of cancer care.

Implementation of International Conference on Harmonisation of Technical Requirements for Registration of Pharmaceuticals for Human Use Good Clinical Practice (ICH GCP) guidelines in 1998 promoted rapid growth of quality control mechanisms for industry-sponsored investigational new drug (IND) cancer trials. However, full compliance with ICH GCP in investigator-initiated non-IND trials still is not regulated in Japan. Therefore, the

---

Figure 57-1. Japan's National Cooperative Groups

- Comprehensive Support Program for Oncology Research (CSPOR)
- Japan Adult Leukemia Study Group (JALSG)
- Japan Clinical Oncology Group (JCOG)
- Japanese Gynecologic Oncology Group (JGOG)
- West Japan Thoracic Oncology Group (WJTOG)

---

cooperative groups have been self-regulated while trying to achieve GCP compliance.

The cooperative groups conduct cancer clinical trials that examine standard end points (i.e., toxicity, tumor response, survival) along with quality of life (QOL) and cost effectiveness. Rarely are nursing research questions incorporated into cooperative group trials. None of these cooperative groups has a nursing committee. Most nurses at participating institutions are involved in clinical trials as clinical research coordinators (CRCs). Some nurses who work for central administration or the data center of study groups assume roles for protocol writing, data management, trial management, and education of CRCs at participating institutions.

Protocol Development

The procedures for protocol development vary among study groups. Often the protocol committee assigns the study chair and cochairs to an approved study concept; usually one or more investigators propose the study concept. The study chair typically collaborates with cochairs, statisticians, and data managers to write the protocol. Opinions from representative CRCs of the member institutions may be solicited before finalizing the protocol.

For the external review, a scientific review committee and/or other disease groups of the study group review the protocol. From there, the protocol is presented to a protocol committee and/or ethics committee that include individuals who have no association with the group. No approval mechanism currently exists for cooperative group studies by the government. Finally, each protocol must have local institutional review board (IRB) approval prior to activation.

Elements of a Protocol

Basically, the elements of protocols are listed in Figure 57-2. Other important information (e.g., pathology review process, surgical guidelines) is provided as appendices to the protocol.

Budgets

In cooperative group trials, financial factors may pose obstacles to study implementation. Budgets for cooperative groups are very limited regardless of their funding sources. Equitable reimbursement is not given to the participating institutions for costs and time/effort. Many cooperative group trials have such minimal reimbursement that the investigators cannot obtain any staff support.

To obtain governmental approval in industry-sponsored IND trials, financial requests of participating institutions are greatly reduced. The institutions can calculate the cost for each study and negotiate with their sponsors. Consideration is given for the *direct* expenses of a trial depending on the phase of the trial, whether it is inpatient or outpatient, the severity of the target disease, and the frequency of the required tests. It also includes *overhead* expenses for personnel, utilities, and administration.

For cooperative group trials using government-approved agents for indication or treatment, the additional costs of tests, medications, and potentially prolonged hospitalizations associated with the trials can be covered by national health insurance. In that case, patients usually need to pay about 30% of the total medical costs.

For industry-sponsored IND trials, the sponsors normally have to carry all expenses for the study drugs, laboratory tests, or diagnostic images directly associated with the trial during the period when the study drug is administered. Other expenses, such as medications to treat adverse events, except for predetermined conditions

with the sponsor, may be covered by national health insurance. The coverage of national health insurance for these certain conditions in combination with uninsured medical expenses in clinical trials is not governmentally approved, whereas for an investigator-initiated indication-directed trial, the coverage requirement for the investigator sponsor is clearly approved by the government; only the expenses of laboratory tests, diagnostic imaging, or medications other than the same sort (i.e., the same indication) as the study drugs will be covered by national health insurance.

Statistical Considerations

A biostatistician is assigned for each trial. This individual is responsible for the study design, sample size calculation, and randomization procedure, including the stratification factors. Rationales for statistical methods used are described in the statistical section of the protocol. The statistician participates from the beginning of the protocol development.

The number of biostatisticians in Japan is much smaller than in the United States. This is especially true for investigator-initiated study groups, where sometimes only one statistician is responsible for all studies of the group.

Assurances

The Pharmaceuticals and Medical Devices Agency (PMDA) was established in 2004. The key services of the PMDA are summarized in Figure 57-3. Inspections for GCP compliance are conducted by the MHLW (PMDA, 2004).

Figure 57-2. Elements of a Protocol

- Background and rationale
- Objectives
- Patient eligibility and exclusion criteria
- Study modalities
- Entry/randomization procedure
- Expected adverse events and treatment
- Treatment modifications
- Stopping rules
- Study parameters, serial observations, and evaluation criteria
- Study duration (both a patient entry period and a follow-up period)
- Study monitoring and reporting procedures
- Statistical considerations
- Publication of results
- Organizational information of the study group
- Bibliography

Figure 57-3. Services of the Pharmaceuticals and Medical Devices Agency

- Adverse health effect relief services, such as payment to the sufferers of adverse drug reactions
- Review and approval of pharmaceuticals and medical devices based on the Pharmaceutical Affairs Law
- Guidance and advice concerning clinical trials
- Collection, analysis, and dissemination of information regarding the quality, efficacy, and safety of pharmaceuticals and medical devices
- Promotion of research necessary for the development of innovative pharmaceuticals and medical devices

Note. Based on information from Pharmaceuticals and Medical Devices Agency, 2004.

Through these activities, the PMDA and MHLW take pivotal roles in quality assurance of clinical trials. However, their concerns are directed more toward registration-directed clinical trials and less toward investigator-initiated clinical trials. Clinical trial nurses (CTNs) and other research professionals advocate for this assurance mechanism to expand to all investigator-initiated clinical trials with the aim of protecting human research participants.

Determining Workload

Several variables must be considered when determining workloads. Institutions determine workload from variables such as the phase of trial, whether it is inpatient or outpatient, the severity of the target disease, and the frequency of the required tests and specialized tests. CRCs routinely are assigned to all registration-directed clinical trials but not to investigator-initiated non-registration-directed trials. Therefore, conducting clinical trials adds to the investigator's workload. More active involvement of CTNs is needed for the care of patients in clinical trials in Japan.

Laboratory Issues

For Japanese institutions participating in clinical trials, most laboratory tests of blood and urine, as well as radiographic image tests such as computed tomography or magnetic resonance imaging, are easily accessible. Most laboratory tests are performed within each institution, and only tests that are not frequently done, such as rare tumor markers, are performed at commercial laboratories outside the institutions.

In registration-directed clinical trials, the sponsor may use a commercial laboratory to centralize the tests and lessen the effects of institutional differences. In investigator-initiated clinical trials, such variation is not strictly checked. The institutions usually report the raw laboratory values, along with the grading, according to evaluation criteria, such as the National Cancer Institute's (NCI's) Common Terminology Criteria for Adverse Events (CTCAE), which is one of the criteria widely used to evaluate toxicity of anticancer agents in clinical trials in Japan.

Sponsoring Agencies

In Japan registration-directed cancer trials are almost completely sponsored by pharmaceutical companies. The very few exceptions are investigator-initiated registration-directed cancer trials, most of which are used to obtain approvals for different disease indications. The PMDA evaluates these protocols before executing the trial.

Resources for investigator-initiated cancer trials sponsored by the government are extremely limited, so most study groups rely heavily on donations from pharmaceutical companies or personal donations.

Intergroup Trials

Intergroup trials are not yet commonly conducted in Japan because of the differences of target diseases and/or group policies. The two largest benefits of participating in intergroup trials are (a) to be able to conduct a clinical trial that requires a large number of accruals to obtain adequate statistical power and (b) to conduct clinical trials for rare tumors. Interest in international collaboration is increasing, especially in the field of gynecologic cancer. The JGOG became a member of Gynecologic Cancer Intergroup in 2003. JGOG currently is conducting a phase III international trial for clear cell carcinoma of the ovary. This is the first clinical trial with international collaboration that is being led by a Japanese trial group. Participating groups are from Japan (JGOG), Korea (KGOG—the Korean Gynecologic Oncology Group), Italy (MITO—the Multicentre Italian Trials in Ovarian cancer), the United Kingdom (SGCTG/UK—the Scottish Gynaecological Cancer Trials Group), and the United States (GOG—the Gynecologic Oncology Group). For international clinical trials, the time difference between participating countries should be considered for patient registration. The JGOG Data Center developed a Web-based registration and randomization system for the trial. Crucial issues during trial preparation include

- Obtaining a consensus for data collection methods (including the case report forms [CRFs])
- Serious adverse event (SAE) reporting procedures
- Tissue collection procedures among the participating groups.

Clinical Research Team/ Interdisciplinary Team

An interdisciplinary approach enhances all aspects of clinical trials, from protocol development to patient care. The opinions from experts in distinct disciplines, such as medical oncologists, radiation oncologists, pathologists, and nurses, are sought when preparing protocols. The degree of interdisciplinary approach varies widely among the study groups.

The *principal investigator* is the leader of the research team and is responsible for the scientific integrity of the study and protection of research participants. Coinvestigators can act as decision makers with the principal investigator for the study. Administration officers, statisticians, and data managers are other key members of clinical trials.

Site investigators implement the study and provide feedback to improve it. CRCs and CTNs have vital roles in implementation, which are outlined in Figure 57-4. In Japan, some CRCs are not nurses but rather are pharmacists or lab technicians. No differences currently exist in the job descriptions of CRCs and CTNs. CTNs have fundamental knowledge of the treatment and emotional support needs of patients and their families. Hence, they are central to the research team, and input from the nursing perspective is highly valued. The roles of CRCs, CTNs, local data managers, and staff nurses

Figure 57-4. Clinical Trial Nurse and Clinical Research Coordinator Roles in Clinical Trial Implementation

- Patient recruitment
- Scheduling patient visits and required tests
- Developing useful tools for trial management
- Collection of relevant clinical data
- Preparation of case report forms
- Education of patients and the research team

overlap depending on organizational structure. Nutritionists, social workers, ethicists, and religion representatives are not routinely part of the research team.

Introduction to Legal and Registration Issues

Since the introduction of ICH GCP into Japanese GCP in 1997, greater attention has been paid to the quality of clinical trials. Clinical trials in Japan traditionally have been divided into two categories: (a) industry-sponsored registration-directed trials, including IND trials, that must follow GCP and (b) investigator-initiated non-registration-directed trials that are not strictly regulated. Investigator-initiated trials were not considered acceptable for drug registration purposes until 2002. At that time, the Japanese government revised the regulations so that investigators could conduct registration-directed trials that may be ignored by pharmaceutical companies. The third category of clinical trials in Japan is investigator-initiated registration-directed clinical trials for which GCP compliance is required. This reform is expected to improve the overall quality of investigator-initiated clinical trials (Ando & Fujiwara, 2005).

Regardless of whether the law mandates it, protection of research participants (based on the Declaration of Helsinki (see Appendix 2) is required in all clinical research. The *Ethical Guidelines for Clinical Research*, issued by the MHLW in 2003, applies to all clinical research. These guidelines clearly state ethical principles such as responsibilities of investigators and institutions, requirements for IRB approval and written informed consents, and protection of privacy.

Institutional Review Boards and Protocol Modification

It is a fundamental rule to obtain IRB approval before conducting a clinical trial, and the local IRB is responsible for initially reviewing the protocols and consent forms. Registration-directed clinical trials are more strictly regulated than others, as per institutional standard operating procedures (SOPs) regarding the IRB reporting procedures, including protocol revision, amendments, termination, and SAE reporting. IRB approval letters are subject to audit.

Although IRBs must follow the *Ethical Guidelines for Clinical Research*, continuous education for members and quality assurance mechanisms for IRBs still are in development in Japan. Many institutions still do not require annual review for investigator-initiated non-registration-directed trials. As of 2006, the central IRB system was approved by regulation but was not yet widely used. The authors believe that education and quality assurance systems for IRBs are necessary, and CTNs in Japan could contribute to such education in the near future.

Informed Consent

The requirements and basic elements of the informed consent process are the same as in the United States. CRCs, especially CTNs, perform vital roles in this process. They provide information about the trials and other options using simple language for patients and their family members. In addition, they ensure that participation is based on the patients' voluntary decisions. Preparation of the consent document for IRB review usually is the job of the CRC.

Illiteracy rates in Japan are very low. According to a study of 85 patients by Sato, Watanabe, Katsumata, and Ohashi (2005), the detailed consent form did not improve patients' understanding of their consent but significantly improved their satisfaction. In Japan, the signature of a witness is not mandatory unless the patient's comprehension ability is questionable. Genetic testing or future use of patients' specimens requires an additional, separate informed consent.

Compassionate Use

The compassionate use of investigational new drugs outside studies is mostly prohibited, except for those drugs that are effective during the study period, and then only if there is a strong demand from patients in the trials. After discussion with the patient about compassionate use, a separate written informed consent is required. In the case of sponsor-initiated registration-directed clinical trials, pharmaceutical companies might consider this as an option. However, it is highly unlikely for pharmaceutical companies to provide for the compassionate use of drugs for investigator-initiated non-registration-directed trials.

No regulation exists to allow for the use of INDs (nonapproved drugs) outside clinical trials in Japan. The patient has to pay all costs for the treatment, including sometimes importing the drugs from abroad. CTNs recognize and accept patients' wishes and serve as an advocate for patients.

Conflict of Interest

The financial disclosure of investigators is not a regulatory requirement in Japan. Conflict-of-interest issues receive less attention in Japan than they do in the United States. As of 2006, the Japanese Society of Medical Oncology and the Japan Society of Clinical Oncology are jointly developing the guideline regarding conflicts of interest in clinical trials. In past decades, personal stockholders were relatively rare in Japan, so the concerns about stockholding investigators might not receive much attention. However, the situation is changing. All research team members, including CTNs, need to be more sensitive to this issue while considering the ethical principles in research. Disclosing personal assets and talking about monetary involvement is an uncomfortable subject for many Japanese people. Traditionally, Japanese people believe that speaking of personal wealth outside of the immediate family or showing interests in others' assets is not proper. However, CTNs need to recognize their own personal values and the ethical implications for their patients when dealing with this issue.

General Publication

The authors of publications for clinical trials must be those who have made a significant contribution to the design and/or implementation of the trial. In many cases, the principal investigator from the institution with the largest number of patient accruals chooses either to be the first author of the manuscript or to be the presenter at a major academic meeting. The second author usually is the study chair or statistician, depending on the trial group policy. Other coauthors include study cochairs and investigators from institutions where significant numbers of patients were enrolled. CRCs and CTNs are not normally listed on publications, but sometimes their names appear in the acknowledgment section.

Psychosocial Considerations

A study regarding stress among patients with cancer in Japan showed relatively similar results to those in the Western countries, where 4%–35% of patients with cancer experienced symptoms of adjustment disorders such as anxiety, and 4%–7% of them developed depression. Many of those who developed adjustment disorders were experiencing a cancer recurrence (Inagaki & Uchitomi, 2001). Many Japanese still consider a diagnosis of cancer as a death sentence. When introducing a clinical trial as a treatment option, it is crucial for CTNs to observe the readiness of patients for new information and to take enough time for the patient's acceptance of treatment.

In Japanese culture, family members play significant roles in the patient's decision-making processes. In a large 1992 survey of the family members of deceased patients with cancer, 36% requested more effective communication with the physician, and 13% requested a consultation system with medical information for them (Saeki, 2004).

Historically in Japanese culture, an apparent paternalistic relationship has existed between physicians, their patients, and their patients' families. The situation is improving, but CTNs should ensure that a coordinated effort is made for effective communication with the patients and their families and that continuous efforts for improvement are made.

Psychosocial issues of patients participating in a clinical trial are not routinely assessed at each hospital visit. CRCs assigned for industry-sponsored trials can take considerable time interviewing and assessing the psychosocial status of the patients. However, very few CRCs are assigned for investigator-initiated clinical trials. For these trials, only when the patients or their family members express concerns or if the investigators observe signs of psychosocial problems will a patient be referred to psychiatrists or other specialists. Psychosocial assessment is an important area of the nursing domain. CTNs in Japan would like to get more involved in this area for all patients, regardless of the difference in clinical trial sponsors. For that purpose, organizational innovation of job assignment for CRCs/CTNs is essential.

Public and Patient Education

Patient educational materials about clinical trials and disease, such as handmade brochures or institutional advertisement videos, mostly are prepared by CRCs. For sponsor-initiated indication-directed trials, the sponsor will provide these materials. They are prepared with sensitivity to clarity of information and visual attraction.

Promotion and Recruitment Strategies

Since 1999, pharmaceutical companies have used media such as newspapers or Internet advertisements to find patients for registration-directed trials. When patients see an advertisement, they call the coordinating center (called a "call center"), which directs them to participating medical centers. By August 2005, more than 200 such advertisements were published. However, many of the patients who applied for the trials through those advertisements did not meet the eligibility criteria. Therefore, efficiency of patient recruitment through media advertisements varies.

Advertisements (such as pamphlets or posters) for patient recruitment for a trial within an institution are relatively efficient, especially for cancer trials. This is based on the premise that eligible candidates for the trials are more readily available. IRB approval is required for any kind of patient recruitment tools for trials.

Unlike in the United States, patients who visit a hospital seeking the opportunity to participate in a clinical trial are rare in Japan because so many patients seek cancer treatment within a close geographic area of their home. However, some patients will traverse the entire country to seek clinical trials with new drugs or new modalities that have already been approved in foreign countries.

CTNs need to be knowledgeable about ways to obtain accurate trial information to help patients to acquire other treatment options. Ongoing registration-directed trials are disclosed on the Web site of the Japanese Pharmaceutical Manufacturers Association, as well as in the clinical trials registration database (described later in "Registries") on the Web.

Recruitment methods for participating institutions vary for each cooperative group. Cooperative groups are responsible for evaluating their participating institutions with regard to the number of accruals and data quality. Although it rarely happens, an institution with low evaluations can be terminated, and new institutions may be recruited after obtaining approval from the steering committee of the study group. Some study groups invite institutions to participate through advertisements of the trial at academic meetings.

Eligibility

The protocols clearly state the eligibility criteria in two sections: inclusion criteria and exclusion criteria. Eligibility criteria are for patients for whom it appears to be reasonable to apply the study treatment. Exclusion criteria are for patients who also belong to the previous group but who are not appropriate to include in the trial because of ethical concerns or other factors that may affect the evaluation and/or safety of the trial.

The eligibility parameters in a cancer clinical trial mainly are specified by factors listed in Figure 57-5. CRCs/CTNs or physicians need to be certain that those parameters are scheduled for evaluation within the study time frame and that the patient fully understands the impact of study participation. The patient registration form is completed and usually is sent by fax to the patient registration.

Figure 57-5. Factors Reviewed for Patient Eligibility

- Cancer type
- Clinical stage
- Performance status
- Existence of measurable disease (based on Response Evaluation Criteria in Solid Tumors [known as RECIST])
- Type of prior treatment
- Existence of past and/or concomitant disease history
- Concomitant drug and/or treatment
- Organ function (such as bone marrow function, liver function, kidney function)

Investigational Agents

Investigational drugs for registration-directed trials are all distributed directly from the sponsor to participating institutions. The drugs are sent to the institution's pharmacy, where a pharmacist is appointed for the receipt, storage, preparation, handling, disposal, and accountability of the study drugs, as well as for maintenance of records of the drug log forms. The investigational agents cannot be substituted without permission from the sponsor.

Administration of Protocol Agents

Practical aspects of drug administration, such as premedications or specific procedures, are detailed in the protocol. Modification criteria, such as dose modifications, treatment delays, and discontinuation criteria, also are stated in the protocol. Usually the first dose of each protocol agent is calculated at the patient registration center and reported to the investigator. The investigators and CRCs/CTNs are responsible for confirming accurate dosing and timing thereafter.

Symptom Management

Physicians who are participating investigators in the study usually perform symptom management during clinical trials. Because nurses have no authority to write prescriptions in Japan, the treating physician prescribes drugs to prevent or treat symptoms after confirming that they do not contradict the protocol treatment.

CTNs can contribute to symptom management in terms of prevention, observation, and education for patients and their families. The treating physician and CTNs usually observe symptoms such as infection or peripheral neuropathy. Special attention is paid to such symptoms for possible attribution to the study treatment. CTNs report the patient's symptoms to the physician and sometimes record them directly on the medical chart. In addition, CTNs record both subjective and objective information regarding the symptoms, often in detail, with assessment and plans on a separate nursing chart. Interventions for loss of appetite, control of bowel movements, prevention of infection, and psychological support are common examples of nursing interventions in symptom management.

Adverse Events

Adverse events for cancer trials are graded according to the NCI CTCAE in Japan. JCOG and the Japan Society of Clinical Oncology translated the most commonly used Japanese translation of the CTCAE. Although investigators are responsible for evaluation of adverse events, CRCs/CTNs support the grading procedure by interviewing patients and reviewing laboratory tests before conferring with the physician.

Each protocol indicates the definition of an SAE. The principal investigator of the participating institution is responsible for reporting SAEs to the institution's IRB, the director of the institution, and the sponsor of the trial according to the institution's SOP. Because SAEs ultimately must be reported to PMDA, CRCs are starting to play a more active role in the preparation of SAE reports to keep to a reporting timeline of 7–15 days.

Compliance in Clinical Trials

Protocol compliance has improved dramatically in Japan since CRCs became involved in registration-directed clinical trials in the late 1990s. Unfortunately, this has not been the case for investigator-initiated clinical trials. Only about 8%–17% of the participating institutions have CRCs available for non-registration-directed cancer cooperative group trials. This low number is the result of very limited resource allocation to institutions and the lack of an official support system for such trials within the institutions (Aotani, 2006; Tamura, 2006). Therefore, minor deviations, such as missing data or delays in the required tests, are not rare. Most of these deviations can be preventable if responsible CRCs/CTNs are assigned.

Quality-of-Life Studies

QOL studies are now becoming more important components of cancer trials in Japan. QOL assessment particularly is important when the primary end points of two arms in a randomized trial have minimal efficacy differences but large differences in toxicity profiles. The most popular QOL assessment method among Japanese study groups is the Functional Assessment of Cancer Therapy (FACT) scale because most FACT scale components have a validated Japanese version.

CRCs/CTNs can affect the future of cancer care by making important contributions to QOL studies. The authors believe that CTNs in Japan have more potential for coordinating QOL studies in which they help patients and gather timely and reliable QOL data.

Pharmacokinetics and Genetics

Pharmacokinetic studies usually are conducted during phase I trials. It is necessary to obtain blood and urine samples a prescribed number of times during and after drug administration. Genetic studies usually are conducted using the tissue samples collected for pathology review. The study purpose for this type of investigation must be clearly written in the protocol and the IRB-approved consent forms.

Genetic Testing and Storage

Genetic testing is a rapidly evolving component of clinical trials. However, it is an extremely sensitive issue in Japanese society. When genetic testing is planned using samples obtained from patients in a study, some local IRBs may reject the study unless the component of future tissue use is eliminated. Other local IRBs require a separate informed consent from patients each time samples or tests are used for purposes beyond the initial clinical trial. Key elements of genetic testing that require particular attention when it is a component of a clinical trial are summarized in Figure 57-6.

Pharmacoeconomic Studies

Recently, the national budget shortage for medical expenses has become apparent. Medical treatment costs are higher, along with the costs of developing new diagnostic and therapeutic measures, such as molecular targeted new anticancer agents. Under such circumstances, pharmacoeconomic studies have gained more attention in Japan but are not yet common.

Methodology for pharmacoeconomic studies is the same as for those conducted in the United States. The most common approach is cost-effect analysis, in which the cost of a treatment is compared in monetary terms with the ef-

fectiveness of the treatment. It usually measures the clinical outcome in terms of number of lives saved or number of toxicities prevented. Keeping personal information confidential is essential. As with other clinical trials, pharmacoeconomic studies also need to obtain IRB approval.

Nursing Companion Studies

Nursing companion studies offer nurses the opportunity to perform independent research while conducting an oncology clinical trial. It offers them benefits, such as easy access to study participants, when compared to an independent nursing study. However, conducting a companion study is a great challenge because obtaining permission and support from the study group may not be easy.

Unfortunately, none of the cancer cooperative groups in Japan currently hold a nursing committee; thus, opportunities for nursing companion studies have not yet matured. CTNs in Japan are expected to take vital roles in promoting recognition of nursing research within the cooperative group. The first step in promoting the recognition of nursing research may be to propose a nursing research concept and make a good presentation with emphasis on the significance of the study and the scientific research methodology to committee members of the cooperative group. Because many investigators have little knowledge about nursing research, it is essential to introduce them to the importance of nursing research for the care of patients with cancer as a science.

Protocol Considerations

Since 1997, protocols for cancer clinical trials in Japan have been written based on ICH GCP guidelines. Protocols must be justified both scientifically and ethically. The elements of a protocol were described earlier in this chapter. A protocol may be revised and amended, but it always serves as the ultimate guide for the trial.

CTNs in Japan must emphasize the data collection and submission schedule, because delay is common, with no penalties to investigators and institutions.

Long-Term Follow-Up

Data centers in Japan mail follow-up forms to participating institutions once or twice a year. Institutions must return these with required information such as survival, progression, and late adverse events data according to the protocols.

At the time of a patient's first visit, the hospital checks the patient's national health insurance card, which includes contact information. Some cancer centers in Japan require submission of the resident's card. When a patient moves and the new address has been lost, the patient's information, such as survival information and the new address, can be tracked by the patient's legal domicile. However, concern exists that extensive reaction to the Act on the Protection of Personal Information in Japan, implemented in 2005, may make future follow-ups difficult.

Figure 57-6. Key Elements of Patient Protection in Genetic Testing

- Informed consent must be obtained prior to disclosure of information to others.
- Information/specimens collected for one purpose should not be used for another purpose without obtaining further consent.
- Personal information that is not relevant for the study should not be used.
- Strict protection should be adopted to minimize the release of personal information to those other than the required research team members.

Off-Treatment Documentation

Investigators are required to retain all medical records and regulatory documents of patients who enter clinical trials. Medical records include original source documents describing basic patient identification information and materials showing that each patient has met eligibility criteria, such as pathology reports, surgery reports, laboratory test data, and/or radiographic image films. Regulatory documents include the signed original informed consent, the protocol and its amendments, and other communications and actions pertaining to the study. These materials and documentations are subject to audit by the trial group or inspection by the MHLW. CRCs are responsible for ensuring that required documents are complete and kept in place.

The Need for Data Management

Accurate and prompt data submission is important for successful clinical trials. CRCs are responsible for local data management in registration-directed trials, whereas the investigators themselves often perform local data management in investigator-initiated clinical trials. Monitoring methods also are different in the two types of trials. Registration-directed trials have on-site monitoring with strict source documentation verification (SDV) by clinical research associates who have a contract with the sponsor. Conversely, non-registration-directed trials have only periodic central monitoring without SDV. Establishing a support system for participating physicians, especially including assignment of CRCs/CTNs for all clinical trials, is the most urgent step that should be taken to improve the quality of clinical trials in Japan.

Data Management Systems

Most CRFs for clinical trials in Japan are paper-based. Each study group or pharmaceutical company develops its own templates for CRFs that are partially modified according to the protocol. CRFs and other supplies, such as the CRF manual and the exam calendar, are distributed to the institutions. Usually, the institutions receive newsletters or e-mails with updates, tips, and reminders.

Kick-off meetings normally take place just before the activation of the trials. The data centers for each study group or study-specific data center at a contract research organization take responsibility for overseeing the data management of the trials.

Remote Data Entry and Electronic Data Capture

Some of the pharmaceutical companies conducting registration-directed clinical trials have already adopted a remote data entry or electronic data capturing (EDC) system. Most use a Web-based data entry system with personal ID and password (Saito, 2006b). However, remote data entry systems are not popular in investigator-initiated trials because of the high cost of preparation and maintenance of the system.

CSPOR uses a universal serial bus (USB) device for remote data entry, and JGOG uses a Web-based data entry system that is only for patient registration. To date, none of the cancer cooperative groups in Japan use a fully activated EDC system.

Cancer Trials Support Unit

No governmental agency similar to the U.S. Cancer Trials Support Unit currently exists in Japan. Increasing physician and patient access to clinical trials, standardizing data collection and reporting, and reducing regulatory and administrative burden on investigators are all responsibilities of the sponsor or study group.

Clinical Trial Registries

Japan has two clinical trial registries. One is the University Hospital Medical Information Network Clinical Trials Registry (UMIN-CTR), and the other is the Japan Pharmaceutical Information Center Clinical Trials Information (JAPIC-CTI). UMIN, a cooperative organization of national medical schools in Japan, is sponsored by the Ministry of Education, Culture, Science, Sports and Technology (MEXT) and is now the largest, most versatile academic network information center for biomedical sciences. JAPIC is a public service corporation approved by the Minister of Health and Welfare to ensure proper clinical use of medicine. This is accomplished by bridging pharmaceutical manufacturers and medical societies by collecting, processing, and offering useful information from domestic and foreign sources.

Most academic investigator-initiated research, including both clinical trials and observational studies, is registered in UMIN-CTR, and most sponsor-initiated trials are registered in JAPIC-CTR. Clinical trial information is provided in Japanese for the public, as well as in English for access to key elements for those in other counties. As of February 2007, the UMIN-CTR database contained 561 clinical research listings, and the JAPIC-CTI database included 488 registration-directed clinical trials that were open to the public. The listings for each are available online (UMIN-CTR: www.umin.ac.jp/ctr/index.htm; JAPIC-CTR: www.clinicaltrials.jp/user/cte_main_e.jsp).

Good Clinical Practice

New GCP was legislated in 1997 as a *ministerial ordinance* in response to the revision of the Pharmaceutical Affairs Law of 1996. Before this, GCP was a *notice of a bureau chief* with no legal force of constraint. It was renewed based on the ICH GCP agreement and on a report from the Task Force Committee on Establishment of Pharmaceutical Safety. This task force was established after "the sorivudine incident," a tragedy that involved the intentional underreporting of drug-related deaths with concomitant administration fluorouracil during the registration-directed trial for herpes, which led to 15 deaths soon after marketing of the drug.

The new GCP conforms to ICH GCP (positioning of step 5, which is the final step of the process for the harmonization guideline for the European Union, the United States, and Japan to move to the regulatory implementation within the country), and the contents also are equivalent. Regulations regarding written informed consent, IRB requirements, and responsibilities of the sponsor (including protocol development, monitoring, and audits) and of the investigator (including obtaining informed consent and submitting data) are all mentioned in the new GCP.

In 2003, the revised GCP was issued, and investigator-initiated registration-directed trials became possible. It currently applies only to registration-directed clinical trials in Japan. Still, some trial groups make continuous efforts to follow the fundamental principles of GCP.

Standard Operating Procedures

Figure 57-7 lists the clinical trial activities for which, according to GCP, the sponsor and the investigator who plan a registration-directed trial must prepare SOPs. SOPs for clinical trials within the institution also have to be developed and maintained. The responsibility for developing such SOPs belongs to the head official of the institution. Usually CRCs at the clinical trial office within the institution assume the task of preparing and maintaining such SOPs.

Figure 57-7. Clinical Trial Activities That Require a Standard Operating Procedure

- Protocol development
- Selection of participating institutions and investigators
- Development of investigator's brochures
- Drug accountability
- Collection of adverse drug reaction information
- Monitoring and audits
- Preparation of clinical trial reports
- Recording of source documents
- Other activities that are related to the trial

Audit Preparation

Audits are essential components in conducting clinical trials to ensure the quality of data obtained during the trials. Audits usually are initiated by (a) notification of the date and the patient numbers to be audited, (b) submission of the curricula vitae of the auditors to the institution, and (c) reservation of a room and necessary equipment for the audit.

The investigators are responsible for preparation of medical records, radiographic imaging films, and regulatory documents, including IRB approval forms, original informed consent forms signed by patients, and protocols and amendment records. The CRCs may help with preparation for the audit.

The audit team of the sponsoring company or the contract research organization can perform audits for registration-directed trials sponsored by pharmaceutical companies. Inspections may be conducted by the PMDA, and violations of GCP can be subject to penalty. Audits for investigator-initiated non-registration-directed trials are not regulated by GCP. However, cancer trial groups such as JCOG and JGOG employ audit mechanisms in which investigators from other participating institutions can audit members for educational purposes.

Off-Site Treatment

Off-site treatment is not permitted in Japan.

Drug Accountability

Drug accountability is strictly enforced for investigational drugs in registration-directed trials in Japan and is subject to inspection by the MHLW. The institution's pharmacy usually is responsible for drug accountability. The items that the pharmacy should record on the drug accountability logbook include (a) date, dose, and lot number of drug received, (b) the patient's initials and identification number, (c) log number and quantity of drugs dispensed for the study, (d) log number and quantity of drugs returned after administration, and (e) balance of the total drug account. The procedures for handling investigational drugs are determined by SOP.

Interdisciplinary Team Review

Interdisciplinary team review is essential to improve the quality of clinical trials. Some Japanese institutions have two different types of review committees. One discusses the scientific part of the protocol, and the other reviews ethical issues. Committee responsibilities include a systematic review of clinical trials before, during, and after each trial.

Interdisciplinary review committee members usually consist of professional members, as well as lay members who can represent the perspective of the community. It is ideal to include professional members who represent an ethics committee, risk management, finance, administration, marketing, multiple medical departments, and co-medical departments such as nursing, laboratory, and radiology. The extent of the interdisciplinary approach to review a clinical trial varies significantly at each institution.

Specialization in Clinical Research Nursing

In Japan, no specialization in clinical research nursing is available. However, recognition of CRCs as clinical research specialists gradually is increasing in research communities. The Japanese Society of Cancer Nursing (JSCN) established 14 special interest groups in 2006. Among those is a special interest group for clinical trial nurses where CTNs working as CRCs at the institutions work together with those working as study coordinators or auditors at the data centers of cooperative groups. They exchange information and nursing skills about clinical trials, maintain a professional network, and may contribute to improved awareness of CTNs/CRCs as a profession. Small group meetings and a mailing list often are utilized for effective communication among members.

Role Justification

It can be a challenge for Japanese CTNs to show their unique contributions to clinical trials "as a nurse." However, being involved in oncology trials as a nurse brings several advantages. Oncology trials require specialized knowledge of cancer treatment and its standardized evaluation criteria. In addition, the study participants are the patients with cancer who face fear of death, which requires ethical judgments and psychological support on the part of the CTN. Furthermore, research teams consist of multidisciplinary professionals surrounding the patients and their families. This requires effective communication and coordination skills so that principles of family nursing can be applied. Patients also expect to receive advice for symptom management. The authors believe that nurses possess the educational background to fulfill those expectations. Therefore, recognition of these advantages by JSCN is important to increase the number of CTNs in Japan.

Mentorship

Currently, no formal mentorship program for CTNs exists in Japan. Most CTNs are educated through on-the-job training with senior CTNs.

Professional Continuing Education

Oncology nurse programs that prepare nurses to be clinical nurse specialists are available at eight universities in Japan. Additionally, the Japanese Nursing Association endorses the programs to produce certified oncology nurses in three areas of oncology nursing: chemotherapy, pain control, and breast cancer (Japanese Nursing Association, 2001).

Several educational programs exist for CRCs. Parts of the Japanese government, such as the MHLW or MEXT, support periodical CRC seminars. Cancer cooperative groups also provide seminars for their members.

Currently, no academic courses are designed especially for CTNs in Japan. Instead, two graduate programs exist that target CRCs and CTNs. The International University of Health and Welfare offers education at both the master's and doctorate levels. Kyoto University offers education for CRCs at the master's level as of February 2007.

Three organizations provide certification for CRCs in Japan. They are the Society of Clinical Research Associates (SoCRA), the Japanese Society of Clinical Pharmacology and Therapeutics, and the Japan Site Management Organization Association. They also provide continuous education and certification exams (Saito, 2006a).

Summary

The role of the CTN in Japanese clinical trials has increased greatly in the past decade. However, much still needs to be done to bring Japanese CTNs to an equivalent level with their foreign peers. Nurse CRCs need to gain nursing perspectives within their current roles to contribute to successful clinical trials.

The authors wish to acknowledge the following professionals for their expert and insightful reviews: Haruhiko Fukuda, MD, Director, JCOG Data Center/National Cancer Center, Japan; Izumi Kohara, RN, MSN, CCRP, National Cancer Center East, Japan; Keiichi Fujiwara, MD, Saitama Medical University, Japan; and Yasuo Ohashi, PhD, University of Tokyo Graduate School, Japan.

References

Ando, M., & Fujiwara, Y. (2005, January). Changes to the clinical trials system in Japan. *ASCO News,* p. 35.

Aotani, E. (2006). Support for the GOG participating institutions. *Proceedings of the 4th Annual Meeting of Japanese Society of Medical Oncology, 4*(SII-5), 135.

Fujimoto, N., & Saijo N. (2003). Clinical practice and clinical trials: Anticancer drugs and clinical trials. *Surgery Frontier, 10,* 99–102.

Inagaki, M., & Uchitomi, Y. (2001). Psychological burden after cancer diagnosis. *Igaku No Ayumi, 197,* 288–289.

Japanese Nursing Association. (2001). *Reports on clinical trial nurse coordinators 2000.* Retrieved December 3, 2007 from http://www.nurse.or.jp/senmon/crc2000.pdf

Ministry of Health, Labour and Welfare. (2003). *Ethical guidelines for clinical research.* Retrieved December 3, 2007, from http://www.mhlw.go.jp/topics/2003/07/tp0730-2b.html

Pharmaceuticals and Medical Devices Agency. (2004). *Summary of annual report.* Tokyo, Japan: Author.

Saeki, T. (2004). Psychosocial intervention for cancer patients and family members. *Japanese Journal of Psychosomatic Medicine, 44,* 496–501.

Saito, Y. (2006a). CRC education and future perspective in cancer clinical trials. *Rinsho Yakuri, 37,* 70–74.

Saito, Y. (2006b). *System development of connections between electric medical chart and EDC system.* Proc. SAS Users Forum 2006. Tokyo: SAS Institute Japan.

Sato, K., Watanabe, T., Katsumata, Y., & Ohashi Y. (2005). Japanese breast cancer patients prefer detailed consent forms: A comparative study of detailed forms vs. standard forms. *Journal of Clinical Oncology, 23*(Suppl. 16), Abstract 6046.

Tamura, K. (2006). Infrastructure of the participating institutions for a cooperative group. *Proceedings of the 4th Annual Meeting of Japanese Society of Medical Oncology, 4*(SII-2), 132.

Tamura, T. (2003). The role of Japan Clinical Oncology Group (JCOG) in the clinical research of lung cancer. *Gan-no-Rinsho, 49,* 1219–1226.

About the Authors

Eriko Aotani, RN, MSN, CCRP, currently is working as a chief study coordinator and the operations manager at the Kitasato Institute in Japan, which is where the data center for JGOG and several other study groups is located. She graduated from the University of California, San Francisco, in 2001 with a master's degree in nursing, specializing in clinical research management and nursing education. Before Ms. Aotani obtained her graduate education in the United States, she had extensive clinical experience, especially in obstetrics and gynecology nursing in Japan for 10 years. She currently is responsible for project management of cancer trials and administration of the data center. Ms. Aotani also has been actively involved in education programs for clinical research professionals in Japan, such as SoCRA and CRC seminars, and has been a lecturer for clinical trial communications and clinical trial nursing at the universities.

Yuko Saito, RN, MS, CCRP, currently is working as the chief clinical research coordinator at Shizuoka Cancer Center in Japan. She graduated from the University of Tokyo, Faculty of Medicine, School of Health Sciences and Nursing in 2000 with a master's degree in science, with specialization in clinical research methods and outcomes research. Ms. Saito worked as a staff nurse at Tokyo University Hospital devoted to nursing care for patients with cancer for two years. She then worked as a clinical research coordinator at National Cancer Center Hospital for five years. She currently is responsible for clinical trial management and education for the nursing staff of Shizuoka Cancer Center. Ms. Saito also participates in protocol development, operations, and other committees of the cooperative groups in Japan, such as JCOG and CSPOR.

CHAPTER 58
European Union Directives

Gabriele Elser, RN, and Jane Bryce, RN, MSN, AOCNS®

Background

The European Union (EU) provides guidance, legislation, and oversight of clinical trials on medicinal products conducted within its member states. Member states as of October 2006 are listed in Figure 58-1. The European Medicines Agency (EMEA) is a decentralized body of the EU responsible for coordinating the evaluation and supervision of medicinal products throughout Europe, both pre- and postregistration (EMEA, 2006).

Member states of the EU agree to conduct clinical trials according to good clinical practice (GCP). Since 1965, the European Commission has provided guidance and standards on the authorization for marketing of medicinal products and the conduct of clinical trials ("Council Directive 65/65/EEC of 26 January 1965; "Council Directive 75/318/EEC of May 20, 1975). The European Commission introduced the International Conference on Harmonisation (ICH) Tripartite Guideline for Good Clinical Practices (GCP) in 1996.

The most recent EU clinical trial directives are reviewed in this chapter. An *EU directive* is a type of legislation that binds member states to specific objectives to be achieved within a given time frame while allowing the national governments of each state to decide the form and means of implementation.

Directive 2001/20/EC of the European Parliament

This directive was passed on April 4, 2001, and sets forth the laws, regulations, and administrative provisions related to the implementation of GCP in the conduct of clinical trials on medicinal products for human use. The EU passed Clinical Trials Directive (CTD) 2001/20/EC (2001) to harmonize European practices in clinical medicinal research. A principal objective of the directive is the *protection of human subjects,* according to the Declaration of Helsinki (see Appendix 2) and ICH GCP guidelines (see Appendix 6). A second objective is to *reduce the delays in activating*

Figure 58-1. Member States of the European Union	
• Austria	• Latvia
• Belgium	• Lithuania
• Bulgaria	• Luxembourg
• Cyprus	• Malta
• Czech Republic	• The Netherlands
• Denmark	• Poland
• Estonia	• Portugal
• Finland	• Romania
• France	• Slovakia
• Germany	• Slovenia
• Greece	• Spain
• Hungary	• Sweden
• Ireland	• United Kingdom
• Italy	

clinical trials in member states through the simplification and harmonization of administrative procedures while reducing the duplication of processes. Member states were to have implemented the CTD 2001/20/EC by May 1, 2004. The key points of the CTD are listed in Figure 58-2. Each member state develops its own system of registering and authorizing ethics committees (ECs). The EC considerations for rendering an opinion on a clinical trial are outlined in Figure 58-3. A single favorable opinion of the EC is required for each member state. Each state also must designate its competent authority (CA), the national or local regulatory authority that provides oversight of clinical trials on medicinal products. Guidance is provided for the evaluation of clinical trials on minors and on incapacitated adults not able to give informed legal consent, with specific restrictions outlined for each case.

The sponsor may not start a clinical trial until the EC has issued a favorable opinion and the CA of the member state concerned has not informed the sponsor of any grounds for nonacceptance. The procedures to reach these decisions can be parallel or not, depending on the sponsor and on national procedures. Figure 58-4 lists the required documentation for EC and CA submission. The sponsor

Figure 58-2. Key Points of the European Union Clinical Trials Directive Implemented in 2004

- The protection of clinical trial subjects
- The creation of a European clinical trials database (EudraCT) for the registration of clinical trials and for safety reporting (EudraVigilance)
- Defining of sponsor, investigator, and ethics committee responsibilities
- Compliance with Good Clinical Practice and Good Manufacturing Practice guidelines
- Standardized labeling of investigational medicinal products
- The requirement of both a favorable opinion of the ethics committee and the authorization of the competent authority of each participating member state
- The provision of study drugs to subjects free of charge
- Clinical trial insurance for indemnity or compensation for injury

Figure 58-3. European Union Ethics Committees' Considerations for Rendering an Opinion

- Protocol relevance, design, risks, and benefits
- Suitability of the investigator(s) and facilities
- The investigator's brochure
- Protection of trial subjects
- The adequacy and completeness of the informed consent (IC) and IC procedures
- Provisions for indemnity or compensation for injury and any insurance coverage
- Agreements between the sponsor and the facility conducting the trial
- Arrangements for the recruitment of subjects

also must obtain a EudraCT number, the procedures for which are available at the EudraCT Web site at http://eudract.emea.europa.eu.

Once a sponsor has submitted a protocol for opinion to the EC, the EC has 60 days to render its decision and to communicate it to the sponsor and CA. An automatic 30-day extension is given for trials with gene therapy, somatic cell therapy, and medicinal products containing genetically modified organisms, with the possibility of an additional 90-day extension if further consultation or committee review is needed. No time limit exists for the review of clinical trials of xenogenic cell therapy.

The EC may make a single request for additional information from the sponsor, during which time the 60-day clock is suspended. In the case of an unfavorable opinion by the EC, a sponsor has only one opportunity to resubmit the protocol after amending the content, taking into account the reasons given for rejection.

A sponsor may submit an application for a clinical trial to different European countries in parallel. A single favorable EC opinion is required for each member state. The sponsor is responsible for providing various language versions of the clinical trial documents per national requirements.

Each member state where the clinical trial takes place is required to enter specific information into the EudraCT database. A list of specific entry points is presented in Figure 58-5.

The sponsor is responsible for obtaining authorization to import the investigational medicinal product (IMP) in accordance with good manufacturing practices (GMP) and EU regulations. The directive outlines the required labeling for the IMP, including the use of the official language of the member state on the outer packaging.

The CTD requires investigators to immediately report serious adverse events (SAEs) to the sponsor and to report adverse events, laboratory evaluations, and any safety reporting to the sponsor as stipulated by the protocol. The sponsor is responsible for maintaining detailed records of *all* reported adverse events.

The sponsor also is responsible for reporting all relevant information about suspected unexpected serious adverse reactions (SUSARs) to the CAs in all the member states concerned and to the ECs. A SUSAR that is life-threatening or results in death must be reported within 7 days of the sponsor's knowledge of the event and within 15 days for all other cases. The sponsor must inform all investigators of *any* SUSAR. Each member state must register SUSARs that are brought to its attention, and all SUSARs are entered into EudraVigilance database. The EudraVigilance Clinical Trial Module (available at http://eudravigilance.emea.europa.eu) facilitates the electronic reporting of SUSARs. The sponsor provides annual reports listing all suspected serious adverse reactions that have occurred, along with a report of the subjects' safety.

The 2001 CTD provides that inspections be carried out to verify compliance with GCP and GMP. CAs of member states appoint inspectors, and the inspections are carried out on behalf of the European Community, with mutual recognition among member states. Several implementation and practical issues were identified after the issue of CTD 2001/20/EC. Much of the discussion centered on the increased clinical trial costs for the nonprofit sponsor related to insurance policies, provision of all medicines in the clinical trial, and monitoring activities to ensure GCP (Crawley, 2004; Habeck, 2003; Meunier et al., 2003; Meunier & Lacombe, 2003; Perrone et al., 2004; Watson, 2003). The increased costs and bureaucracy created concern that academic clinical trials in the EU could be jeopardized by a lack of competitiveness with non-EU trials. A subsequent clinical trial directive was issued in 2005 to, in part, address some of these issues, as well as to provide further guidance on the 2001 directive.

Directive 2005/28/EC of the European Parliament

Directive 2005/28/EC (2005), passed on April 9, 2005, states principles and detailed guidelines for GCP regarding IMPs for human use and the authorization requirements for the manufacturing or importing of such products. The issues that CTD 2005/28/EC addresses are summarized in Figure 58-6. Member states were to implement this directive

Figure 58-4. Checklist of Information for European Union Member States Competent Authority and Ethics Committees*

General
- Receipt of confirmation of EudraCT number
- Covering letter
- Application form
- List of competent authorities within the community to which the application has been submitted and details of decisions
- Copy of ethics committee opinion in the member state concerned, when available
- Copy/summary of any scientific advice
- If the applicant is not the sponsor, a letter of authorization enabling the applicant to act on behalf of the sponsor

Subject related
- Informed consent form
- Subject information leaflet
- Arrangements for recruitment of subjects

Protocol related
- Clinical trial protocol with all current amendments
- Summary of the protocol in the national language
- Peer review of trial when available
- Ethical assessment made by the principal/coordinating investigator, if not given in the application form or protocol

Investigational Medicinal Product Related
- Investigator's brochure
- Investigational Medicinal Product Dossier (IMPD)
- Simplified IMPD for known products
- Summary of Product Characteristics (SmPC) for products with marketing authorization in the community
- Outline of all active trials with the same IMP
- If IMP is manufactured in the European Union (EU) and if there is no marketing authorization in EU: A copy of the manufacturing authorization referred to in Article 13.1 of the Directive stating the scope of this authorization.
- If IMP is not manufactured in the EU and if there is no marketing authorization in EU: Certification of the Qualified Person that the manufacturing site works in compliance with good manufacturing practice (GMP) at least equivalent to EU GMP, or that each production batch has undergone all relevant analyses, tests or checks necessary to confirm its quality; certification of GMP status of active biologic substance; and copy of the importer's manufacturing authorization
- Certificate of analysis for test product in exceptional cases
- Viral studies, when applicable
- Applicable authorizations to cover trials or products with special characteristics (e.g., GMOs, radiopharmaceuticals)
- Examples of the labels in the national language

Facilities and Staff Related
- Facilities for the trial
- Curriculum vitae (CV) of the coordinating investigator in the member state concerned (for multicenter trials)
- CV of each investigator responsible for the conduct of a trial in a site in the member state concerned (principal investigator)
- Information about supporting staff

Finance Related
- Provision for indemnity or compensation in the event of injury or death attributable to the clinical trial
- Any insurance or indemnity to cover the liability of the sponsor or investigator
- Compensation to investigators
- Compensation to subjects
- Agreement between the sponsor and the trial site
- Agreement between the investigators and the trial sites
- Certificate of agreement between sponsor and investigator when not in the protocol

*Refer to detailed guidance documents for specific member state requirements.

Note. From *Detailed Guidance for the Request for Authorisation of a Clinical Trial on a Medicinal Product for Human Use to the Competent Authorities, Notification of Substantial Amendments and Declaration of the End of the Trial* (pp. 47–48), by European Commission, October 2005, Brussels, Belgium: Author. Retrieved February 10, 2006, from http://eudract.emea.europa.eu/docs/Detailed%20guidance%20CTA.pdf. Copyright 2005 by European Commission. Adapted with permission.

Figure 58-5. Clinical Trial Information in EudraCT Required by Each Member State

- Request for authorization
- Any amendments to the request
- Any substantial protocol amendments
- The favorable opinion of the ethics committee
- The declaration of the end of the clinical trial
- A reference to any good clinical practice–related inspections

---

Figure 58-6. Key Issues of Clinical Trials Directive 2005/28/EC

- The principles of good clinical practice referred to in the 2001 directive with specific consideration to noncommercial trials
- The authorization requirements for the manufacture or importation of investigational medicinal products, as noted in Clinical Trial Directive (CTD) 2001/20/EC
- Documentation-related guidelines to clinical trials and its archiving
- Inspectors' qualifications and inspection procedures in accordance with CTD 2001/20/EC

---

by January 29, 2006. The directive clarifies that member states can introduce modalities to take into account noncommercial clinical trials (nonprofit-sponsored trials, often referred to as academic trials) in which the pharmaceutical industry does not participate, while still applying the principles of GCP.

Further, the provision and labeling of already-licensed medicinal products may be simplified according to GMP. Import authorization is outlined and must be provided by the CA within 90 days.

The directive outlines minimal educational requirements for inspectors and provides that GCP inspections may take place at any time before, during, or after the conduct of a clinical trial and during or after the marketing authorization process. Member states must establish the framework for GCP inspectors and inspections, such as providing adequate resources and procedures. The CTD foresees joint training and inspections by the commission and agency and the provision of guidance documents for inspections.

Resources for Clinical Trial Application and Registration

Request for authorization of a clinical trial on a medicinal product for human use to the CA and for an opinion of the EC in the community is available at http://eudract.emea.europa.eu. Additional forms are available for the required notification of amendments, including the declaration of the end of a trial. Other relevant EU guidance documents are accessible on the EudraCT Web site and include

- European CTDs 2001/20/EC and 2005/28/EC
- Detailed guidance for the request for authorization of a clinical trial on a medicinal product for human use to

the CAs, notification, and substantial amendments, and declaration of the end of the trial
- Detailed guidance on the European clinical trials database (EudraCT)
- Detailed guidance on the European database of SUSARs (the EudraVigilance Clinical Trial Module)
- Detailed guidance on the collection, verification, and presentation of adverse reaction reports arising from clinical trials on medicinal products for human use.

Other Clinical Trials Nursing Resources

The European Oncology Nursing Society (EONS) is an organization of professional nurses throughout Europe dedicated to the care of patients with cancer. EONS collaborates with national oncology nursing societies, and individual nurses, as well as professional, political, and patient advocacy organizations across Europe, with the mission of promoting and developing healthy communities through research and education. EONS seeks to "add value to the work of its individual members and societies in delivering care to patients with cancer" (EONS, 2006).

EONS represents European oncology nurses at the Federation of European Cancer Societies (FECS), providing a voice for patient advocacy and nursing excellence. The *European Journal of Oncology Nursing (EJON)* is the official journal of EONS. EONS participates in the biannual European Cancer Congress with a scientific nursing program, as well as a biannual spring convention. EONS develops and promotes many research and educational and projects. Membership and other information is available at www.cancerworld.org.

The European School of Oncology (ESO) was established in 1982 as a nonprofit organization, which seeks to increase the knowledge of healthcare professionals in cancer care (ESO, 2006). ESO provides nursing, physician, and multidisciplinary continuing education and specialization courses in cancer care. The courses are available in English and other national languages in Europe, Russia, the Balkans, the Middle East, and Latin America. ESO courses are clinically oriented and place a special focus on patient advocacy. A wide range of both basic and advanced courses is offered across many topics. ESO sponsors a course for clinical trial nurses, which was based on a European curriculum and first offered in 2005. Information about ESO events, publications, fellowships, and other activities is available at www.cancerworld.org.

The European Organisation for Research and Treatment of Cancer (EORTC), founded in 1962, is a private, nonprofit international organization that aims to promote and conduct research to improve cancer care. Its core activity is conducting clinical trials that develop new treatments or define new standards (EORTC, 2006).

Clinical trials are international, multidisciplinary and independent. The EORTC aims to provide a European platform

- To develop and conduct quality research
- To facilitate collaboration across countries
- To promote clinically oriented research through education and policy.

The EORTC has a network of more than 200 institutions from more than 30 countries. The EORTC clinical research division is composed of many tumor-site-specific research groups, as well as radiotherapy and quality-of-life groups. The EORTC quality-of-life questionnaires are available in many languages and are widely used in European clinical trials. The EORTC offers multidisciplinary educational courses on the topic of clinical research. Information regarding EORTC protocols, groups, publications, educational offerings, and other information can be found at www.eortc.be.

Summary

The European CTD 2001/20/EC was aimed at harmonizing clinical research practices in Europe and protecting clinical trial participants. Although commercial sponsors of clinical trials have realized the simplification of authorization procedures, many European academic researchers have identified the opposite effect for noncommercial sponsors. Member states are responding on a national level to some of the identified barriers for noncommercial sponsors of research, such as insurance coverage and the provision of study drugs free of charge. Both types of research are important in addressing clinical issues in oncology and in providing greater benefits to patients with cancer.

References

Commission directive 2001/20/EC of the European Parliament and of the Council of 4 April 2001 on the approximation of the laws, regulations and administrative provisions of the member states relating to the implementation of good clinical practice in the conduct of clinical trials on medicinal products for human use. (2001, May 1). *Official Journal of the European Union, L121,* 34–44.

Commission directive 2005/28/EC of the European Parliament and of the Council of 9 April 2005 laying down principles and detailed guidelines for good clinical practice as regards investigational medicinal products for human use, as well as the requirements for authorisation of the manufacturing or importation of such products. (2005, April 9). *Official Journal of the European Union, L91,* 13–19.

Council directive 65/65/EEC of 26 Janurary 1965 on the approximation of provisions laid down by law, regulation or administrative action relating to proprietary medicinal products. *Official Journal of the European Union, L126,* 2148.

Council directive 75/318/EEC of 20 May 1975 on the approximation of the laws of member states relating to analytical, pharmaco-toxicological and clinical standards and protocols in respect of the testing of proprietary medicinal products. *Official Journal of the European Union, L147,* 1–12.

Crawley, F.P. (2004). New European clinical trials directive: Is European research possible? *BMJ, 328,* 522.

European Commission. (2005, October). *Detailed guidance for the request for authorisation of a clinical trial on a medicinal product for human use to the competent authorities, notification of substantial amendments and declaration of the end of the trial.* Retrieved February 10, 2006, from http://eudract.emea.europa.eu/docs/Detailed%20guidance%20CTA.pdf

European Medicines Agency. (2006). *Overview.* Retrieved February 20, 2006, from http://www.emea.eu.int/htms/aboutus/emeaoverview.htm

European Oncology Nursing Society. (2006). *EONS mission statement.* Retrieved February 20, 2006, from http://www.cancerworld.org

European Organisation for Research and Treatment of Cancer. (2006). *EORTC aims and mission.* Retrieved February 20, 2006, from http://www.eortc.be

European School of Oncology. (2006). *Mission statement.* Retrieved February 20, 2006, from http://www.cancerworld.org

Habeck, M. (2003). Gloomy prospects for European cancer research. *Lancet Oncology, 4,* 66.

Meunier, F., Dubois, N., Negrouk, A., Rea, L.A., Saghatchian, M., Tursz, T., et al. (2003). Throwing a wrench in the works? *Lancet Oncology, 4,* 717–719.

Meunier, F., & Lacombe, D. (2003). The European Organisation for the Research and Treatment of Cancer's point of view. *Lancet, 362,* 663.

Perrone, F., Marangolo, M., Di Costanzo, F., Colucci, G., Repeto, L., Merlano, M., et al. (2004). Insurance for independent cancer trials. *Annals of Oncology, 15,* 1722–1723.

Watson, R. (2003). EU legislation threatens clinical trials. *BMJ, 326,* 1348.

About the Authors

Gabriele Elser, RN, attended nursing school in the General Hospital of Backnang, receiving a certificate in 1984 from the regional board of Baden-Wuerttemberg, Germany. She has several years of experience in the field of accident surgery and gynecology. Ms. Elser also has two years of additional training at the School of Medical Documentalists in Bad Cannstatt (bfw). From 1993 to 1999, she worked part-time as a study nurse and part-time as a study coordinator in the field of gynecologic oncology for Arbeitsgemeinschaft Gynaekologische Onkologie (AGO) and the Ovarian Cancer Study Group at the Saint Vincentius Hospital in Karlsruhe. Since 1999, Ms. Elser has worked in Wiesbaden (Hessen) as the head of the study office of the AGO Study Group. The main aspects of her work are protocol development, establishment of clinical trials, dealing with regulatory issues, and providing support of education for study nurses. Internationally, Ms. Elser is a representative of the AGO Study Group in the Gynecologic Cancer Intergroup harmonization working group.

Jane Bryce, RN, MSN, AOCNS®, has been a registered nurse since 1980. She received her BSN and MSN from the University of Pittsburgh. Ms. Bryce worked at the University of Pittsburgh Medical Center for 14 years, and began working as an oncology clinical nurse specialist and clinical trials nurse for the National Cancer Institute in Naples, Italy in 1997. She is a member of ONS and the Clinical Trial Nurses Special Interest Group, Italian Oncology Nursing Association, EONS, and the Italian Clinical Research Nurse Group. Ms. Bryce teaches in undergraduate and graduate oncology and research nursing programs of Italian universities and is codirector of the Research Nursing Course of the European School of Oncology.

CHAPTER 59
Austria

Johanna Ulmer, PhD, SC

Introduction

The European Union Clinical Trials Directive (EUCTD) ("Directive 2001/20/EC," 2001) was implemented into Austrian national legislation on April 29, 2004 (BGBl.I 35/2004). Any clinical trial initiated after that date must be performed according to new Austrian medicinal products legislation (known as AMG). Trials that were started before this date are to be continued according to the previously valid laws (BGBl.I 85/1983; BGBl.I 12/2003).

This means that numerous ongoing trials currently are performed according to both old and new regulations. Furthermore, new legislation has led to much uncertainty regarding national submission procedures and approval procedures. The prevailing diversification and uncertainty must progress to unity and harmonization.

Background

Austrian oncology centers increasingly are performing and participating in multicenter clinical trials, as more and more evidence surfaces that patients benefit from better therapies (Janni et al., 2005) and have a higher survival rate (DuBois, 2002). Numerous academic trial centers have been founded, and with the assistance of well-trained study personnel of nurses, administrative assistants, and specially trained study coordinators (SCs), effective coordinating centers have been established. Such coordinating units have become essential because medical doctors alone can no longer manage the constantly increasing administrative workload. Currently, much of this administrative workload is a result of evolving procedures; although the author expects that in the immediate future, high-quality trial performance can only be ensured by intense efforts of compliance with all valid rules and regulations.

Submission Procedures

Four governing bodies exist to which clinical trials have to be submitted in Austria. These are listed in Figure 59-1. Approval from all of these must be issued before a

---

Figure 59-1. Government Agencies That Review Clinical Trials

- Regulatory authorities (RAs)
- Ethics committees (ECs)
- Medical university research boards (MURBs)
- Hospital management boards (HMBs)

---

trial can begin. All respective institutions have defined submission procedures according to national legislation and local demands. Thus, each trial center currently has its own specific procedure based on national and local regulation.

Regulatory Authority

The official competent regulatory authority (RA) for submission of all clinical trials performed in Austria is the Austrian Ministry of Health and Women (*Bundesministerium für Gesundheit und Frauen*). All clinical trials must be submitted to the RA according to defined procedures before commencing. Submission procedures and essential documents are defined on the home page, www.bmgf.gv.at. As soon as all the required documents are submitted, an official statement of submission is issued to the sponsor/investigator. Then, if no further query is issued from the RA within 35 days, the trial can be initiated. This procedure is part of the new legislation.

Ethics Committees

According to the Austrian medicinal product legislation (AMG), as of April 29, 2004, multicenter clinical trials need one national approval of a lead ethics committee (EC) (BGBl.I 35/2004). The status of lead EC was originally given to four major national ECs that have sufficient experience and competence in evaluating clinical trial protocols, including the ECs at Vienna city hospitals, Medical University of Vienna, Medical University of Graz, and Medical University of Innsbruck.

The sponsor/investigator may select one lead EC for submission, and subsequent approval of the selected lead EC is valid for all the participating trial centers listed on the approval. Respective local ECs are to be informed of the planned trial by the sponsor simultaneously. Submission to the lead EC and reporting to the local ECs must be done three weeks before the lead EC meets, so that local ECs have sufficient time to intervene or issue a statement or query to the lead EC. This three-week time frame is intended to allow communication between the local EC and the lead EC (Poznanski, 2004). The investigator/SC continues to request updates of approval status until final permission is given.

To eliminate uncertainties concerning the validity of lead EC approvals for local centers, previously local ECs were nominated to become lead ECs in June 2005. As a result, seven lead ECs in Austria currently are authorized to give approval for multicenter trials (see Figure 59-2).

Figure 59-2. Lead Ethics Committees in Austria

- Vienna city hospitals
- Medical University of Vienna
- Medical University of Graz
- Medical University of Innsbruck
- Salzburg county
- Oberösterreich county
- Niederösterreich county

Medical University Research Boards

In 2004, three medical universities (MUs) were established in Austria, evolving from the faculties of the Austrian state universities. These new MUs in Vienna, Graz, and Innsbruck became autonomous because of legislation in 2002 (BGBl.I 96/2004). One of the central issues of the new MUs is promotion of research. Realizing the increasing scientific importance of clinical trials, MUs encourage investigators to participate not only in preclinical research but also in clinical trials.

For the purpose of supporting investigators, MUs set up Departments of Research Organization (DROs). The aim of the DROs is to assist all interested investigators with trial-specific procedures, such as providing legal expertise for research agreements and assistance with legal requirements for research staff and administrative staff.

The services offered by DROs are not free of charge. For a calculation of costs, a sponsor now has to submit all trial-specific information required by the respective DRO. This procedure differs for each MU in Austria. Whereas the University of Vienna requires a five-sheet form and a detailed cost evaluation, the DRO at the University of Innsbruck makes its own cost calculation on the basis of the financial agreement between the sponsor and investigator. Uncertainty remains concerning payment for services of academic trials when there is no financial support from a sponsor.

Unfortunately, common procedures do not yet exist concerning the submission of essential documents and the timeline for approving projects and issuing permission documents. According to national legislation, the investigator is not allowed to initiate a trial at an MU center until the DRO has issued a statement of "non-prohibition." Each university states submission requirements and procedures on its Web site (www.meduniwien.ac.at, www.i-med.ac.at, and www.medunigraz.ac.at). Procedures and details differ in each case.

Hospital Management Boards

All hospital management boards (HMB) require reporting of clinical trials before initiation. Throughout Austria, no standardized reporting procedure to HMBs exists. Some HMBs have forms that need to be submitted together with certain essential documents, whereas others require only a cover letter with the protocol and locally adapted informed consent document. Some HMBs do not require any reporting from the sponsor/investigator; instead, they are notified by the respective EC about all planned trials.

Most HMBs differentiate between commercial and academic trials. In general, for commercial trials, an extensive cost calculation needs to be completed, and expenses are charged for all extra services of the planned trial. Some HMBs charge expenses before initiation, whereas others charge expenses after recruitment of a certain number of patients. Other HMBs charge one overall fee before permission is issued to start the trial. Academic trials are, in most cases, free of charge, unless extra services are extensive. Usually, inquiries concerning the academic character of the trial are done by the HMB.

Before the investigator can start patient accrual, it is essential for the sponsor/investigator to ensure that the HMB has all the required documents and that permission is given. The investigator is well advised to have proof of submission because some boards do not issue any written statement of acknowledgment or permission. Only some HMBs issue official letters permitting the investigator to start.

Practice and Management

As current submission procedures lack transparency and cohesiveness, it is essential for a trial center to have qualified staff to ensure quality performance. Most medical centers have reduced the number of staff in recent years to contain explosive costs of medical care. Therefore, investigators are considering new models of establishing trial teams. Various models of trial-specific procedures are evolving, always depending on local resources and structures. Select models are summarized in Figure 59-3.

It is the responsibility of the department head to select studies, to set up a team, and to evaluate performance. Depending on local resources, the principal investigator (PI) may perform all trial-specific duties, or the PI may work

---

Figure 59-3. Austrian Trial Team Models

- Investigator only
- Investigator plus any or all of the following:
  - Nurses
  - Lab assistants
  - Administrative assistants
  - Study coordinators

---

together with one or more subinvestigators to manage the performance of a trial. Recently, new procedure models have been installed in most oncologic trial centers so that investigators may delegate more and more duties to nurses, lab assistants, administrative assistants, or SCs. The situation differs in almost every trial center, depending on the authority of the investigator and the available staff.

The Investigator

The investigator could manage all of the trial-specific duties only when protocols are less complicated and where there are few procedures in addition to standard treatment. However, in oncologic trials, close observation of trial patients for toxicities, dose adjustments, and other issues make them difficult for the investigator to manage alone. Therefore, this investigator-only model has become quite rare in oncologic trials.

Investigators who individually manage patients with cancer receiving chemotherapy treatment are more likely to manage trial procedures and documentation themselves. This is not the case with other investigators, such as oncologic surgeons, who do not have the time to contact ambulatory and hospitalized patients at every visit. In this model, to keep the trial patient under sufficient observation and to comply with regulatory requirements, trial duties are delegated to authorized personnel.

In recent years, MUs and HMBs have not allowed investigators to receive compensation for trial-specific work. Investigators must disclose financial agreements. Part of the compensation is used to cover hospital and university expenses, and the rest goes to an account of the department for purposes of general scientific and research activities. This has encouraged investigators to develop trial teams.

Nurses

The basis of nurses' responsibilities is defined by national legislation (BGBl.I 108/1997; *Gesundheits und Krankenpflegegesetz*, 2004) and local agreements between hospital administration and staff. Nurses' duties are explicitly stated in their contracts. However, there are three models of nurses' active participation in clinical trial-specific activities.

First, nurses are designated by the department head or investigator to perform certain trial-specific duties *in addition to their general duties* in the unit where they work. Such clearly defined additional trial-specific duties must be described, and a written agreement must exist between the nurse and the responsible authority at the HMB. Thus, the HMBs can evaluate which duties nurses perform outside of their general duty agreement. Compensation for trial-specific tasks must be drawn from trial sponsorship.

Second, the department head or investigator can hire nurses *exclusively* for trial-specific duties. The department head and the PI are responsible for educating trial nurses and assigning them with clearly defined duties. Most nurses in such positions have contracts that are limited to one or more projects for a specified period of time.

Third, in some centers, investigators have *separate arrangements with employed nurses on a private basis* for specific trial work. These nurses are regularly employed with clearly defined tasks at the hospital, but they have an additional agreement with an investigator to support him or her in performing trial-related work. In this case, nurses can be assigned to assess toxicities, set up schedules, organize fluid and tissue shipping, enter data into CRFs, or manage drug supply, and more. Currently, clinical trial forms are not computerized. Although no registry of Austrian-specific clinical trials currently exists, the EUDRACT registry is widely used.

The more competent and experienced nurses may assume more delegated duties, always depending on the local provisions and agreements. How much the PI delegates to whom is key; only the very competent nurses who have been assigned to perform trial-specific work may assess toxicity, draw blood, and assess performance status and vital signs, among other responsibilities. Nurses are able to perform only what is delegated to them, and this may vary from PI to PI.

Although the investigator primarily manages the informed consent process, nurses may inform patients about upcoming procedures. The PI may delegate parts of the patient communication process to the nurse, such as informing the patient about the trial-specific procedures involved, the duration of the trial, the duration of the follow-up period, the medication intake, and visit planning when children are involved. All patients, regardless of age or social status, receive the same considerations in the informed consent process.

Medical Students

Many trial centers or investigators hire medical students to perform trial-specific work. Such work can include data transcription onto CRFs or preparation of documents and patient charts for monitoring. Because medical students usually only participate on an irregular basis, they need to work under the supervision of permanent trial staff to ensure current knowledge of all amendments and changes.

Administrative Assistants

Administrative assistants frequently are involved with administrative trial tasks that do not necessarily need to be separately authorized by the PI, such as claiming outstanding documents or forwarding them to the sponsor, investigator, or other institutions. Administrative assistants rarely are involved in trial-specific processes other than general clerical tasks.

Study Coordinators

The full-time SC position in Austria is new, and only a few large trial centers have established a trial unit with this position. SCs can be former nurses, administrative assistants, employees in the pharmaceutical industry, or staff from laboratory research institutions (private or public), as long as they are qualified, willing, capable of continuous trial-specific training, and constantly aware of legislative changes and local requirements. Perfect English skills are essential, as protocols usually are written in English. Because most Austrian nurses do not have adequate English skills, most SCs are non-nurses.

Initial educational programs, including local procedures, good clinical practice, and national legislation, along with participation in regular educational programs, are essential. These are offered by private organizations or enterprises, such as pharmaceutical companies with expertise.

Full-time SCs are essential in large oncologic centers participating in multiple clinical trials. They manage all trial-specific procedures at the center, usually for a number of trials. SCs guarantee continuity and have an overview of all ongoing procedures and all accrued patients. They manage the trial center where all documents are stored, all patients are randomized/registered, all protocol medication is stored, and drug accounts are kept. SCs survey all trial-specific therapies and check all trial-specific entries in charts. Furthermore, they are involved with the screening process, the accrual process, randomizations and registrations, ongoing treatment, data management, and serious adverse event reporting. The extent of involvement on the part of the SC depends on the specific trial and on the individual arrangement between the SC and the investigator.

Summary

With new legislation and encouragement on the part of universities and medical departments to increase participation in clinical trials, a state of transition concerning initiation and performance of trials exists in the Austrian clinical trial landscape. Numerous high-quality educational programs are ongoing to overcome obstacles and establish premium trial centers. Full-time SCs are key to maintaining the integrity of the study and the safety of the patient.

References

BGBl.I 85/1983. Retrieved October 12, 2007, from *Federal Law Gazette (Bundesgesetzblatt)* online: http://www.ris.bka.gv.at/bgbl

BGBl.I 108/1997. Retrieved October 12, 2007, from *Federal Law Gazette (Bundesgesetzblatt)* online: http://www.ris.bka.gv.at/bgbl

BGBl.I 12/2003. Retrieved October 12, 2007, from *Federal Law Gazette (Bundesgesetzblatt)* online: http://www.ris.bka.gv.at/ bgbl

BGBl.I 96/2004. Retrieved October 12, 2007, from *Federal Law Gazette (Bundesgesetzblatt)* online: http://ris1.bka.gv.at/authentic/index.aspx?page=doc&docnr=1

BGBl.I 35/2004. Retrieved October 12, 2007, from *Federal Law Gazette (Bundesgesetzblatt)* online: http://www.ris.bka.gv.at

Directive 2001/20/EC of the European Parliament and of the council of 4 April 2001 on the approximation of the laws, regulations and administrative provisions of the member states relating to the implementation of good clinical practice in the conduct of clinical trials on medicinal products for human use. (2001). *Official Journal of the European Union, 44*(L 121), 34–44.

DuBois, A. (2002). Klinische studien und ihr einfluss auf die versorgungsqualität. *GynSpectrum, 10,* 3–5.

Gesundheits und Krankenpflegegesetz (GuKG). (2004). *Gesundheits und krankenpflegegesetz.* Retrieved October 12, 2007, from http://www.oegkv.at

Janni, W., Kiechle, M., Sommer, H., Rack, B., Gauger, K., Heinrigs, M., et al. (2005). Studienteilnahme verbessert therapiestrategien und individuelle patientenversorgung in teilnehmenden zentren. *Geburtsh Frauenheilk, 65,* 955–973.

Poznanski, U. (2004). Ethikkommissionen: Zum schutz der patientinnen. *Krebshilfe, 4,* 78–79.

About the Author

Johanna Ulmer, PhD, SC, was born in Innsbruck, Austria, in 1952 and moved to Chicago, IL, at age 16. She went to high school and college there, receiving a Bachelor of Arts in liberal arts and sciences at the age of 21. Upon returning to Austria, Dr. Ulmer taught English at a high school in Austria for three years. She was married at the age of 24 and has two children. At age 30, Dr. Ulmer worked as a medical administrative assistant at a gynaecologist's practice and was employed there for 15 years. During the latter years, she began studies at the University of Innsbruck, where she received a PhD in philosophy (medical ethics).

In 1995, Dr. Ulmer began working as an administrative research assistant at the University of Innsbruck, Department of Obstetrics and Gynecology. The AGO Trial Center was established at the Medical University of Innsbruck in 2001. Since that time, Dr. Ulmer has held the position of trial manager for AGO trials in Austria and study coordinator for local trial participation at the Medical University of Innsbruck, Department of Obstetrics and Gynecology.

CHAPTER 60
Denmark

Fie Budtz, RN

History and Background

Denmark, the world's oldest kingdom, is a small country with approximately 5.4 million inhabitants and has been a democracy since 1849 (Danmarks Statistik, n.d.; "Denmark," 2006). Health services are financed through taxes; therefore, equal and free medical treatment is offered to everyone. Five oncology centers exist, in addition to several minor oncology departments within general hospitals.

In this country, 32,802 people are diagnosed with cancer annually, and 15,452 people die from cancer. The lifetime risk for developing cancer before the age of 75 is 34% for both men and women. As of 2003, 4.3% of the population, or 229,535 people, were living with cancer (Kraeft i Danmark, n.d.; Kraeftens Bekaempelse, n.d.).

Apart from skin cancer, lung, prostate, urinary bladder, and colorectal cancers are the most commonly diagnosed cancers in Danish men. Regarding women, the incidence of breast cancer outnumbers skin cancer and is the most commonly occuring cancer disease among women. After breast cancer, skin, colorectal, and lung cancers are the most common cancers in Danish women (Kraeft i Danmark, n.d.; Kraeftens Bekaempelse, n.d.).

Protocol Development

Denmark has 30–50 academic groups that are involved in conducting clinical trials, some of them more formal than others. Through networking with the European Organisation for Research and Treatment of Cancer, more clinical research activity occurs in the oncology field than in any other specialty.

All clinical trial protocols in Denmark that involve testing drugs on human beings are approved by the Danish Medicines Agency, which reports to the Ministry of Health. An ethical committee system addresses the ethical questions in clinical trials (*Den Centrale Videnskabsetiske Komité*, n.d.-a; "*Forsøg Med Habile Personer*," n.d.; "*Vejledning om Anmeldelse m.v. af et Biomedicinsk Forskningsprojekt til de Videnskabsetiske*

Komité System," n.d.). Figure 60-1 lists the Danish protocol requirements for written patient information and informed consent (IC).

Ethics Committees

Denmark has one national and eight regional ethics committees (RECs), plus one for the Faroe Islands and one for Greenland. The Faroe Islands have been an autonomous region of the Kingdom of Denmark since 1948 (Faroe Islands, n.d.). Greenland has been an integral part of Denmark since 1953 and was granted self-government in 1979 by the Danish Parliament (Gronland, n.d.).

The system of RECs was established in 1980 and became statutory in 1992. Each of these RECs has a minimum of seven and a maximum of 15 members. Approximately half of the members are medical professionals, but the majority must be laypeople.

International guidelines and ethical standards, as well as Danish law (*Den Centrale Videnskabsetiske Komité*, n.d.-b), regulate the responsibilities of the ethics committee. The REC must ensure that a trial will comply with the Declaration of Helsinki (see Appendix 2) and with the European Union directive ("Commission Directive 2001/20/EC," 2001; "Commission Directive 2005/28/EC," 2005), accord-

---

Figure 60-1. Danish Protocol Requirements for Written Patient Information and Informed Consent

Every clinical trial protocol must describe the following procedures in detail.
- How the patient will be informed
- How informed consent will be obtained
- How the above guidelines apply to the person giving the information, on behalf of the investigator

Note. Based on information from "Bekendtgørelse om Information og Samtykke ved Inddragelse af Forsøgspersoner i Biomedicinske Forskningsprojekter," n.d.; "Forsøg Med Habile Personer," n.d.; "Vejledning om Anmeldelse m.v. af et Biomedicinsk Forskningsprojekt til de Videnskabsetiske Komité System," n.d.

---

ing to Danish law (*Den Centrale Videnskabsetiske Komité*, n.d.-a, n.d.-b; *Lov om et Videnskabsetisk Komitésystem og Behandling af Biomedicinske Forskningsprojekter*, 2003). The reader is referred to Chapter 58 for additional information regarding the European Union Directive.

Because of the high number of laypeople in the REC, a protocol written in a foreign language has to be translated into Danish before the REC will review it. This procedure frequently delays further action.

A registry of studies is available in Danish at the following Web site: www.skaccd.org/ABC%20Catalog/Customized/Index.asp. It is available, however, only to citizens of Denmark, Greenland, and the Faroe Islands. Physicians, nurses, and patients use online registries only for specific protocols and only when a physician is listed as a coinvestigator.

Informed Consent

The written patient information and IC form have to be identical in all participating centers in multicenter trials. To avoid disputes among centers concerning the terminology, the special interest group (SIG) for clinical trial nurses (CTNs) in Denmark has developed a manual, which should be used when writing the document. The author of an IC form is encouraged to follow the manual to ensure that the IC form will comply with directives and with the law. The manual is widely recognized by both investigators and CTNs. Although CTNs are skilled in creating IC forms, they rarely obtain IC themselves. Physician investigators generally obtain a patient's consent to participate in a clinical trial.

The REC assesses and approves the written patient information and the IC form. Danish law requires that the protocol describe specific procedures in detail, including how the patient will be informed, how informed consent will be obtained, and how the guidelines for informing the patient and obtaining the consent apply to the person that acts on the physician's behalf (*Bekendtgørelse om Information og Samtykke ved Inddragelse af Forsøgspersoner i Biomedicinske Forskningsprojekter*, n.d.). The investigator may delegate any trial-related task to other staff, provided that the staff members are well informed and have received adequate instructions (*Vejledning om Anmeldelse m.v. af et Biomedicinsk Forskningsprojekt til de Videnskabsetiske Komité System*, n.d.; *Forsøg Med Habile Personer*, n.d.).

Patients are referred to the oncology clinic from other departments (i.e., surgical, medical) and usually are already diagnosed. The oncologist reviews the patients' medical files and the information given by the referring department. The oncology clinic sends a letter to the patients with a time for an appointment, which briefly addresses that the patients might be asked to participate in a clinical trial when they come to the clinic. When the patient arrives for his or her first consultation with the oncologist (not necessarily the investigator), the clinic provides complete verbal information about the clinical

trial and written information to take home. Usually, a nurse will be present during the verbal presentation of information by the physician. The patient also will be given general information on his or her rights as participant in a clinical trial. These rights are detailed at www.aaa.dk/aaa/rettigheder_som_forsoegsperson.pdf.

The patient is given *at least* 24 hours to consider the option of participating in the trial; however, usually two days to one week is standard. A follow-up appointment is made for the patient with the physician to address any questions so that he or she can make an informed decision.

The physician is required to inform the patient that he or she may leave a study at any time and without any explanation if the individual wishes to do so. Patient rights should be stressed in all written and verbal communication. The physician also emphasizes that should the patient choose to leave the trial, this will not negatively affect the patient's relationship with the staff in the oncology clinic or the possibility of receiving other treatments. During the second consultation, the physician usually can determine if a person has understood the implications of participating in a specific trial.

If a person younger than 18 years of age is asked to participate in a clinical trial, certain precautionary measures should be observed. These measures are defined by the EC and are found in sections 20 and 21 of chapter 3 in *Bekendtgørelse om Information og Samtykke ved Inddragelse af Forsøgspersoner i Biomedicinske Forskningsprojekter* at www.retsinformation.dk/Forms/R0710.aspx?id=9930. The minor must receive verbal information adapted to the individual's age. This information shall include the risks and advantages of participating in the trial. A person with clear communication skills and knowledge of minors and their perception of words should give the information. If the minor is 15–18 years of age, this information should also be presented in writing. The written information must be adapted to the age group.

All participants, regardless of age and social status, receive the same rights during a clinical trial. If a person has difficulties understanding the written information, the verbal information must be adapted and may be repeated.

The Role of the Clinical Trial Nurse

CTNs work within a clearly defined infrastructure with a multifarious role. CTNs encourage the staff to take ownership of clinical research within the department. The purpose of a clinical trial as it relates to a specific patient may not always be clear to staff. CTNs reinforce the ethical conduct of the research, the protection of patients' rights, and the important role that clinical trials play in treating patients in the future. By implementing these values and encouraging commitment to them, CTNs help to solidify a relationship of trust with the staff. CTNs support adjusting staff assignments to ensure that the staff working with a patient enrolled in a clinical trial has received adequate training. The staff must be trained with regard to the protocol, protocol tools, and professional conduct to safeguard the patient and the integrity of the protocol.

At the same time, the CTNs will consider the information needed among the staff and their education levels. CTNs have a vital role in educating staff about specific protocols. Thus, it is important that they assess the information that the staff needs. It is equally important for them to assess the educational level of each staff member so that protocol information is presented at a level that is easily understood.

Each of the responsibilities of the CTN supports the integrity of the protocol, as well as the safety of the patient. The tools developed by the CTN extract essential information, such as the protocol summary, flowchart, schema, and patient diary, from the protocol so that staff can access it easily. Specific aspects of the CTN role in Denmark are listed in Figure 60-2.

Figure 60-2. Role of the Clinical Trial Nurse in Denmark

- Developing standard operating procedures (SOPs)
- Developing templates to ensure uniformity for administrative tools based on SOPs
- Providing the staff with tools for the day-to-day handling of clinical trials
  - Schema
  - Flowchart
  - Guidelines on specific observations
  - Guidelines for dose modification
  - Patient diary
  - Drug accountability schema for patients receiving oral treatment to use at home

---

When preparing for the start of a clinical trial, the CTN meets representatives of the nurses' protocol group, who represent each of the different oncology wards or clinics in their hospital that will treat and care for patients included in the protocol. The group discusses implications of the protocol and arranges for the implementation and staff education.

Trial Conduct

The delegation of tasks and procedures will differ among the various clinical trial units in Denmark. Normally, the physician will assess the patient for eligibility criteria. The CTN rarely administers the treatment, mainly because of the trial unit's organization. The CTN is more involved in patient care and the administration of medicines only when conducting phase I trials. As the physician assesses toxicity symptoms, the tools prepared by the CTN guide toxicity scoring, evaluation of treatment, blood work, and dose reduction. During the conversation with the patient, the physician will address the subject of psychosocial issues and will document this in the patient's record/file.

Sponsoring Agencies

Agency involvement in clinical trials depends on the nature of the study. Most agencies conduct registration studies internationally. These studies are centrally activated by the company and involve many oncology centers. Agency-sponsored studies add extra regulatory concerns, and all involved have to follow the good clinical practice guidelines (International Conference on Harmonisation of Technical Requirements for Registration of Pharmaceuticals for Human Use, 1996) for clinical research. The medical department in the agency is responsible for monitoring the trial.

Agencies support investigator-initiated studies on different levels, most often local studies with registered new drugs. Both the investigators and the agency want the study carried out per GCP guidelines, but regulatory concerns and monitoring will not be at the same level as registration (i.e., investigational new drug) studies. These studies will be observed by the local agencies, and the investigators will have their own database and case report forms. Often, the investigator and the agency will have an agreement to ensure feedback and reports on side effects and results.

Quality Assurance

In Denmark, industry-sponsored studies are monitored and audited by representatives from the sponsoring companies. The national health authorities also conduct audits in the Ministry of Health. During the performance of the studies, RECs are expected to review ongoing ethical management, although they do not have time to do this regularly. Investigator-sponsored studies are monitored. During the past few years, the university hospitals have established GCP units that employ staff to monitor studies.

Professional Development

The primary function of the CTN is to be a catalyst to all of the processes throughout the trial. The investigator and the CTN are responsible for ensuring that all staff receive tools to manage the protocol and patient care correctly. An exception to this is the caregiving role of the CTN in phase I studies. So far, phase I studies have been performed in only one or two centers in Denmark. Typically, the CTN performs data management, as well.

The SIG for CTNs in Denmark was established in 1994. As of 2006, the SIG had 10 members, with all five oncology centers represented. All are members of the Danish Cancer Nursing Society, also called FSK (*Faglig Sammenslutning af Kræftsygeplejersker*), which is a group member of the European Oncology Nursing Society. All members take part in the regular meetings and bring news and education to all other oncology nurses by writing for the *Fokus på kræft og sygepleje* newsletter or arranging sessions or workshops at the Danish Cancer Nursing Society's annual congress.

In 1997, the CTN SIG created an educational course for CTNs, which is supported by sponsors from the pharmaceutical industry. The topics are taught over six days (42 hours) in three two-day modules, with six months between the modules. The courses take place in a hotel setting, and the participants stay overnight. This gives them the opportunity to socialize with colleagues and create a professional network that is very helpful when conducting multicenter trials. The SIG has been maintaining and updating the education course ever since. The course is very popular among novice CTNs. The SIG group is currently considering a fourth module tailored for experienced CTNs. Specific topics presented in the course are shown in Figure 60-3.

Figure 60-3. Danish Clinical Trial Nurse Special Interest Group Educational Course Topics

- Cell biology
- Development of drugs, future possibility of development, problems related to development of drugs
- Preclinical process
- Study phases
- Foreseeable problems regarding clinical trials and strategies for treatment
- Scientific theories and research methods
- Good clinical practice
- Valid data
- Quality-of-life questionnaires
- Quality development, quality improvement
- The future tasks of the clinical trial nurse
- Ethics of science
- Protection of the patient
- The written patient information and informed consent
- Discussion of ethical issues and problems regarding clinical trials, including patients' rights and duties when participating in a clinical trial
- Essential statistical problems in clinical trials
- Critical reading of scientific results and articles

Summary

Denmark has a sophisticated clinical trial model for the conduct of cancer research studies. CTNs have a pivotal role in clinical trial research that includes patient safety, protocol integrity, data collection, and patient and staff education. Danish CTNs work collaboratively throughout the country, sharing skills and expertise to train both novice and expert CTNs.

References

Bekendtgørelse om information og samtykke ved inddragelse af forsøgspersoner i biomedicinske forskningsprojekter. (n.d.). Retrieved January 16, 2008, from https://www.retsinformation.dk/Forms/R0710.aspx?id=9930

Commission directive 2001/20/EC of the European Parliament and of the Council of 4 April 2001 on the approximation of the laws, regulations and administrative provisions of the member states relating to the implementation of good clinical practice in the conduct of clinical trials on medicinal products for human use. (2001, May 1). *Official Journal of the European Union, L 121,* 34–44.

Commission directive 2005/28/EC of the European Parliament and of the Council of 9 April 2005 laying down principles and detailed guidelines for good clinical practice as regards investigational medicinal products for human use, as well as the requirements for authorisation of the manufacturing or importation of such products. (2005, April 9). *Official Journal of the European Union, L 91,* 13–19.

Danmarks Statistik [Statistics Denmark]. (n.d.). Retrieved January 16, 2008, from http://www.dst.dk/Statistik/seneste/Befolkning/Folketal_kvartal.aspx

Den Centrale Videnskabsetiske Komité. (n.d.-a). *English.* Retrieved January 16, 2008, from http://www.cvk.im.dk/cvk/site.aspx?p=119

Den Centrale Videnskabsetiske Komité. (n.d.-b). *Om komitésystemet.* Retrieved January 16, 2008, from http://www.cvk.im.dk/cvk/site.aspx?p=47

Denmark—a demokratic society founded on the rule of law. (2006, December 20). Retrieved January 16, 2008, from http://www.nyidanmark.dk/en-us/citizenship/citizen_in_denmark/denmark_demokratic_society_founded_on_the_rule_of_law/Danmark_et_demokratisk_samfund.htm

Faroe Islands. (n.d.). *Lov nr. 137 af 23. marts 1948 om Færøernes Hjemmestyre.* Retrieved January 16, 2008, from http://www.stm.dk/Index/dokumenter.asp?o=19&n=0&h=19&d=2299&s=5

Forsøg med habile personer 4.1.3.1. Retningslinjer for mundtligt deltagerinformation. (n.d.). Retrieved January 16, 2008, from http://www.cvk.im.dk/cvk/site.aspx?p=421

Grønland [Greenland]. (n.d.). Retrieved January 16, 2008, from http://da.wikipedia.org/wiki/Gr%C3%B8nland

International Conference on Harmonisation of Technical Requirements for Registration of Pharmaceuticals for Human Use. (1996). *Guidance for industry: E6 good clinical practice: Consolidated guidance.* Retrieved August 15, 2005, from http://www.ich.org/cache/compo/276-254-1.html

Kraeft i Danmark—en opslagsbog. (n.d.). Retrieved January 16, 2008, from http://www.cancer.dk/NR/rdonlyres/FE4EAE10-A3AD-45DD-9D7A-E175D60FC538/0/kraefttaldkokt2006.pdf

Kraeftens Bekaempelse. (n.d.). *Viden om kraeft.* Retrieved January 16, 2008, from http://www.cancer.dk/Cancer/forside+cancerdk.htm

Lov om et videnskabsetisk komitésystem og behandling af biomedicinske forskningsprojekter. (2003). Retrieved January 16, 2008, from https://www.retsinformation.dk/Forms/R0710.aspx?id=29142

Vejledning om anmeldelse m.v. af et biomedicinsk forskningsprojekt til de videnskabsetiske komité system. (n.d.). Retrieved January 16, 2008, from http://www.cvk.im.dk/cvk/site.aspx?p=405

About the Author

Fie Budtz, RN, is a CTN at the University Hospital of Aarhus in Denmark. She became an RN in 1978 and worked in oncology for 10 years prior to becoming a CTN in 1998.

Ms. Budtz has attended various courses in oncology and research, including a postgraduate course in oncology for oncology nurses (1997–1998) and coursework for hematology-oncology nurses (1999–2000), decision making and methods of research (2000), and good clinical practice and clinical cancer research (2005). Ms. Budtz attended a diploma course for Good Clinical Practice for Clinical Trial Nurses, an inclusive program with a pharmacologic component, in 2007.

CHAPTER 61
France

Bénédicte Votan, MSc, Post Graduate, and Brigitte Nadeau-Vaissade, BA, Sp.

Background

Cancer clinical trials in France are very important, and many of them are sponsored by nonprofit organizations. Oncology center staff are well versed in performing clinical trials, and most of the larger centers are structured with a clinical trial department, clinical research associates (CRAs), and study nurses.

Protocol Development

Clinical studies may be sponsored by pharmaceutical companies, nonprofit organizations, or cancer centers. In France, all clinical trial protocols that involve testing drugs on humans are sent to a national ethics committee (EC) for submission. A total of 40 ECs exist throughout the French Territory. ECs are independent from the competent authorities (CAs); they have no ties to or relationship with one another. The Minister of Health oversees the proper functioning of the activities of ECs and authorizes them to pursue their operations.

Although the EC generally is attached to a hospital or a clinic, some are completely independent from any institution. By design, all ECs function in the same required manner, with the same number of members and responsibilities. The sponsor of the study can submit the dossier to whichever EC he or she prefers. Sponsors often will submit their new protocols to the same EC. Once a relationship is established, the turnaround time for a favorable opinion may be influenced greatly.

Each EC has a minimum of 14 members, including medical professionals, pharmacists, laypeople, and nurses. The EC reviews and approves the protocol, patient information, and the informed consent (IC) form. It also verifies that the sponsor has arranged for appropriate trial insurance.

IC is accepted as a process by both patients and doctors; in France, only a medical doctor involved with a given trial is permitted to review the information contained in the IC form with the patient. Eligible patients are approached to assess their interest and opinion regarding trial participation. The doctor reviews all of the essential medical information contained in the IC form, as well as the benefits and possible adverse events. Patients take the form home and are asked to review it at their leisure and to return it for the next appointment with a list of questions related to the study or their conditions. Then, if after answering all queries that arise the patient is satisfied and willing to participate, a signature is requested and a copy of the IC form is given to the patient.

Meanwhile, the protocol must be forwarded to the CA, the Agence Française de Sécurité Sanitaire des Produits de Santé (AFSSAPS), to obtain national approval. With the new European directive, the ethics application and the CA application may be submitted simultaneously. A clinical trial may not begin until it has obtained authorizations from *both* the EC and the French CA.

A clinical trial can occur in one center, known as a *monocenter trial*, or in several centers, known as a *multicenter trial*.

Eligibility

Eligibility criteria are clearly stated in all protocols, and the investigators are responsible for checking all of the criteria before inclusion of a patient. IC, as approved by the EC, must always be obtained prior to the first trial-related procedures. Laboratory, x-ray, and other baseline tests must be obtained within the protocol-stated time frames and within specified acceptable limits.

Active Treatment

A pharmaceutical company supplies investigational agents, which are shipped to the pharmacy of each center. The center's pharmacy is responsible for storing, preparing, handling, dispensing, and accounting for the trial drugs. The pharmacy must receive the protocol and other trial-related documents that direct the pharmacy in the trial.

In some trials, treatment can be *blinded* by using a placebo with the same appearance and management as the investigational drug.

During treatment, patients are assessed for adverse reactions. All adverse reactions/events and serious adverse events must be reported to the EC and CA. The clinical trial team in the hospital must ensure that accurate details of the patient's toxicities and side effects are recorded in the case report forms (CRFs). It is important to record symptoms and assess their relationship to the treatment.

Tumor response assessments are performed per protocol. Most trials will seek disease-free survival at a minimum, but many will challenge for a response. As there are many trials in oncology, the study end points and goals will vary from study to study. For trials that require radiology response assessments, computed tomography is used alone; positron-emission tomography is not very widely used in France.

Ancillary Studies

Most clinical studies include a method of evaluating a patient's quality of life (QOL) during treatment, as it is well known that the QOL maintenance is very important for patients with cancer. The most common QOL tools used in France are the European Organisation for Research and Treatment of Cancer general and disease-specific assessments, followed by the Functional Assessment of Cancer Therapy. These questionnaires are administered as part of the original investigations, as nurses in France conduct very few "nursing-oriented" studies. Patients are referred to a psycho-oncologist at the time of their initial diagnosis and as needed, but rarely more than once or twice during treatment.

Follow-Up

In general, patients are evaluated until deceased, independent of the objectives of the trial (i.e., response rate or progression-free survival). Centers are asked to make every effort to fulfil the follow-up reporting required to complete the analyses. Unfortunately, no national database currently exists to locate patients that have moved out of the area or are deemed "lost to follow-up." Centers can, however, contact the local town hall where a patient originally lived to obtain survival information or date of death. The new regulations plan for a system to be put in place soon to serve this purpose.

Quality Assurance

All clinical trials and personnel involved must adhere to the International Conference on Harmonisation of Technical Requirements for Registration of Pharmaceuticals for Human Use (ICH) Good Clinical Practice (GCP). Clinical studies, industry sponsored or not, are monitored by CRAs. They determine if the study personnel followed GCP by verifying the integrity of the data and ensuring the

patient's rights. This is done via a full review of the source documents and the information in the CRFs. Electronic CRFs and e-Trial Master files are gaining in popularity in France, as they result in a substantial decrease in the heavy trial-associated paperwork. The frequency of monitoring is dependent on the terms of the study.

Audits from the quality assurance department of the pharmaceutical companies or from the national CA can occur at any time. Centers are expected to archive all study patients' records and documentation for a minimum of 15 years after the results have been published and the study considered officially closed.

Ethics

All clinical trials are subject to the regulations of *La Loi Huriet*, as has been the code of biomedical research ethics in France since 1988. In 2004, this regulation was updated to the *Loi de Santé Publique* ("Loi N° 2004-806 du 9 Août 2004," 2004). The key points of this revision are the integration of the new European Directive 2001/20/CE and its direct application in France, including the new pharmacovigilance safety measures. Furthermore, it attributes a new role to the French agency in that the previous process of simply notifying the agency to the commencement of a clinical trial was changed to require prior approval from the agency, thus moving from a notification process to an approval process. This law also defined in greater detail the role of the parties involved in a clinical research study (investigator, sponsor, study coordinator). Responsibilities of each member of the clinical research study team are shown in Table 61-1.

Information Systems

Per the reviewed legislation currently applicable in France, two new systems became effective in 2007. The first is a repertoire for patients and their families of all trials conducted that provided basic details on eligibility criteria, primary end points, and investigator contact information. Currently, the only information available pertains to trials in hepatitis or for orphan drugs. The Web site where this information can be found is http://afssaps.sante.fr/htm/5/repec/repec0.htm.

The second is a national registry of all patients participating in a clinical trial, a tool for investigators and clinical study personnel. At press time, the authorities had not yet set forth how these systems will be implemented.

Professional Development

In France, nurses follow a minimum curriculum of three years and have a variety of professional role possibilities from which to choose, including the field of clinical research. No official nursing society exists, and credentials need not be updated once a student has graduated from the basic nursing program. The titles of study nurse or coordinator just recently have been recognized in France,

Table 61-1. Responsibilities of Personnel Actively Involved in Clinical Trials in France		
Clinical Study Role	Legal Obligations	Restrictions
Sponsor	Oversees the setup, conduct, and finances of the study and the results published Must ensure adequate clinical trial indemnity throughout the duration of study Submits to local ethics committees (EC) and authorities to obtain approval prior to commencing the study	May not have any direct interactions with patients participating in the study
Study coordinator	Is an investigator selected by the sponsor to act as a representative of the study in a multi-center trial Often writes the final publications of the study	May not have any direct interactions with the health authorities with respect to the study
Investigator	Is a physician participating in the trial responsible for a given center and its staff.	May not have any direct interactions with the EC or the authorities with respect to the study
Co-investigator	Is synonymous with subinvestigator in the United States and Canada; is always a physician	May not perform any other task than those delegated to by the investigator
Study nurse	–	May not present the informed consent document to a patient May not prescribe any meds

protocol procedures, and patients will refer to the nurse for questions or problems concerning treatment or other study-related issues. The role of the oncology study nurse within the hospital setting often features an array of activities, including bedside care, treatment administration, toxicity assessments, and more. The oncology nurse working in a cancer center will carry out those same tasks, however with a smaller number of patients, thus allowing him or her to have more time to complete CRFs and perform other trial-related functions. The support function of the study nurse is key in the successful recruitment and conduct of a study at a given research center. Furthermore, academic trials designed with study nurses' collaboration often yield a smoother process throughout the duration of the study, as nurses tend to have more practical approaches to logistics issues.

Summary

In conclusion, centers that utilize study nurses for trials yield fewer study deviations. A study nurse can positively affect a center by being more acquainted with the specifics of trials where the data generated (source documents and CRFs) are of higher quality. Patients appreciate the availability of a study nurse, as he or she is almost always present during their treatment and is a readily available contact for questions and answers. Study nurses do not replace the medical oncologist in a trial; however, given the complexity of today's trials, they are a definite advantage to have within a team of clinical trial staff.

Reference

Loi N° 2004-806 du 9 août 2004 relative à la politique de santé publique. (2004). *Journal Officiel, 185,* 14277.

About the Authors

Bénédicte Votan is a graduate from Lyon University, France, where she obtained her master's degree in science. She is post-graduate in industrial pharmacy since 1989. She has worked in various positions for 14 years in clinical research departments of pharmaceutical companies. She currently works as general manager of an operational team of a collaborative group in Paris dedicated to clinical research in oncology.

Brigitte Nadeau-Vaissade is a graduate from Concordia University, Montreal, where she obtained her bachelor's degree in neuropharmacology, with a specialty in experimental research, in 1993. She has since worked at the bench and moved to the pharmaceutical industry in 1999, where she began as a CRA in oncology trials.

as a result of the ever-increasing number of clinical trials in the hospital and private setting. Although there has been some discussion about creating a specific training program for study nurses, no organization has undertaken this project.

Specifically, the study nurse's role is to act as the communication liaison between doctor and patient. Investigators rely on the study nurse to review the required

CHAPTER 62
Germany

Gabriele Elser, RN, Heike Busse, RN, and Belinda Thorwirth, RN

History and Background

Clinical oncologic research in Germany is based on the oldest and biggest scientific association in oncology, the German Cancer Society, known as *Deutsche Krebsgesellschaft e.V.*, which began around 1900. Detailed information about the German Cancer Society may be accessed at www.deutsche-krebsgesellschaft.de. Split into 23 working groups, physicians and scientists are searching to identify the basic mechanism of cancer, to develop new diagnostic and therapeutic methods, and to prevent and follow malignant diseases.

Several independent academic research organizations (scientific study groups) were established that specialize in different tumor entities (e.g., the AGO-OVAR study group [gynecologic tumors], the NOGGO [gynecologic tumors], and the GBG [German Breast Group]). Networks, such as the Competence Network/Malignant Lymphomas, that focus on various tumor types also were established. The scientific study group named the *Deutsches Krebsforschungsinstitut* (German Cancer Research Center), found at www.dkfz.de, systematically investigates the mechanisms of cancer development and works on the identification of cancer risk factors. Most of the academic research organizations are supported by the pharmaceutical industry and/or receive subsidies from different institutions and contributors.

Elements of a Protocol

Based on the nature of a protocol (e.g., national trial, international collaboration, including European Union [EU] and non-EU collaboration, pharmaceutical company trial), the elements are checked according to the recommendation of the German Cancer Society, which provides a "master protocol" template on its Web page at www.krebsgesellschaft.de/download/Masterprotokoll.doc.

Additionally, the principal investigator's team checks the protocol for formal, scientific, and statistical aspects, as well as for feasibility. The major elements of a protocol are listed in Figure 62-1.

Figure 62-1. Protocol Elements

- Design and objectives of the study (phase, primary, secondary end points)
- Scientific background and rationale for the trial
- Patient selection (inclusion and exclusion criteria)
- Study parameters and safety parameters
- Assessment of side effects, assessment of response criteria
- Treatment (dose, schedule, dose adjustments)
- Statistical considerations for analyses
- Ethical considerations
- Publication statement
- Signatures and responsibilities
- References
- Informed consent form and patient information form

In protocols where the German academic research groups or the principal investigator were not part of the protocol writing team, it becomes more difficult to make changes.

Budget

Based on the nature of a protocol, costs are assessed according to the study requirements. Calculations must be made to ascertain that the trial is sufficiently equipped. Additional financial support may be needed for documentation materials and staff; additional examinations for imaging, laboratory, or other tests that will not be covered as standard by the health insurance; costs for the ethical review board; and trial insurance. Negotiations with the various partners must be done prior to agreements to ensure that the trial is opened at all applicable centers.

Statistical Considerations

Statistical considerations are based on the nature of a protocol and must be carefully checked. The primary areas of the statistical section of a protocol are listed in Figure 62-2.

Assurances

Depending on the type of clinical trial that is being proposed, either the *Arzneimittelgesetz* (German Medi-

---

Figure 62-2. Required Statistical Protocol Elements

- Sample size calculation, power, and hypothesis (e.g., inferiority/noninferiority)
- Primary, secondary, and tertiary end points
- Randomization and stratification procedures
- Definition of end points
  - Stopping rules
  - Statistical analysis plan, statistical methods, and/or tests
  - International Data Monitoring and Safety Committee established (yes/no)
  - Writing and timing of final report

---

cines Law) or the *Medizinproduktegesetz* (Medical Device Directive) applies. The focus of these laws varies with the products that will be investigated. German Medicines Law covers all medicinal products or *active substances*, whereas the Medical Device Directive covers all medicinal devices. Whether the approval of the Federal Radiation Protection Office is required for a clinical trial is determined on an individual basis. All aspects of the Federal Data Protection Law must be respected in every clinical trial.

Most pharmaceutical company-sponsored trials are monitored and audited by representatives of the sponsoring companies. Nevertheless, in accord with the EU directive (see Chapter 58), the local German authorities perform more inspections and the competent authority (CA) performs more audits at clinical trial sites than before the directive went into effect. Also, U.S. Food and Drug Administration (FDA) and European Medicines Agency inspections are performed more often in agreement with international regulations.

Local authorities monitor involved sites, including investigator and site staff, for conducting the trial according to good clinical practice (GCP), reporting high-quality data, and accurately accounting for trial drugs. The location of the investigator's residence and study site determines which local authority will monitor the site.

Audits can be performed by the Federal Health Authority or initiated by a pharmaceutical company or an academic research organization.

Determining Workload

Determining trial manageability takes into account the workload for documentation (paper, electronic), patient examinations (physical, imaging, special exams), preparation of tumor samples or blood samples (who is involved), determination of treating units' availability (unit census), and patient compliance. Overall, GCP criteria must be achieved, and staffing is adjusted accordingly.

Laboratory Issues

Whether a designated central laboratory unit or each site laboratory is used must be taken into consideration. If the trial is using a central laboratory, the protocol must clearly describe processes for sample preparation and

transportation, including packaging, overseas transportation, billing, documentation, and needed equipment. The same considerations are true for tumor tissue or any other human specimen samples.

The Data Protection Act and good laboratory practice must be considered, and the laboratory certification and normal values must be provided to the sponsor. The Data Protection Act protects the patient against data misuse; therefore, only patient identifiers, excluding the full name, are allowed for trial documentation.

Sponsoring Agencies

Agency involvement in clinical trials depends on the nature of the study. Most agencies run international registration studies with a new drug. These trials are centrally activated by the company and involve several oncology sites. The trials are organized using a high level of experience and manpower of the involved sponsoring team. Conversely, local staff organize local investigator-sponsored trials (ISTs).

Intergroup Trials

The research in clinical oncology trials grows more important as the number of newly diagnosed patients with cancer increases. Questions regarding prognostic factors, which help to identify patients who will benefit from treatment and determine further development of the best state-of-the-art therapies, should be addressed expediently. Therefore, network research through international collaboration is the best approach to get answers.

The examples of Gynecological Cancer InterGroup (GCIG) trials in gynecologic malignancies show an impressive overview of how intergroup trials' results can influence cancer treatment.

One very important issue in intergroup trials is the scientific independence; these trials are not conducted by the pharmaceutical companies but are supported by them.

Collaboration of several scientific study groups requires a "leading" group. All participating groups have to follow the policies and guidelines for a specific trial as determined by the leading group. The written intergroup agreement describes the roles and responsibilities among the groups. Centers can participate in a clinical trial through the cooperative group with which they are affiliated. The cooperative group governs its centers according to national requirements and in compliance with the leading group.

Potential Accrual Base

The recruitment base in oncology trials is broad because the diagnosis of cancer makes patients want the best treatment. On the other hand, not all sites have the capability to take part in a clinical trial because of a lack of manpower, trained staff, or support of their administration regarding department issues (Sehouli, Kostromitskaia, Stengel, & Bois, 2005). The investigator exerts an important influence on the recruitment of patients (Harter et al., 2005). Thus, the investigator is the most important person in conducting a clinical trial. The investigator oversees the number of eligible patients in the institution and has the ability, together with the clinical staff, to educate all potential patients. More and more, patients are obtaining information about clinical trials from the Internet.

Of concern is whether older adult patients can take part in clinical trials, as most studies have a cut-off of 75–80 years of age. When planning clinical trials, a process of rethinking the view of older adult patients should be taken into account.

Public and Patient Education

The German Cancer Society offers several programs for the public including nutrition and smoking cessation programs. Selected information regarding clinical trials for a specific kind of cancer is offered to the public community. However, no public adult education activity occurs within academic research organizations. *Krebsinformationsdienst* (Cancer Information Service, www.krebsinformationsdienst. de), an institution of the German Cancer Research Center in Heidelberg, develops the bulk of all patient education materials related to clinical trials. A minor portion is prepared by industry sponsors and distributed by nurses at clinical trial research sites. Medical physicians and the investigator of each clinical trial approve all patient education materials.

Clinical Research Team and Interdisciplinary Team

The clinical trial team consists ideally of the principal investigator (PI), coinvestigator(s), nurses, a pharmacist, laboratory personnel, and, depending on the clinical trial, additional physicians and specialized staff. All staff involved in clinical trials must have a high level of knowledge of oncology and GCP. This must be demonstrated and documented, for example, in a curriculum vitae.

Prior to starting the clinical trial, the PI delegates the responsibilities for the specific study, including obtaining patient consent, administering treatment, assessing toxicity, documenting, reporting, and much more. Normally, this will be listed on a signature list where every involved person must sign. The sponsor or monitor usually conducts the training program for the clinical research team during the initiation visit.

Legal and Regulatory Issues

For an in-depth discussion of legal and regulatory issues in Germany, please refer to Chapter 58, which presents the European Union directives.

Institutional Review Boards

The ethics committee (EC) is comparable to the institutional review board. Every clinical research site has a local EC that governs and monitors the conduct of research at that site. Regarding the latest German Medicines Law and GCP–Verordnung (directive), the EC must be respected. A clinical trial may not start until the EC has issued a favorable opinion and the sponsor has not been informed by the CA of any grounds for nonacceptance.

Informed Consent

The informed consent (IC) document contains specific, required information about the clinical trial. It is a legal document, which must be reviewed and approved by the EC. The IC document must be written for laypeople in understandable language. The main elements of the IC form are outlined in Figure 62-3.

Figure 62-3. Elements of an Informed Consent Document

- An explanation about purpose of the research
- Treatment schedule
- Risks and benefits for the human subject
- Alternative treatments
- Explanation that participation is voluntary and refusal to participate causes no penalty or loss of benefits for the patients
- Statement about insurance, including address and insurance number
- Statement about data protection in association with the patient's confidential data

---

All trial-related examinations and procedures can begin only if the patient understands the implications of the clinical trial and has given written IC. The consent is effective as long as the patient does not withdraw from the clinical trial. The investigator may delegate obtaining IC to a designee who is also a physician. Special consideration has to be taken for children in clinical trials; the consent of their legal representative is required. The consent of a legal representative or authorized representative also is required for adult patients who are not able to understand the nature, impact, and consequences of a clinical trial.

Conflicts of Interest

The terms of GCP principles must be followed: "The rights, safety, and well-being of the trial subjects are the most important considerations and should prevail over interests of science and society" (International Conference on Harmonisation of Technical Requirements for Registration of Pharmaceuticals for Human Use, 1996, p. 13). Centers are advised to avoid having more than one active clinical trial in the same population set. Also, investigators are required to disclose if they have financial interests in a company-sponsored trial.

General Publication

The study protocol should include a chapter about publication rules. Generally, publication of results depends on the sponsor of a trial, the guidelines of the specific protocol, and the agreement between sponsor and investigator. In ISTs the same procedures are valid. For final publication, authors have to respect the guidelines of the selected journal and the author's disclosure declaration and contribution form. Usually, these aspects apply to investigators and not to research nurses.

Psychosocial Considerations

The psychosocial aspect is an important factor that is underrepresented at the moment in Germany. At the time of protocol treatment completion, patients have follow-up examinations, but psychosocial aspects are not routinely addressed. However, comprehensive cancer centers provide psychosocial support for some patients. For example, patients with breast cancer are offered psycho-oncologic support from the time of first diagnosis until departure from the hospital. After treatment completion, self-care groups generally continue the program. The establishment of a breast cancer nurse position, who supports patients, has come into force over the past two years. In the future, this support should be offered to all patients with cancer in Germany.

Recruitment Strategies

Recruitment strategies are based on the nature of the clinical trial. The majority of patients in oncology trials are seen in clinical departments and hospitals specialized according to the tumor being treated. The available patient medical charts are screened to select eligible patients. Normally, no advertising in the public media is necessary.

Eligibility

Identifying patients for clinical trials is primarily the role of investigator or coinvestigator. Study nurses, if established at the site, help in the screening period. If a patient seems to be eligible, he or she will be asked to take part in a clinical trial, after a full explanation of the treatment, benefits and risks, or any other behavior associated with the clinical trial.

Procedures as postulated in the clinical trial protocol can begin only if a patient gives written IC.

Cancer Prevention and Control Studies

Only a few cancer prevention studies are currently active. Identification of subjects who might be eligible is the main obstacle. It takes more investigator time in the screening period and in the introduction of a trial to a healthy human subject, regardless of high-risk factors, than in a person with cancer. As a result, few healthy individuals are approached; therefore, few are enrolled in cancer prevention clinical trials.

Investigational Agents

The logistics of the clinical trial protocol have to be checked prior to initiation, as well as the facilities for storage (e.g., temperature control, locked rooms). If drugs will be provided to a site or investigator, the staff (including pharmacists) must be instructed about their nature, handling, and side effect profile. An investigator's brochure or summary of products characteristics sheet should be available for the staff. The shipping/transportation plan must be stated clearly and request receipt documentation for clinical supplies. If a pharmaceutical company located in the United States provides an investigational new drug, the FDA form 1572, signed by the individual investigator, must be completed. All received and used/unused drugs have to be reported in the specified documents for study drug accountability.

Administration of Protocol Agents

Physicians prescribe study drugs according to the clinical trial protocol. Drug dosages have to be calculated and recalculated according to the protocol-specific guidelines (e.g., mg/qm). Compliance with described formulas for dose calculation should be documented in the patient record. Research professionals, mostly physicians and pharmacists, then recheck the calculations. All guidelines for dose reduction and dose interruption must be observed.

The specific laboratory or physical values, and any reported side effects, must be evaluated prior to each calculation and scheduling of the study treatment. The pharmacist prepares most cytotoxic agents. The treating staff must be trained in administration of the drugs and observation of the patient during treatment. For documentation purposes, all treatment data should be kept in the medical record.

Symptom Management

Before starting the study treatment, patients are informed about specific side effects and instructed in the handling of those. Patients are informed about examinations during the treatment interval (e.g., weekly blood drawing). Additionally, the use of supporting agents, such as antiemetics or growth factors, is explained to the patient. A patient diary can be helpful for recording and reporting symptoms. Symptoms must be recorded in the trial documentation according to the protocol guidelines.

Adverse Events

Adverse events experienced by a patient in a clinical trial should be reported according to the protocol-specific assessment scales. The recent toxicity criteria of the U.S. National Cancer Institute (NCI), the Common Terminology Criteria for Adverse Events (NCI Cancer Therapy Evaluation Program, 2003), currently are used for grading and reporting toxicities in German clinical trials.

The specific definitions for adverse event, serious adverse event (SAE), significant adverse event (SIAE), and suspected unexpected serious adverse reactions (SUSARs) have to be taken into consideration.

The investigator or designee must report an SAE, SUSAR, or SIAE to the sponsor within 24 hours after becoming aware of it. Also, follow-up reports should be given in cases of initially unresolved SAEs. All further obligations regarding the reporting and recording of any adverse events have to be respected by the trial's sponsor.

Patient and Family Education

The investigator, along with the trial staff at the treating institution, informs the patient and the patient's relatives about expected discomforts or complaints during the study treatment, as well as how to deal with them. Verbal and written instructions regarding medication (if the patient has to take medication at home) should be given to the patient. Communication with the general practitioner is always a great help to the patient during treatment and follow-up. Therefore, it is important for the clinical trial investigator to confer with the patient's general practitioner throughout the patient's time on the study.

Compliance in Clinical Trials

The more the patient and family are involved in the activities of the clinical trial, the better the patient compliance will be. However, the clinical staff that is taking care of a patient is responsible to ensure this involvement.

Quality-of-Life Studies

Depending on the phase (i.e., phase III) of the primary clinical trial, a quality-of-life (QOL) study is included. Usually, the QOL studies use the European Organisation for Research and Treatment of Cancer QOL questionnaires. The study assistant teaches the patient about the completion and meaningfulness of compliance with this portion of a trial.

Pharmacokinetics and Genetics

The evaluation of pharmacokinetics and genetics in clinical trials in Germany is planned carefully with consideration to time and effort. Ethics and data protection must be taken into serious consideration and respected. Study site personnel assist the investigators in sample preparation and processing. Even the technical requirements (e.g., dry ice, liquid nitrogen) and logistics (e.g., shipping procedures) have to be checked together with the investigating and laboratory staff to ensure compliance.

Genetic Testing and Storage

Genetic testing and storage usually is possible at sites located in university hospitals. If clinical trials are running in smaller institutions, the equipment often is not available. Whenever genetic testing and storage is completed, the process for transportation should be defined very clearly.

Pharmacoeconomic Studies

The evaluation of pharmacoeconomics in Germany is not commonly included in cancer trials. Only a very few clinical trials are investigating issues, such as cost benefit or cost effectiveness.

Long-Term Follow-Up

Documentation of long-term follow-up is an issue associated with unsatisfying results. The crucial factors are two-fold: (a) patients' contactability and (b) the dedication of site personnel. Depending on the accreditation of a site in Germany, patients can routinely have follow-up examinations at the principal site or go to a medical specialist at an outpatient practice.

Off-Treatment Documentation

All required patient data should be kept in the hospital record as source documentation for the study-specific case report forms (CRFs). According to protocol, the documentation has to be provided from the time the patient is registered into a clinical trial for as long as the patient is participating.

Data Management, Documentation, Forms Submission, and Electronic Data Capture

When participating in clinical trials, study assistants are responsible for data entry using either paper CRFs or electronic CRFs (e-CRFs). They are required to follow the guidelines given for each specific protocol. Training begins with initiation visits with the monitoring team and is continued on an ongoing basis. Regarding e-CRFs, different systems may be used depending on the sponsor. Knowledge and experience in technical and software skills are required more often now than in the past.

The site/hospital internal systems must be compatible with the study system (for example, firewalls can be a huge problem). Online training sessions are provided and noted in an education record for each participant. Study assistants should learn the steps of reporting, changing of data entries, and query processing.

Even in intergroup trials, the coordinating (or lead) group is responsible to establish the set of master CRFs, which are used by all groups and adapted for international conditions. As done in the GCIG, the definition of common data elements should be recommended and instructions for data collection established.

Clinical Trials Registries and Resources

"The purpose of a Clinical Trials Registry is to promote the public good by ensuring that everyone can locate key information about clinical trials whose principal aims are to shape medical decision-making" (DeAngelis et al., 2005a, p. 2928).

According to the recommendations of the International Committee of Medical Journal Editors (DeAngelis et al., 2005b), clinical trials will be listed at the Web page of www.clinicaltrials.gov. It is recommended to register a randomized trial on the Web site of current controlled trials at www.controlled-trials.com.

A widespread use of Web sites occurs for the registration of trials nationally. The main one is the Web page of the German Cancer Society in the German Cancer Trials Register. It may be accessed at www.studien.de.

Standard Operating Procedures

All parties involved in clinical trial conduct should have training according to local and German standard operating procedures. These may vary depending on the role that each person or team plays in the specific trial. Training also varies by the definition of roles and responsibilities established for each project.

Audit Preparation

The criteria for auditing and monitoring must be described in the German language as a separate section of the protocol. Monitoring encompasses the routine source data verification and checking of protocol compliance. It may include checking the investigator's site files, IC documents, and drug accountability documentation. Personnel of the study sponsor of the trial conduct the study closure visit. Depending on the protocol and the monitoring plan, these visits can take place routinely, such as at 8–12-month intervals.

An audit is the review by authorized sponsor personnel of the entire study documentation, including the investigator's site files, IC form, institutional review board regulatory files, and drug accountability records. Occasionally, audits are initiated upon the authority of the Ministry of Health CA. An FDA inspection, or inspection conditional upon the local regulatory body, may be initiated for international trials.

Both monitoring and audit visits are arranged with the investigator and study team to be sure that all involved persons are available.

Off-Site Treatment

The investigator is obliged to administer treatment only at the dedicated site unless otherwise specified in the contractual agreements. Off-site treatment could involve phase I–II trials, or phase III trials where new investigational drugs are to be tested. Additionally, many clinical trials are initiated in centers of excellence where patients are identified for a study but can be treated off-site. The study team must ensure that the treatment complies with protocol specifications and that all staff are trained. The advantage is greater for a patient to undergo treatment nearer to home, but it complicates documentation, source data validation, and drug accountability.

Drug Accountability

Usually, the pharmacy department at a site is responsible for drug receipt, storage, accountability, and preparation. The investigational staff includes the pharmacists in their decision making. The study assistants order the drugs for patients from the trial-specific distributor. Pharmacists must agree with the documentation of received, dispensed,

and destroyed drugs, as well as the balance, lot numbers, and expiration dates that are reported on the study-specific documentation.

Specialization in Clinical Research Nursing

The role of German clinical research nurses is not as clear as in other countries. Differentiation into a research nurse, data manager, or nurse researcher is not clear. The majority of nurses caring for patients with cancer are associates in the *Konferenz Onkologischer Kranken und Kinderkrankenpflege*, the national society for oncology nurses in Germany. More information may be accessed at www.kok-krebsgesellschaft.de.

A variety of educational offerings from institutions and companies with different learning content about clinical research are available. One of these is the study assistant training offered by the German Cancer Society together with the coordinating centers for clinical trials.

The coordinating centers for clinical trials are a network for clinical trials (KKS-Netzwerk) and were consolidated in 2005. Today, 12 locations exist in Germany (see Table 62-1). Their aim is to encourage cooperation among university disciplines, maintenance units, and the pharmaceutical and medicine-technological industry, as well as to provide educational training to investigators and study site staff.

Summary

Conducting clinical trials in Germany includes struggles with bureaucracy, regulations, and finances. The support of non-pharmaceutical-sponsored trials through public institutions should receive more appreciation. The definition of a clinical trial nurse is not established commonly

Table 62-1. KKS-Netzwerk Locations in Germany	
City	Internet Address
Berlin	www.kks.charite.de
Dresden	www.kksdresden.de
Duesseldorf	www.uniklinik-duesseldorf.de/kks
Freiburg	www.zks.uni-freiburg.de
Halle	www.kks-halle.de
Heidelberg	www.kks-hd.de
Cologne	www.kksk.de
Leipzig	www.kksl.uni-leipzig.de
Mainz	www.kks-mainz.de
Marburg	www.kks-mr.de
Muenster	www.kks-ms.de
Tubingen	www.kks-ukt.de

as it is in many other European and overseas countries. The more common terms of *study nurse, research nurse*, and *study assistant* frequently are used in Germany. Nevertheless, the nurses all work within the same broad domain of cancer research. Widely varying views on education exist. Thus, it would be preferable to establish a more structured education and culture in this professional field worldwide. Increasing specialization not only in nursing but also in technical and language skills is becoming essential.

References

DeAngelis, C.D., Drazen, J.M., Frizelle, F.A., Haug, C., Hoey, J., Horton, R., et al. (2005a). Is this clinical trial fully registered? A statement from the International Committee of Medical Journal Editors. *JAMA, 293,* 2927–2929.

DeAngelis, C.D., Drazen, J.M., Frizelle, F.A., Haug, C., Hoey, J., Horton, R., et al. (2005b). Is this clinical trial fully registered? A statement from the International Committee of Medical Journal Editors. *New England Journal of Medicine, 352,* 2436–2438.

Harter, P., du Bois, A., Schade-Brittinger, C., Burges, A., Wollschlaeger, K., Gropp, M., et al. (2005). Non-enrollment of ovarian cancer patients in clinical trials: Reasons and backgrounds. *Annals of Oncology, 16,* 1801–1805.

International Conference on Harmonisation of Technical Requirements for Registration of Pharmaceuticals for Human Use. (1996). *ICH: E6 (R1) note for guidance on good clinical practice (CPMP/ICH/135/95).* Retrieved October 31, 2007, from http://www.emea.europa.eu/pdfs/human/ich/013595en.pdf

National Cancer Institute Cancer Therapy Evaluation Program. (2003). *Common terminology criteria of adverse events,* (version 3.0). Bethesda, MD: National Cancer Institute.

Sehouli, J., Kostromitskaia, J., Stengel, D., & Bois, A. (2005). Why institutions do not participate in ovarian cancer trials—Results from a survey in Germany. *Onkologie, 28,* 13–17.

About the Authors

Gabriele Elser, RN, attended nursing school in the General Hospital of Backnang, receiving a certificate in 1984 from the regional board of Baden-Wuerttemberg, Germany. She has several years of experience in the field of accident surgery and gynecology. Ms. Elser also has two years of additional training at the school of medical documentalists in Bad Cannstatt (bfw). From 1993 to 1999, she worked part-time as a study nurse and part-time as a study coordinator in the field of gynecologic oncology for AGO Ovarian Cancer Study Group at the Saint Vincentius Hospital in Karlsruhe. Since 1999, Ms. Elser has worked in Wiesbaden (Hessen) as the head of the study office of the AGO Study Group. The main aspects of her work are developing protocols, establishing a clinical trial dealing with regulatory issues, and providing support of education for study nurses. Internationally, Ms. Elser is a representative of the AGO Study Group in the GCIG harmonization working group.

Heike Busse, RN, attended nursing school in the DKR-Schwesternschaft Oranien e.V., receiving a certificate in 1990 from the regional board of Hessen, Germany. Since 1990, she has worked in the field of gynecology while completing postgraduate studies in business management with a focus on hospital economics. Ms. Busse has been employed since 1999 as a study nurse at Dr. Horst Schmidt Hospital, Department of Gynecology and Gynecologic Oncology in Wiesbaden. She continued her education as a study nurse through the German Cancer Society in 2000. The main aspect of Ms. Busse's work is organization of clinical trials with a focus on administrative issues, documentation, and patient management.

Belinda Thorwirth, RN, attended nursing school in Bristol, United Kingdom, and received a certificate in 1981. She worked at the University of Mainz Intensive Care Unit for Cardiology from 1983 to 1997. Between 1997 and 2003, Ms. Thorwirth gained international experience in private nursing in Hong Kong, experience as a data recorder at the Cancer Registry Rhineland-Palatinate, and practical training as a study assistant. She has also continued her professional education as a study nurse through the German Cancer Society. Since 2003, Ms. Thorwirth has been employed as a study nurse in Wiesbaden at Dr. Horst Schmidt Hospital, Department of Gynecology and Gynecologic Oncology. The main aspect of her work is organization of clinical trials with a focus on documentation and patient management.

CHAPTER 63

Italy

Jane Bryce, RN, MSN, AOCNS®, Marianna Connola, BSN, and Marzia Falanga, BSN

History and Background

Cancer is a significant problem in Italy, and incidence and mortality rates are similar to those of other Western industrialized nations (Zanetti, Gafa, Pannelli, Conti, & Rosso, 2002). Italy also has the potential healthcare burden of an aging population with the largest and fastest-growing proportion of older adults in Europe (Statistical Office of the European Communities, 2005).

The Italian national healthcare system guarantees healthcare services to all residents. This care is provided within both public healthcare institutes and private hospitals that have an agreement with the national healthcare system. Italians also may choose to pay for health care in completely private institutes. Oncology care is given in both public and private hospital settings. Several national cancer institutes exist throughout Italy, which practice independently from one another. An alliance of these institutes (*Alleanza contro il Cancro*) was formed in 2002, with one of its goals being to increase national and international oncology research collaboration.

Oversight of clinical research in Italy is mandated by national law and determined by the Health Ministry. In 1997, Italy received the European Union (EU) guidelines for good clinical practice (GCP) in medicinal clinical trials (Decreto Ministeriale, 1997) and in 1998 set guidelines for the establishment and functions of independent ethics committees (Decreto Ministeriale, 1998). The Italian National Medicines Agency (*Agenzia Italiana del Farmaco* [AIFA]) began operating the National Monitoring Centre for Clinical Trials (*Osservatorio Nazionale della Sperimentazione Clinica* [OsSC]) in 1999. The primary functions of OsSC are summarized in Figure 63-1.

Italy was then well positioned for the European strategy of collaboration and harmonization of clinical trial procedures and transmission of data to the European clinical trials database (EudraCT). The country was one of the first member states to implement European Directive 2001/20/EC on clinical trials of medicinal products (Decreto Legislativo, 2003).

Figure 63-1. Primary Functions of the *Osservatorio Nazionale della Sperimentazione Clinica* (National Monitoring Centre for Clinical Trials)

- Guarantee the epidemiologic surveillance of clinical trials of drugs conducted in Italy
- Serve as a national registry of ethics committees, clinical trials, and private clinics accredited for conduction of clinical trials

Data from the OsSC are published regularly and can be accessed online (https://oss-sper-clin.agenziafarmaco.it). The following data reflect activity from 2000 through 2004. During that period, 2,838 clinical trials were registered, and the vast majority of studies were multicenter (81.2%), international (64.9%), phase II or III (33.6% and 55%, respectively), and sponsored by pharmaceutical companies (75%) (AIFA, 2005). Most of the trials are conducted under the specialty of oncology, and antineoplastic and immunomodulatory drugs account for the largest therapeutic category (31.9%). Unlike other categories, however, nonprofit groups sponsor the majority (58.7%) of antineoplastic and immunomodulatory drug trials (AIFA).

Protocol Development

Proposals for new trials come from a variety of sources within oncology institutes, cooperative groups, universities, and pharmaceutical companies. Proposals then are evaluated for scientific merit and feasibility. Some groups have established scientific committees. Once a proposal is accepted, a study chair, principal investigator (PI), or steering committee is designated, and a multidisciplinary writing committee is formed. The writing committee can be composed of oncology physicians and trialists, clinical trial nurses (CTNs), biostatisticians, data managers, and other specialists to provide input for specific trials. The protocol is written following the essential protocol elements as outlined in GCP.

Toxicity and response criteria are based on international standards. The most often used toxicity criteria are the

Common Terminology Criteria for Adverse Events, version 3.0 (National Cancer Institute Cancer Therapy Evaluation Program, 2003), and the most often used response criteria are the Response Evaluation Criteria in Solid Tumors (Therasse et al., 2000). Performance status most often is measured using the World Health Organization, Eastern Cooperative Oncology Group, and Karnofsky scales. Protocols may be written in Italian or English, and because of the high number of international trials conducted in Italy, many protocols are written directly in English. A synopsis of the protocol and the patient informed consent (IC) must be prepared in Italian.

CTNs are involved in the development and content review of the IC form: When a different language version of the informed consent is needed, CTNs work with the study sponsor to facilitate translation using the standard forward-backward method. This method requires translation from the original language to the new language, and then translation of the new document back to the original language by a different translator. The two original-language documents then are compared for semantic equivalence.

Ancillary studies are formulated concurrently with the protocol using the same development and review process, although members may be added to the writing committee to provide expertise according to the study objectives. Protocol amendments are written with the same process as that of the protocol.

The plan for statistical analysis is written in the protocol according to GCP. The protocol details the rules for interrupting the trial and for excluding single subjects, which are reflected in the IC form. The statistical methodology of ancillary studies is detailed in the companion protocol.

Case report forms (CRFs) are developed concurrently with the protocol and generally are trial-specific, although some groups such as the European Organisation for Research and Treatment of Cancer (EORTC) have an established standard format. CRFs are developed by the sponsor in pharmaceutical industry–sponsored studies and by central data managers in clinical trial units in nonprofit-sponsored studies.

For profit or nonprofit studies, sponsors cover the costs of conducting clinical trials. According to EU Directive 2001/20/EC ("Commission Directive 2001/20/EC," 2001), the sponsor should provide an insurance policy for each clinical trial, provide medicines used in the trial (whether investigational or already registered), and provide the monitoring activities to ensure GCP compliance. This directive raised discussion about increased costs throughout Europe, where oncology trials frequently are promoted by nonprofit sponsors (Crawley, 2004; Habeck, 2003; Meunier et al., 2003; Meunier & Lacombe, 2003; Perrone et al., 2004; Watson, 2003).

Italy issued a decree regarding noncommercial clinical trials addressing the increased burdens placed on the nonprofit sponsors and promoting research that aims to enhance clinical practices (Decreto Ministeriale, 2004).

This decree established that the national health system will cover the cost of registered drugs used in noncommercial clinical trials, that the ethics committees fees be waived, and that an institution's general insurance policy could be used to cover patients being treated in clinical trials within that institute.

The issue of adequate insurance coverage is evaluated by the ethics committee prior to protocol approval, and the nonprofit sponsor may still be required to provide an insurance policy if the institute's policy is not considered adequate or if it excludes patients enrolled in clinical trials. The sponsor will develop the budget together with the study chair or PI. The CTN evaluates the costs related to nursing and trial coordination activity. The investigator and sponsor sign research agreements, including financial agreements. Authorship and ownership of data should be clearly delineated in the agreement and may be written directly in the protocol.

Preparation

The sponsor and each single investigator are responsible for signing agreements to conduct a trial according to GCP and the governing Italian and European laws regarding clinical research and privacy. Specific assurances may be required for trials originating outside of Europe. Many Italian institutions have registered their ethics committees with the U.S. Office for Human Research Protections and have obtained a federalwide assurance to participate in U.S. federally funded trials.

Before protocol activation, a multidisciplinary team is assembled that includes physicians, nurses, pharmacists, data managers, laboratory professionals, radiologists, and other specialists depending on the institution and type of trial. CTNs and data managers have emerging roles in Italy, and although becoming increasingly present in the multidisciplinary team, they are not yet represented in every research group.

The CTN has an important role in evaluating the protocol for its feasibility of implementation within the work environment considering the patient population, staff, workload created by the protocol, additional technical and human resources that may be necessary, and any special training required by the protocol. The Italian CTN often acts as research coordinator, helps to establish channels of communication within the research team, and collaborates in the development of a *protocol pathway* or map that demonstrates the coordination and continuity of trial participants' care within the institution (Bryce, Bell, Colussi, De Maio, & Rossi, 2003).

The CTN must identify aspects of the protocol that directly affect nursing care. Developing a *nursing summary* (Di Giulio et al., 1996) is a standard approach of the Italian CTN to summarize the research protocol and guide the treatment and care of patients participating in clinical trials. Nursing summaries are being established as an effective collaborative tool within nursing (Gilger, Groben, & Hinds, 2002; Max et al., 2003; Price, Spencer, Mayor, & Boyle, 2003). The nursing summary or protocol is adapted from the trial protocol and describes the steps of the research process. Figure 63-2 describes the contents of a nursing summary.

Figure 63-2. Nursing Summary Key Points

- Background information
- Toxicity observed in preclinical research
- Goals of the trial
- Selection criteria
- Drug information (including distribution, reconstitution, stability, storage, metabolism and excretion, measures for spillage and extravasation, and hypersensitivity reactions)
- Treatment administration and scheduling
- Logistics
- Toxicity checklists or tools
- Patient self-report tools
- Study testing and follow-up schema
- Nursing care plan with strategies for patient education and symptom management

---

The CTN evaluates the adequacy of source documents to capture required data and works within the institution's standards to facilitate complete documentation within the patient's medical records. CTNs often collaborate in the development of paper or electronic charting systems that permit more complete and accurate documentation in both the inpatient and outpatient settings. Patient education materials are reviewed by the PI and approved by the ethics committee. Additionally, specific testing, such as pharmacokinetic testing, is addressed with the development of appropriate documentation tools for such testing, including shipping and handling information (see the "Ancillary Studies" section).

In this phase, the CTN considers strategies for recruitment of patients into the trial and identifies potential barriers to participation. After evaluation of the protocol and development of a nursing summary, the CTN educates the appropriate staff on patient care issues and provides information to colleagues who have contacts with the accrual base so that referrals can occur. The CTN works with the PI and sponsor to organize site start-up visits and may be involved in training of other sites.

Legal and Regulatory Issues

The procedures for gaining approval and activating a protocol are detailed in the Italian decree enacting the 2001 European directive and its successive integrations (Decreto Legislativo, 2003). The sponsor must obtain a favorable opinion from the ethics committee for a monocentric trial or from the coordinating center's ethics committee for a multicenter trial. The sponsor obtains a financial agreement with the legal officer of the healthcare facility where the trial will be conducted. The sponsor must obtain special permission from the Health Institute (ISS) for all phase I

studies and for trials involving the use of medicinal products for gene therapy, somatic cell (including xenogenic cell) therapy, and all medicinal products containing genetically modified organisms.

The minimum requirements for the institution, organization, and functioning of ethics committees were updated with a decree in 2006 (Decreto Ministeriale, 2006). To render an opinion, the ethics committee evaluates trial relevance and design, risks and benefits, the protocol, the suitability of the investigator, support staff and facilities, the investigator brochure, the IC, insurance policy, and financial agreements. After the single favorable opinion is obtained by the coordinating ethics committees in multicenter studies, ethics committees of satellite sites may either accept or reject the opinion in its entirety. IC forms may be modified and approved by the satellite center for use only with patients treated in that center. Ethics committees render opinions in a timely manner adhering to time limits as established by the legislative decree. Protocol amendments are processed in the same way as the original protocol and are applicable to all sites. Sponsors of medicinal clinical trials must register their trials with the OsSC.

Physicians may request the compassionate use of nonregistered therapeutic agents. The pharmaceutical company (or producer of the drug) is responsible for providing the necessary documentation regarding the use of the agent (e.g., clinical motivation, efficacy and tolerability data, patient information, plan for monitoring data relative to compassionate use). The requesting physician presents the documentation to the ethics committee and to the National Medicines Agency. After the ethics committee grants its approval, the drug is provided free of charge. The requesting physician is responsible for providing data relative to the use of the agent; these data are used for pharmacovigilance rather than registrative purposes (Decreto Ministeriale, 2003).

The structure of Italian oncology clinical trials described in this chapter, with independent ethics committees, adherence to international GCP standards, and transparent research and financial agreements, is designed to avoid conflicts of interest among the researchers, sponsors, and institutes where clinical research is undertaken. Despite this, conflicts of interest—real or perceived—still may exist.

The Italian Society of Medical Oncology (*Associazione Italiana di Oncologia Medica* [AIOM]) published recommendations to avoid conflicts of interests with the pharmaceutical industry (AIOM, 2005a) and has undertaken a study to determine oncology patients' perceptions of conflict of interest (AIOM, 2005b). Italian investigators provide financial disclosure to sponsors of investigational new drug trials as required by the U.S. Food and Drug Administration.

Italian CTNs are guided by the deontologic code for nurses, which is founded on the ethical and nonprejudicial treatment of all patients (Italian National Federation of Nursing, 1999). The Italian CTN has a two-fold responsibility in this regard: to act as a patient advocate and raise awareness of any ethical issues, including potential conflicts of interest, and to ensure IC (discussed in the next section).

Promotion and Recruitment

Promotion of clinical trials is the sponsor's responsibility in terms of content and costs. Individual investigators should get sponsor approval of local published or broadcasted publicity spots. Most promotional activities of clinical trials are geared toward physicians who treat patients in a target group. Many Italian cooperative oncology groups exist; some are united by disease site (e.g., Multicenter Italian Trials in Ovarian Cancer), some by geography (e.g., Gruppo Oncologico del Nord-Ovest), and some by special interest (e.g., Gruppo Italiano di Oncologia Geriatrica). These groups play an important role both in protocol development and in promotion and enrollment into clinical trials, and CTNs have an increasingly active role in many of these groups.

Many Italian patients with cancer are informed protagonists in health care who actively seek information about clinical trials on the Internet and from advocacy organizations and healthcare professionals. Self-referral is becoming more common. Apolone and Mosconi (2002), in a survey of healthy Italians, reported that the public had limited knowledge in general about clinical trials and was reluctant to participate in prevention trials. Promotional campaigns that were focused on both healthcare professionals and patients have been successful in recruiting high-risk patients in Italian prevention and screening trials. Rotmensz, Robertson, Maisonneuve, and Boyle (1998), in reviewing the Italian Tamoxifen Breast Cancer Prevention Trial, suggested a relationship between external events, including negative media coverage, on a decrease in recruitment and problematic early voluntary withdrawal of subjects.

The Italian CTN recruits potential participants in clinical trials from the institution or referring groups by evaluating the target population, examining the inclusion and exclusion criteria, and being cognizant of the timelines and protocol-specific testing that may be required. The CTN ensures that patients have signed the IC form prior to undergoing protocol-specific tests that otherwise would not have been part of standard care. Screening tools and eligibility checklists sometimes are developed with the protocol to assist in evaluating potential participants and to track the enrollment process while ensuring that eligibility requirements are met.

The IC process begins with the first contact with the patient by study staff, and the investigator and/or CTN explain the study to the patient and family/caregivers. The CTN ensures that adequate time is provided to the patient to ask questions and consider whether to participate and documents this process in the clinical record. The patient receives a copy of the consent and a letter for the primary care physician; these can be reviewed and discussed before the patient's next visit with the study team. The CTN plays

an important role in enhancing the patient's understanding of participation in the clinical trial through follow-up discussions with the patient and family. When a patient chooses to participate in a clinical trial, the investigator and patient sign the IC form. The IC process continues throughout the patient's participation in the clinical trial and can be viewed as an ongoing relationship between the patient and the research team. Patient assessment and education also are ongoing responsibilities of the CTN (Bryce et al., 2003).

Once eligibility is confirmed, the CTN or data manager submits the necessary documents for enrolling the patient, usually by fax, phone, or the Internet. CTNs may be involved in requesting protocol waivers in particular circumstances, communicating the request to the study sponsor. The CTN informs the patient of the result of the request to enroll/randomize in the study and schedules study visits per the trial's protocol.

Active Treatment

In this phase, the CTN engages in administering (or overseeing the administration of) the experimental therapy according to the protocol. The CTN works with the pharmacist and staff nurse to ensure adequate receipt, conservation, accountability, preparation, administration, and destruction of the study drug according to the study protocol.

Experimental drugs are received and dispensed by the pharmacist. Drug reconstitution is done in the pharmacy unit (where this service is available) or by the CTN or clinical nurse. Drug dosages are prescribed by the physician and confirmed by the CTN and administering nurse. Depending on the local structure, the CTN or clinical nurse administers the study drug. The CTN and the pharmacist document drug accountability and order drugs from the sponsor. Depending on the protocol requirements, the pharmacist either returns expired or unused drug to the sponsor or destroys it according to local institutional procedures.

Another key CTN responsibility during the treatment phase is the assessment of the patient for crucial toxicity information and the grading and reporting of adverse events. The CTN reports serious adverse events to both the sponsor and the ethics committee. The CTN provides patient education (e.g., by patient information sheets) regarding expected effects of therapy, symptom management, completion of patient diary cards, and study-specific quality-of-life evaluations. The CTN is well positioned for early identification of patient symptoms (toxicities) and for prompt intervention. Poor symptom control can lessen patient compliance with therapy and willingness to continue study therapy and can lead to dose modifications or changes in the treatment plan that may have been avoidable. The CTN assists patients in managing symptoms within the parameters of the protocol when feasible.

The Italian CTN has an important role in coordinating the care of the patient within this phase and is a key liaison between the patient and the investigator. The CTN often is the patient's point of contact for all study-related issues and continues to provide education and support to the patient and family/caregivers. The CTN ensures that evaluations are scheduled according to the protocol to assess patient response to the experimental therapy and for any other study end points.

The CTN also is the communication link between the sponsor and the investigator. The CTN maintains source documentation, provides for CRF completion and transmission, monitors data, and coordinates monitor visits. The CTN submits updates regarding study progress to the ethics committee and clinical staff and helps to coordinate and implement protocol amendments.

Ancillary Studies

The Italian CTN has an active role in the development and conduct of ancillary studies. Studies that involve obtaining patient specimens, such as bioavailability and genetic studies, require specific IC. The specimen may be used for only the purpose(s) indicated in the IC document. Whether results of specimen evaluation will be disclosed to patients must be specified in the consent form. The CTN refers the patient for genetic counseling when indicated. CTN responsibilities include ensuring that the patient is adequately informed and has given consent.

The CTN also must ensure adequate planning for these special studies, assessing for proper documentation tools, supplies, coordination of sampling, shipping, and costs. The CTN provides or oversees the necessary documentation required in the clinical record and study forms and ensures tracking of specimens from collection to storage and shipping, according to protocol specifications and within national and international safety standards. Specimens generally are shipped through a courier, and Italy adheres to international safety standards for biologic and infectious materials (International Air Transport Association, 2005). The date format used in Italy is day, month, year, and time is documented using the 24-hour clock. It is Italian practice and the sponsor's responsibility to request special permission from the Ministry of Health to import and export biologic materials.

Quality-of-life studies are conducted using validated Italian language instruments. The EORTC QLC-C30 and subinstruments often are used. CTNs may contribute to the validation of translated instruments (e.g., Bell, Del Mastro, Marchetti, Bryce, & Costantini, 2003; Piccinelli, Bisoffi, Bon, Cunico, & Tansella, 1993) and be involved in the design and implementation of quality-of-life and companion studies (e.g., ICAI [*Ischemia Cronica degli Arti Inferiori*] Nursing, 1996; Italian Group for the Study of Survival After Infarct Nursing, 1995). The number of nursing companion studies and independent nursing research is growing in Italy, with increased attention to multicenter nursing intervention trials promoted by nursing cooperative groups and within oncology cooperative groups.

Off Treatment

Long-term follow up of patients may be required by the protocol for evaluating survival, time to recurrence, and late or long-term toxicities. In Italy, the CTN continues to have an important role during this time to not only assess and report this data but also to provide emotional and educational support to patients who are no longer on active treatment. Patients may stop experimental therapy in a clinical trial for various reasons, such as those shown in Figure 63-3.

Figure 63-3. Reasons Patients Stop Experimental Therapy in Clinical Trials

- Conclusion of planned therapy
- Voluntary withdrawal
- Withdrawal because of events such as disease recurrence or progression or unacceptable toxicity
- Trial interruption for safety or efficacy reasons

Patients may have different reactions and psychosocial and medical needs once they enter the off-treatment phase, and CTNs can assist patients as they transition to the next phase of care. This ongoing nurse-patient relationship also enhances the patient's compliance with responding to inquiries or requests for follow-up. CTNs document patient follow-up within the patient medical record and provide relevant data in the CRF to the study sponsor. CTNs participate in data query resolution, study closure, and audits. Patient clinical records are maintained permanently and indefinitely within the healthcare institution in which the patient participates in the trial. Clinical trial documents are the responsibility of the PI and the sponsor and are maintained according to GCP and local institutional requirements.

The Italian Clinical Research Nurse Working Group (2005) (*Gruppo Italiano Infermieri di Ricerca Clinica*) advocates the public registration and disclosure of clinical trial results. In Italy, CTNs participate in communicating the study results to patients who participated in the trial (e.g., Bryce, Connola, Salzano de Luna, Caraco, & Chiofalo, 2006; D'Aiuto, Oliviero, & Bryce, 2003), to the ethics committee, and to the primary care physicians. CTNs also participate in the scientific publication of study results (e.g., Del Mastro et al., 2006). CTNs are responsible for helping patients to understand information about clinical trials and research results.

Data Management and Clinical Trial Units

Data management strategies are described in the protocol and include the method (using the CRF is most common), timing, and mode (fax and electronic submissions are most common) of data transmission. Source data documentation and protocol data entry occur distinctly and separately. The CTN is responsible for ensuring complete and accurate source documentation. Data managers (DMs) and/or CTNs, depending on the local structure, transcribe, verify, and transmit data.

The DM role is being defined in Italy (Italian Data Manager Group, 2005). Local DMs may be involved in transcribing and reporting source data, in query resolution, and in administrative, supportive, or coordinative functions related to the clinical trial. Central DMs collaborate with protocol planning and are involved with CRF development, database design, and data entry, validation, and analysis. Central DMs create standard operating procedures (SOPs) for paper or Web-based data collection, transmit data to the OsSC, and provide training to individual research sites (Andreuccetti, 2005).

Some institutes have clinical trial units dedicated to the support of clinical trials. These units generally comprise physicians, biostatisticians, central DMs, CTNs, pharmacists, monitors, and informatics specialists, who are involved in all aspects of the clinical trial. Figure 63-4 outlines the reponsibilities of the clinical trial unit.

Figure 63-4. Responsibilities of the Clinical Trial Unit Team*

- Protocol development and submission for approval
- Coordination of trial activity
- Data management
- Statistical analysis
- Training of sites
- Communication and publication of results
- Quality assurance

* The clinical trials unit team comprises physicians, biostatisticians, central data managers, clinical trial nurses, pharmacists, monitors, and informatics specialists.

Quality Assurance

Assuring adherence to GCP and Italian law is a responsibility of both the PI and the study sponsor. On a practical level, adherence is ensured through the collaboration of the study monitors (the clinical research associate [CRA] or central DM) with the CTN and local DM. The sponsor provides monitoring of the study to ensure GCP and protocol adherence, to verify data, and to assist with resolving any quality improvement issues. Directive 2005/28/EC further underlined the importance of quality data (accurate and verified) and the necessity of qualified personnel in clinical trials ("Commission Directive 2005/28/EC," 2005). The investigator is responsible for assembling a qualified research team, and the sponsor provides any additional training specific to certain trials.

Sites may develop tools such as screening tools, eligibility checklists, timelines, protocol maps, and adequate source documents to assist with protocol adherence. The local DM or CTN can use electronic tools, such as databases, to
- Follow individual cases

- Provide an overview of all patients enrolled in the protocol
- Evaluate study progress, trends, and deviations from the protocol or other quality issues.

The research team writes local SOPs that designate specific functions and activities related to research protocols within the institute, such as dose verification procedures. The CTN reviews deviations from the protocol and safety issues and works with the PI and the CRA to identify and resolve any issues that affect quality.

Independent audits may be used to assess overall compliance and may be requested by the sponsor to evaluate a specific trial. Alternatively, an audit may be performed as part of an overall assessment by the participating healthcare institution, oncology cooperative group, or clinical trial unit. The CTN is involved in preparing for and assisting with audits and in engaging an action plan to resolve any quality issues identified during the audit.

Inspections in Italy may be carried out by the National Medicines Agency, the European Medicines Agency, or the U.S. Food and Drug Administration before, during, or after the conduct of a clinical trial and may be part of the verification process during the application for registration. EU Directive 2005/28/EC provides guidelines for the qualification of inspectors and for inspection procedures ("Commission Directive 2005/28/EC," 2005).

Professional Development

The specialized role of the oncology nurse in clinical trials has evolved alongside the growth of clinical research in oncology. Complex and diverse responsibilities of the CTN have been well described in European and North American literature (Klimaszewski et al., 2000; Ocker & Pawlik-Plank, 2000; Van Wijk, Batchelor, & Dubbelman, 2001). However, this role in Italy is relatively new, and educational and competency requirements have not been established.

The title of CTN is only beginning to be used within the Italian public healthcare system, although nurses have performed this role as contractors and collaborators for more than a decade. A group of CTNs from several cancer institutes in Italy began collaborating in late 2002 to define the responsibilities of the CTN as practiced in Italy and to develop strategies for the preparation, implementation, and evaluation of CTNs within the network of Italian cancer institutes. This group identified two primary barriers to the use of CTNs: the lack of recognition of the CTN role within the Italian public healthcare system and the lack of preparation for this role at the basic and postgraduate level (Bryce et al., 2003).

A strategy for role validation and education should include delineation of responsibilities and role structure, processes for education and research, and policy evaluation and forecasting (Ehrenberger & Lillington, 2004; Mueller, 2001; Shedlock, 2000). The oncology CTN group focused on the following initial objectives.

- To define the responsibilities of Italian CTNs
- To develop an education program for CTNs
- To obtain institutional recognition of the CTN role
- To establish a network of oncology CTNs

This work has continued with Italian Clinical Research Nurse Working Group. CTN responsibilities have been generally categorized as shown in Figure 63-5.

Figure 63-5. Components of the Clinical Trial Nurse Role in Italy

- Protocol development
- Patient education and advocacy
- Patient care and coordination of care
- Consultation and staff education
- Management of patient records and data
- Evaluation of clinical trial performance

Competency-based job descriptions are being revised delineating specific responsibilities along the continuum of care of patients in clinical research (Bryce, Bell, Colussi, De Maio, & Gini, 2004; Italian Clinical Research Nurse Working Group, 2005). Other roles of nurses in clinical research, such as membership on ethics committees and participation in evaluation of protocols and results, also are described ("Guideline of the Italian Ministry of Health," 2004).

A postgraduate clinical trial nursing course developed by the CTN group and sponsored by the European School of Oncology (see www.cancerworld.org) has been available since 2005. The course provides continuing education credits (CEM) from the Italian Health Ministry. Specific objectives for the course, which expand upon the core curriculum proposed by the EORTC Oncology Nurse Group (2003), are listed in Figure 63-6.

Figure 63-6. Objectives of a Clinical Trial Nursing Course in Italy

- To understand the elements of and the basis for a trial protocol in order to participate more fully in all aspects of a clinical trial, from its design and conduct to discussion of the results
- To improve data collection in clinical trials
- To be able to write and implement nursing summaries according to the medical protocol
- To identify patients' and family members' educational needs and take appropriate action
- To have an enhanced awareness of the ethical and legal implications and requirements of a clinical trial
- To be able to assess the impact and workload of the protocol on nursing care
- To identify resources for networking and professional development
- To explore opportunities for nursing research

AIOM regularly offers multidisciplinary CEM courses in oncology clinical research, and the CTN role and responsibilities are part of the curriculum. Several Italian universities began enrollment in 2004 in master's programs in clinical research nursing (encompassing both nursing research and clinical trials nursing) and in clinical research coordination (open to both clinicians and nonclinicians).

Oncology nurses working in clinical research (CTNs and nurse researchers) have a special interest group within the Italian Oncology Nursing Association (AIIO). The AIIO special interest group is very active in increasing the visibility of the CTN within the healthcare and general communities. This is accomplished by presenting the CTN role and responsibilities at conferences and workshops sponsored by AIIO, AIOM, cooperative oncology and DM groups, and patient advocacy associations. AIIO members also belong to the European Oncology Nursing Society, where further networking is possible.

The AIIO and Italian Clinical Research Nurse Working Group CTN working groups are collaborating to realize the objective of gaining widespread institutional recognition of the CTN role, beginning with a prototype job description proposal within oncology and aiming toward validation of the role within the national health system. A CTN role study is in progress to delineate the dimensions of the role in Italy using the validated Clinical Trials Nursing Questionnaire® (CTNQ) developed by Ehrenberger and Lillington (2004), which was adapted and validated in the Italian language by G. Catania and colleagues (personal communication, January 12, 2006). The working groups also are collaborating to increase multicenter interventional nursing research in both companion and independent studies.

Summary

The CTN has an increasingly more active and recognized role in Italy. The CTN is involved in all aspects of clinical research, including protocol development, screening, informed consent, active treatment, study conclusion, and communication of results. The CTN often is the link between the patient, the clinical area, and the PI and has responsibilities both to the clinical trial participant and to the research team. The primary responsibilities toward the patient are to ensure his or her safety and to be an advocate and a caregiver, which are realized through the multiple activities of the CTN throughout the continuum of clinical research. With respect to the research team, CTN activities along the continuum are aimed toward maintaining the integrity of the protocol and quality of research data. The complex and specialized role of the oncology CTN continues to evolve alongside advances in basic and health sciences. The CTN is a key partner of the healthcare research team and with patients enrolled in clinical trials.

The author wishes to thank the following professionals for their expertise and insightful reviews: Gianluca Catania, CTN, Istituto Nazionale di Ricerca sul Cancro, Genova; Anna Maria Colussi, CTN, Centro Riferimento Oncologico, Aviano; Paola Di Giulio, Associate Professor of Nursing, Turin University; Massimo Di Maio, MD, Clinical Trials Unit, National Cancer Institute, Napoli.

References

Agenzia Italiana del Farmaco. (2005). *Bulletin clinical trials of drugs in Italy (n. 6 July 2005)*. Retrieved December 2, 2005, from https://oss-sper-clin.agenziafarmaco.it/dati_pubblicazioni.htm

Andreuccetti, M. (2005, October). *The data manager*. Paper presented at the VII Annual Congress of the Italian Association of Medical Oncology (AIOM), Naples, Italy.

Apolone, G., & Mosconi, P. (2002). Knowledge and opinions about clinical research: A cross-sectional survey in a sample of Italian citizens. *Journal of Ambulatory Care Management, 26*, 83–87.

Associazione Italiana di Oncologia Medica. (2005a, October). *AIOM recommendations on the relationship between medical oncologists and the pharmaceutical industry*. Retrieved December 14, 2005, from http://www.aiom.it/

Associazione Italiana di Oncologia Medica. (2005b, October). *Prospective observational study of oncology patients' perceptions of conflict of interest between physicians and the pharmaceutical industry*. Retrieved December 14, 2005, from http://www.aiom.it/

Bell, C., Del Mastro, L., Marchetti, M., Bryce, J., & Costantini, M. (2003). Psychometric properties of the Italian version of the Brief Fatigue Inventory [Abstract 206]. *Oncology Nursing Forum, 30*(Part 2), 158.

Bryce, J., Bell, C., Colussi, A.M., De Maio, G., & Rossi, V. (2003). The clinical trial nurse in Italy: Strategies for role preparation, implementation and evaluation. *European Journal of Oncology Supplements, 1*, S370.

Bryce, J., Bell, C., Colussi, A.M., De Maio, G., & Gini, S. (2004). *Clinical trial nursing: Strategies for developing role competencies and role recognition in Italy*. Paper presented at the Oncology Nursing Society 29th Annual Congress, Anaheim, CA.

Bryce, J., Connola, M., Salzano de Luna, A., Caraco, C., & Chiofalo, M.G. (2006). Participating patients' reactions to early closure of a clinical trial for negative results [Abstract 22]. *Oncology Nursing Forum, 33*, 459.

Commission directive 2001/20/EC of the European Parliament and of the Council of 4 April 2001 on the approximation of the laws, regulations and administrative provisions of the member states relating to the implementation of good clinical practice in the conduct of clinical trials on medicinal products for human use. (2001). *Official Journal of the European Union, L 121*, 34–44.

Commission directive 2005/28/EC of 9 April 2005 laying down principles and detailed guidelines for good clinical practice as regards investigational medicinal products for human use, as well as the requirements for authorisation of the manufacturing or importation of such products. (2005). *Official Journal of the European Union, L 91*, 13–19.

Crawley, F.P. (2004). New European clinical trials directive: Is European research possible? *BMJ, 328*, 522.

D'Aiuto, G., Oliviero, P., & Bryce, J. (2003, May). *Results of the Italian tamoxifen breast cancer prevention study*. Meeting of the clinical trial participants Progetto Donna: Risultati and prospective, Naples, Italy.

Decreto Legislativo (Italian Legislative Decree). (2003, September 8). Transposition of directive 2001/20/EC relating to the implementation of good clinical practice in the conduct of clinical trials of medicinal products for clinical use. Legislative decree n. 211 of 24/06/2003 published in the *Official Gazette of the Italian Republic*, n. 184, Suppl. 130.

Decreto Ministeriale (Italian Ministerial Decree). (1997, August 18). Transposition of the guidelines of the European Union for good clinical practice in the conduct of clinical trials with medicines. D.M. 15/7/97 published in the *Official Gazette of the Italian Republic*, n. 191, Suppl. 162.

Decreto Ministeriale (Italian Ministerial Decree). (1998, May 28). Guidelines for the institution and functions of independent ethics committees. D.M. 18/3/98 published in the *Official Gazette of the Italian Republic*, n. 122.

Decreto Ministeriale (Italian Ministerial Decree). (2003, July 28). Therapeutic use of experimental drugs. D.M. 8/05/2003 published in the *Official Gazette of the Italian Republic*, n. 173.

Decreto Ministeriale (Italian Ministerial Decree). (2004). Prescriptions and general conditions of a general nature referring to the conduct of clinical trials of medicines with special reference to those designed to enhance clinical practice as an integral part of health and medical care. D.M. 17/12/2004 published in the *Official Gazette of the Italian Republic*, n. 43.

Decreto Ministeriale (Italian Ministerial Decree). (2006, August 22). Minimal requirements for the institution, organization and functioning of ethics committees for clinical trials of medicines. D.M. 12/05/2006 published in the *Official Gazette of the Italian Republic*, n. 194.

Del Mastro, L., Catzeddu, T., Boni, L., Bell, C., Sertoli, M.R., Bighin, C., et al. (2006). Prevention of chemotherapy-induced menopause by temporary ovarian suppression with goserelin in young, early breast cancer patients. *Annals of Oncology, 17*, 74–78.

Di Giulio, P., Arrigo, C., Gall, H., Molin, C., Nieweg, R., & Strohbucker, B. (1996). Expanding the role of the nurse in clinical trials: The nursing summaries. *Cancer Nursing, 19*, 343–347.

Ehrenberger, H.E., & Lillington, L. (2004). Development of a measure to delineate the clinical trials nursing role. *Oncology Nursing Forum, 31*, E64–E68.

European Organisation for Research and Treatment of Cancer Oncology Nurse Group. (2003). *A core curriculum on cancer clinical trials for oncology nurses*. Brussels, Belgium: European Organisation for Research and Treatment of Cancer.

Gilger, E.A., Groben, V.J., & Hinds, P.S. (2002). Osteosarcoma nursing care guidelines: A tool to enhance the nursing care of children and adolescents enrolled on a medical research protocol. *Journal of Pediatric Oncology Nursing, 19*, 172–181.

Guideline of the Italian Ministry of Health for the implementation of the European Directive. (2004). *Assistenza Infermieristica e Ricerca, 23*, 93–95.

Habeck, M. (2003). Gloomy prospects for European cancer research. *Lancet Oncology, 4*, 66.

International Air Transport Association. (2005, January). *IATA dangerous goods regulations* (46th ed.). Retrieved December 14, 2005, from http://www.iata.org

Ischemia Cronica degli Arti Inferiori (ICAI) Nursing. (1996). [Use of drugs in patients with critical leg ischemia]. *Rivista dell'Infermiere, 15*, 14–21.

Italian Clinical Research Nurse Working Group (Gruppo Italiano Infermieri di Ricerca Clinica). (2005, December). Unpublished proceedings from GIRC national meeting, Milan, Italy.

Italian Data Manager Group (Gruppo Italiano Data Manager). (2005). *What is a data manager?* Retrieved January 9, 2006, from http://www.gidm.org

Italian Group for the Study of Survival After Infarct Nursing. (1995). Evaluation of the perception of the quality of health of the patient with myocardial infarct. Final report of the study. *Rivista dell'Infermiere, 14*, 16–29.

Italian National Federation of Nursing. (1999, May). *Il codice deontologico degli infermieri*. Retrieved December 28, 2005, from http://www.ipasvi.it

Klimaszewski, A., Aikin, J., Bacon, M., Distasio, S., Ehrenberger, H., & Ford, B. (Eds.). (2000). *Manual for clinical trials nursing*. Pittsburgh, PA: Oncology Nursing Society.

Max, A., Gattuso, J., Hinds, P., Norman, G., Price, R., Whitmore-Sisco, L., et al. (2003). Developing nursing care guidelines for children with Hodgkin's disease. *European Journal of Oncology Nursing, 7*, 253–258.

Meunier, F., Dubois, N., Negrouk, A., Rea, L.A., Saghatchian, M., Tursz, T., et al. (2003). Throwing a wrench in the works? *Lancet Oncology, 4*, 717–719.

Meunier, F., & Lacombe, D. (2003). The European Organisation for the Research and Treatment of Cancer's point of view. *Lancet, 362*, 663.

Mueller, M.R. (2001). From delegation to specialization: Nurses and clinical trial co-ordination. *Nursing Inquiry, 8*, 182–190.

National Cancer Institute Cancer Therapy Evaluation Program. (2003). *Common terminology criteria for adverse events* (version 3.0). Bethesda, MD: National Cancer Institute. Retrieved December 1, 2005, from http://ctep.cancer.gov

Ocker, B., & Pawlik-Plank, D. (2000). The research nurse role in a clinic-based oncology research center. *Cancer Nursing, 23*, 286–292.

Perrone, F., Marangolo, M., Di Costanzo, F., Colucci, G., Repeto, L., Merlano, M., et al. (2004). Insurance for independent cancer trials. *Annals of Oncology, 15,* 1722–1723.

Piccinelli, M., Bisoffi, G., Bon, M.G., Cunico, L., & Tansella, M. (1993). Validità and test-retest reliability of the Italian version of the 12-item General Health Questionnaire in general practice: A comparison between three scoring methods. *Comprehensive Psychiatry, 34,* 98–205.

Price, L., Spencer, H., Mayor, P., & Boyle, P. (2003). Using clinical research summaries to aid research nurses. *Professional Nurse, 19,* 223–226.

Rotmensz, N., Robertson, C., Maisonneuve, P., & Boyle, P. (1998, May). *The effect of external events on a large double blind chemoprevention trial.* Paper presented at the 19th Annual Meeting of the Society for Clinical Trials, Atlanta, GA.

Shedlock, K. (2000). Role validation. In A. Klimaszewski, J. Aikin, M. Bacon, S. Distasio, H. Ehrenberger, & B. Ford (Eds.), *Manual for clinical trials nursing* (pp. 279–282). Pittsburgh, PA: Oncology Nursing Society.

Statistical Office of the European Communities. (2005). *Proportion of population aged 65 and over.* Retrieved December 20, 2005, from http://epp.eurostat.cec.eu.int

Therasse, P., Arbuck, S.G., Eisenhauer, E.A., Wanders, J., Kaplan, R.S., Rubinstein, L., et al. (2000). New guidelines to evaluate the response to treatment in solid tumors. European Organization for Research and Treatment of Cancer, National Cancer Institute of the United States, National Cancer Institute of Canada. *Journal of the National Cancer Institute, 92,* 205–216.

Van Wijk, A., Batchelor, D., & Dubbelman, A. (Eds.). (2001). *Manual for research nurses.* Amsterdam: Early Clinical Studies Group Research Nurses.

Watson, R. (2003). EU legislation threatens clinical trials. *BMJ, 326,* 1348.

Zanetti, R., Gafa, L., Pannelli, F., Conti, E., & Rosso, S. (Eds.). (2002). *Cancer in Italy: Incidence data from cancer registries* (Vol. 3, 1993–1998). Rome: Il Pensiero Scientifico Editore.

About the Authors

Jane Bryce, RN, MSN, AOCNS®, has been a registered nurse since 1980. She received her BSN and MSN from the University of Pittsburgh. Ms. Bryce worked at the University of Pittsburgh Medical Center for 14 years and began working as an oncology clinical nurse specialist and clinical trials nurse in the National Cancer Institute in Naples, Italy, in 1997. She is a member of the Oncology Nursing Society and its CTN Special Interest Group, AIIO, the European Oncology Nursing Society, and the Italian Clinical Research Nurse Group (GIRC). Ms. Bryce teaches in undergraduate and graduate oncology and research nursing programs of Italian universities and is codirector of the Research Nursing Course of the European School of Oncology.

Marianna Connola, BSN, graduated from the Second University of Naples in 2003 and immediately began working as a CTN in the National Cancer Institute in Naples. She is a member of the Oncology Nursing Society and its CTN Special Interest Group, AIIO, and GIRC.

Marzia Falanga, BSN, graduated from the Second University of Naples in 2003 and began working in oncology clinical trials in 2004. She is a member of the Oncology Nursing Society and its CTN Special Interest Group, AIIO, and GIRC. She is working as a CTN in the Oncology Division of San Giuseppe Moscati Hospital of Avellino, Italy.

CHAPTER 64
United Kingdom

Karen Carty, CCR, and Andrea Harkin, BA, CCR

Background

In the United Kingdom (UK), the National Health Service (NHS) was established in 1948 to provide health care to all citizens. The NHS is funded by the UK taxpayers and managed by the UK government's Department of Health (DOH). Since its foundation, the NHS has seen many changes to its organizational structure and the format of provision of patient services administration.

The 10-Year Plan

A major milestone occurred in July 2000 for the modernization of NHS when a 10-year plan was published. The plan for investment and reform across NHS was to develop an NHS for the 21st century by offering fast, convenient, high-quality care, with patients at the center. The aim was to create a patient-led health service.

The 10-year NHS plan identified cancer treatment and services as high priority and promised progress in prevention, research, and improved access to services (DOH, 2000). On the basis of this, the NHS cancer plan for England was published in September 2000. One of the key areas identified in this plan was investment in cancer research.

National Cancer Research Institute

At that time, the infrastructure for cancer clinical research within the UK was highlighted as a weakness with insufficient planning and coordination among the existing funding partners. This led to the formation of the National Cancer Research Institute (NCRI). The NCRI is a partnership between the UK government, charitable organizations, and private sectors. By April 2001, the NCRI formally was established as a key element of the English national cancer plan. The NCRI objectives are summarized in Figure 64-1. To meet these objectives, the NCRI concentrated its activities in three areas: strategic reviews, national infrastructure, and international collaborations.

Figure 64-1. National Cancer Research Institute Objectives

- Perform strategic oversight of cancer research in the United Kingdom.
- Identify gaps and opportunities in cancer research.
- Facilitate collaboration among cancer research funding bodies.
- Monitor progress.

Strategic Reviews

Strategic planning of cancer research was impossible because of a lack of assessable and comparable data on the activities of the major funders of cancer research. The Cancer Research Database (CRD) was set up to provide this functionality. This database contains up-to-date and accurate information on all of the directly supported cancer research in the UK by the NCRI member organizations. It allows researchers to plan new trials strategically, undertake a review of the current trial portfolio in the UK, and identify specific areas where research is lacking (e.g., specific types of cancer or stages in treatment for specific cancers).

National Infrastructure

National infrastructure is being addressed by the NCRI in three areas of cancer research: bioinformatics, tissue sample collection, and clinical trial registers. Work is currently ongoing in this respect.

International Collaborations

Because it is crucial to develop national approaches to cancer research, the NCRI recognized that this must occur with the knowledge of what is happening internationally. Work is ongoing, and the number of international interactions is growing (e.g., European Bioinformatics Council, U.S. National Cancer Institute, European Union [EU]).

In addition to clinical research, the translation of basic laboratory research into new therapies is a major area of interest for the NCRI. The National Translational Cancer

Research Network (NTRAC) was established in May 2001, taking the lead in coordinating the NHS infrastructure support for translational cancer research. The main aim of NTRAC is to speed up the development of novel anticancer therapies and diagnostics from the laboratory to the patient and to test their promise in early clinical trials. Currently, 14 NTRAC-funded centers of scientific and clinical excellence in translational cancer research are operating throughout the UK and Northern Ireland.

Within the NCRI framework, clinical studies groups have been established to provide a route through which new ideas for cancer clinical trials in the UK are developed. Currently, 22 NCRI Clinical Studies Groups (CSGs) exist, including 15 cancer site-specific groups (see Figure 64-2), one radiotherapy group, five development groups (see Figure 64-3), and one consumer liaison group. The primary role of the CSGs is to develop and maintain a balanced and relevant portfolio of studies.

In addition to the implementation of the NCRI in April 2001, the National Cancer Research Network (NCRN) for England was established. It is funded by DOH and overseen by the NCRI. The three main aims of the NCRN are delineated in Figure 64-4. Most new academic trials in the UK have the support of the relevant NCRI CSG prior to being awarded funding from the NCRI member organizations. Funded trials or those from international cooperative groups that are reviewed receive "badging" and are included in the NCRN portfolio.

Within England, 34 cancer *treatment* networks already existed. The objective was to establish them as cancer *research* networks. The NCRN provided funds to establish the neces-

---

Figure 64-2. United Kingdom Cancer Site-Specific Clinical Studies Groups

- Bladder
- Brain
- Breast
- Colorectal
- Gynecologic
- Hematologic
- Head and neck
- Lung
- Lymphoma
- Melanoma
- Prostate
- Renal
- Sarcoma
- Testis
- Upper gastrointestinal

Figure 64-3. United Kingdom Cancer Development Clinical Studies Groups

- Complementary therapies
- Palliative care development
- Primary care development
- Psychosocial oncology
- Teenagers and young adults

Figure 64-4. 2001 Goals of the National Cancer Research Network

- Benefit patients by improving the coordination, integration, quality, inclusiveness, and speed of cancer research.
- Develop a world-class infrastructure in cancer research.
- Double the number of patients with cancer entered into clinical trials and other well-designed studies by April 2004.

---

sary infrastructure support to achieve this objective. A clinical lead and research network manager were appointed for each research network. Additionally, funds were given to employ the necessary research support staff, including data managers and research nurses, in each network.

In March 2004, the DOH formally reviewed the performance of the NCRN in the first three years of its existence. The DOH identified seven key areas against which performance was assessed (see Figure 64-5).

Figure 64-5. Performance Measures for the National Cancer Research Network

- Recruiting patients with cancer to academic trials
- Improving patient care
- Improving the coordination of research
- Improving the speed of research
- Maintaining and enhancing the quality of research
- Widening participation in research
- Providing a world-class health service infrastructure to support cancer research

---

The Annual Report of the NCRN for 2003–2004 reported the following areas for assessment (NCRN, 2004).

1. Recruiting trial participants—The target was to double the number of patients with cancer entering academic trials within three years. The baseline accrual against which this was measured was 3.75% of patients. The overall accrual rate at the end of the three-year review was 10.9% (NCRN, 2004).

2. Improving patient care—The target was to speed up access to the best treatment and care for people in all parts of the country. The rapid increase of accrual into clinical trials and widened participation across the country geographically and through different areas of activity provided evidence of an increase in the dissemination of high-quality patient care.

3. Improving the coordination of research—The target was to provide an effective and efficient mechanism for conducting research in areas identified as priorities. The establishment of 34 cancer research networks that provide coordination of research at a local and national level substantially has improved the coordination. Furthermore, the establishment of the CSGs enabled this to be accomplished in a more strategic and systematic manner.

4. Improving the speed of research—The target was to increase the number of patients in research and the rate

at which they are recruited. The increase in the overall accrual rate underpins this achievement and results in the faster completion of clinical trials.

5. Maintaining and enhancing the quality of research—The target was to provide the systems necessary to develop high-quality research protocols and the infrastructure necessary to deliver them. Although the volume of activity increased, the quality of research was maintained via the requirement for external peer review and the establishment of a structured system of review of NCRN studies.

6. Widening participation in research—The target was to increase the number of NHS organizations, professionals, and patients participating in research studies. The establishment of the cancer research networks, particularly in areas not previously known to have a research tradition, achieved this. In addition, the increased involvement of consumers in clinical trial research has affected this achievement.

7. Providing a world-class health service infrastructure to support cancer research—The NCRN is building toward this objective.

The review panel concluded that the "NCRN had satisfactorily addressed and achieved the criteria set out" (NCRN, 2004, p. 4).

In addition to the establishment of the NCRN in England, the remaining three countries that make up the UK (Scotland, Wales, and Northern Ireland) have their own cancer research networks (see Figure 64-6). These are partners of the NCRN.

Figure 64-6. United Kingdom Cancer Research Network Partners

- England—National Cancer Research Network
- Scotland—Scottish Cancer Research Network
- Ireland—All Ireland Cooperative Cancer Research Group
- Wales—Wales Cancer Trials Network

The Scottish Cancer Research Network

In March 2002, the DOH announced additional funds to support the development of the Scottish Cancer Research Network, supported by Cancer in Scotland, the Chief Scientist Office (CSO), and the Information Services Division (ISD) Cancer Programme. The target of the SCRN was to at least *double* the number of patients recruited to cancer clinical trials in Scotland. The SCRN is made up of three cancer research networks—north region, south east region, and west region. The SCRN was fully established as of December 2003, and recruitment figures from 2004–2005 show that they have at least doubled since the baseline figures from 2001.

The All Ireland Cooperative Oncology Research Group

The All Ireland Cooperative Oncology Research Group was established in October 1996 and is a joint collabora-

tion between the Irish Clinical Oncology Research Group in Dublin, the Clinical Research Support Centre in Belfast, and oncology professionals throughout Northern Ireland and the Republic of Ireland. The aim of the group is to promote, design, conduct and facilitate clinical cancer research in Northern Ireland and the Republic of Ireland.

The Wales Cancer Trials Network

The Wales Cancer Trials Network (WCTN) was set up in 1998 as a jointly funded collaboration between Cancer Research UK (CR-UK) and the Welsh Assembly Government. The aims of the WCTN are to support patients and relatives entering cancer clinical trials, to promote a research environment within the NHS in Wales, to make clinical trials more accessible in Welsh hospitals, to support specialists and teams who contribute to research, to provide an infrastructure for the research, to develop and manage trials coordinated in Wales, and to provide training and information to health professionals involved in cancer clinical trials. Since the WCTN was established, the recruitment to cancer trials has more than doubled annually.

International Partners

In addition to the national partners, the NCRN also has international partners: the European Organisation for Research and Treatment of Cancer (EORTC), the National Cancer Institute (NCI) in the United States, and the National Cancer Institute of Canada.

With the increase in recruitment to cancer clinical trials and a more strategic approach to coordination of these trials in the UK, it was acknowledged that clinical trial units (CTUs) have a central role in the development and successful completion of clinical trials. Prior to the establishment of the NCRI, the approach to the management of these trials evolved in an ad hoc manner, with little coordination between CTUs and with little or no strategy.

One of the key recommendations of the NCRI Strategic Review was to identify a network of NCRI-accredited CTUs in the UK. These CTUs must display key competencies in the coordination of cancer clinical trials (see Figure 64-7).

To date, nine NCRI-accredited units exist in the UK: seven based in England, one in Scotland, and one in Wales. In the future, it is expected that all national cancer clinical trials will feed through one of the NCRI-accredited units. Potential benefits for cancer clinical trials in the UK include that potential researchers and research groups will have

---

Figure 64-7. Key Competencies of Clinical Trial Units in the United Kingdom

- Display a track record in the coordination of phase III multi-center trials.
- Employ a core team of expert staff.
- Implement quality-assurance and archiving systems.
- Show evidence of long-term viability.
- Contribute to the national program of cancer trials.

---

access to and links with relevant national expertise and confidence in working with a nationally accredited unit. Good communication between the accredited units also provides benefits, such as the development of central resources and systems, discussion of information technology–related issues, sharing of expertise, working practice, and standardization of data between units.

Within the UK, the licensing of medications is regulated by the Medicines and Healthcare Products Regulatory Agency (MHRA). The agency was formed in 2003 from a merger of the previous regulatory bodies, including the Medicines Control Agency and the Medical Devices Agency. MHRA is the government agency that is responsible for ensuring that medicines and medical devices work and are acceptably safe. It assesses the safety, quality, and efficacy of medicines and authorizes the sale or supply in the UK for human use. As such, the MHRA is responsible the regulating clinical trials of medicines and medical devices in the UK.

Medicinal products need to have a marketing authorization granted before they can be prescribed or sold to patients. Before this is granted, clinical trials are undertaken to collect data on the safety and efficacy of new products. A clinical trial authorization (CTA) is required from the MHRA for a product and trial before the product can be tested on human subjects. Further detail regarding the application of CTAs for clinical trials is detailed in the "Ethics and Regulations" section.

Clinical trials in the UK must abide by several regulations, including the International Conference on Harmonisation of Technical Requirements for Registration of Pharmaceuticals for Human Use Good Clinical Practice (ICH GCP) guidelines. The objective of these guidelines is to provide and maintain unified standards of care. All clinical trials within the UK and other EU countries must be run according to ICH GCP standards.

The UK also must abide by EU Clinical Trials Directive (CTD) 2001/20/EC. Figure 64-8 identifies the goals of that directive, and a complete overview of the EU CTD and its impact on clinical trials in Europe appears in Chapter 58.

Each EU member state (country) is responsible for the implementation of the directive within its national laws. The UK regulations took effect on May 1, 2004, and all clinical trials from that point must adhere to the regulations. The directive only applies to trials involving an investigational medicinal product. In addition, all trials in the UK should follow the NHS Research Governance Framework. The MHRA is responsible for ensuring that all clinical trials

that fall under the EU CTD are conducted according to this regulatory standard.

The directive has had a major effect on the clinical trial activity in the UK, particularly within the academic sector. All trials need a legal sponsor who is responsible for the conduct of the study and patient safety. The more stringent laws have resulted in increased costs and activity for CTUs where the support may not be available to handle this additional work. The major research groups within the UK, including NCRI/NCRN, CR-UK, and the Medical Research Council (MRC), have all undertaken investigations to review and report on the impact of the implementation of the EU CTD.

All clinical trials in the UK must obtain ethics committee approval prior to commencement of the study (see the section on "Ethics and Regulations" for more protocol-specific details). Within the UK, the Central Office for Research Ethics Committees (COREC) provides help and leadership for local research ethics committees (RECs) and the ethics system by coordinating the development of operational and infrastructure arrangements in the UK. This includes the implementation of standards to ensure national consistency and the provision of training for committee members.

To meet the requirements of the EU CTD, which standardizes regulatory and approval procedures, the COREC introduced new standard operating procedures (SOPs) for RECs. The procedures became effective on March 1, 2004. All NHS RECs in the UK are required to operate in accordance with these SOPs. The complexity of conducting clinical trials has increased significantly, and, as a result, trials have become more expensive. Guidelines on the processes involved in setting up and managing trials under the new regulations are clearly summarized at www.ct-toolkit.ac.uk.

Protocol Development

As with most countries, ideas for new cancer clinical trials in the UK can be initiated by a number of sources, including industry (e.g., pharmaceutical companies), research groups (e.g., Scottish Gynaecological Cancer Trials Group, NCRI CSG), or a single investigator at a hospital site. They can be a completely new idea or concept, such as a feasibility study, or can be the result of a line of previous research trials.

Before the protocol is actually drafted, a proposal commonly is generated. Investigator-led studies may be reviewed internally by the hospital clinical trial committee or by the study group. Investigators are encouraged to work with a CTU at an early stage to develop the protocol and grant application, if applicable. Investigator-led protocols from industry often are prepared in-house initially and then circulated to known experts in the field for review.

Peer review of clinical trials is an important aspect of protocol development in the UK. It is important for noncommercial trials to obtain support from the appropriate NCRI CSG. The CSG will be made up of leading investi-

---

Figure 64-8. Goals of the European Union Clinical Trials Directive

- Protect the rights, safety, and well-being of trial participants.
- Simplify and harmonize the administrative provisions governing trials.
- Establish a transparent procedure that will harmonize trial conduct in the European Union and ensure the credibility of results.

gators from across the UK who come together under the CSG chair. CSGs have a central role in the development of a balanced national portfolio and are the preferred route for the generation of new noncommercial cancer clinical trials in the UK.

The MRC and CR-UK, the two leading public-sector funders of cancer trials and supporters of CTUs in the UK, developed a joint committee, the Clinical Trials Advisory and Awards Committee (CTAAC), to streamline and speed up the peer-review process of cancer trial proposals. Proposals to CTAAC are assessed and scored under the criteria listed in Figure 64-9.

Figure 64-9. Clinical Trials Advisory and Awards Committee Criteria to Assess and Score Proposals

- Clinical and scientific importance of the research question
- Adequacy of the background and preliminary data
- Study design and statistics
- Expected interest to patients and potential accrual
- Fit with current National Cancer Research Network trial portfolio

---

Many of the applications to CTAAC are expected to be developed or endorsed by the NCRI CSG, although applications are accepted via other routes. If successful, protocols accepted by CTAAC are included on the NCRN portfolio and, if requested, also can be awarded grant funding.

With the growing importance of well-designed translational studies in cancer research, the Translational Research in Clinical Trials Committee was formed by the MRC and CR-UK in 2004. This committee provides the same facility as CTAAC but for translational research associated with cancer clinical trials.

Protocols normally are drafted by the lead clinician for the study, known in the UK as the chief investigator. Most study groups and CTUs have an SOP for their protocols that provides a template of the expected sections to be included in the protocol and outlines the review process. Following the implementation of the EU CTD, a number of items must be included in the clinical trial protocol, such as the definition of the end of study, expected adverse events, and a list of study responsibilities.

Once the first draft of the protocol completed, it is normal for this to be reviewed and amended by the *study team*. This should include the study coordinator (or data manager) and study statistician.

Currently in the UK, the sponsor commonly will assess risks for clinical trial protocols in accordance with EU CTD. Controls must be in place to offset the associated risks. The level of monitoring often is determined as a result of the risk assessment. The risk assessment of a protocol can result in changes being made to the draft protocol.

Once the final draft of the protocol is produced, it must be given a version number and dated to enable version control of the protocol. Although a great deal of work is put into the final version of the protocol, it is very difficult to avoid future amendments to it. These can be simple amendments for administrative errors or changes or can be the result of new findings in relation to the study drug or regimen. It is at this point that *version control* of the protocol becomes vital.

Preparation

Preparation for any clinical trial in the UK, whether it is commercial (pharmaceutical/industry sponsored) or noncommercial (academic), is essentially similar. Recruitment to a clinical trial cannot begin until the necessary ethics and regulatory approvals have been granted. Beyond the ethics and regulatory approvals, a large amount of preparatory work must be completed before the commencement of the trial.

For commercial trials, pharmaceutical companies often conduct visits with potential sites to assess a site's suitability to participate in the trial. The company will check the site for the necessary qualified staff, facilities, and resources to conduct the trial. When it is agreed that a site will participate in a clinical trial, financial agreements are drawn up between the site and the company (sponsor) that documents the financial aspects of the trial. In addition, a signed agreement is drawn up between each party that states their responsibilities in relation to the trial.

The relevant essential documents for conducting a trial in accordance with ICH GCP guidelines are collected before the commencement of the trial. These are "those documents which individually and collectively permit evaluation of the conduct of the trial and the quality of the data produced. They serve to demonstrate the compliance of the investigator, sponsor and monitor with the standards of Good Clinical Practice and with all applicable regulatory requirements" (European Medicines Agency, 2002, p. 47).

The curricula vitae for the staff involved in the trial, laboratory normal ranges and accreditation certificates for laboratory tests and procedures to be carried out in the trial, site responsibility log, and necessary ethical and regulatory approvals are included among the essential documents.

Normally, the sponsor will conduct site initiation visits with the hospital research team to ensure that the staff involved understands the trial and the required procedures. At the time of the initiation visit, an investigator site *master file* and *pharmacy file* will be provided, which house all of the required essential documents for the conduct of the trial.

The preparation for noncommercial (academic) trials is similar to the preparation of a commercial trial. A noncommercial trial is a non-pharmaceutical company–sponsored trial. These trials tend to be investigator-led and generally are in collaboration with other hospitals or research groups. As with commercial trials, the sponsor of the trial and each participating site prepare agreements. The coordinating site must collect the necessary documents from each site.

In addition to the previously mentioned documents, a lot of preparation work goes into the design and development of both paper and electronic case report forms (CRFs) for the trial to ensure they capture the required data of the protocol. CRFs and the CRF completion guidelines are reviewed and approved by the trial team.

Promotion and Recruitment

Trials often are promoted through the members of cancer trials groups, research organizations, or pharmaceutical companies, if a company sponsors the trial. Depending on the size of the trial, this could be at a local, national, or international level. The trial may be presented at trials group meetings to generate interest or presented at international conferences to encourage collaboration from other trial groups. Alternatively, investigators who have previously participated in trials of academic groups or pharmaceutical companies may be approached directly.

Promotion of cancer trials in the UK tends to be aimed at investigators and research groups as opposed to patients. Patients have access to information regarding clinical trials in the UK via various Web sites from organizations, such as CR-UK and Cancerbackup. Cancerbackup is a cancer information charity that provides up-to-date cancer information, practical advice, and support for patients with cancer, their families, and caregivers. A list of useful Web sites is provided at the end of this chapter. These Web sites provide support and information to patients about cancer, treatments for cancer, and clinical trials.

Recruitment to trials is performed at a local level in cancer centers and smaller associated cancer units within the network. The type of trial undertaken is dependent on the population covered by the network and its local strategy.

Throughout the UK, managed clinical networks exist for specific disease types (e.g., gynecology). Staff multidisciplinary teams hold meetings, often on a weekly basis, in their region to make decisions regarding the diagnosis and treatment of individual patients. These teams include surgical, medical/clinical oncology, pathology, radiology, and nursing staff, as well as clinical trial staff, who may advise on any current trials that might be appropriate for the patient.

Eligibility

Protocols for any clinical trial conducted in the UK clearly state the eligibility criteria for the trial, outlining the inclusion and exclusion criteria. The eligibility criteria are an important aspect of the protocol; they define the group of patients who are eligible for the trial. Many factors need to be taken into account when considering a patient for a trial. Written informed consent (IC) must be obtained for all patients, and this must be done prior to the commencement of any trial-specific procedures. IC generally is taken by the local principal investigator or coinvestigator for the study. On occasions, this duty may be delegated to a research nurse, depending on the type of study. Patients'

understanding of the information sheet and consent form for the clinical trial is ascertained by verbal questioning.

The majority of protocols have a table of investigations that summarizes the investigations, procedures, and required time points. Before patients can be registered or randomized to the trial, the required baseline investigations, as dictated in the protocol, must be carried out.

The principal investigator or a delegated member of the research team is responsible for taking written IC from the patient, assessing the patient's eligibility for the trial, and ensuring that the necessary investigations have been carried out. A registration or randomization form is completed at this point, confirming that the patient fulfills the eligibility criteria for the trial. If a research nurse or data manager is assigned to the trial, this person may complete the registration or randomization form, but ultimately the principal investigator or coinvestigator checks the patient's eligibility for the trial and signs the registration or randomization form.

The study sponsor or coordinating site then completes registration or randomization by telephone, fax, or the Internet. Patients are given a unique trial identifier. If the trial is randomized, the patient is assigned to a treatment arm. If the purpose of the trial is dose finding, the dose is determined at this point.

In exceptional circumstances, a waiver may be granted to allow entry of a patient who is otherwise ineligible for the trial. On this rare occasion, the chief investigator, coordinators, or sponsor of the trial will grant a waiver only when a valid explanation or reason exists. Common requests for waivers often are related to hematology or biochemistry baseline results, which may be slightly outside of the eligibility criteria or time frame. A waiver does not require approval by the ethics committee. In instances where the same waiver has been granted on several circumstances, a protocol amendment may be considered.

Active Treatment

The investigational agents used in clinical trials are either supplied by the pharmaceutical company sponsor to the hospital pharmacy of each participating site or, as may be the case in noncommercial trials, are taken from the hospital pharmacy's own stock.

When the investigational agent is received on site, it is the responsibility of the hospital pharmacy to ensure the correct storage, preparation, handling, accountability, disposal, and destruction of the investigational agent. The majority of hospital pharmacies now have clinical trial pharmacists and technicians dedicated to work on clinical trials.

These staff must be involved in the trial from an early stage to ensure that any practical issues related to the dispensing of the investigational agent are addressed before commencement of the trial. Often, the premedication, hydration, or antiemetic regimens specified in the protocol will differ from the standard regimens used at sites. It may be possible for an agreement to be made for sites to use their own regimen. The premedication regimens specified in the protocol are often included as guidance.

The treatment schedule for the trial is clearly stated in the protocol with details on the method to be used for calculating the dose of drug where applicable. The protocol also provides specification and information on dose adjustments, dose modifications, treatment delays, expected side effects, management of side effects, time points of investigations, response assessment, and discontinuation of protocol treatment. The protocol for the clinical trial must be strictly adhered to at all times. If this is not done, it is deemed a protocol violation and may render the patient ineligible for the trial. Whether the patient's treatment is changed or the patient's data are considered ineligible for analysis of the trial will be dependent on the severity of the protocol violation. An example of a violation is where a patient was given the wrong treatment arm regimen.

Patients generally are reviewed before each course of treatment by the responsible clinician. Prior to treatment, the clinician assesses the patient's current medical condition, taking into consideration any toxicities that have occurred during the previous cycle, to establish whether treatment can be given, and if so, at what dose.

In the UK, either a chemotherapy nurse (IV nurse) or research nurse commonly administers the treatment. Clinicians and research nurses regularly assess the patients during the treatment cycle and document in their hospital case notes any side effects or reactions, known as adverse events (AEs), experienced by the patient, regardless of whether they are related to trial treatment.

For the majority of cancer trials in the UK, AEs are graded in accordance with the NCI Common Toxicity Criteria, version 2.0 (NCI Cancer Therapy Evaluation Program [CTEP], 1998) or Common Terminology Criteria for Adverse Events, version 3.0 (NCI CTEP, 2003). These provide standard terminology to name and describe the severity (grade) of AEs that occur in the treatment of cancer (see http://ctep.cancer.gov/reporting/index.html). The protocol specifies which version is to be used.

Serious adverse events (SAEs) occurring during treatment and up to 30 days from the last administration of the protocol treatment are required to be reported within 24 hours of the site becoming aware of the event. SAEs are reported by fax or telephone, normally by the data manager or research nurse, to the pharmacovigilance department of the trial sponsor or the coordinating site. This department is responsible for determining whether the SAE is a suspected unexpected serious adverse reaction. If so, it must be reported to the competent authority, which is the MHRA in the UK, and to the ethics committees within the correct timelines. The protocol provides clear guidance on the reporting of SAEs.

Many trials have trial steering committees and data monitoring committees (DMCs). Trial steering committees are independent bodies, which include a majority of members not involved in running the trial. Their role is to monitor and supervise the progress of the trial toward its interim and overall objectives. They also regularly review relevant information from other sources and consider recommendations of the DMC (MRC, 1998).

DMCs are independent bodies whose members are not involved in the trial. Generally, DMCs require a minimum of three members, including one or more clinicians and one or more statisticians with experience in trials. DMC members are the only people to see the data during the trial. They are independent and look at the trial from the point of view of trial participants. The members are responsible for protecting patients from exposure to any excess risk by recommending that the trial stop early if the safety or efficacy results are sufficiently convincing.

Ancillary Studies

Ancillary studies, commonly known as add-on studies, are incorporated into many of the cancer clinical trials in the UK. Examples of these studies include quality-of-life questionnaires, neurologic questionnaires, economics, translational research, pharmacokinetics, and nursing. The types of ancillary studies incorporated are dependent on the protocol and the objectives of the trial.

Patients are fully informed of any additional studies in the patient information sheet for the trial and often will sign an additional consent form for these. These studies usually are optional.

Off-Treatment Follow-Up

Clear guidance is provided in the protocol for when a patient is considered to be off protocol treatment, as well as regarding follow-up intervals and their duration as required for the trial.

The duration of the follow-up period of a trial depends on the phase of the trial. Follow-up for phase I trials tends to be relatively short, whereas phase III trials, which look for survival data, may require patients to be followed until death. The patient's continued consent (to collect data in this period) is required. If the patient withdraws his or her consent for participation in the trial, no further data will be collected. Sometimes a patient is lost to follow-up. This can happen for a variety of reasons, such as moving away or continuing follow-up at a local hospital. Every effort is made to collect follow-up data on patients. It may be possible to obtain information from the patient's general practitioner or via the Office of National Statistics in the UK, although this incurs a cost.

Quality Assurance

For any clinical trial, the appropriate quality assurance procedures and systems must be in place to ensure the trial is run according to the appropriate regulatory standards. It is important that the company, group, and trial unit running the clinical trial can be assured of the participants' safety and of producing good-quality data that provide the answers to the research questions posed.

When the study is in the set-up phase and also during the course of the study, *version control* of study documents is very important. Protocols, patient information sheets, consent forms, and investigator's drug brochures should display the version number and date on all pages of the document. When the study is approved by the ethics committee, the committee will note which version of the documents it has approved and should be used as reference. This is particularly important for the protocol and patient information sheet, as these documents can often change during the course of the study. Staff members must be able to identify the current version in use.

Site selection is very important to ensure good quality research. Participating sites must have the appropriate expertise available to participate in the study, including clinical, nursing, and research support staff (e.g., data management). Site initiation takes place before a patient can be recruited by the site, and at this time, a number of documents will be collected. (See the "Preparation" section for further details.)

Once the study is under way, a number of different systems typically are put in place to ensure quality, including the following.
- *Source data verification (SDV):* The study data are compared and verified with the patients' medical notes to ensure that all the appropriate information has been collected. This can range from 10% SDV to a full 100% check of study data. As outlined in the "Protocol Development" section, the level of monitoring often is determined by the risk assessment of the protocol.
- *Checking of patient consent:* It is normal practice for the consent forms to be checked for *all* patients recruited to the study. As well as checking that the consent has been signed, the monitor will check that the correct version of the consent was signed.

In addition to SDV of patient data, the coordinating site may carry out a number of checks on the quality of data returned by the participating site. Manual and computer-generated checks on the data are produced, and any subsequent data queries will be created and returned to site. Any sites that continually produce a large amount of queries and poor quality of data may be examined more closely, leading to an increase in the level of SDV for that site. A system also is in place to monitor the return of data within the timelines set, and any problem sites will be identified and the appropriate action taken.

In addition to the previously described quality checks carried out by the study coordinator, it is common practice for CTUs, companies, and groups to have quality assurance staff in place to internally audit the trial. As per the SOPs for the department, an internal member of the quality assurance staff will carry out various checks to ensure the study coordinator and on-site staff are running the trial

according to SOPs. This includes checks to ensure that the data have been checked and queried appropriately, that SDV is performed correctly, and that the sites have been initiated correctly and all of the relevant documentation is in place.

On occasion, the trial sponsor will delegate much of the day-to-day running of the trial to a CTU. In this case, the sponsor also may undertake an audit of the study to ensure that the CTU is carrying out its responsibilities as outlined in the clinical trial agreement. The sponsor may decide to audit participating sites to ensure they are also meeting their responsibilities.

Finally, as the licensing and regulatory body of clinical trials in the UK, the MHRA also may perform an audit of any specific trials or research units in the UK. The MHRA may notify a CTU of a forthcoming audit at very short notice. The audits can range from small study-specific audits to large audits of the complete set-up and practice of a unit.

Safety and Environment

The Health and Safety Commission and the Health and Safety Executive (HSE) are government advisory bodies in the UK responsible for the regulation of almost all the risks to health and safety arising from work activity in the UK.

The HSE (n.d.) provides guidelines for Control of Substances Hazardous to Health (see www.hse.gov.uk/coshh). The HSE, DOH, and Her Majesty's Inspectorate of Pollution provide guidance on the safe handling of cytotoxic drugs, radiation therapy, radioactive substances, and specimens.

All hospitals and institutions involved in the handling of cytotoxic drugs and radiation therapy work to the guidelines provided by the HSE and the other noted governing bodies. Each hospital will also have its own SOPs. Biologic specimens are handled according to the SOPs of the hospital. Specimens requiring shipment by air are shipped in accordance with the International Air Transport Association guidelines.

The safety and protection of staff, patients, and their relatives is paramount. Staff must be fully educated on all aspects of safety to achieve a safe working environment. Education of staff is repeated and updated as required, particularly in instances where changes are made to guidelines.

Ethics and Regulations

All clinical trials in the UK are conducted in accordance with the Declaration of Helsinki and ICH GCP guidelines. The purpose of RECs in the UK is to protect the dignity, rights, safety, and well-being of research participants. An essential aspect of any clinical trial is the *IC process*. In compliance with the recommendations of the Declaration of Helsinki, each patient must be fully informed of the aims, methods, benefits, and potential risks of the trial.

RECs and clinical research in general in the UK have undergone significant changes following the EU CTD. One of the aims of the directive was to standardize regulatory and approval procedures for the conduct of clinical trials. The requirements of the directive in relation to ethical review were

- Decisions on a valid application must be delivered within 60 days.
- One decision is to be valid for the whole UK.
- Applicants are restricted to one written request for clarification or further information.

The chief investigator of the trial is responsible for applying for ethical approval. This is done by COREC, which allocates the trial to an REC for review. COREC has a common electronic application form, which is mandatory for all applications. All sites participating in the trial require approval from their local REC; this is known as *site-specific assessment*.

In addition to ethical approval, any clinical trial involving an investigational medicinal product requires a CTA prior to commencement of the trial. An application for a CTA is submitted to the MHRA. Set time frames for the assessment of the application exist, as well as applicable fees for the CTA, which can be costly.

All clinical trials conducted in the UK require research management and governance approval, usually referred to as research and development (R&D) approval from the R&D department of each hospital participating in the trial. R&D departments establish the likely impact and cost implications that participating in the trial will have on the hospital. Generally, hospitals will fund the extra treatment and service costs of NCRN-badged trials. They receive an income for this research activity in an R&D budget from the DOH.

Depending on the type of trial, additional approvals or licenses may be required before the trial can commence. An example of this is a license from the Administration of Radioactive Substances Advisory Committee required for any trial involving the administration of radioactive medicinal products to humans, such as multigated acquisition scans or bone scans.

Trials involving the use of gene therapy require approval from the Gene Therapy Advisory Committee (GTAC). GTAC is a government advisory body that considers and advises on the ethical acceptability of proposals for gene therapy research in patients, taking account of the scientific merits of the proposals and the potential benefits and risks (www.advisorybodies.doh.gov.uk/genetics/gtac/index.htm) (DOH, n.d.). These trials do not need COREC approval, as the committee reviews the ethical consideration of the protocol.

Data Management Tools and Systems

The provision of accurate data in clinical trials is vital, as the data determine the results of a clinical trial. The protocol for the trial defines the required data and timing of collection.

When a site is activated to begin recruitment to the trial, the site is provided with the necessary study materials for conducting the trial, including the CRFs and, where applicable, quality-of-life questionnaires, neurotoxicity questionnaires, patient diary cards, and any other required study materials.

CRF completion guidelines that provide step-by-step instructions for the completion of the CRFs often are provided to sites. During site initiation visits, time is spent reviewing the data management aspects of the trial.

The data manager or the clinical research nurse for the trial normally completes the CRFs and subsequent queries. Sites involved in clinical trials tend to have methods to ensure that the required data are collected, including creating trial-specific worksheets to ensure the investigations and procedures are carried out at the specified times or adding prompts to a patient's case notes to remind the investigator when investigations are required or to be arranged at each patient visit. Copies of the table of investigations from the protocol also may be inserted in the patient's case notes, confirming that protocols are readily available in treatment areas. The investigator, co-investigator, or research nurse requests the investigations required for the trial.

Various formats of CRFs exist. The most commonly used are paper and electronic. The paper CRF format is generally in the form of ring binders or books. Multiple no-carbon-required papers are used, which allow the study site, sponsor, or coordinating site to each have an original copy of the data.

The electronic CRF format is carried out by data entry to a database on a laptop at sites or via an Internet Web site. This method is becoming more widely used. The electronic format is beneficial to the sponsors, as they have quicker access to the data. The disadvantages of this type of system are that more training is required and the set-up costs can be high.

Commercial trials generally are fully monitored. Monitoring visits to sites are conducted either by a clinical research associate (CRA) from the pharmaceutical company or by a CRA from a clinical research organization employed by the company. SDV is completed at monitoring visits by checking the data recorded on the CRF with the patient's case notes to ensure the accuracy of the data recorded. Protocol compliance is checked at monitoring visits, as well as the sites' compliance with GCP and necessary regulatory requirements. The amount of monitoring will depend on performing an initial risk assessment of the study and assessing the compliance and data quality of participating centers.

Academic trials do not routinely involve full monitoring; this is mainly because of a lack of resources. Following the implementation of the EU CTD, it has now become more common for academic trials to have some form of monitoring to meet the directive's requirements.

Trials are required to have quality assurance measures in place to ensure the trial meets the standards for safety, reliability, and completeness. Actions will be taken if, for any reason, the data returned from a site raise concern regarding accuracy, consistency, completeness, or timelines, or if it is felt that any serious deficiencies exist in the reporting of SAEs. Generally, recruitment will be suspended from the site until a selection of CRFs is been checked against the original patients' case notes.

Information Systems Resources

The World Wide Web provides a great resource for education and information on current clinical research in the UK. Many CTUs have established their own Web sites to provide information about their unit and research activities, such as the CR-UK Clinical Trials Unit Glasgow, www.crukctuglasgow.co.uk. Larger groups and organizations, such as CR-UK, COREC, NCRN, and MHRA, have their own Web sites that are used regularly by research professionals. Some Web sites, such as the COREC Web site, also provide a question-and-answer facility that allows researchers to ask the experts within COREC for advice on ethical issues and regulations.

Patients also can access a great deal of information at these sites. In addition to the sites already mentioned, a number of charities and research groups in the UK provide information for patients. Cancerbackup and Cancerhelp UK are two of the main providers of information and support to patients with cancer in the UK. Cancerbackup provides information to patients via telephone and information booklets. Cancerhelp UK has a Web site that, where possible, allows patients to see what research and trials are being carried out in different hospitals in the UK. Tumor-specific patient support groups also exist, such as Ovacome, Breakthrough Breast Cancer, and Colon Concern. See Figure 64-10 for useful Web sites within the UK.

Figure 64-10. Useful Web Sites in the United Kingdom

Patient Support Web sites
- Bowel Cancer UK: www.bowelcanceruk.org.uk
- Breakthrough Breast Cancer: www.breakthrough.org.uk
- Cancerbackup Charity: www.cancerbackup.org.uk
- Cancerhelp, Cancer Research UK: www.cancerhelp.org.uk
- The Ovarian Cancer Support Network: www.ovacome.org.uk

Regulatory Web sites
- Central Office for Research Ethics Committee, Department of Health: www.corec.org.uk
- Clinical Trials Unit Glasgow, Cancer Research UK: www.crukctuglasgow.org.uk
- Medicine and Healthcare Products Regulatory Agency, Department of Health: www.mhra.gov.uk
- National Cancer Research Institute: www.ncri.org.uk
- National Cancer Research Network, National Cancer Research Institute: www.ncrn.org.uk

---

Professional Development

Within the UK clinical research environment, a number of sources are available for the professional development of research nurses, trial coordinators, and data managers. Most CTUs and hospitals provide ongoing in-house training for staff by making use of the on-site experts in their field, such as oncology and tumor-related education sessions, treatment (chemotherapy and radiotherapy) education

sessions, update sessions on current research in various tumor areas, and pathology presentations.

A number of organizations are located throughout UK communities that provide training and development, including

- Institute of Clinical Research
- British Oncology Data Managers' Association
- Royal College of Nursing
- UK Oncology Nursing Society.

These organizations hold annual general meetings where members can participate and vote on issues, as well as attend a forum for education. Regular training courses are available on topics such as data management, GCP, and presentation skills, to name but a few. The ICR sponsors longer-term courses held at universities in the UK: master's degrees in clinical research, postgraduate diplomas, and certificates in clinical research. Also, within the UK, the NCRN and MHRA conduct training courses on issues such as GCP, audit, pharmacovigilance, and SOPs.

Internationally, the EORTC organizes training courses for staff involved in cancer clinical research. Conferences held by the American Society of Clinical Oncology and the European Convention of Clinical Oncology allow staff to keep up-to-date with developments in diagnosis and treatment in oncology.

Summary

Following the implementation of the EU CTD in May 2004, academic units slowly have been adapting to the more regulated processes required to undertake clinical research in the UK. By 2008, most large academic CTUs should be meeting the majority of the regulatory requirements. This will be credited to a tremendous amount of work by the clinical research staff, as well as support from organizations such as NCRI and NCRN. In addition, funding from support bodies (e.g., CR-UK) has had a major impact on allowing the units to develop as required.

Clinical research is a rapidly changing environment, and all staff involved must be aware of and keep up-to-date with the current regulations. Within the UK, the ethics and R&D approval structure currently is under review and will be updated in the near future.

The authors wish to acknowledge the expert opinion and review of Dr. Jonathan Ledermann, Cancer Research UK and UCL Cancer Trials Centre, London, UK.

References

Department of Health. (2000). *The NHS cancer plan: A plan for investment, a plan for reform.* London: Author.

Department of Health. (n.d.). *Gene Therapy Advisory Committee.* Retrieved May 2, 2007, from http://www.advisorybodies.doh.gov.uk/genetics/gtac/index.htm

European Medicines Agency. (2002, July). *ICH topic E6 (R1): Guideline for good clinical practice: ICH harmonised tripartite guideline.* Retrieved November, 14, 2007, from http://www.emea.europa.eu/pdfs/human/ich/013595en.pdf

Health and Safety Executive. (n.d.). *Control of substances hazardous to health (COSHH)*. Retrieved May 2, 2007, from http://www.hse.gov.uk/coshh

Medical Research Council. (1998). *Guidelines for good clinical practice.* London: Author.

National Cancer Institute Cancer Therapy Evaluation Program. (1998). *Common toxicity criteria* (version 2.0). Bethesda, MD: National Cancer Institute.

National Cancer Institute Cancer Therapy Evaluation Program. (2003). *Common terminology criteria for adverse events* (version 3.0). Bethesda, MD: National Cancer Institute.

National Cancer Research Network. (2004). *Annual report of NCRN 2003–2004*. Leeds, UK: Author.

About the Authors

The authors of this chapter both work in the CR-UK Clinical Trials Unit in Glasgow. This is one of nine NCRI-accredited Cancer Trials Units in the UK.

Karen Carty, CCR, has been working in clinical research for six-and-a-half years. Prior to this, she worked in health records information and management for six years. Ms. Carty was initially employed as a clinical trial coordinator, which involved coordinating and managing a broad portfolio of phase I, II, and III clinical trials in oncology. After six years in this role, she was promoted to the post of project manager. In addition, Ms. Carty has held the position of secretary of the Scottish Gynaecological Cancer Trials Group for the last two-and-a-half years and is the data management representative for the group at the Gynecologic Cancer Intergroup.

Andrea Harkin, BA, CCR, has worked in the field of clinical research for 10 years. She was initially employed in the CR-UK Clinical Trials Unit, Glasgow, in 1997 as a clinical trial coordinator. In this role, she coordinated and managed clinical trials in gynecologic oncology. In 2001, Ms. Harkin was promoted to the post of senior clinical trial coordinator. As well as continuing to coordinate clinical trials in the unit, she was responsible for the day-to-day management of all the clinical trial coordinators employed there. Ms. Harkin continued in this role until 2004, when she was promoted to the post of head of trial coordination, overseeing all trial coordination activity with the unit. This role encompasses quality assurance, monitoring, administration (financial and regulatory), and project management, as well as trial coordination. Additionally, Ms. Harkin previously held the position of secretary of the Scottish Gynaecological Cancer Trials Group and chair of the Harmonization Group of the Gynecologic Cancer Intergroup. She is currently the NCRI portfolio coordinator for the NCRI Gynaecological Clinical Studies Group and will hold this post until November 2010.

Appendices

Appendix 1. Nuremberg Code

Directives for Human Experimentation

NUREMBERG CODE

1. The voluntary consent of the human subject is absolutely essential. This means that the person involved should have legal capacity to give consent; should be so situated as to be able to exercise free power of choice, without the intervention of any element of force, fraud, deceit, duress, over-reaching, or other ulterior form of constraint or coercion; and should have sufficient knowledge and comprehension of the elements of the subject matter involved as to enable him to make an understanding and enlightened decision. This latter element requires that before the acceptance of an affirmative decision by the experimental subject there should be made known to him the nature, duration, and purpose of the experiment; the method and means by which it is to be conducted; all inconveniences and hazards reasonable to be expected; and the effects upon his health or person which may possibly come from his participation in the experiment.

   The duty and responsibility for ascertaining the quality of the consent rests upon each individual who initiates, directs or engages in the experiment. It is a personal duty and responsibility which may not be delegated to another with impunity.

2. The experiment should be such as to yield fruitful results for the good of society, unprocurable by other methods or means of study, and not random and unnecessary in nature.

3. The experiment should be so designed and based on the results of animal experimentation and a knowledge of the natural history of the disease or other problem under study that the anticipated results will justify the performance of the experiment.

4. The experiment should be so conducted as to avoid all unnecessary physical and mental suffering and injury.

5. No experiment should be conducted where there is an a priori reason to believe that death or disabling injury will occur; except, perhaps, in those experiments where the experimental physicians also serve as subjects.

6. The degree of risk to be taken should never exceed that determined by the humanitarian importance of the problem to be solved by the experiment.

7. Proper preparations should be made and adequate facilities provided to protect the experimental subject against even remote possibilities of injury, disability, or death.

8. The experiment should be conducted only by scientifically qualified persons. The highest degree of skill and care should be required through all stages of the experiment of those who conduct or engage in the experiment.

9. During the course of the experiment the human subject should be at liberty to bring the experiment to an end if he has reached the physical or mental state where continuation of the experiment seems to him to be impossible.

10. During the course of the experiment the scientist in charge must be prepared to terminate the experiment at any stage, if he has probable cause to believe, in the exercise of the good faith, superior skill and careful judgment required of him that a continuation of the experiment is likely to result in injury, disability, or death to the experimental subject.

Note. From *Trials of War Criminals Before the Nuremberg Military Tribunals Under Control Council Law No. 10* (Vol. 2, pp. 181–182). Washington, DC: U.S. Government Printing Office, 1949.

Appendix 2. Declaration of Helsinki

WORLD MEDICAL ASSOCIATION DECLARATION OF HELSINKI
Ethical Principles for Medical Research Involving Human Subjects

Adopted by the 18th WMA General Assembly, Helsinki, Finland, June 1964, and amended by the
29th WMA General Assembly, Tokyo, Japan, October 1975
35th WMA General Assembly, Venice, Italy, October 1983
41st WMA General Assembly, Hong Kong, September 1989
48th WMA General Assembly, Somerset West, Republic of South Africa, October 1996
and the 52nd WMA General Assembly, Edinburgh, Scotland, October 2000
Note of Clarification on Paragraph 29 added by the WMA General Assembly, Washington 2002
Note of Clarification on Paragraph 30 added by the WMA General Assembly, Tokyo 2004

A. INTRODUCTION
   1. The World Medical Association has developed the Declaration of Helsinki as a statement of ethical principles to provide guidance to physicians and other participants in medical research involving human subjects. Medical research involving human subjects includes research on identifiable human material or identifiable data.
   2. It is the duty of the physician to promote and safeguard the health of the people. The physician's knowledge and conscience are dedicated to the fulfillment of this duty.
   3. The Declaration of Geneva of the World Medical Association binds the physician with the words, "The health of my patient will be my first consideration," and the International Code of Medical Ethics declares that, "A physician shall act only in the patient's interest when providing medical care which might have the effect of weakening the physical and mental condition of the patient."
   4. Medical progress is based on research which ultimately must rest in part on experimentation involving human subjects.
   5. In medical research on human subjects, considerations related to the well-being of the human subject should take precedence over the interests of science and society.
   6. The primary purpose of medical research involving human subjects is to improve prophylactic, diagnostic and therapeutic procedures and the understanding of the aetiology and pathogenesis of disease. Even the best proven prophylactic, diagnostic, and therapeutic methods must continuously be challenged through research for their effectiveness, efficiency, accessibility and quality.
   7. In current medical practice and in medical research, most prophylactic, diagnostic and therapeutic procedures involve risks and burdens.
   8. Medical research is subject to ethical standards that promote respect for all human beings and protect their health and rights. Some research populations are vulnerable and need special protection. The particular needs of the economically and medically disadvantaged must be recognized. Special attention is also required for those who cannot give or refuse consent for themselves, for those who may be subject to giving consent under duress, for those who will not benefit personally from the research and for those for whom the research is combined with care.
   9. Research Investigators should be aware of the ethical, legal and regulatory requirements for research on human subjects in their own countries as well as applicable international requirements. No national ethical, legal or regulatory requirement should be allowed to reduce or eliminate any of the protections for human subjects set forth in this Declaration.
B. BASIC PRINCIPLES FOR ALL MEDICAL RESEARCH
   10. It is the duty of the physician in medical research to protect the life, health, privacy, and dignity of the human subject.
   11. Medical research involving human subjects must conform to generally accepted scientific principles, be based on a thorough knowledge of the scientific literature, other relevant sources of information, and on adequate laboratory and, where appropriate, animal experimentation.
   12. Appropriate caution must be exercised in the conduct of research which may affect the environment, and the welfare of animals used for research must be respected.
   13. The design and performance of each experimental procedure involving human subjects should be clearly formulated in an experimental protocol. This protocol should be submitted for consideration, comment, guidance, and where appropriate, approval to a specially appointed ethical review committee, which must be independent of the investigator, the sponsor or any other kind of undue influence. This independent committee should be in conformity with the laws and regulations of the country in which the research experiment is performed. The committee has the right to monitor ongoing trials. The researcher has the obligation to provide monitoring information to the committee, especially any serious adverse events. The researcher should also submit to the committee, for review, information regarding funding, sponsors, institutional affiliations, other potential conflicts of interest and incentives for subjects.
   14. The research protocol should always contain a statement of the ethical considerations involved and should indicate that there is compliance with the principles enunciated in this Declaration.
   15. Medical research involving human subjects should be conducted only by scientifically qualified persons and under the supervision of a clinically competent medical person. The responsibility for the human subject must always rest with a medically qualified person and never rest on the subject of the research, even though the subject has given consent.
   16. Every medical research project involving human subjects should be preceded by careful assessment of predictable risks and burdens in comparison with foreseeable benefits to the subject or to others. This does not preclude the participation of healthy volunteers in medical research. The design of all studies should be publicly available.
   17. Physicians should abstain from engaging in research projects involving human subjects unless they are confident that the risks involved have been adequately assessed and can be satisfactorily managed. Physicians should cease any investigation if the risks are found to outweigh the potential benefits or if there is conclusive proof of positive and beneficial results.
   18. Medical research involving human subjects should only be conducted if the importance of the objective outweighs the inherent risks and burdens to the subject. This is especially important when the human subjects are healthy volunteers.
   19. Medical research is only justified if there is a reasonable likelihood that the populations in which the research is carried out stand to benefit from the results of the research.

(Continued on next page)

Appendix 2. Declaration of Helsinki *(Continued)*

20. The subjects must be volunteers and informed participants in the research project.

21. The right of research subjects to safeguard their integrity must always be respected. Every precaution should be taken to respect the privacy of the subject, the confidentiality of the patient's information and to minimize the impact of the study on the subject's physical and mental integrity and on the personality of the subject.

22. In any research on human beings, each potential subject must be adequately informed of the aims, methods, sources of funding, any possible conflicts of interest, institutional affiliations of the researcher, the anticipated benefits and potential risks of the study and the discomfort it may entail. The subject should be informed of the right to abstain from participation in the study or to withdraw consent to participate at any time without reprisal. After ensuring that the subject has understood the information, the physician should then obtain the subject's freely-given informed consent, preferably in writing. If the consent cannot be obtained in writing, the non-written consent must be formally documented and witnessed.

23. When obtaining informed consent for the research project the physician should be particularly cautious if the subject is in a dependent relationship with the physician or may consent under duress. In that case the informed consent should be obtained by a well-informed physician who is not engaged in the investigation and who is completely independent of this relationship.

24. For a research subject who is legally incompetent, physically or mentally incapable of giving consent or is a legally incompetent minor, the investigator must obtain informed consent from the legally authorized representative in accordance with applicable law. These groups should not be included in research unless the research is necessary to promote the health of the population represented and this research cannot instead be performed on legally competent persons.

25. When a subject deemed legally incompetent, such as a minor child, is able to give assent to decisions about participation in research, the investigator must obtain that assent in addition to the consent of the legally authorized representative.

26. Research on individuals from whom it is not possible to obtain consent, including proxy or advance consent, should be done only if the physical/mental condition that prevents obtaining informed consent is a necessary characteristic of the research population. The specific reasons for involving research subjects with a condition that renders them unable to give informed consent should be stated in the experimental protocol for consideration and approval of the review committee. The protocol should state that consent to remain in the research should be obtained as soon as possible from the individual or a legally authorized surrogate.

27. Both authors and publishers have ethical obligations. In publication of the results of research, the investigators are obliged to preserve the accuracy of the results. Negative as well as positive results should be published or otherwise publicly available. Sources of funding, institutional affiliations and any possible conflicts of interest should be declared in the publication. Reports of experimentation not in accordance with the principles laid down in this Declaration should not be accepted for publication.

C. ADDITIONAL PRINCIPLES FOR MEDICAL RESEARCH COMBINED WITH MEDICAL CARE

28. The physician may combine medical research with medical care, only to the extent that the research is justified by its potential prophylactic, diagnostic or therapeutic value. When medical research is combined with medical care, additional standards apply to protect the patients who are research subjects.

29. The benefits, risks, burdens and effectiveness of a new method should be tested against those of the best current prophylactic, diagnostic, and therapeutic methods. This does not exclude the use of placebo, or no treatment, in studies where no proven prophylactic, diagnostic or therapeutic method exists.[1]

30. At the conclusion of the study, every patient entered into the study should be assured of access to the best proven prophylactic, diagnostic and therapeutic methods identified by the study.[2]

31. The physician should fully inform the patient which aspects of the care are related to the research. The refusal of a patient to participate in a study must never interfere with the patient-physician relationship.

32. In the treatment of a patient, where proven prophylactic, diagnostic and therapeutic methods do not exist or have been ineffective, the physician, with informed consent from the patient, must be free to use unproven or new prophylactic, diagnostic and therapeutic measures, if in the physician's judgement it offers hope of saving life, re-establishing health or alleviating suffering. Where possible, these measures should be made the object of research, designed to evaluate their safety and efficacy. In all cases, new information should be recorded and, where appropriate, published. The other relevant guidelines of this Declaration should be followed.

[1]**Note**: Note of clarification on paragraph 29 of the WMA Declaration of Helsinki

The WMA hereby reaffirms its position that extreme care must be taken in making use of a placebo-controlled trial and that in general this methodology should only be used in the absence of existing proven therapy. However, a placebo-controlled trial may be ethically acceptable, even if proven therapy is available, under the following circumstances:

- Where for compelling and scientifically sound methodological reasons its use is necessary to determine the efficacy or safety of a prophylactic, diagnostic or therapeutic method; or
- Where a prophylactic, diagnostic or therapeutic method is being investigated for a minor condition and the patients who receive placebo will not be subject to any additional risk of serious or irreversible harm.

All other provisions of the Declaration of Helsinki must be adhered to, especially the need for appropriate ethical and scientific review.

[2]**Note**: Note of clarification on paragraph 30 of the WMA Declaration of Helsinki

The WMA hereby reaffirms its position that it is necessary during the study planning process to identify post-trial access by study participants to prophylactic, diagnostic and therapeutic procedures identified as beneficial in the study or access to other appropriate care. Post-trial access arrangements or other care must be described in the study protocol so the ethical review committee may consider such arrangements during its review.

The Declaration of Helsinki (Document 17.C) is an official policy document of the World Medical Association, the global representative body for physicians. It was first adopted in 1964 (Helsinki, Finland) and revised in 1975 (Tokyo, Japan), 1983 (Venice, Italy), 1989 (Hong Kong), 1996 (Somerset-West, South Africa) and 2000 (Edinburgh, Scotland). Note of clarification on Paragraph 29 added by the WMA General Assembly, Washington 2002.
9.10.2004

Appendix 3. National Research Act, Public Law 93-348, July 12, 1974

Institutional Review Boards; Ethics Guidance Program

Sec. 212. (a) Part I of title IV of the Public Health Service Act, as amended by section 103 of this Act, is amended by adding at the end of the following new section:

"Institutional Review Boards; Ethics Guidance Program"

"Sec. 474. (a) The Secretary shall by regulation require that each entity which applies for a grant or contract under this Act for any project or program which involves the conduct of biomedical or behavioral research involving human subjects submit in or with its application for such grant or contract assurances satisfactory to the Secretary that it has established (in accordance with regulations which the Secretary shall prescribe) a board (to be known as an 'Institutional Review Board') to review biomedical and behavioral research involving human subjects conducted at or sponsored by such entity in order to protect the rights of the human subjects of such research."

"(b) The Secretary shall establish a program within the Department under which requests for clarification and guidance with respect to ethical issues raised in connection with biomedical or behavioral research involving human subjects are responded to promptly and appropriately."

(b) The Secretary of Health, Education, and Welfare shall within 240 days of the date of the enactment of this Act promulgate such regulations as may be required to carry out section 474(a) of the Public Health Service Act. Such regulations shall apply with respect to applications for grants and contracts under such Act submitted after promulgation of such regulations.

The Code of Federal Regulations, 45 CFR 46, Implements these Amendments to the Public Health Service Act.

Appendix 4. The Belmont Report

Office of the Secretary
Ethical Principles and Guidelines for the Protection of Human Subjects of Research
The National Commission for the Protection of Human Subjects of Biomedical and Behavioral Research
April 18, 1979

AGENCY: Department of Health, Education, and Welfare.

ACTION: Notice of Report for Public Comment.

SUMMARY: On July 12, 1974, the National Research Act (Pub. L. 93-348) was signed into law, there-by creating the National Commission for the Protection of Human Subjects of Biomedical and Behavioral Research. One of the charges to the Commission was to identify the basic ethical principles that should underlie the conduct of biomedical and behavioral research involving human subjects and to develop guidelines which should be followed to assure that such research is conducted in accordance with those principles. In carrying out the above, the Commission was directed to consider: **(i)** the boundaries between biomedical and behavioral research and the accepted and routine practice of medicine, **(ii)** the role of assessment of risk-benefit criteria in the determination of the appropriateness of research involving human subjects, **(iii)** appropriate guidelines for the selection of human subjects for participation in such research and **(iv)** the nature and definition of informed consent in various research settings.

The Belmont Report attempts to summarize the basic ethical principles identified by the Commission in the course of its deliberations. It is the outgrowth of an intensive four-day period of discussions that were held in February 1976 at the Smithsonian Institution's Belmont Conference Center supplemented by the monthly deliberations of the Commission that were held over a period of nearly four years. It is a statement of basic ethical principles and guidelines that should assist in resolving the ethical problems that surround the conduct of research with human subjects. By publishing the Report in the Federal Register, and providing reprints upon request, the Secretary intends that it may be made readily available to scientists, members of Institutional Review Boards, and Federal employees. The two-volume Appendix, containing the lengthy reports of experts and specialists who assisted the Commission in fulfilling this part of its charge, is available as DHEW Publication No. (OS) 78-0013 and No. (OS) 78-0014, for sale by the Superintendent of Documents, U.S. Government Printing Office, Washington, D.C. 20402.

Unlike most other reports of the Commission, the Belmont Report does not make specific recommendations for administrative action by the Secretary of Health, Education, and Welfare. Rather, the Commission recommended that the Belmont Report be adopted in its entirety, as a statement of the Department's policy. The Department requests public comment on this recommendation.

National Commission for the Protection of Human Subjects of Biomedical and Behavioral Research
Members of the Commission
Kenneth John Ryan, M.D., Chairman, Chief of Staff, Boston Hospital for Women.
Joseph V. Brady, Ph.D., Professor of Behavioral Biology, Johns Hopkins University.
Robert E. Cooke, M.D., President, Medical College of Pennsylvania.
Dorothy I. Height, President, National Council of Negro Women, Inc.
Albert R. Jonsen, Ph.D., Associate Professor of Bioethics, University of California at San Francisco.
Patricia King, J.D., Associate Professor of Law, Georgetown University Law Center.
Karen Lebacqz, Ph.D., Associate Professor of Christian Ethics, Pacific School of Religion.
*** David W. Louisell, J.D., Professor of Law, University of California at Berkeley.
Donald W. Seldin, M.D., Professor and Chairman, Department of Internal Medicine, University of Texas at Dallas.
***Eliot Stellar, Ph.D., Provost of the University and Professor of Physiological Psychology, University of Pennsylvania.
*** Robert H. Turtle, LL.B., Attorney, VomBaur, Coburn, Simmons & Turtle, Washington, D.C.
*** Deceased.

Table of Contents

Ethical Principles and Guidelines for Research Involving Human Subjects
A. Boundaries Between Practice and Research
B. Basic Ethical Principles
    1. Respect for Persons
    2. Beneficence
    3. Justice
C. Applications
    1. Informed Consent
    2. Assessment of Risk and Benefits
    3. Selection of Subjects

(Continued on next page)

Appendix 4. The Belmont Report *(Continued)*

Ethical Principles & Guidelines for Research Involving Human Subjects

Scientific research has produced substantial social benefits. It has also posed some troubling ethical questions. Public attention was drawn to these questions by reported abuses of human subjects in biomedical experiments, especially during the Second World War. During the Nuremberg War Crime Trials, the Nuremberg code was drafted as a set of standards for judging physicians and scientists who had conducted biomedical experiments on concentration camp prisoners. This code became the prototype of many later codes(1) intended to assure that research involving human subjects would be carried out in an ethical manner.

The codes consist of rules, some general, others specific, that guide the investigators or the reviewers of research in their work. Such rules often are inadequate to cover complex situations; at times they come into conflict, and they are frequently difficult to interpret or apply. Broader ethical principles will provide a basis on which specific rules may be formulated, criticized and interpreted.

Three principles, or general prescriptive judgments, that are relevant to research involving human subjects are identified in this statement. Other principles may also be relevant. These three are comprehensive, however, and are stated at a level of generalization that should assist scientists, subjects, reviewers and interested citizens to understand the ethical issues inherent in research involving human subjects. These principles cannot always be applied so as to resolve beyond dispute particular ethical problems. The objective is to provide an analytical framework that will guide the resolution of ethical problems arising from research involving human subjects.

This statement consists of a distinction between research and practice, a discussion of the three basic ethical principles, and remarks about the application of these principles.

Part A. Boundaries Between Practice and Research

It is important to distinguish between biomedical and behavioral research, on the one hand, and the practice of accepted therapy on the other, in order to know what activities ought to undergo review for the protection of human subjects of research. The distinction between research and practice is blurred partly because both often occur together (as in research designed to evaluate a therapy) and partly because notable departures from standard practice are often called "experimental" when the terms "experimental" and "research" are not carefully defined. For the most part, the term "practice" refers to interventions that are designed solely to enhance the well-being of an individual patient or client and that have a reasonable expectation of success. The purpose of medical or behavioral practice is to provide diagnosis, preventive treatment or therapy to particular individuals.(2) By contrast, the term "research" designates an activity designed to test an hypothesis, permit conclusions to be drawn, and thereby to develop or contribute to generalizable knowledge (expressed, for example, in theories, principles, and statements of relationships). Research is usually described in a formal protocol that sets forth an objective and a set of procedures designed to reach that objective.

When a clinician departs in a significant way from standard or accepted practice, the innovation does not, in and of itself, constitute research. The fact that a procedure is "experimental," in the sense of new, untested or different, does not automatically place it in the category of research. Radically new procedures of this description should, however, be made the object of formal research at an early stage in order to determine whether they are safe and effective. Thus, it is the responsibility of medical practice committees, for example, to insist that a major innovation be incorporated into a formal research project.(3)

Research and practice may be carried on together when research is designed to evaluate the safety and efficacy of a therapy. This need not cause any confusion regarding whether or not the activity requires review; the general rule is that if there is any element of research in an activity, that activity should undergo review for the protection of human subjects.

Part B. Basic Ethical Principles

The expression "basic ethical principles" refers to those general judgments that serve as a basic justification for the many particular ethical prescriptions and evaluations of human actions. Three basic principles, among those generally accepted in our cultural tradition, are particularly relevant to the ethics of research involving human subjects: the principles of respect of persons, beneficence and justice.

1. **Respect for Persons.** -- Respect for persons incorporates at least two ethical convictions: first, that individuals should be treated as autonomous agents, and second, that persons with diminished autonomy are entitled to protection. The principle of respect for persons thus divides into two separate moral requirements: the requirement to acknowledge autonomy and the requirement to protect those with diminished autonomy.

   An autonomous person is an individual capable of deliberation about personal goals and of acting under the direction of such deliberation. To respect autonomy is to give weight to autonomous persons' considered opinions and choices while refraining from obstructing their actions unless they are clearly detrimental to others. To show lack of respect for an autonomous agent is to repudiate that person's considered judgments, to deny an individual the freedom to act on those considered judgments, or to withhold information necessary to make a considered judgment, when there are no compelling reasons to do so.

   However, not every human being is capable of self-determination. The capacity for self-determination matures during an individual's life, and some individuals lose this capacity wholly or in part because of illness, mental disability, or circumstances that severely restrict liberty. Respect for the immature and the incapacitated may require protecting them as they mature or while they are incapacitated.

   Some persons are in need of extensive protection, even to the point of excluding them from activities which may harm them; other persons require little protection beyond making sure they undertake activities freely and with awareness of possible adverse consequence. The extent of protection afforded should depend upon the risk of harm and the likelihood of benefit. The judgment that any individual lacks autonomy should be periodically reevaluated and will vary in different situations.

(Continued on next page)

Appendix 4. The Belmont Report *(Continued)*

In most cases of research involving human subjects, respect for persons demands that subjects enter into the research voluntarily and with adequate information. In some situations, however, application of the principle is not obvious. The involvement of prisoners as subjects of research provides an instructive example. On the one hand, it would seem that the principle of respect for persons requires that prisoners not be deprived of the opportunity to volunteer for research. On the other hand, under prison conditions they may be subtly coerced or unduly influenced to engage in research activities for which they would not otherwise volunteer. Respect for persons would then dictate that prisoners be protected. Whether to allow prisoners to "volunteer" or to "protect" them presents a dilemma. Respecting persons, in most hard cases, is often a matter of balancing competing claims urged by the principle of respect itself.

2. **Beneficence.** -- Persons are treated in an ethical manner not only by respecting their decisions and protecting them from harm, but also by making efforts to secure their well-being. Such treatment falls under the principle of beneficence. The term "beneficence" is often understood to cover acts of kindness or charity that go beyond strict obligation. In this document, beneficence is understood in a stronger sense, as an obligation. Two general rules have been formulated as complementary expressions of beneficent actions in this sense: **(1)** do not harm and **(2)** maximize possible benefits and minimize possible harms.

The Hippocratic maxim "do no harm" has long been a fundamental principle of medical ethics. Claude Bernard extended it to the realm of research, saying that one should not injure one person regardless of the benefits that might come to others. However, even avoiding harm requires learning what is harmful; and, in the process of obtaining this information, persons may be exposed to risk of harm. Further, the Hippocratic Oath requires physicians to benefit their patients "according to their best judgment." Learning what will in fact benefit may require exposing persons to risk. The problem posed by these imperatives is to decide when it is justifiable to seek certain benefits despite the risks involved, and when the benefits should be foregone because of the risks.

The obligations of beneficence affect both individual investigators and society at large, because they extend both to particular research projects and to the entire enterprise of research. In the case of particular projects, investigators and members of their institutions are obliged to give forethought to the maximization of benefits and the reduction of risk that might occur from the research investigation. In the case of scientific research in general, members of the larger society are obliged to recognize the longer term benefits and risks that may result from the improvement of knowledge and from the development of novel medical, psychotherapeutic, and social procedures.

The principle of beneficence often occupies a well-defined justifying role in many areas of research involving human subjects. An example is found in research involving children. Effective ways of treating childhood diseases and fostering healthy development are benefits that serve to justify research involving children -- even when individual research subjects are not direct beneficiaries. Research also makes it possible to avoid the harm that may result from the application of previously accepted routine practices that on closer investigation turn out to be dangerous. But the role of the principle of beneficence is not always so unambiguous. A difficult ethical problem remains, for example, about research that presents more than minimal risk without immediate prospect of direct benefit to the children involved. Some have argued that such research is inadmissible, while others have pointed out that this limit would rule out much research promising great benefit to children in the future. Here again, as with all hard cases, the different claims covered by the principle of beneficence may come into conflict and force difficult choices.

3. **Justice.** -- Who ought to receive the benefits of research and bear its burdens? This is a question of justice, in the sense of "fairness in distribution" or "what is deserved." An injustice occurs when some benefit to which a person is entitled is denied without good reason or when some burden is imposed unduly. Another way of conceiving the principle of justice is that equals ought to be treated equally. However, this statement requires explication. Who is equal and who is unequal? What considerations justify departure from equal distribution? Almost all commentators allow that distinctions based on experience, age, deprivation, competence, merit and position do sometimes constitute criteria justifying differential treatment for certain purposes. It is necessary, then, to explain in what respects people should be treated equally. There are several widely accepted formulations of just ways to distribute burdens and benefits. Each formulation mentions some relevant property on the basis of which burdens and benefits should be distributed. These formulations are **(1)** to each person an equal share, **(2)** to each person according to individual need, **(3)** to each person according to individual effort, **(4)** to each person according to societal contribution, and **(5)** to each person according to merit.

Questions of justice have long been associated with social practices such as punishment, taxation and political representation. Until recently these questions have not generally been associated with scientific research. However, they are foreshadowed even in the earliest reflections on the ethics of research involving human subjects. For example, during the 19th and early 20th centuries the burdens of serving as research subjects fell largely upon poor ward patients, while the benefits of improved medical care flowed primarily to private patients. Subsequently, the exploitation of unwilling prisoners as research subjects in Nazi concentration camps was condemned as a particularly flagrant injustice. In this country, in the 1940's, the Tuskegee syphilis study used disadvantaged, rural black men to study the untreated course of a disease that is by no means confined to that population. These subjects were deprived of demonstrably effective treatment in order not to interrupt the project, long after such treatment became generally available.

Against this historical background, it can be seen how conceptions of justice are relevant to research involving human subjects. For example, the selection of research subjects needs to be scrutinized in order to determine whether some classes (e.g., welfare patients, particular racial and ethnic minorities, or persons confined to institutions) are being systematically selected simply because of their easy availability, their compromised position, or their manipulability, rather than for reasons directly related to the problem being studied. Finally, whenever research supported by public funds leads to the development of therapeutic devices and procedures, justice demands both that these not provide advantages only to those who can afford them and that such research should not unduly involve persons from groups unlikely to be among the beneficiaries of subsequent applications of the research.

(Continued on next page)

Appendix 4. The Belmont Report *(Continued)*

Part C. Applications

Applications of the general principles to the conduct of research leads to consideration of the following requirements: informed consent, risk/benefit assessment, and the selection of subjects of research.

1. **Informed Consent.** -- Respect for persons requires that subjects, to the degree that they are capable, be given the opportunity to choose what shall or shall not happen to them. This opportunity is provided when adequate standards for informed consent are satisfied.

   While the importance of informed consent is unquestioned, controversy prevails over the nature and possibility of an informed consent. Nonetheless, there is widespread agreement that the consent process can be analyzed as containing three elements: information, comprehension and voluntariness.

   Information. Most codes of research establish specific items for disclosure intended to assure that subjects are given sufficient information. These items generally include: the research procedure, their purposes, risks and anticipated benefits, alternative procedures (where therapy is involved), and a statement offering the subject the opportunity to ask questions and to withdraw at any time from the research. Additional items have been proposed, including how subjects are selected, the person responsible for the research, etc. However, a simple listing of items does not answer the question of what the standard should be for judging how much and what sort of information should be provided. One standard frequently invoked in medical practice, namely the information commonly provided by practitioners in the field or in the locale, is inadequate since research takes place precisely when a common understanding does not exist. Another standard, currently popular in malpractice law, requires the practitioner to reveal the information that reasonable persons would wish to know in order to make a decision regarding their care. This, too, seems insufficient since the research subject, being in essence a volunteer, may wish to know considerably more about risks gratuitously undertaken than do patients who deliver themselves into the hand of a clinician for needed care. It may be that a standard of "the reasonable volunteer" should be proposed: the extent and nature of information should be such that persons, knowing that the procedure is neither necessary for their care nor perhaps fully understood, can decide whether they wish to participate in the furthering of knowledge. Even when some direct benefit to them is anticipated, the subjects should understand clearly the range of risk and the voluntary nature of participation.

   A special problem of consent arises where informing subjects of some pertinent aspect of the research is likely to impair the validity of the research. In many cases, it is sufficient to indicate to subjects that they are being invited to participate in research of which some features will not be revealed until the research is concluded. In all cases of research involving incomplete disclosure, such research is justified only if it is clear that **(1)** incomplete disclosure is truly necessary to accomplish the goals of the research, **(2)** there are no undisclosed risks to subjects that are more than minimal, and **(3)** there is an adequate plan for debriefing subjects, when appropriate, and for dissemination of research results to them. Information about risks should never be withheld for the purpose of eliciting the cooperation of subjects, and truthful answers should always be given to direct questions about the research. Care should be taken to distinguish cases in which disclosure would destroy or invalidate the research from cases in which disclosure would simply inconvenience the investigator.

   Comprehension. The manner and context in which information is conveyed is as important as the information itself. For example, presenting information in a disorganized and rapid fashion, allowing too little time for consideration or curtailing opportunities for questioning, all may adversely affect a subject's ability to make an informed choice.

   Because the subject's ability to understand is a function of intelligence, rationality, maturity and language, it is necessary to adapt the presentation of the information to the subject's capacities. Investigators are responsible for ascertaining that the subject has comprehended the information. While there is always an obligation to ascertain that the information about risk to subjects is complete and adequately comprehended, when the risks are more serious, that obligation increases. On occasion, it may be suitable to give some oral or written tests of comprehension.

   Special provision may need to be made when comprehension is severely limited -- for example, by conditions of immaturity or mental disability. Each class of subjects that one might consider as incompetent (e.g., infants and young children, mentally disable patients, the terminally ill and the comatose) should be considered on its own terms. Even for these persons, however, respect requires giving them the opportunity to choose to the extent they are able, whether or not to participate in research. The objections of these subjects to involvement should be honored, unless the research entails providing them a therapy unavailable elsewhere. Respect for persons also requires seeking the permission of other parties in order to protect the subjects from harm. Such persons are thus respected both by acknowledging their own wishes and by the use of third parties to protect them from harm.

   The third parties chosen should be those who are most likely to understand the incompetent subject's situation and to act in that person's best interest. The person authorized to act on behalf of the subject should be given an opportunity to observe the research as it proceeds in order to be able to withdraw the subject from the research, if such action appears in the subject's best interest.

   Voluntariness. An agreement to participate in research constitutes a valid consent only if voluntarily given. This element of informed consent requires conditions free of coercion and undue influence. Coercion occurs when an overt threat of harm is intentionally presented by one person to another in order to obtain compliance. Undue influence, by contrast, occurs through an offer of an excessive, unwarranted, inappropriate or improper reward or other overture in order to obtain compliance. Also, inducements that would ordinarily be acceptable may become undue influences if the subject is especially vulnerable.

(Continued on next page)

Appendix 4. The Belmont Report *(Continued)*

Unjustifiable pressures usually occur when persons in positions of authority or commanding influence -- especially where possible sanctions are involved -- urge a course of action for a subject. A continuum of such influencing factors exists, however, and it is impossible to state precisely where justifiable persuasion ends and undue influence begins. But undue influence would include actions such as manipulating a person's choice through the controlling influence of a close relative and threatening to withdraw health services to which an individual would otherwise be entitled.

2. **Assessment of Risks and Benefits.** -- The assessment of risks and benefits requires a careful arrayal of relevant data, including, in some cases, alternative ways of obtaining the benefits sought in the research. Thus, the assessment presents both an opportunity and a responsibility to gather systematic and comprehensive information about proposed research. For the investigator, it is a means to examine whether the proposed research is properly designed. For a review committee, it is a method for determining whether the risks that will be presented to subjects are justified. For prospective subjects, the assessment will assist the determination whether or not to participate.

    The Nature and Scope of Risks and Benefits. The requirement that research be justified on the basis of a favorable risk/benefit assessment bears a close relation to the principle of beneficence, just as the moral requirement that informed consent be obtained is derived primarily from the principle of respect for persons. The term "risk" refers to a possibility that harm may occur. However, when expressions such as "small risk" or "high risk" are used, they usually refer (often ambiguously) both to the chance (probability) of experiencing a harm and the severity (magnitude) of the envisioned harm.

    The term "benefit" is used in the research context to refer to something of positive value related to health or welfare. Unlike, "risk," "benefit" is not a term that expresses probabilities. Risk is properly contrasted to probability of benefits, and benefits are properly contrasted with harms rather than risks of harm. Accordingly, so-called risk/benefit assessments are concerned with the probabilities and magnitudes of possible harm and anticipated benefits. Many kinds of possible harms and benefits need to be taken into account. There are, for example, risks of psychological harm, physical harm, legal harm, social harm and economic harm and the corresponding benefits. While the most likely types of harms to research subjects are those of psychological or physical pain or injury, other possible kinds should not be overlooked.

    Risks and benefits of research may affect the individual subjects, the families of the individual subjects, and society at large (or special groups of subjects in society). Previous codes and Federal regulations have required that risks to subjects be outweighed by the sum of both the anticipated benefit to the subject, if any, and the anticipated benefit to society in the form of knowledge to be gained from the research. In balancing these different elements, the risks and benefits affecting the immediate research subject will normally carry special weight. On the other hand, interests other than those of the subject may on some occasions be sufficient by themselves to justify the risks involved in the research, so long as the subjects' rights have been protected. Beneficence thus requires that we protect against risk of harm to subjects and also that we be concerned about the loss of the substantial benefits that might be gained from research.

    The Systematic Assessment of Risks and Benefits. It is commonly said that benefits and risks must be "balanced" and shown to be "in a favorable ratio." The metaphorical character of these terms draws attention to the difficulty of making precise judgments. Only on rare occasions will quantitative techniques be available for the scrutiny of research protocols. However, the idea of systematic, nonarbitrary analysis of risks and benefits should be emulated insofar as possible. This ideal requires those making decisions about the justifiability of research to be thorough in the accumulation and assessment of information about all aspects of the research, and to consider alternatives systematically. This procedure renders the assessment of research more rigorous and precise, while making communication between review board members and investigators less subject to misinterpretation, misinformation and conflicting judgments. Thus, there should first be a determination of the validity of the presuppositions of the research; then the nature, probability and magnitude of risk should be distinguished with as much clarity as possible. The method of ascertaining risks should be explicit, especially where there is no alternative to the use of such vague categories as small or slight risk. It should also be determined whether an investigator's estimates of the probability of harm or benefits are reasonable, as judged by known facts or other available studies.

    Finally, assessment of the justifiability of research should reflect at least the following considerations: **(i)** Brutal or inhumane treatment of human subjects is never morally justified. **(ii)** Risks should be reduced to those necessary to achieve the research objective. It should be determined whether it is in fact necessary to use human subjects at all. Risk can perhaps never be entirely eliminated, but it can often be reduced by careful attention to alternative procedures. **(iii)** When research involves significant risk of serious impairment, review committees should be extraordinarily insistent on the justification of the risk (looking usually to the likelihood of benefit to the subject -- or, in some rare cases, to the manifest voluntariness of the participation). **(iv)** When vulnerable populations are involved in research, the appropriateness of involving them should itself be demonstrated. A number of variables go into such judgments, including the nature and degree of risk, the condition of the particular population involved, and the nature and level of the anticipated benefits. **(v)** Relevant risks and benefits must be thoroughly arrayed in documents and procedures used in the informed consent process.

3. **Selection of Subjects.** -- Just as the principle of respect for persons finds expression in the requirements for consent, and the principle of beneficence in risk/benefit assessment, the principle of justice gives rise to moral requirements that there be fair procedures and outcomes in the selection of research subjects.

(Continued on next page)

Appendix 4. The Belmont Report *(Continued)*

Justice is relevant to the selection of subjects of research at two levels: the social and the individual. Individual justice in the selection of subjects would require that researchers exhibit fairness: thus, they should not offer potentially beneficial research only to some patients who are in their favor or select only "undesirable" persons for risky research. Social justice requires that distinction be drawn between classes of subjects that ought, and ought not, to participate in any particular kind of research, based on the ability of members of that class to bear burdens and on the appropriateness of placing further burdens on already burdened persons. Thus, it can be considered a matter of social justice that there is an order of preference in the selection of classes of subjects (e.g., adults before children) and that some classes of potential subjects (e.g., the institutionalized mentally infirm or prisoners) may be involved as research subjects, if at all, only on certain conditions.

Injustice may appear in the selection of subjects, even if individual subjects are selected fairly by investigators and treated fairly in the course of research. Thus injustice arises from social, racial, sexual and cultural biases institutionalized in society. Thus, even if individual researchers are treating their research subjects fairly, and even if IRBs are taking care to assure that subjects are selected fairly within a particular institution, unjust social patterns may nevertheless appear in the overall distribution of the burdens and benefits of research. Although individual institutions or investigators may not be able to resolve a problem that is pervasive in their social setting, they can consider distributive justice in selecting research subjects.

Some populations, especially institutionalized ones, are already burdened in many ways by their infirmities and environments. When research is proposed that involves risks and does not include a therapeutic component, other less burdened classes of persons should be called upon first to accept these risks of research, except where the research is directly related to the specific conditions of the class involved. Also, even though public funds for research may often flow in the same directions as public funds for health care, it seems unfair that populations dependent on public health care constitute a pool of preferred research subjects if more advantaged populations are likely to be the recipients of the benefits.

One special instance of injustice results from the involvement of vulnerable subjects. Certain groups, such as racial minorities, the economically disadvantaged, the very sick, and the institutionalized may continually be sought as research subjects, owing to their ready availability in settings where research is conducted. Given their dependent status and their frequently compromised capacity for free consent, they should be protected against the danger of being involved in research solely for administrative convenience, or because they are easy to manipulate as a result of their illness or socioeconomic condition.

(1) Since 1945, various codes for the proper and responsible conduct of human experimentation in medical research have been adopted by different organizations. The best known of these codes are the Nuremberg Code of 1947, the Helsinki Declaration of 1964 (revised in 1975), and the 1971 Guidelines (codified into Federal Regulations in 1974) issued by the U.S. Department of Health, Education, and Welfare, Codes for the conduct of social and behavioral research have also been adopted, the best known being that of the American Psychological Association, published in 1973.

(2) Although practice usually involves interventions designed solely to enhance the well-being of a particular individual, interventions are sometimes applied to one individual for the enhancement of the well-being of another (e.g., blood donation, skin grafts, organ transplants) or an intervention may have the dual purpose of enhancing the well-being of a particular individual, and, at the same time, providing some benefit to others (e.g., vaccination, which protects both the person who is vaccinated and society generally). The fact that some forms of practice have elements other than immediate benefit to the individual receiving an intervention, however, should not confuse the general distinction between research and practice. Even when a procedure applied in practice may benefit some other person, it remains an intervention designed to enhance the well-being of a particular individual or groups of individuals; thus, it is practice and need not be reviewed as research.

(3) Because the problems related to social experimentation may differ substantially from those of biomedical and behavioral research, the Commission specifically declines to make any policy determination regarding such research at this time. Rather, the Commission believes that the problem ought to be addressed by one of its successor bodies.

Appendix 5. Code of Federal Regulations

TITLE 45
PUBLIC WELFARE
DEPARTMENT OF HEALTH AND HUMAN SERVICES
PART 46
PROTECTION OF HUMAN SUBJECTS
* * *
Revised June 23, 2005
Effective June 23, 2005
* * *

(Continued on next page)

Appendix 5. Code of Federal Regulations *(Continued)*

46.406	Research involving greater than minimal risk and no prospect of direct benefit to individual subjects, but likely to yield generalizable knowledge about the subject's disorder or condition.
46.407	Research not otherwise approvable which presents an opportunity to understand, prevent, or alleviate a serious problem affecting the health or welfare of children.
46.408	Requirements for permission by parents or guardians and for assent by children.
46.409	Wards.

Authority: 5 U.S.C. 301; 42 U.S.C. 289(a).

Editorial Note: The Department of Health and Human Services issued a notice of waiver regarding the requirements set forth in part 46, relating to protection of human subjects, as they pertain to demonstration projects, approved under section 1115 of the Social Security Act, which test the use of cost--sharing, such as deductibles, copayment and coinsurance, in the Medicaid program. For further information see 47 FR 9208, Mar. 4, 1982.

Note: As revised, Subpart A of the HHS regulations incorporates the Federal Policy for the Protection of Human Subjects (56 FR 28003). Subpart D of the HHS regulations has been amended at Section 46.401(b) to reference the revised Subpart A.

The Federal Policy for the Protection of Human Subjects is also codified at

7 CFR Part 1c	Department of Agriculture
10 CFR Part 745	Department of Energy
14 CFR Part 1230	National Aeronautics and Space Administration
15 CFR Part 27	Department of Commerce
16 CFR Part 1028	Consumer Product Safety Commission
22 CFR Part 225	International Development Cooperation Agency, Agency for International Development
24 CFR Part 60	Department of Housing and Urban Development
28 CFR Part 46	Department of Justice
32 CFR Part 219	Department of Defense
34 CFR Part 97	Department of Education
38 CFR Part 16	Department of Veterans Affairs
40 CFR Part 26	Environmental Protection Agency
45 CFR Part 690	National Science Foundation
49 CFR Part 11	Department of Transportation

* * *

Subpart A	**Basic HHS Policy for Protection of Human Research Subjects**
	Authority: 5 U.S.C. 301; 42 U.S.C. 289(a); 42 U.S.C. 300v-1(b).
	Source: 56 FR 28003, June 18, 1991; 70 FR 36325, June 23, 2005.

§46.101 To what does this policy apply?

(a) Except as provided in paragraph (b) of this section, this policy applies to all research involving human subjects conducted, supported or otherwise subject to regulation by any federal department or agency which takes appropriate administrative action to make the policy applicable to such research. This includes research conducted by federal civilian employees or military personnel, except that each department or agency head may adopt such procedural modifications as may be appropriate from an administrative standpoint. It also includes research conducted, supported, or otherwise subject to regulation by the federal government outside the United States.

(1) Research that is conducted or supported by a federal department or agency, whether or not it is regulated as defined in §46.102(e), must comply with all sections of this policy.

(2) Research that is neither conducted nor supported by a federal department or agency but is subject to regulation as defined in §46.102(e) must be reviewed and approved, in compliance with §46.101, §46.102, and §46.107 through §46.117 of this policy, by an institutional review board (IRB) that operates in accordance with the pertinent requirements of this policy.

(b) Unless otherwise required by department or agency heads, research activities in which the only involvement of human subjects will be in one or more of the following categories are exempt from this policy:

(1) Research conducted in established or commonly accepted educational settings, involving normal educational practices, such as (i) research on regular and special education instructional strategies, or (ii) research on the effectiveness of or the comparison among instructional techniques, curricula, or classroom management methods.

(2) Research involving the use of educational tests (cognitive, diagnostic, aptitude, achievement), survey procedures, interview procedures or observation of public behavior, unless:

(i) information obtained is recorded in such a manner that human subjects can be identified, directly or through identifiers linked to the subjects; and (ii) any disclosure of the human subjects' responses outside the research could reasonably place the subjects at risk of criminal or civil liability or be damaging to the subjects' financial standing, employability, or reputation.

(3) Research involving the use of educational tests (cognitive, diagnostic, aptitude, achievement), survey procedures, interview procedures, or observation of public behavior that is not exempt under paragraph (b)(2) of this section, if:

(i) the human subjects are elected or appointed public officials or candidates for public office; or (ii) federal statute(s) require(s) without exception that the confidentiality of the personally identifiable information will be maintained throughout the research and thereafter.

(Continued on next page)

Appendix 5. Code of Federal Regulations *(Continued)*

(4) Research involving the collection or study of existing data, documents, records, pathological specimens, or diagnostic specimens, if these sources are publicly available or if the information is recorded by the investigator in such a manner that subjects cannot be identified, directly or through identifiers linked to the subjects.

(5) Research and demonstration projects which are conducted by or subject to the approval of department or agency heads, and which are designed to study, evaluate, or otherwise examine:

    (i) Public benefit or service programs; (ii) procedures for obtaining benefits or services under those programs; (iii) possible changes in or alternatives to those programs or procedures; or (iv) possible changes in methods or levels of payment for benefits or services under those programs.

(6) Taste and food quality evaluation and consumer acceptance studies, (i) if wholesome foods without additives are consumed or (ii) if a food is consumed that contains a food ingredient at or below the level and for a use found to be safe, or agricultural chemical or environmental contaminant at or below the level found to be safe, by the Food and Drug Administration or approved by the Environmental Protection Agency or the Food Safety and Inspection Service of the U.S. Department of Agriculture.

(c) Department or agency heads retain final judgment as to whether a particular activity is covered by this policy.

(d) Department or agency heads may require that specific research activities or classes of research activities conducted, supported, or otherwise subject to regulation by the department or agency but not otherwise covered by this policy, comply with some or all of the requirements of this policy.

(e) Compliance with this policy requires compliance with pertinent federal laws or regulations which provide additional protections for human subjects.

(f) This policy does not affect any state or local laws or regulations which may otherwise be applicable and which provide additional protections for human subjects.

(g) This policy does not affect any foreign laws or regulations which may otherwise be applicable and which provide additional protections to human subjects of research.

(h) When research covered by this policy takes place in foreign countries, procedures normally followed in the foreign countries to protect human subjects may differ from those set forth in this policy. [An example is a foreign institution which complies with guidelines consistent with the World Medical Assembly Declaration (Declaration of Helsinki amended 1989) issued either by sovereign states or by an organization whose function for the protection of human research subjects is internationally recognized.] In these circumstances, if a department or agency head determines that the procedures prescribed by the institution afford protections that are at least equivalent to those provided in this policy, the department or agency head may approve the substitution of the foreign procedures in lieu of the procedural requirements provided in this policy. Except when otherwise required by statute, Executive Order, or the department or agency head, notices of these actions as they occur will be published in the FEDERAL REGISTER or will be otherwise published as provided in department or agency procedures.

(i) Unless otherwise required by law, department or agency heads may waive the applicability of some or all of the provisions of this policy to specific research activities or classes or research activities otherwise covered by this policy. Except when otherwise required by statute or Executive Order, the department or agency head shall forward advance notices of these actions to the Office for Human Research Protections, Department of Health and Human Services (HHS), or any successor office, and shall also publish them in the FEDERAL REGISTER or in such other manner as provided in Department or Agency procedures.[1]

[1] Institutions with HHS-approved assurances on file will abide by provisions of Title 45 CFR part 46 subparts A-D. Some of the other departments and agencies have incorporated all provisions of Title 45 CFR Part 46 into their policies and procedures as well. However, the exemptions at 45 CFR 46.101(b) do not apply to research involving prisoners, subpart C. The exemption at 45 CFR 46.101(b)(2), for research involving survey or interview procedures or observation of public behavior, does not apply to research with children, <u>subpart D</u>, except for research involving observations of public behavior when the investigator(s) do not participate in the activities being observed.

[56 FR 38012, 28022, June 18, 1991; 56 FR 29756, June 28, 1991; 70 FR 36325, June 23, 2005]

§46.102 Definitions.

(a) *Department or agency head* means the head of any federal department or agency and any other officer or employee of any department or agency to whom authority has been delegated.

(b) *Institution* means any public or private entity or agency (including federal, state, and other agencies).

(c) *Legally authorized representative* means an individual or judicial or other body authorized under applicable law to consent on behalf of a prospective subject to the subject's participation in the procedure(s) involved in the research.

(d) *Research* means a systematic investigation, including research development, testing and evaluation, designed to develop or contribute to generalizable knowledge. Activities which meet this definition constitute research for purposes of this policy, whether or not they are conducted or supported under a program which is considered research for other purposes. For example, some demonstration and service programs may include research activities.

(e) *Research subject to regulation*, and similar terms are intended to encompass those research activities for which a federal department or agency has specific responsibility for regulating as a research activity, (for example, Investigational New Drug requirements administered by the Food and Drug Administration). It does not include research activities which are incidentally regulated by a federal department or agency solely as part of the department's or agency's broader responsibility to regulate certain types of activities whether research or non-research in nature (for example, Wage and Hour requirements administered by the Department of Labor).

(f) *Human subject* means a living individual about whom an investigator (whether professional or student) conducting research obtains

    (1) Data through intervention or interaction with the individual, or

    (2) Identifiable private information.

    Intervention includes both physical procedures by which data are gathered (for example, venipuncture) and manipulations of the subject or the subject's environment that are performed for research purposes. Interaction includes communication or interpersonal contact between investigator and subject. *Private information* includes information about behavior that occurs in a context in which an individual can reasonably expect that no observation or recording is taking place, and information which has been provided for specific purposes by an individual and which the individual can reasonably expect will not be made public (for example, a medical record). Private information must be individually identifiable (i.e., the identity of the subject is or may readily be ascertained by the investigator or associated with the information) in order for obtaining the information to constitute research involving human subjects.

(Continued on next page)

Appendix 5. Code of Federal Regulations *(Continued)*

(g) *IRB* means an institutional review board established in accord with and for the purposes expressed in this policy.

(h) *IRB approval* means the determination of the IRB that the research has been reviewed and may be conducted at an institution within the constraints set forth by the IRB and by other institutional and federal requirements.

(i) *Minimal risk* means that the probability and magnitude of harm or discomfort anticipated in the research are not greater in and of themselves than those ordinarily encountered in daily life or during the performance of routine physical or psychological examinations or tests.

(j) *Certification* means the official notification by the institution to the supporting department or agency, in accordance with the requirements of this policy, that a research project or activity involving human subjects has been reviewed and approved by an IRB in accordance with an approved assurance.

§46.103 Assuring compliance with this policy -- research conducted or supported by any Federal Department or Agency.

(a) Each institution engaged in research which is covered by this policy and which is conducted or supported by a federal department or agency shall provide written assurance satisfactory to the department or agency head that it will comply with the requirements set forth in this policy. In lieu of requiring submission of an assurance, individual department or agency heads shall accept the existence of a current assurance, appropriate for the research in question, on file with the Office for Human Research Protections, HHS, or any successor office, and approved for federal-wide use by that office. When the existence of an HHS-approved assurance is accepted in lieu of requiring submission of an assurance, reports (except certification) required by this policy to be made to department and agency heads shall also be made to the Office for Human Research Protections, HHS, or any successor office.

(b) Departments and agencies will conduct or support research covered by this policy only if the institution has an assurance approved as provided in this section, and only if the institution has certified to the department or agency head that the research has been reviewed and approved by an IRB provided for in the assurance, and will be subject to continuing review by the IRB. Assurances applicable to federally supported or conducted research shall at a minimum include:

(1) A statement of principles governing the institution in the discharge of its responsibilities for protecting the rights and welfare of human subjects of research conducted at or sponsored by the institution, regardless of whether the research is subject to Federal regulation. This may include an appropriate existing code, declaration, or statement of ethical principles, or a statement formulated by the institution itself. This requirement does not preempt provisions of this policy applicable to department- or agency-supported or regulated research and need not be applicable to any research exempted or waived under §46.101 (b) or (i).

(2) Designation of one or more IRBs established in accordance with the requirements of this policy, and for which provisions are made for meeting space and sufficient staff to support the IRB's review and recordkeeping duties.

(3) A list of IRB members identified by name; earned degrees; representative capacity; indications of experience such as board certifications, licenses, etc., sufficient to describe each member's chief anticipated contributions to IRB deliberations; and any employment or other relationship between each member and the institution; for example: full-time employee, part-time employee, member of governing panel or board, stockholder, paid or unpaid consultant. Changes in IRB membership shall be reported to the department or agency head, unless in accord with §46.103(a) of this policy, the existence of an HHS-approved assurance is accepted. In this case, change in IRB membership shall be reported to the Office for Human Research Protections, HHS, or any successor office.

(4) Written procedures which the IRB will follow (i) for conducting its initial and continuing review of research and for reporting its findings and actions to the investigator and the institution; (ii) for determining which projects require review more often than annually and which projects need verification from sources other than the investigators that no material changes have occurred since previous IRB review; and (iii) for ensuring prompt reporting to the IRB of proposed changes in a research activity, and for ensuring that such changes in approved research, during the period for which IRB approval has already been given, may not be initiated without IRB review and approval except when necessary to eliminate apparent immediate hazards to the subject.

(5) Written procedures for ensuring prompt reporting to the IRB, appropriate institutional officials, and the department or agency head of

(i) any unanticipated problems involving risks to subjects or others or any serious or continuing noncompliance with this policy or the requirements or determinations of the IRB; and (ii) any suspension or termination of IRB approval.

(c) The assurance shall be executed by an individual authorized to act for the institution and to assume on behalf of the institution the obligations imposed by this policy and shall be filed in such form and manner as the department or agency head prescribes.

(d) The Department or Agency head will evaluate all assurances submitted in accordance with this policy through such officers and employees of the department or agency and such experts or consultants engaged for this purpose as the department or agency head determines to be appropriate. The department or agency head's evaluation will take into consideration the adequacy of the proposed IRB in light of the anticipated scope of the institution's research activities and the types of subject populations likely to be involved, the appropriateness of the proposed initial and continuing review procedures in light of the probable risks, and the size and complexity of the institution.

(e) On the basis of this evaluation, the department or agency head may approve or disapprove the assurance, or enter into negotiations to develop an approvable one. The department or agency head may limit the period during which any particular approved assurance or class of approved assurances shall remain effective or otherwise condition or restrict approval.

(f) Certification is required when the research is supported by a federal department or agency and not otherwise exempted or waived under §46.101 (b) or (i). An institution with an approved assurance shall certify that each application or proposal for research covered by the assurance and by §46.103 of this Policy has been reviewed and approved by the IRB. Such certification must be submitted with the application or proposal or by such later date as may be prescribed by the department or agency to which the application or proposal is submitted. Under no condition shall research covered by §46.103 of the Policy be supported prior to receipt of the certification that the research has been reviewed and approved by the IRB. Institutions without an approved assurance covering the research shall certify within 30 days after receipt of a request for such a certification from the department or agency, that the application or proposal has been approved by the IRB. If the certification is not submitted within these time limits, the application or proposal may be returned to the institution.

(Approved by the Office of Management and Budget under control number 0990-0260.)

(Continued on next page)

Appendix 5. Code of Federal Regulations *(Continued)*

[56 FR 38012, 28022, June 18, 1991; 56 FR 29756, June 28, 1991; 70 FR 36325, June 23, 2005]

§§46.104--46.106 [Reserved]

§46.107 IRB membership.

(a) Each IRB shall have at least five members, with varying backgrounds to promote complete and adequate review of research activities commonly conducted by the institution. The IRB shall be sufficiently qualified through the experience and expertise of its members, and the diversity of the members, including consideration of race, gender, and cultural backgrounds and sensitivity to such issues as community attitudes, to promote respect for its advice and counsel in safeguarding the rights and welfare of human subjects. In addition to possessing the professional competence necessary to review specific research activities, the IRB shall be able to ascertain the acceptability of proposed research in terms of institutional commitments and regulations, applicable law, and standards of professional conduct and practice. The IRB shall therefore include persons knowledgeable in these areas. If an IRB regularly reviews research that involves a vulnerable category of subjects, such as children, prisoners, pregnant women, or handicapped or mentally disabled persons, consideration shall be given to the inclusion of one or more individuals who are knowledgeable about and experienced in working with these subjects.

(b) Every nondiscriminatory effort will be made to ensure that no IRB consists entirely of men or entirely of women, including the institution's consideration of qualified persons of both sexes, so long as no selection is made to the IRB on the basis of gender. No IRB may consist entirely of members of one profession.

(c) Each IRB shall include at least one member whose primary concerns are in scientific areas and at least one member whose primary concerns are in nonscientific areas.

(d) Each IRB shall include at least one member who is not otherwise affiliated with the institution and who is not part of the immediate family of a person who is affiliated with the institution.

(e) No IRB may have a member participate in the IRB's initial or continuing review of any project in which the member has a conflicting interest, except to provide information requested by the IRB.

(f) An IRB may, in its discretion, invite individuals with competence in special areas to assist in the review of issues which require expertise beyond or in addition to that available on the IRB. These individuals may not vote with the IRB.

§46.108 IRB functions and operations.

In order to fulfill the requirements of this policy each IRB shall:

(a) Follow written procedures in the same detail as described in §46.103(b)(4) and to the extent required by §46.103(b)(5).

(b) Except when an expedited review procedure is used (see §46.110), review proposed research at convened meetings at which a majority of the members of the IRB are present, including at least one member whose primary concerns are in nonscientific areas. In order for the research to be approved, it shall receive the approval of a majority of those members present at the meeting.

§46.109 IRB review of research.

(a) An IRB shall review and have authority to approve, require modifications in (to secure approval), or disapprove all research activities covered by this policy.

(b) An IRB shall require that information given to subjects as part of informed consent is in accordance with §46.116. The IRB may require that information, in addition to that specifically mentioned in §46.116, be given to the subjects when in the IRB's judgment the information would meaningfully add to the protection of the rights and welfare of subjects.

(c) An IRB shall require documentation of informed consent or may waive documentation in accordance with §46.117.

(d) An IRB shall notify investigators and the institution in writing of its decision to approve or disapprove the proposed research activity, or of modifications required to secure IRB approval of the research activity. If the IRB decides to disapprove a research activity, it shall include in its written notification a statement of the reasons for its decision and give the investigator an opportunity to respond in person or in writing.

(e) An IRB shall conduct continuing review of research covered by this policy at intervals appropriate to the degree of risk, but not less than once per year, and shall have authority to observe or have a third party observe the consent process and the research.

(Approved by the Office of Management and Budget under control number 0990-0260.)

§46.110 Expedited review procedures for certain kinds of research involving no more than minimal risk, and for minor changes in approved research.

(a) The Secretary, HHS, has established, and published as a Notice in the FEDERAL REGISTER, a list of categories of research that may be reviewed by the IRB through an expedited review procedure. The list will be amended, as appropriate, after consultation with other departments and agencies, through periodic republication by the Secretary, HHS, in the FEDERAL REGISTER. A copy of the list is available from the Office for Human Research Protections, HHS, or any successor office.

(b) An IRB may use the expedited review procedure to review either or both of the following:

   (1) some or all of the research appearing on the list and found by the reviewer(s) to involve no more than minimal risk,

   (2) minor changes in previously approved research during the period (of one year or less) for which approval is authorized.
   Under an expedited review procedure, the review may be carried out by the IRB chairperson or by one or more experienced reviewers designated by the chairperson from among members of the IRB. In reviewing the research, the reviewers may exercise all of the authorities of the IRB except that the reviewers may not disapprove the research. A research activity may be disapproved only after review in accordance with the non-expedited procedure set forth in §46.108(b).

(c) Each IRB which uses an expedited review procedure shall adopt a method for keeping all members advised of research proposals which have been approved under the procedure.

(d) The department or agency head may restrict, suspend, terminate, or choose not to authorize an institution's or IRB's use of the expedited review procedure.

(Continued on next page)

Appendix 5. Code of Federal Regulations *(Continued)*

§46.111 Criteria for IRB approval of research.

(a) In order to approve research covered by this policy the IRB shall determine that all of the following requirements are satisfied:

    (1) Risks to subjects are minimized: (i) By using procedures which are consistent with sound research design and which do not unnecessarily expose subjects to risk, and (ii) whenever appropriate, by using procedures already being performed on the subjects for diagnostic or treatment purposes.

    (2) Risks to subjects are reasonable in relation to anticipated benefits, if any, to subjects, and the importance of the knowledge that may reasonably be expected to result. In evaluating risks and benefits, the IRB should consider only those risks and benefits that may result from the research (as distinguished from risks and benefits of therapies subjects would receive even if not participating in the research). The IRB should not consider possible long-range effects of applying knowledge gained in the research (for example, the possible effects of the research on public policy) as among those research risks that fall within the purview of its responsibility.

    (3) Selection of subjects is equitable. In making this assessment the IRB should take into account the purposes of the research and the setting in which the research will be conducted and should be particularly cognizant of the special problems of research involving vulnerable populations, such as children, prisoners, pregnant women, mentally disabled persons, or economically or educationally disadvantaged persons.

    (4) Informed consent will be sought from each prospective subject or the subject's legally authorized representative, in accordance with, and to the extent required by §46.116.

    (5) Informed consent will be appropriately documented, in accordance with, and to the extent required by §46.117.

    (6) When appropriate, the research plan makes adequate provision for monitoring the data collected to ensure the safety of subjects.

    (7) When appropriate, there are adequate provisions to protect the privacy of subjects and to maintain the confidentiality of data.

(b) When some or all of the subjects are likely to be vulnerable to coercion or undue influence, such as children, prisoners, pregnant women, mentally disabled persons, or economically or educationally disadvantaged persons, additional safeguards have been included in the study to protect the rights and welfare of these subjects.

§46.112 Review by institution.

Research covered by this policy that has been approved by an IRB may be subject to further appropriate review and approval or disapproval by officials of the institution. However, those officials may not approve the research if it has not been approved by an IRB.

§46.113 Suspension or termination of IRB approval of research.

An IRB shall have authority to suspend or terminate approval of research that is not being conducted in accordance with the IRB's requirements or that has been associated with unexpected serious harm to subjects. Any suspension or termination of approval shall include a statement of the reasons for the IRB's action and shall be reported promptly to the investigator, appropriate institutional officials, and the department or agency head.

(Approved by the Office of Management and Budget under control number 0990-0260.)

§46.114 Cooperative research.

Cooperative research projects are those projects covered by this policy which involve more than one institution. In the conduct of cooperative research projects, each institution is responsible for safeguarding the rights and welfare of human subjects and for complying with this policy. With the approval of the department or agency head, an institution participating in a cooperative project may enter into a joint review arrangement, rely upon the review of another qualified IRB, or make similar arrangements for avoiding duplication of effort.

§46.115 IRB records.

(a) An institution, or when appropriate an IRB, shall prepare and maintain adequate documentation of IRB activities, including the following:

    (1) Copies of all research proposals reviewed, scientific evaluations, if any, that accompany the proposals, approved sample consent documents, progress reports submitted by investigators, and reports of injuries to subjects.

    (2) Minutes of IRB meetings which shall be in sufficient detail to show attendance at the meetings; actions taken by the IRB; the vote on these actions including the number of members voting for, against, and abstaining; the basis for requiring changes in or disapproving research; and a written summary of the discussion of controverted issues and their resolution.

    (3) Records of continuing review activities.

    (4) Copies of all correspondence between the IRB and the investigators.

    (5) A list of IRB members in the same detail as described in §46.103(b)(3).

    (6) Written procedures for the IRB in the same detail as described in §46.103(b)(4) and §46.103(b)(5).

    (7) Statements of significant new findings provided to subjects, as required by §46.116(b)(5).

(b) The records required by this policy shall be retained for at least 3 years, and records relating to research which is conducted shall be retained for at least 3 years after completion of the research. All records shall be accessible for inspection and copying by authorized representatives of the department or agency at reasonable times and in a reasonable manner.

(Approved by the Office of Management and Budget under control number 0990-0260.)

§46.116 General requirements for informed consent.

Except as provided elsewhere in this policy, no investigator may involve a human being as a subject in research covered by this policy unless the investigator has obtained the legally effective informed consent of the subject or the subject's legally authorized representative. An investigator shall seek such consent only under circumstances that provide the prospective subject or the representative sufficient opportunity to consider whether or not to participate and that minimize the possibility of coercion or undue influence. The information that is given to the subject or the representative shall be in language understandable to the subject or the representative. No informed consent, whether oral or written, may include any exculpatory language through which the subject or the representative is made to waive or appear to waive any of the subject's legal rights, or releases or appears to release the investigator, the sponsor, the institution or its agents from liability for negligence.

(Continued on next page)

Appendix 5. Code of Federal Regulations *(Continued)*

(a) Basic elements of informed consent. Except as provided in paragraph (c) or (d) of this section, in seeking informed consent the following information shall be provided to each subject:

(1) A statement that the study involves research, an explanation of the purposes of the research and the expected duration of the subject's participation, a description of the procedures to be followed, and identification of any procedures which are experimental;

(2) A description of any reasonably foreseeable risks or discomforts to the subject;

(3) A description of any benefits to the subject or to others which may reasonably be expected from the research;

(4) A disclosure of appropriate alternative procedures or courses of treatment, if any, that might be advantageous to the subject;

(5) A statement describing the extent, if any, to which confidentiality of records identifying the subject will be maintained;

(6) For research involving more than minimal risk, an explanation as to whether any compensation and an explanation as to whether any medical treatments are available if injury occurs and, if so, what they consist of, or where further information may be obtained;

(7) An explanation of whom to contact for answers to pertinent questions about the research and research subjects' rights, and whom to contact in the event of a research-related injury to the subject; and

(8) A statement that participation is voluntary, refusal to participate will involve no penalty or loss of benefits to which the subject is otherwise entitled, and the subject may discontinue participation at any time without penalty or loss of benefits to which the subject is otherwise entitled.

(b) Additional elements of informed consent. When appropriate, one or more of the following elements of information shall also be provided to each subject:

(1) A statement that the particular treatment or procedure may involve risks to the subject (or to the embryo or fetus, if the subject is or may become pregnant) which are currently unforeseeable;

(2) Anticipated circumstances under which the subject's participation may be terminated by the investigator without regard to the subject's consent;

(3) Any additional costs to the subject that may result from participation in the research;

(4) The consequences of a subject's decision to withdraw from the research and procedures for orderly termination of participation by the subject;

(5) A statement that significant new findings developed during the course of the research which may relate to the subject's willingness to continue participation will be provided to the subject; and

(6) The approximate number of subjects involved in the study.

(c) An IRB may approve a consent procedure which does not include, or which alters, some or all of the elements of informed consent set forth above, or waive the requirement to obtain informed consent provided the IRB finds and documents that:

(1) The research or demonstration project is to be conducted by or subject to the approval of state or local government officials and is designed to study, evaluate, or otherwise examine: (i) public benefit or service programs; (ii) procedures for obtaining benefits or services under those programs; (iii) possible changes in or alternatives to those programs or procedures; or (iv) possible changes in methods or levels of payment for benefits or services under those programs; and

(2) The research could not practicably be carried out without the waiver or alteration.

(d) An IRB may approve a consent procedure which does not include, or which alters, some or all of the elements of informed consent set forth in this section, or waive the requirements to obtain informed consent provided the IRB finds and documents that:

(1) The research involves no more than minimal risk to the subjects;

(2) The waiver or alteration will not adversely affect the rights and welfare of the subjects;

(3) The research could not practicably be carried out without the waiver or alteration; and

(4) Whenever appropriate, the subjects will be provided with additional pertinent information after participation.

(e) The informed consent requirements in this policy are not intended to preempt any applicable federal, state, or local laws which require additional information to be disclosed in order for informed consent to be legally effective.

(f) Nothing in this policy is intended to limit the authority of a physician to provide emergency medical care, to the extent the physician is permitted to do so under applicable federal, state, or local law.

(Approved by the Office of Management and Budget under control number 0990-0260.)

§46.117 Documentation of informed consent.

(a) Except as provided in paragraph (c) of this section, informed consent shall be documented by the use of a written consent form approved by the IRB and signed by the subject or the subject's legally authorized representative. A copy shall be given to the person signing the form.

(b) Except as provided in paragraph (c) of this section, the consent form may be either of the following:

(1) A written consent document that embodies the elements of informed consent required by §46.116. This form may be read to the subject or the subject's legally authorized representative, but in any event, the investigator shall give either the subject or the representative adequate opportunity to read it before it is signed; or

(2) A short form written consent document stating that the elements of informed consent required by §46.116 have been presented orally to the subject or the subject's legally authorized representative. When this method is used, there shall be a witness to the oral presentation. Also, the IRB shall approve a written summary of what is to be said to the subject or the representative. Only the short form itself is to be signed by the subject or the representative. However, the witness shall sign both the short form and a copy of the summary, and the person actually obtaining consent shall sign a copy of the summary. A copy of the summary shall be given to the subject or the representative, in addition to a copy of the short form.

(c) An IRB may waive the requirement for the investigator to obtain a signed consent form for some or all subjects if it finds either:

(1) That the only record linking the subject and the research would be the consent document and the principal risk would be potential harm resulting from a breach of confidentiality. Each subject will be asked whether the subject wants documentation linking the subject with the research, and the subject's wishes will govern; or

(Continued on next page)

Appendix 5. Code of Federal Regulations *(Continued)*

(2)   That the research presents no more than minimal risk of harm to subjects and involves no procedures for which written consent is normally required outside of the research context.

In cases in which the documentation requirement is waived, the IRB may require the investigator to provide subjects with a written statement regarding the research.

(Approved by the Office of Management and Budget under control number 0990-0260.)

§46.118 Applications and proposals lacking definite plans for involvement of human subjects.

Certain types of applications for grants, cooperative agreements, or contracts are submitted to departments or agencies with the knowledge that subjects may be involved within the period of support, but definite plans would not normally be set forth in the application or proposal. These include activities such as institutional type grants when selection of specific projects is the institution's responsibility; research training grants in which the activities involving subjects remain to be selected; and projects in which human subjects' involvement will depend upon completion of instruments, prior animal studies, or purification of compounds. These applications need not be reviewed by an IRB before an award may be made. However, except for research exempted or waived under §46.101 (b) or (i), no human subjects may be involved in any project supported by these awards until the project has been reviewed and approved by the IRB, as provided in this policy, and certification submitted, by the institution, to the department or agency.

§46.119 Research undertaken without the intention of involving human subjects.

In the event research is undertaken without the intention of involving human subjects, but it is later proposed to involve human subjects in the research, the research shall first be reviewed and approved by an IRB, as provided in this policy, a certification submitted, by the institution, to the department or agency, and final approval given to the proposed change by the department or agency.

§46.120 Evaluation and disposition of applications and proposals for research to be conducted or supported by a Federal Department or Agency.

(a)   The department or agency head will evaluate all applications and proposals involving human subjects submitted to the department or agency through such officers and employees of the department or agency and such experts and consultants as the department or agency head determines to be appropriate. This evaluation will take into consideration the risks to the subjects, the adequacy of protection against these risks, the potential benefits of the research to the subjects and others, and the importance of the knowledge gained or to be gained.

(b)   On the basis of this evaluation, the department or agency head may approve or disapprove the application or proposal, or enter into negotiations to develop an approvable one.

§46.121 [Reserved]

§46.122 Use of Federal funds.

Federal funds administered by a department or agency may not be expended for research involving human subjects unless the requirements of this policy have been satisfied.

§46.123 Early termination of research support: Evaluation of applications and proposals.

(a)   The department or agency head may require that department or agency support for any project be terminated or suspended in the manner prescribed in applicable program requirements, when the department or agency head finds an institution has materially failed to comply with the terms of this policy.

(b)   In making decisions about supporting or approving applications or proposals covered by this policy the department or agency head may take into account, in addition to all other eligibility requirements and program criteria, factors such as whether the applicant has been subject to a termination or suspension under paragraph (a) of this section and whether the applicant or the person or persons who would direct or has/have directed the scientific and technical aspects of an activity has/have, in the judgment of the department or agency head, materially failed to discharge responsibility for the protection of the rights and welfare of human subjects (whether or not the research was subject to federal regulation).

§46.124 Conditions.

With respect to any research project or any class of research projects the department or agency head may impose additional conditions prior to or at the time of approval when in the judgment of the department or agency head additional conditions are necessary for the protection of human subjects.

Subpart B	Additional Protections for Pregnant Women, Human Fetuses and Neonates Involved in Research
	Source: 66 FR 56778, Nov. 13, 2001, unless otherwise noted.

§46.201 To what do these regulations apply?

(a)   Except as provided in paragraph (b) of this section, this subpart applies to all research involving pregnant women, human fetuses, neonates of uncertain viability, or nonviable neonates conducted or supported by the Department of Health and Human Services (DHHS). This includes all research conducted in DHHS facilities by any person and all research conducted in any facility by DHHS employees.

(b)   The exemptions at §46.101(b)(1) through (6) are applicable to this subpart.

(c)   The provisions of §46.101(c) through (i) are applicable to this subpart. Reference to State or local laws in this subpart and in §46.101(f) is intended to include the laws of federally recognized American Indian and Alaska Native Tribal Governments.

(d)   The requirements of this subpart are in addition to those imposed under the other subparts of this part.

(Continued on next page)

Appendix 5. Code of Federal Regulations *(Continued)*

§46.202 Definitions.

The definitions in §46.102 shall be applicable to this subpart as well. In addition, as used in this subpart:

(a) Dead fetus means a fetus that exhibits neither heartbeat, spontaneous respiratory activity, spontaneous movement of voluntary muscles, nor pulsation of the umbilical cord.

(b) Delivery means complete separation of the fetus from the woman by expulsion or extraction or any other means.

(c) Fetus means the product of conception from implantation until delivery.

(d) Neonate means a newborn.

(e) Nonviable neonate means a neonate after delivery that, although living, is not viable.

(f) Pregnancy encompasses the period of time from implantation until delivery. A woman shall be assumed to be pregnant if she exhibits any of the pertinent presumptive signs of pregnancy, such as missed menses, until the results of a pregnancy test are negative or until delivery.

(g) Secretary means the Secretary of Health and Human Services and any other officer or employee of the Department of Health and Human Services to whom authority has been delegated.

(h) Viable, as it pertains to the neonate, means being able, after delivery, to survive (given the benefit of available medical therapy) to the point of independently maintaining heartbeat and respiration. The Secretary may from time to time, taking into account medical advances, publish in the FEDERAL REGISTER guidelines to assist in determining whether a neonate is viable for purposes of this subpart. If a neonate is viable then it may be included in research only to the extent permitted and in accordance with the requirements of subparts A and D of this part.

§46.203 Duties of IRBs in connection with research involving pregnant women, fetuses, and neonates.

In addition to other responsibilities assigned to IRBs under this part, each IRB shall review research covered by this subpart and approve only research which satisfies the conditions of all applicable sections of this subpart and the other subparts of this part.

§46.204 Research involving pregnant women or fetuses.

Pregnant women or fetuses may be involved in research if all of the following conditions are met:

(a) Where scientifically appropriate, preclinical studies, including studies on pregnant animals, and clinical studies, including studies on non-pregnant women, have been conducted and provide data for assessing potential risks to pregnant women and fetuses;

(b) The risk to the fetus is caused solely by interventions or procedures that hold out the prospect of direct benefit for the woman or the fetus; or, if there is no such prospect of benefit, the risk to the fetus is not greater than minimal and the purpose of the research is the development of important biomedical knowledge which cannot be obtained by any other means;

(c) Any risk is the least possible for achieving the objectives of the research;

(d) If the research holds out the prospect of direct benefit to the pregnant woman, the prospect of a direct benefit both to the pregnant woman and the fetus, or no prospect of benefit for the woman nor the fetus when risk to the fetus is not greater than minimal and the purpose of the research is the development of important biomedical knowledge that cannot be obtained by any other means, her consent is obtained in accord with the informed consent provisions of subpart A of this part;

(e) If the research holds out the prospect of direct benefit solely to the fetus then the consent of the pregnant woman and the father is obtained in accord with the informed consent provisions of subpart A of this part, except that the father's consent need not be obtained if he is unable to consent because of unavailability, incompetence, or temporary incapacity or the pregnancy resulted from rape or incest.

(f) Each individual providing consent under paragraph (d) or (e) of this section is fully informed regarding the reasonably foreseeable impact of the research on the fetus or neonate;

(g) For children as defined in §46.402(a) who are pregnant, assent and permission are obtained in accord with the provisions of subpart D of this part;

(h) No inducements, monetary or otherwise, will be offered to terminate a pregnancy;

(i) Individuals engaged in the research will have no part in any decisions as to the timing, method, or procedures used to terminate a pregnancy; and

(j) Individuals engaged in the research will have no part in determining the viability of a neonate.

§46.205 Research involving neonates.

(a) Neonates of uncertain viability and nonviable neonates may be involved in research if all of the following conditions are met:

  (1) Where scientifically appropriate, preclinical and clinical studies have been conducted and provide data for assessing potential risks to neonates.

  (2) Each individual providing consent under paragraph (b)(2) or (c)(5) of this section is fully informed regarding the reasonably foreseeable impact of the research on the neonate.

  (3) Individuals engaged in the research will have no part in determining the viability of a neonate.

  (4) The requirements of paragraph (b) or (c) of this section have been met as applicable.

(b) Neonates of uncertain viability. Until it has been ascertained whether or not a neonate is viable, a neonate may not be involved in research covered by this subpart unless the following additional conditions have been met:

  (1) The IRB determines that:

    (i) The research holds out the prospect of enhancing the probability of survival of the neonate to the point of viability, and any risk is the least possible for achieving that objective, or

    (ii) The purpose of the research is the development of important biomedical knowledge which cannot be obtained by other means and there will be no added risk to the neonate resulting from the research; and

  (2) The legally effective informed consent of either parent of the neonate or, if neither parent is able to consent because of unavailability, incompetence, or temporary incapacity, the legally effective informed consent of either parent's legally authorized representative is obtained in accord with subpart A of this part, except that the consent of the father or his legally authorized representative need not be obtained if the pregnancy resulted from rape or incest.

(Continued on next page)

Appendix 5. Code of Federal Regulations *(Continued)*

(c) Nonviable neonates. After delivery nonviable neonate may not be involved in research covered by this subpart unless all of the following additional conditions are met:

(1) Vital functions of the neonate will not be artificially maintained;

(2) The research will not terminate the heartbeat or respiration of the neonate;

(3) There will be no added risk to the neonate resulting from the research;

(4) The purpose of the research is the development of important biomedical knowledge that cannot be obtained by other means; and

(5) The legally effective informed consent of both parents of the neonate is obtained in accord with subpart A of this part, except that the waiver and alteration provisions of §46.116(c) and (d) do not apply. However, if either parent is unable to consent because of unavailability, incompetence, or temporary incapacity, the informed consent of one parent of a nonviable neonate will suffice to meet the requirements of this paragraph (c)(5), except that the consent of the father need not be obtained if the pregnancy resulted from rape or incest. The consent of a legally authorized representative of either or both of the parents of a nonviable neonate will not suffice to meet the requirements of this paragraph (c)(5).

(d) Viable neonates. A neonate, after delivery, that has been determined to be viable may be included in research only to the extent permitted by and in accord with the requirements of subparts A and D of this part.

§46.206 Research involving, after delivery, the placenta, the dead fetus or fetal material.

(a) Research involving, after delivery, the placenta; the dead fetus; macerated fetal material; or cells, tissue, or organs excised from a dead fetus, shall be conducted only in accord with any applicable federal, state, or local laws and regulations regarding such activities.

(b) If information associated with material described in paragraph (a) of this section is recorded for research purposes in a manner that living individuals can be identified, directly or through identifiers linked to those individuals, those individuals are research subjects and all pertinent subparts of this part are applicable.

§46.207 Research not otherwise approvable which presents an opportunity to understand, prevent, or alleviate a serious problem affecting the health or welfare of pregnant women, fetuses, or neonates.

The Secretary will conduct or fund research that the IRB does not believe meets the requirements of §46.204 or §46.205 only if:

(a) The IRB finds that the research presents a reasonable opportunity to further the understanding, prevention, or alleviation of a serious problem affecting the health or welfare of pregnant women, fetuses or neonates; and

(b) The Secretary, after consultation with a panel of experts in pertinent disciplines (for example: science, medicine, ethics, law) and following opportunity for public review and comment, including a public meeting announced in the FEDERAL REGISTER, has determined either:

(1) That the research in fact satisfies the conditions of §46.204, as applicable; or

(2) The following:

(i) The research presents a reasonable opportunity to further the understanding, prevention, or alleviation of a serious problem affecting the health or welfare of pregnant women, fetuses or neonates;

(ii) The research will be conducted in accord with sound ethical principles; and

(iii) Informed consent will be obtained in accord with the informed consent provisions of subpart A and other applicable subparts of this part.

Subpart C	Additional Protections Pertaining to Biomedical and Behavioral Research Involving Prisoners as Subjects
	Source: 43 FR 53655, Nov. 16, 1978, unless otherwise noted.

§46.301 Applicability.

(a) The regulations in this subpart are applicable to all biomedical and behavioral research conducted or supported by the Department of Health and Human Services involving prisoners as subjects.

(b) Nothing in this subpart shall be construed as indicating that compliance with the procedures set forth herein will authorize research involving prisoners as subjects, to the extent such research is limited or barred by applicable State or local law.

(c) The requirements of this subpart are in addition to those imposed under the other subparts of this part.

§46.302 Purpose.

Inasmuch as prisoners may be under constraints because of their incarceration which could affect their ability to make a truly voluntary and uncoerced decision whether or not to participate as subjects in research, it is the purpose of this subpart to provide additional safeguards for the protection of prisoners involved in activities to which this subpart is applicable.

§46.303 Definitions.

As used in this subpart:

(a) *Secretary* means the Secretary of Health and Human Services and any other officer or employee of the Department of Health and Human Services to whom authority has been delegated.

(b) *DHHS* means the Department of Health and Human Services.

(c) *Prisoner* means any individual involuntarily confined or detained in a penal institution. The term is intended to encompass individuals sentenced to such an institution under a criminal or civil statute, individuals detained in other facilities by virtue of statutes or commitment procedures which provide alternatives to criminal prosecution or incarceration in a penal institution, and individuals detained pending arraignment, trial, or sentencing.

(d) *Minimal risk* is the probability and magnitude of physical or psychological harm that is normally encountered in the daily lives, or in the routine medical, dental, or psychological examination of healthy persons.

(Continued on next page)

Appendix 5. Code of Federal Regulations *(Continued)*

§46.304 Composition of Institutional Review Boards where prisoners are involved.

In addition to satisfying the requirements in §46.107 of this part, an Institutional Review Board, carrying out responsibilities under this part with respect to research covered by this subpart, shall also meet the following specific requirements:

(a) A majority of the Board (exclusive of prisoner members) shall have no association with the prison(s) involved, apart from their membership on the Board.

(b) At least one member of the Board shall be a prisoner, or a prisoner representative with appropriate background and experience to serve in that capacity, except that where a particular research project is reviewed by more than one Board only one Board need satisfy this requirement.

[43 FR 53655, Nov. 16, 1978, as amended at 46 FR 8366, Jan. 26, 1981]

§46.305 Additional duties of the Institutional Review Boards where prisoners are involved.

(a) In addition to all other responsibilities prescribed for Institutional Review Boards under this part, the Board shall review research covered by this subpart and approve such research only if it finds that:

    (1) The research under review represents one of the categories of research permissible under §46.306(a)(2);

    (2) Any possible advantages accruing to the prisoner through his or her participation in the research, when compared to the general living conditions, medical care, quality of food, amenities and opportunity for earnings in the prison, are not of such a magnitude that his or her ability to weigh the risks of the research against the value of such advantages in the limited choice environment of the prison is impaired;

    (3) The risks involved in the research are commensurate with risks that would be accepted by nonprisoner volunteers;

    (4) Procedures for the selection of subjects within the prison are fair to all prisoners and immune from arbitrary intervention by prison authorities or prisoners. Unless the principal investigator provides to the Board justification in writing for following some other procedures, control subjects must be selected randomly from the group of available prisoners who meet the characteristics needed for that particular research project;

    (5) The information is presented in language which is understandable to the subject population;

    (6) Adequate assurance exists that parole boards will not take into account a prisoner's participation in the research in making decisions regarding parole, and each prisoner is clearly informed in advance that participation in the research will have no effect on his or her parole; and

    (7) Where the Board finds there may be a need for follow-up examination or care of participants after the end of their participation, adequate provision has been made for such examination or care, taking into account the varying lengths of individual prisoners' sentences, and for informing participants of this fact.

(b) The Board shall carry out such other duties as may be assigned by the Secretary.

(c) The institution shall certify to the Secretary, in such form and manner as the Secretary may require, that the duties of the Board under this section have been fulfilled.

§46.306 Permitted research involving prisoners.

(a) Biomedical or behavioral research conducted or supported by DHHS may involve prisoners as subjects only if:

    (1) The institution responsible for the conduct of the research has certified to the Secretary that the Institutional Review Board has approved the research under §46.305 of this subpart; and

    (2) In the judgment of the Secretary the proposed research involves solely the following:

        (i) Study of the possible causes, effects, and processes of incarceration, and of criminal behavior, provided that the study presents no more than minimal risk and no more than inconvenience to the subjects;

        (ii) Study of prisons as institutional structures or of prisoners as incarcerated persons, provided that the study presents no more than minimal risk and no more than inconvenience to the subjects;

        (iii) Research on conditions particularly affecting prisoners as a class (for example, vaccine trials and other research on hepatitis which is much more prevalent in prisons than elsewhere; and research on social and psychological problems such as alcoholism, drug addiction, and sexual assaults) provided that the study may proceed only after the Secretary has consulted with appropriate experts including experts in penology, medicine, and ethics, and published notice, in the FEDERAL REGISTER, of his intent to approve such research; or

        (iv) Research on practices, both innovative and accepted, which have the intent and reasonable probability of improving the health or well-being of the subject. In cases in which those studies require the assignment of prisoners in a manner consistent with protocols approved by the IRB to control groups which may not benefit from the research, the study may proceed only after the Secretary has consulted with appropriate experts, including experts in penology, medicine, and ethics, and published notice, in the FEDERAL REGISTER, of the intent to approve such research.

(b) Except as provided in paragraph (a) of this section, biomedical or behavioral research conducted or supported by DHHS shall not involve prisoners as subjects.

Subpart D	Additional Protections for Children Involved as Subjects in Research
	Source: 48 FR 9818, March 8, 1983, unless otherwise noted.

§46.401 To what do these regulations apply?

(a) This subpart applies to all research involving children as subjects, conducted or supported by the Department of Health and Human Services.

    (1) This includes research conducted by Department employees, except that each head of an Operating Division of the Department may adopt such nonsubstantive, procedural modifications as may be appropriate from an administrative standpoint.

(Continued on next page)

Appendix 5. Code of Federal Regulations *(Continued)*

(2)   It also includes research conducted or supported by the Department of Health and Human Services outside the United States, but in appropriate circumstances, the Secretary may, under paragraph (i) of §46.101 of subpart A, waive the applicability of some or all of the requirements of these regulations for research of this type.

(b)   Exemptions at §46.101(b)(1) and (b)(3) through (b)(6) are applicable to this subpart. The exemption at §46.101(b)(2) regarding educational tests is also applicable to this subpart. However, the exemption at §46.101(b)(2) for research involving survey or interview procedures or observations of public behavior does not apply to research covered by this subpart, except for research involving observation of public behavior when the investigator(s) do not participate in the activities being observed.

(c)   The exceptions, additions, and provisions for waiver as they appear in paragraphs (c) through (i) of §46.101 of subpart A are applicable to this subpart.

[48 FR 9818, Mar.8, 1983; 56 FR 28032, June 18, 1991; 56 FR 29757, June 28, 1991.]

§46.402 Definitions.

The definitions in §46.102 of subpart A shall be applicable to this subpart as well. In addition, as used in this subpart:

(a)   *Children* are persons who have not attained the legal age for consent to treatments or procedures involved in the research, under the applicable law of the jurisdiction in which the research will be conducted.

(b)   *Assent* means a child's affirmative agreement to participate in research. Mere failure to object should not, absent affirmative agreement, be construed as assent.

(c)   *Permission* means the agreement of parent(s) or guardian to the participation of their child or ward in research.

(d)   *Parent* means a child's biological or adoptive parent.

(e)   *Guardian* means an individual who is authorized under applicable State or local law to consent on behalf of a child to general medical care.

§46.403 IRB duties.

In addition to other responsibilities assigned to IRBs under this part, each IRB shall review research covered by this subpart and approve only research which satisfies the conditions of all applicable sections of this subpart.

§46.404 Research not involving greater than minimal risk.

HHS will conduct or fund research in which the IRB finds that no greater than minimal risk to children is presented, only if the IRB finds that adequate provisions are made for soliciting the assent of the children and the permission of their parents or guardians, as set forth in §46.408.

§46.405 Research involving greater than minimal risk but presenting the prospect of direct benefit to the individual subjects.

HHS will conduct or fund research in which the IRB finds that more than minimal risk to children is presented by an intervention or procedure that holds out the prospect of direct benefit for the individual subject, or by a monitoring procedure that is likely to contribute to the subject's well-being, only if the IRB finds that:

(a)   The risk is justified by the anticipated benefit to the subjects;

(b)   The relation of the anticipated benefit to the risk is at least as favorable to the subjects as that presented by available alternative approaches; and

(c)   Adequate provisions are made for soliciting the assent of the children and permission of their parents or guardians, as set forth in §46.408.

§46.406 Research involving greater than minimal risk and no prospect of direct benefit to individual subjects, but likely to yield generalizable knowledge about the subject's disorder or condition.

HHS will conduct or fund research in which the IRB finds that more than minimal risk to children is presented by an intervention or procedure that does not hold out the prospect of direct benefit for the individual subject, or by a monitoring procedure which is not likely to contribute to the well-being of the subject, only if the IRB finds that:

(a)   The risk represents a minor increase over minimal risk;

(b)   The intervention or procedure presents experiences to subjects that are reasonably commensurate with those inherent in their actual or expected medical, dental, psychological, social, or educational situations;

(c)   The intervention or procedure is likely to yield generalizable knowledge about the subjects' disorder or condition which is of vital importance for the understanding or amelioration of the subjects' disorder or condition; and

(d)   Adequate provisions are made for soliciting assent of the children and permission of their parents or guardians, as set forth in §46.408.

§46.407 Research not otherwise approvable which presents an opportunity to understand, prevent, or alleviate a serious problem affecting the health or welfare of children.

HHS will conduct or fund research that the IRB does not believe meets the requirements of §46.404, §46.405, or §46.406 only if:

(a)   The IRB finds that the research presents a reasonable opportunity to further the understanding, prevention, or alleviation of a serious problem affecting the health or welfare of children; and

(b)   The Secretary, after consultation with a panel of experts in pertinent disciplines (for example: science, medicine, education, ethics, law) and following opportunity for public review and comment, has determined either:

   (1)   That the research in fact satisfies the conditions of §46.404, §46.405, or §46.406, as applicable, or (2) the following:

      (i)   The research presents a reasonable opportunity to further the understanding, prevention, or alleviation of a serious problem affecting the health or welfare of children;

      (ii)   The research will be conducted in accordance with sound ethical principles;

      (iii) Adequate provisions are made for soliciting the assent of children and the permission of their parents or guardians, as set forth in §46.408.

(Continued on next page)

Appendix 5. Code of Federal Regulations *(Continued)*

§46.408 Requirements for permission by parents or guardians and for assent by children.

(a) In addition to the determinations required under other applicable sections of this subpart, the IRB shall determine that adequate provisions are made for soliciting the assent of the children, when in the judgment of the IRB the children are capable of providing assent. In determining whether children are capable of assenting, the IRB shall take into account the ages, maturity, and psychological state of the children involved. This judgment may be made for all children to be involved in research under a particular protocol, or for each child, as the IRB deems appropriate. If the IRB determines that the capability of some or all of the children is so limited that they cannot reasonably be consulted or that the intervention or procedure involved in the research holds out a prospect of direct benefit that is important to the health or well-being of the children and is available only in the context of the research, the assent of the children is not a necessary condition for proceeding with the research. Even where the IRB determines that the subjects are capable of assenting, the IRB may still waive the assent requirement under circumstances in which consent may be waived in accord with §46.116 of Subpart A.

(b) In addition to the determinations required under other applicable sections of this subpart, the IRB shall determine, in accordance with and to the extent that consent is required by §46.116 of Subpart A, that adequate provisions are made for soliciting the permission of each child's parents or guardian. Where parental permission is to be obtained, the IRB may find that the permission of one parent is sufficient for research to be conducted under §46.404 or §46.405. Where research is covered by §46.406 and §46.407 and permission is to be obtained from parents, both parents must give their permission unless one parent is deceased, unknown, incompetent, or not reasonably available, or when only one parent has legal responsibility for the care and custody of the child.

(c) In addition to the provisions for waiver contained in §46.116 of subpart A, if the IRB determines that a research protocol is designed for conditions or for a subject population for which parental or guardian permission is not a reasonable requirement to protect the subjects (for example, neglected or abused children), it may waive the consent requirements in Subpart A of this part and paragraph (b) of this section, provided an appropriate mechanism for protecting the children who will participate as subjects in the research is substituted, and provided further that the waiver is not inconsistent with federal, state, or local law. The choice of an appropriate mechanism would depend upon the nature and purpose of the activities described in the protocol, the risk and anticipated benefit to the research subjects, and their age, maturity, status, and condition.

(d) Permission by parents or guardians shall be documented in accordance with and to the extent required by §46.117 of subpart A.

(e) When the IRB determines that assent is required, it shall also determine whether and how assent must be documented.

§46.409 Wards.

(a) Children who are wards of the state or any other agency, institution, or entity can be included in research approved under §46.406 or §46.407 only if such research is:

(1) Related to their status as wards; or

(2) Conducted in schools, camps, hospitals, institutions, or similar settings in which the majority of children involved as subjects are not wards.

(b) If the research is approved under paragraph (a) of this section, the IRB shall require appointment of an advocate for each child who is a ward, in addition to any other individual acting on behalf of the child as guardian or in loco parentis. One individual may serve as advocate for more than one child. The advocate shall be an individual who has the background and experience to act in, and agrees to act in, the best interests of the child for the duration of the child's participation in the research and who is not associated in any way (except in the role as advocate or member of the IRB) with the research, the investigator(s), or the guardian organization.

Appendix 6. International Conference on Harmonisation Guideline for Good Clinical Practice

INTERNATIONAL CONFERENCE ON HARMONISATION OF TECHNICAL REQUIREMENTS FOR REGISTRATION OF PHARMACEUTICALS FOR HUMAN USE

ICH Harmonised Tripartite Guideline

Guideline for Good Clinical Practice
E6(R1)

Current *Step 4* version
dated 10 June 1996

(including the Post Step 4 corrections)

This Guideline has been developed by the appropriate ICH Expert Working Group and has been subject to consultation by the regulatory parties, in accordance with the ICH Process. At Step 4 of the Process the final draft is recommended for adoption to the regulatory bodies of the European Union, Japan and USA.

E6(R1) Document History			
First Codification	**History**	**Date**	**New Codification November 2005**
E6	Approval by the Steering Committee under *Step 2* and release for public consultation.	27 April 1995	E6
E6	Approval by the Steering Committee under *Step 4* and recommended for adoption to the three ICH regulatory bodies.	1 May 1996	E6
Current *Step 4* version			
E6	Approval by the Steering Committee of *Post-Step 4* editorial corrections.	10 June 1996	E6(R1)

Guideline for Good Clinical Practice
ICH Harmonised Tripartite Guideline
Having reached *Step 4* of the ICH Process at the ICH Steering Committee meeting
on 1 May 1996, this guideline is recommended for
adoption to the three regulatory parties to ICH
(*This document includes the Post Step 4 corrections agreed by the Steering Committee on 10 June 1996*)

TABLE OF CONTENTS

(Continued on next page)

Appendix 6. International Conference on Harmonisation Guideline for Good Clinical Practice *(Continued)*

(Continued on next page)

Appendix 6. International Conference on Harmonisation Guideline for Good Clinical Practice (Continued)

Guideline for Good Clinical Practice
INTRODUCTION

Good Clinical Practice (GCP) is an international ethical and scientific quality standard for designing, conducting, recording and reporting trials that involve the participation of human subjects. Compliance with this standard provides public assurance that the rights, safety and well-being of trial subjects are protected, consistent with the principles that have their origin in the Declaration of Helsinki, and that the clinical trial data are credible.

The objective of this ICH GCP Guideline is to provide a unified standard for the European Union (EU), Japan and the United States to facilitate the mutual acceptance of clinical data by the regulatory authorities in these jurisdictions.

The guideline was developed with consideration of the current good clinical practices of the European Union, Japan, and the United States, as well as those of Australia, Canada, the Nordic countries and the World Health Organization (WHO).

This guideline should be followed when generating clinical trial data that are intended to be submitted to regulatory authorities.
The principles established in this guideline may also be applied to other clinical investigations that may have an impact on the safety and well-being of human subjects.

1.   GLOSSARY

1.1   Adverse Drug Reaction (ADR)

In the pre-approval clinical experience with a new medicinal product or its new usages, particularly as the therapeutic dose(s) may not be established: all noxious and unintended responses to a medicinal product related to any dose should be considered adverse drug reactions. The phrase responses to a medicinal product means that a causal relationship between a medicinal product and an adverse event is at least a reasonable possibility, i.e. the relationship cannot be ruled out.
Regarding marketed medicinal products: a response to a drug which is noxious and unintended and which occurs at doses normally used in man for prophylaxis, diagnosis, or therapy of diseases or for modification of physiological function (see the ICH Guideline for Clinical Safety Data Management: Definitions and Standards for Expedited Reporting).

1.2   Adverse Event (AE)

Any untoward medical occurrence in a patient or clinical investigation subject administered a pharmaceutical product and which does not necessarily have a causal relationship with this treatment. An adverse event (AE) can therefore be any unfavourable and unintended sign (including an abnormal laboratory finding), symptom, or disease temporally associated with the use of a medicinal (investigational) product, whether or not related to the medicinal (investigational) product (see the ICH Guideline for Clinical Safety Data Management: Definitions and Standards for Expedited Reporting).

1.3   Amendment (to the protocol)
See Protocol Amendment.

1.4   Applicable Regulatory Requirement(s)
Any law(s) and regulation(s) addressing the conduct of clinical trials of investigational products.

1.5   Approval (in relation to Institutional Review Boards)
The affirmative decision of the IRB that the clinical trial has been reviewed and may be conducted at the institution site within the constraints set forth by the IRB, the institution, Good Clinical Practice (GCP), and the applicable regulatory requirements.

1.6   Audit
A systematic and independent examination of trial related activities and documents to determine whether the evaluated trial related activities were conducted, and the data were recorded, analyzed and accurately reported according to the protocol, sponsor's standard operating procedures (SOPs), Good Clinical Practice (GCP), and the applicable regulatory requirement(s).

1.7   Audit Certificate
A declaration of confirmation by the auditor that an audit has taken place.

1.8   Audit Report
A written evaluation by the sponsor's auditor of the results of the audit.

1.9   Audit Trail
Documentation that allows reconstruction of the course of events.

(Continued on next page)

Appendix 6. International Conference on Harmonisation Guideline for Good Clinical Practice *(Continued)*

1.10   Blinding/Masking

A procedure in which one or more parties to the trial are kept unaware of the treatment assignment(s). Single-blinding usually refers to the subject(s) being unaware, and double-blinding usually refers to the subject(s), investigator(s), monitor, and, in some cases, data analyst(s) being unaware of the treatment assignment(s).

1.11   Case Report Form (CRF)

A printed, optical, or electronic document designed to record all of the protocol required information to be reported to the sponsor on each trial subject.

1.12   Clinical Trial/Study

Any investigation in human subjects intended to discover or verify the clinical, pharmacological and/or other pharmacodynamic effects of an investigational product(s), and/or to identify any adverse reactions to an investigational product(s), and/or to study absorption, distribution, metabolism, and excretion of an investigational product(s) with the object of ascertaining its safety and/or efficacy. The terms clinical trial and clinical study are synonymous.

1.13   Clinical Trial/Study Report

A written description of a trial/study of any therapeutic, prophylactic, or diagnostic agent conducted in human subjects, in which the clinical and statistical description, presentations, and analyses are fully integrated into a single report (see the ICH Guideline for Structure and Content of Clinical Study Reports).

1.14   Comparator (Product)

An investigational or marketed product (i.e., active control), or placebo, used as a reference in a clinical trial.

1.15   Compliance (in relation to trials)

Adherence to all the trial-related requirements, Good Clinical Practice (GCP) requirements, and the applicable regulatory requirements.

1.16   Confidentiality

Prevention of disclosure, to other than authorized individuals, of a sponsor's proprietary information or of a subject's identity.

1.17   Contract

A written, dated, and signed agreement between two or more involved parties that sets out any arrangements on delegation and distribution of tasks and obligations and, if appropriate, on financial matters. The protocol may serve as the basis of a contract.

1.18   Coordinating Committee

A committee that a sponsor may organize to coordinate the conduct of a multicentre trial.

1.19   Coordinating Investigator

An investigator assigned the responsibility for the coordination of investigators at different centres participating in a multicentre trial.

1.20   Contract Research Organization (CRO)

A person or an organization (commercial, academic, or other) contracted by the sponsor to perform one or more of a sponsor's trial-related duties and functions.

1.21   Direct Access

Permission to examine, analyze, verify, and reproduce any records and reports that are important to evaluation of a clinical trial. Any party (e.g., domestic and foreign regulatory authorities, sponsor's monitors and auditors) with direct access should take all reasonable precautions within the constraints of the applicable regulatory requirement(s) to maintain the confidentiality of subjects' identities and sponsor's proprietary information.

1.22   Documentation

All records, in any form (including, but not limited to, written, electronic, magnetic, and optical records, and scans, x-rays, and electrocardiograms) that describe or record the methods, conduct, and/or results of a trial, the factors affecting a trial, and the actions taken.

1.23   Essential Documents

Documents which individually and collectively permit evaluation of the conduct of a study and the quality of the data produced (see 8. Essential Documents for the Conduct of a Clinical Trial).

1.24   Good Clinical Practice (GCP)

A standard for the design, conduct, performance, monitoring, auditing, recording, analyses, and reporting of clinical trials that provides assurance that the data and reported results are credible and accurate, and that the rights, integrity, and confidentiality of trial subjects are protected.

1.25   Independent Data-Monitoring Committee (IDMC) (Data and Safety Monitoring Board, Monitoring Committee, Data Monitoring Committee)

An independent data-monitoring committee that may be established by the sponsor to assess at intervals the progress of a clinical trial, the safety data, and the critical efficacy endpoints, and to recommend to the sponsor whether to continue, modify, or stop a trial.

1.26   Impartial Witness

A person, who is independent of the trial, who cannot be unfairly influenced by people involved with the trial, who attends the informed consent process if the subject or the subject's legally acceptable representative cannot read, and who reads the informed consent form and any other written information supplied to the subject.

1.27   Independent Ethics Committee (IEC)

An independent body (a review board or a committee, institutional, regional, national, or supranational), constituted of medical professionals and non-medical members, whose responsibility it is to ensure the protection of the rights, safety and well-being of human subjects involved in a trial and to provide public assurance of that protection, by, among other things, reviewing and approving / providing favourable opinion on, the trial protocol, the suitability of the investigator(s), facilities, and the methods and material to be used in obtaining and documenting informed consent of the trial subjects.

The legal status, composition, function, operations and regulatory requirements pertaining to Independent Ethics Committees may differ among countries, but should allow the Independent Ethics Committee to act in agreement with GCP as described in this guideline.

(Continued on next page)

Appendix 6. International Conference on Harmonisation Guideline for Good Clinical Practice *(Continued)*

1.28	Informed Consent
	A process by which a subject voluntarily confirms his or her willingness to participate in a particular trial, after having been informed of all aspects of the trial that are relevant to the subject's decision to participate. Informed consent is documented by means of a written, signed and dated informed consent form.
1.29	Inspection
	The act by a regulatory authority(ies) of conducting an official review of documents, facilities, records, and any other resources that are deemed by the authority(ies) to be related to the clinical trial and that may be located at the site of the trial, at the sponsor's and/or contract research organization's (CRO's) facilities, or at other establishments deemed appropriate by the regulatory authority(ies).
1.30	Institution (medical)
	Any public or private entity or agency or medical or dental facility where clinical trials are conducted.
1.31	Institutional Review Board (IRB)
	An independent body constituted of medical, scientific, and non-scientific members, whose responsibility is to ensure the protection of the rights, safety and well-being of human subjects involved in a trial by, among other things, reviewing, approving, and providing continuing review of trial protocol and amendments and of the methods and material to be used in obtaining and documenting informed consent of the trial subjects.
1.32	Interim Clinical Trial/Study Report
	A report of intermediate results and their evaluation based on analyses performed during the course of a trial.
1.33	Investigational Product
	A pharmaceutical form of an active ingredient or placebo being tested or used as a reference in a clinical trial, including a product with a marketing authorization when used or assembled (formulated or packaged) in a way different from the approved form, or when used for an unapproved indication, or when used to gain further information about an approved use.
1.34	Investigator
	A person responsible for the conduct of the clinical trial at a trial site. If a trial is conducted by a team of individuals at a trial site, the investigator is the responsible leader of the team and may be called the principal investigator. See also Subinvestigator.
1.35	Investigator/Institution
	An expression meaning "the investigator and/or institution, where required by the applicable regulatory requirements".
1.36	Investigator's Brochure
	A compilation of the clinical and nonclinical data on the investigational product(s) which is relevant to the study of the investigational product(s) in human subjects (see 7. Investigator's Brochure).
1.37	Legally Acceptable Representative
	An individual or juridical or other body authorized under applicable law to consent, on behalf of a prospective subject, to the subject's participation in the clinical trial.
1.38	Monitoring
	The act of overseeing the progress of a clinical trial, and of ensuring that it is conducted, recorded, and reported in accordance with the protocol, Standard Operating Procedures (SOPs), Good Clinical Practice (GCP), and the applicable regulatory requirement(s).
1.39	Monitoring Report
	A written report from the monitor to the sponsor after each site visit and/or other trial-related communication according to the sponsor's SOPs.
1.40	Multicentre Trial
	A clinical trial conducted according to a single protocol but at more than one site, and therefore, carried out by more than one investigator.
1.41	Nonclinical Study
	Biomedical studies not performed on human subjects.
1.42	Opinion (in relation to Independent Ethics Committee)
	The judgement and/or the advice provided by an Independent Ethics Committee (IEC).
1.43	Original Medical Record
	See Source Documents.
1.44	Protocol
	A document that describes the objective(s), design, methodology, statistical considerations, and organization of a trial. The protocol usually also gives the background and rationale for the trial, but these could be provided in other protocol referenced documents. Throughout the ICH GCP Guideline the term protocol refers to protocol and protocol amendments.
1.45	Protocol Amendment
	A written description of a change(s) to or formal clarification of a protocol.
1.46	Quality Assurance (QA)
	All those planned and systematic actions that are established to ensure that the trial is performed and the data are generated, documented (recorded), and reported in compliance with Good Clinical Practice (GCP) and the applicable regulatory requirement(s).
1.47	Quality Control (QC)
	The operational techniques and activities undertaken within the quality assurance system to verify that the requirements for quality of the trial-related activities have been fulfilled.
1.48	Randomization
	The process of assigning trial subjects to treatment or control groups using an element of chance to determine the assignments in order to reduce bias.

(Continued on next page)

Appendix 6. International Conference on Harmonisation Guideline for Good Clinical Practice *(Continued)*

1.49   Regulatory Authorities

Bodies having the power to regulate. In the ICH GCP guideline the expression Regulatory Authorities includes the authorities that review submitted clinical data and those that conduct inspections (see 1.29). These bodies are sometimes referred to as competent authorities.

1.50   Serious Adverse Event (SAE) or Serious Adverse Drug Reaction (Serious ADR)

Any untoward medical occurrence that at any dose:

- results in death,
- is life-threatening,
- requires inpatient hospitalization or prolongation of existing hospitalization,
- results in persistent or significant disability/incapacity,

or

- is a congenital anomaly/birth defect

(see the ICH Guideline for Clinical Safety Data Management: Definitions and Standards for Expedited Reporting).

1.51   Source Data

All information in original records and certified copies of original records of clinical findings, observations, or other activities in a clinical trial necessary for the reconstruction and evaluation of the trial. Source data are contained in source documents (original records or certified copies).

1.52   Source Documents

Original documents, data, and records (e.g., hospital records, clinical and office charts, laboratory notes, memoranda, subjects' diaries or evaluation checklists, pharmacy dispensing records, recorded data from automated instruments, copies or transcriptions certified after verification as being accurate copies, microfiches, photographic negatives, microfilm or magnetic media, x-rays, subject files, and records kept at the pharmacy, at the laboratories and at medico-technical departments involved in the clinical trial).

1.53   Sponsor

An individual, company, institution, or organization which takes responsibility for the initiation, management, and/or financing of a clinical trial.

1.54   Sponsor-Investigator

An individual who both initiates and conducts, alone or with others, a clinical trial, and under whose immediate direction the investigational product is administered to, dispensed to, or used by a subject. The term does not include any person other than an individual (e.g., it does not include a corporation or an agency). The obligations of a sponsor-investigator include both those of a sponsor and those of an investigator.

1.55   Standard Operating Procedures (SOPs)

Detailed, written instructions to achieve uniformity of the performance of a specific function.

1.56   Subinvestigator

Any individual member of the clinical trial team designated and supervised by the investigator at a trial site to perform critical trial-related procedures and/or to make important trial-related decisions (e.g., associates, residents, research fellows). See also Investigator.

1.57   Subject/Trial Subject

An individual who participates in a clinical trial, either as a recipient of the investigational product(s) or as a control.

1.58   Subject Identification Code

A unique identifier assigned by the investigator to each trial subject to protect the subject's identity and used in lieu of the subject's name when the investigator reports adverse events and/or other trial related data.

1.59   Trial Site

The location(s) where trial-related activities are actually conducted.

1.60   Unexpected Adverse Drug Reaction

An adverse reaction, the nature or severity of which is not consistent with the applicable product information (e.g., Investigator's Brochure for an unapproved investigational product or package insert/summary of product characteristics for an approved product) (see the ICH Guideline for Clinical Safety Data Management: Definitions and Standards for Expedited Reporting).

1.61   Vulnerable Subjects

Individuals whose willingness to volunteer in a clinical trial may be unduly influenced by the expectation, whether justified or not, of benefits associated with participation, or of a retaliatory response from senior members of a hierarchy in case of refusal to participate. Examples are members of a group with a hierarchical structure, such as medical, pharmacy, dental, and nursing students, subordinate hospital and laboratory personnel, employees of the pharmaceutical industry, members of the armed forces, and persons kept in detention. Other vulnerable subjects include patients with incurable diseases, persons in nursing homes, unemployed or impoverished persons, patients in emergency situations, ethnic minority groups, homeless persons, nomads, refugees, minors, and those incapable of giving consent.

1.62   Well-being (of the trial subjects)

The physical and mental integrity of the subjects participating in a clinical trial.

2.   THE PRINCIPLES OF ICH GCP

2.1   Clinical trials should be conducted in accordance with the ethical principles that have their origin in the Declaration of Helsinki, and that are consistent with GCP and the applicable regulatory requirement(s).

2.2   Before a trial is initiated, foreseeable risks and inconveniences should be weighed against the anticipated benefit for the individual trial subject and society. A trial should be initiated and continued only if the anticipated benefits justify the risks.

2.3   The rights, safety, and well-being of the trial subjects are the most important considerations and should prevail over interests of science and society.

(Continued on next page)

Appendix 6. International Conference on Harmonisation Guideline for Good Clinical Practice *(Continued)*

2.4   The available nonclinical and clinical information on an investigational product should be adequate to support the proposed clinical trial.

2.5   Clinical trials should be scientifically sound, and described in a clear, detailed protocol.

2.6   A trial should be conducted in compliance with the protocol that has received prior institutional review board (IRB)/independent ethics committee (IEC) approval/favourable opinion.

2.7   The medical care given to, and medical decisions made on behalf of, subjects should always be the responsibility of a qualified physician or, when appropriate, of a qualified dentist.

2.8   Each individual involved in conducting a trial should be qualified by education, training, and experience to perform his or her respective task(s).

2.9   Freely given informed consent should be obtained from every subject prior to clinical trial participation.

2.10   All clinical trial information should be recorded, handled, and stored in a way that allows its accurate reporting, interpretation and verification.

2.11   The confidentiality of records that could identify subjects should be protected, respecting the privacy and confidentiality rules in accordance with the applicable regulatory requirement(s).

2.12   Investigational products should be manufactured, handled, and stored in accordance with applicable good manufacturing practice (GMP). They should be used in accordance with the approved protocol.

2.13   Systems with procedures that assure the quality of every aspect of the trial should be implemented.

3.   INSTITUTIONAL REVIEW BOARD/INDEPENDENT ETHICS COMMITTEE (IRB/IEC)

3.1   Responsibilities

3.1.1   An IRB/IEC should safeguard the rights, safety, and well-being of all trial subjects. Special attention should be paid to trials that may include vulnerable subjects.

3.1.2   The IRB/IEC should obtain the following documents: trial protocol(s)/amendment(s), written informed consent form(s) and consent form updates that the investigator proposes for use in the trial, subject recruitment procedures (e.g. advertisements), written information to be provided to subjects, Investigator's Brochure (IB), available safety information, information about payments and compensation available to subjects, the investigator's current curriculum vitae and/or other documentation evidencing qualifications, and any other documents that the IRB/IEC may need to fulfil its responsibilities.

The IRB/IEC should review a proposed clinical trial within a reasonable time and document its views in writing, clearly identifying the trial, the documents reviewed and the dates for the following:

- approval/favourable opinion;

- modifications required prior to its approval/favourable opinion;

- disapproval/negative opinion; and

- termination/suspension of any prior approval/favourable opinion.

3.1.3   The IRB/IEC should consider the qualifications of the investigator for the proposed trial, as documented by a current curriculum vitae and/or by any other relevant documentation the IRB/IEC requests.

3.1.4   The IRB/IEC should conduct continuing reviews of each ongoing trial at intervals appropriate to the degree of risk to human subjects, but at least once per year.

3.1.5   The IRB/IEC may request more information than is outlined in paragraph 4.8.10 be given to subjects when, in the judgement of the IRB/IEC, the additional information would add meaningfully to the protection of the rights, safety and/or well-being of the subjects.

3.1.6   When a non-therapeutic trial is to be carried out with the consent of the subject's legally acceptable representative (see 4.8.12, 4.8.14), the IRB/IEC should determine that the proposed protocol and/or other document(s) adequately addresses relevant ethical concerns and meets applicable regulatory requirements for such trials.

3.1.7   Where the protocol indicates that prior consent of the trial subject or the subject's legally acceptable representative is not possible (see 4.8.15), the IRB/IEC should determine that the proposed protocol and/or other document(s) adequately addresses relevant ethical concerns and meets applicable regulatory requirements for such trials (i.e. in emergency situations).

3.1.8   The IRB/IEC should review both the amount and method of payment to subjects to assure that neither presents problems of coercion or undue influence on the trial subjects. Payments to a subject should be prorated and not wholly contingent on completion of the trial by the subject.

3.1.9   The IRB/IEC should ensure that information regarding payment to subjects, including the methods, amounts, and schedule of payment to trial subjects, is set forth in the written informed consent form and any other written information to be provided to subjects. The way payment will be prorated should be specified.

3.2   Composition, Functions and Operations

3.2.1   The IRB/IEC should consist of a reasonable number of members, who collectively have the qualifications and experience to review and evaluate the science, medical aspects, and ethics of the proposed trial. It is recommended that the IRB/IEC should include:

(a)   At least five members.

(b)   At least one member whose primary area of interest is in a nonscientific area.

(c)   At least one member who is independent of the institution/trial site.

Only those IRB/IEC members who are independent of the investigator and the sponsor of the trial should vote/provide opinion on a trial-related matter.

A list of IRB/IEC members and their qualifications should be maintained.

3.2.2   The IRB/IEC should perform its functions according to written operating procedures, should maintain written records of its activities and minutes of its meetings, and should comply with GCP and with the applicable regulatory requirement(s).

3.2.3   An IRB/IEC should make its decisions at announced meetings at which at least a quorum, as stipulated in its written operating procedures, is present.

(Continued on next page)

Appendix 6. International Conference on Harmonisation Guideline for Good Clinical Practice (Continued)

3.2.4 Only members who participate in the IRB/IEC review and discussion should vote/provide their opinion and/or advise.

3.2.5 The investigator may provide information on any aspect of the trial, but should not participate in the deliberations of the IRB/IEC or in the vote/opinion of the IRB/IEC.

3.2.6 An IRB/IEC may invite nonmembers with expertise in special areas for assistance.

3.3 Procedures

The IRB/IEC should establish, document in writing, and follow its procedures, which should include:

3.3.1 Determining its composition (names and qualifications of the members) and the authority under which it is established.

3.3.2 Scheduling, notifying its members of, and conducting its meetings.

3.3.3 Conducting initial and continuing review of trials.

3.3.4 Determining the frequency of continuing review, as appropriate.

3.3.5 Providing, according to the applicable regulatory requirements, expedited review and approval/favourable opinion of minor change(s) in ongoing trials that have the approval/favourable opinion of the IRB/IEC.

3.3.6 Specifying that no subject should be admitted to a trial before the IRB/IEC issues its written approval/favourable opinion of the trial.

3.3.7 Specifying that no deviations from, or changes of, the protocol should be initiated without prior written IRB/IEC approval/favourable opinion of an appropriate amendment, except when necessary to eliminate immediate hazards to the subjects or when the change(s) involves only logistical or administrative aspects of the trial (e.g., change of monitor(s), telephone number(s)) (see 4.5.2).

3.3.8 Specifying that the investigator should promptly report to the IRB/IEC:

(a) Deviations from, or changes of, the protocol to eliminate immediate hazards to the trial subjects (see 3.3.7, 4.5.2, 4.5.4).

(b) Changes increasing the risk to subjects and/or affecting significantly the conduct of the trial (see 4.10.2).

(c) All adverse drug reactions (ADRs) that are both serious and unexpected.

(d) New information that may affect adversely the safety of the subjects or the conduct of the trial.

3.3.9 Ensuring that the IRB/IEC promptly notify in writing the investigator/institution concerning:

(a) Its trial-related decisions/opinions.

(b) The reasons for its decisions/opinions.

(c) Procedures for appeal of its decisions/opinions.

3.4 Records

The IRB/IEC should retain all relevant records (e.g., written procedures, membership lists, lists of occupations/affiliations of members, submitted documents, minutes of meetings, and correspondence) for a period of at least 3 years after completion of the trial and make them available upon request from the regulatory authority(ies).

The IRB/IEC may be asked by investigators, sponsors or regulatory authorities to provide its written procedures and membership lists.

4. INVESTIGATOR

4.1 Investigator's Qualifications and Agreements

4.1.1 The investigator(s) should be qualified by education, training, and experience to assume responsibility for the proper conduct of the trial, should meet all the qualifications specified by the applicable regulatory requirement(s), and should provide evidence of such qualifications through up-to-date curriculum vitae and/or other relevant documentation requested by the sponsor, the IRB/IEC, and/or the regulatory authority(ies).

4.1.2 The investigator should be thoroughly familiar with the appropriate use of the investigational product(s), as described in the protocol, in the current Investigator's Brochure, in the product information and in other information sources provided by the sponsor.

4.1.3 The investigator should be aware of, and should comply with, GCP and the applicable regulatory requirements.

4.1.4 The investigator/institution should permit monitoring and auditing by the sponsor, and inspection by the appropriate regulatory authority(ies).

4.1.5 The investigator should maintain a list of appropriately qualified persons to whom the investigator has delegated significant trial-related duties.

4.2 Adequate Resources

4.2.1 The investigator should be able to demonstrate (e.g., based on retrospective data) a potential for recruiting the required number of suitable subjects within the agreed recruitment period.

4.2.2 The investigator should have sufficient time to properly conduct and complete the trial within the agreed trial period.

4.2.3 The investigator should have available an adequate number of qualified staff and adequate facilities for the foreseen duration of the trial to conduct the trial properly and safely.

4.2.4 The investigator should ensure that all persons assisting with the trial are adequately informed about the protocol, the investigational product(s), and their trial-related duties and functions.

4.3 Medical Care of Trial Subjects

4.3.1 A qualified physician (or dentist, when appropriate), who is an investigator or a sub-investigator for the trial, should be responsible for all trial-related medical (or dental) decisions.

4.3.2 During and following a subject's participation in a trial, the investigator/institution should ensure that adequate medical care is provided to a subject for any adverse events, including clinically significant laboratory values, related to the trial. The investigator/institution should inform a subject when medical care is needed for intercurrent illness(es) of which the investigator becomes aware.

4.3.3 It is recommended that the investigator inform the subject's primary physician about the subject's participation in the trial if the subject has a primary physician and if the subject agrees to the primary physician being informed.

4.3.4 Although a subject is not obliged to give his/her reason(s) for withdrawing prematurely from a trial, the investigator should make a reasonable effort to ascertain the reason(s), while fully respecting the subject's rights.

4.4 Communication with IRB/IEC

(Continued on next page)

Appendix 6. International Conference on Harmonisation Guideline for Good Clinical Practice *(Continued)*

4.4.1 Before initiating a trial, the investigator/institution should have written and dated approval/favourable opinion from the IRB/IEC for the trial protocol, written informed consent form, consent form updates, subject recruitment procedures (e.g., advertisements), and any other written information to be provided to subjects.

4.4.2 As part of the investigator's/institution's written application to the IRB/IEC, the investigator/institution should provide the IRB/IEC with a current copy of the Investigator's Brochure. If the Investigator's Brochure is updated during the trial, the investigator/institution should supply a copy of the updated Investigator's Brochure to the IRB/IEC.

4.4.3 During the trial the investigator/institution should provide to the IRB/IEC all documents subject to review.

4.5 Compliance with Protocol

4.5.1 The investigator/institution should conduct the trial in compliance with the protocol agreed to by the sponsor and, if required, by the regulatory authority(ies) and which was given approval/favourable opinion by the IRB/IEC. The investigator/institution and the sponsor should sign the protocol, or an alternative contract, to confirm agreement.

4.5.2 The investigator should not implement any deviation from, or changes of the protocol without agreement by the sponsor and prior review and documented approval/favourable opinion from the IRB/IEC of an amendment, except where necessary to eliminate an immediate hazard(s) to trial subjects, or when the change(s) involves only logistical or administrative aspects of the trial (e.g., change in monitor(s), change of telephone number(s)).

4.5.3 The investigator, or person designated by the investigator, should document and explain any deviation from the approved protocol.

4.5.4 The investigator may implement a deviation from, or a change of, the protocol to eliminate an immediate hazard(s) to trial subjects without prior IRB/IEC approval/favourable opinion. As soon as possible, the implemented deviation or change, the reasons for it, and, if appropriate, the proposed protocol amendment(s) should be submitted:

    (a)   to the IRB/IEC for review and approval/favourable opinion,

    (b)   to the sponsor for agreement and, if required,

    (c)   to the regulatory authority(ies).

4.6 Investigational Product(s)

4.6.1 Responsibility for investigational product(s) accountability at the trial site(s) rests with the investigator/institution.

4.6.2 Where allowed/required, the investigator/institution may/should assign some or all of the investigator's/institution's duties for investigational product(s) accountability at the trial site(s) to an appropriate pharmacist or another appropriate individual who is under the supervision of the investigator/institution.

4.6.3 The investigator/institution and/or a pharmacist or other appropriate individual, who is designated by the investigator/institution, should maintain records of the product's delivery to the trial site, the inventory at the site, the use by each subject, and the return to the sponsor or alternative disposition of unused product(s). These records should include dates, quantities, batch/serial numbers, expiration dates (if applicable), and the unique code numbers assigned to the investigational product(s) and trial subjects. Investigators should maintain records that document adequately that the subjects were provided the doses specified by the protocol and reconcile all investigational product(s) received from the sponsor.

4.6.4 The investigational product(s) should be stored as specified by the sponsor (see 5.13.2 and 5.14.3) and in accordance with applicable regulatory requirement(s).

4.6.5 The investigator should ensure that the investigational product(s) are used only in accordance with the approved protocol.

4.6.6 The investigator, or a person designated by the investigator/institution, should explain the correct use of the investigational product(s) to each subject and should check, at intervals appropriate for the trial, that each subject is following the instructions properly.

4.7 Randomization Procedures and Unblinding

The investigator should follow the trial's randomization procedures, if any, and should ensure that the code is broken only in accordance with the protocol. If the trial is blinded, the investigator should promptly document and explain to the sponsor any premature unblinding (e.g., accidental unblinding, unblinding due to a serious adverse event) of the investigational product(s).

4.8 Informed Consent of Trial Subjects

4.8.1 In obtaining and documenting informed consent, the investigator should comply with the applicable regulatory requirement(s), and should adhere to GCP and to the ethical principles that have their origin in the Declaration of Helsinki. Prior to the beginning of the trial, the investigator should have the IRB/IEC's written approval/favourable opinion of the written informed consent form and any other written information to be provided to subjects.

4.8.2 The written informed consent form and any other written information to be provided to subjects should be revised whenever important new information becomes available that may be relevant to the subject's consent. Any revised written informed consent form, and written information should receive the IRB/IEC's approval/favourable opinion in advance of use. The subject or the subject's legally acceptable representative should be informed in a timely manner if new information becomes available that may be relevant to the subject's willingness to continue participation in the trial. The communication of this information should be documented.

4.8.3 Neither the investigator, nor the trial staff, should coerce or unduly influence a subject to participate or to continue to participate in a trial.

4.8.4 None of the oral and written information concerning the trial, including the written informed consent form, should contain any language that causes the subject or the subject's legally acceptable representative to waive or to appear to waive any legal rights, or that releases or appears to release the investigator, the institution, the sponsor, or their agents from liability for negligence.

4.8.5 The investigator, or a person designated by the investigator, should fully inform the subject or, if the subject is unable to provide informed consent, the subject's legally acceptable representative, of all pertinent aspects of the trial including the written information and the approval/favourable opinion by the IRB/IEC.

4.8.6 The language used in the oral and written information about the trial, including the written informed consent form, should be as nontechnical as practical and should be understandable to the subject or the subject's legally acceptable representative and the impartial witness, where applicable.

(Continued on next page)

Appendix 6. International Conference on Harmonisation Guideline for Good Clinical Practice *(Continued)*

4.8.7 Before informed consent may be obtained, the investigator, or a person designated by the investigator, should provide the subject or the subject's legally acceptable representative ample time and opportunity to inquire about details of the trial and to decide whether or not to participate in the trial. All questions about the trial should be answered to the satisfaction of the subject or the subject's legally acceptable representative.

4.8.8 Prior to a subject's participation in the trial, the written informed consent form should be signed and personally dated by the subject or by the subject's legally acceptable representative, and by the person who conducted the informed consent discussion.

4.8.9 If a subject is unable to read or if a legally acceptable representative is unable to read, an impartial witness should be present during the entire informed consent discussion. After the written informed consent form and any other written information to be provided to subjects, is read and explained to the subject or the subject's legally acceptable representative, and after the subject or the subject's legally acceptable representative has orally consented to the subject's participation in the trial and, if capable of doing so, has signed and personally dated the informed consent form, the witness should sign and personally date the consent form. By signing the consent form, the witness attests that the information in the consent form and any other written information was accurately explained to, and apparently understood by, the subject or the subject's legally acceptable representative, and that informed consent was freely given by the subject or the subject's legally acceptable representative.

4.8.10 Both the informed consent discussion and the written informed consent form and any other written information to be provided to subjects should include explanations of the following:

(a) That the trial involves research.

(b) The purpose of the trial.

(c) The trial treatment(s) and the probability for random assignment to each treatment.

(d) The trial procedures to be followed, including all invasive procedures.

(e) The subject's responsibilities.

(f) Those aspects of the trial that are experimental.

(g) The reasonably foreseeable risks or inconveniences to the subject and, when applicable, to an embryo, fetus, or nursing infant.

(h) The reasonably expected benefits. When there is no intended clinical benefit to the subject, the subject should be made aware of this.

(i) The alternative procedure(s) or course(s) of treatment that may be available to the subject, and their important potential benefits and risks.

(j) The compensation and/or treatment available to the subject in the event of trial-related injury.

(k) The anticipated prorated payment, if any, to the subject for participating in the trial.

(l) The anticipated expenses, if any, to the subject for participating in the trial.

(m) That the subject's participation in the trial is voluntary and that the subject may refuse to participate or withdraw from the trial, at any time, without penalty or loss of benefits to which the subject is otherwise entitled.

(n) That the monitor(s), the auditor(s), the IRB/IEC, and the regulatory authority(ies) will be granted direct access to the subject's original medical records for verification of clinical trial procedures and/or data, without violating the confidentiality of the subject, to the extent permitted by the applicable laws and regulations and that, by signing a written informed consent form, the subject or the subject's legally acceptable representative is authorizing such access.

(o) That records identifying the subject will be kept confidential and, to the extent permitted by the applicable laws and/or regulations, will not be made publicly available. If the results of the trial are published, the subject's identity will remain confidential.

(p) That the subject or the subject's legally acceptable representative will be informed in a timely manner if information becomes available that may be relevant to the subject's willingness to continue participation in the trial.

(q) The person(s) to contact for further information regarding the trial and the rights of trial subjects, and whom to contact in the event of trial-related injury.

(r) The foreseeable circumstances and/or reasons under which the subject's participation in the trial may be terminated.

(s) The expected duration of the subject's participation in the trial.

(t) The approximate number of subjects involved in the trial.

4.8.11 Prior to participation in the trial, the subject or the subject's legally acceptable representative should receive a copy of the signed and dated written informed consent form and any other written information provided to the subjects. During a subject's participation in the trial, the subject or the subject's legally acceptable representative should receive a copy of the signed and dated consent form updates and a copy of any amendments to the written information provided to subjects.

4.8.12 When a clinical trial (therapeutic or non-therapeutic) includes subjects who can only be enrolled in the trial with the consent of the subject's legally acceptable representative (e.g., minors, or patients with severe dementia), the subject should be informed about the trial to the extent compatible with the subject's understanding and, if capable, the subject should sign and personally date the written informed consent.

4.8.13 Except as described in 4.8.14, a non-therapeutic trial (i.e., a trial in which there is no anticipated direct clinical benefit to the subject), should be conducted in subjects who personally give consent and who sign and date the written informed consent form.

4.8.14 Non-therapeutic trials may be conducted in subjects with consent of a legally acceptable representative provided the following conditions are fulfilled:

(a) The objectives of the trial cannot be met by means of a trial in subjects who can give informed consent personally.

(b) The foreseeable risks to the subjects are low.

(c) The negative impact on the subject's well-being is minimized and low.

(d) The trial is not prohibited by law.

(e) The approval/favourable opinion of the IRB/IEC is expressly sought on the inclusion of such subjects, and the written approval/favourable opinion covers this aspect.

Such trials, unless an exception is justified, should be conducted in patients having a disease or condition for which the investigational product is intended. Subjects in these trials should be particularly closely monitored and should be withdrawn if they appear to be unduly distressed.

(Continued on next page)

Appendix 6. International Conference on Harmonisation Guideline for Good Clinical Practice *(Continued)*

4.8.15   In emergency situations, when prior consent of the subject is not possible, the consent of the subject's legally acceptable representative, if present, should be requested. When prior consent of the subject is not possible, and the subject's legally acceptable representative is not available, enrollment of the subject should require measures described in the protocol and/or elsewhere, with documented approval/favourable opinion by the IRB/IEC, to protect the rights, safety and well-being of the subject and to ensure compliance with applicable regulatory requirements. The subject or the subject's legally acceptable representative should be informed about the trial as soon as possible and consent to continue and other consent as appropriate (see 4.8.10) should be requested.

4.9   Records and Reports

4.9.1   The investigator should ensure the accuracy, completeness, legibility, and timeliness of the data reported to the sponsor in the CRFs and in all required reports.

4.9.2   Data reported on the CRF, that are derived from source documents, should be consistent with the source documents or the discrepancies should be explained.

4.9.3   Any change or correction to a CRF should be dated, initialed, and explained (if necessary) and should not obscure the original entry (i.e., an audit trail should be maintained); this applies to both written and electronic changes or corrections (see 5.18.4 (n)). Sponsors should provide guidance to investigators and/or the investigators' designated representatives on making such corrections. Sponsors should have written procedures to assure that changes or corrections in CRFs made by sponsor's designated representatives are documented, are necessary, and are endorsed by the investigator. The investigator should retain records of the changes and corrections.

4.9.4   The investigator/institution should maintain the trial documents as specified in Essential Documents for the Conduct of a Clinical Trial (see 8.) and as required by the applicable regulatory requirement(s). The investigator/institution should take measures to prevent accidental or premature destruction of these documents.

4.9.5   Essential documents should be retained until at least 2 years after the last approval of a marketing application in an ICH region and until there are no pending or contemplated marketing applications in an ICH region or at least 2 years have elapsed since the formal discontinuation of clinical development of the investigational product. These documents should be retained for a longer period however if required by the applicable regulatory requirements or by an agreement with the sponsor. It is the responsibility of the sponsor to inform the investigator/institution as to when these documents no longer need to be retained (see 5.5.12).

4.9.6   The financial aspects of the trial should be documented in an agreement between the sponsor and the investigator/institution.

4.9.7   Upon request of the monitor, auditor, IRB/IEC, or regulatory authority, the investigator/institution should make available for direct access all requested trial-related records.

4.10   Progress Reports

4.10.1   The investigator should submit written summaries of the trial status to the IRB/IEC annually, or more frequently, if requested by the IRB/IEC.

4.10.2   The investigator should promptly provide written reports to the sponsor, the IRB/IEC (see 3.3.8) and, where applicable, the institution on any changes significantly affecting the conduct of the trial, and/or increasing the risk to subjects.

4.11   Safety Reporting

4.11.1   All serious adverse events (SAEs) should be reported immediately to the sponsor except for those SAEs that the protocol or other document (e.g., Investigator's Brochure) identifies as not needing immediate reporting. The immediate reports should be followed promptly by detailed, written reports. The immediate and follow-up reports should identify subjects by unique code numbers assigned to the trial subjects rather than by the subjects' names, personal identification numbers, and/or addresses. The investigator should also comply with the applicable regulatory requirement(s) related to the reporting of unexpected serious adverse drug reactions to the regulatory authority(ies) and the IRB/IEC.

4.11.2   Adverse events and/or laboratory abnormalities identified in the protocol as critical to safety evaluations should be reported to the sponsor according to the reporting requirements and within the time periods specified by the sponsor in the protocol.

4.11.3   For reported deaths, the investigator should supply the sponsor and the IRB/IEC with any additional requested information (e.g., autopsy reports and terminal medical reports).

4.12   Premature Termination or Suspension of a Trial

If the trial is prematurely terminated or suspended for any reason, the investigator/institution should promptly inform the trial subjects, should assure appropriate therapy and follow-up for the subjects, and, where required by the applicable regulatory requirement(s), should inform the regulatory authority(ies). In addition:

4.12.1   If the investigator terminates or suspends a trial without prior agreement of the sponsor, the investigator should inform the institution where applicable, and the investigator/institution should promptly inform the sponsor and the IRB/IEC, and should provide the sponsor and the IRB/IEC a detailed written explanation of the termination or suspension.

4.12.2   If the sponsor terminates or suspends a trial (see 5.21), the investigator should promptly inform the institution where applicable and the investigator/institution should promptly inform the IRB/IEC and provide the IRB/IEC a detailed written explanation of the termination or suspension.

4.12.3   If the IRB/IEC terminates or suspends its approval/favourable opinion of a trial (see 3.1.2 and 3.3.9), the investigator should inform the institution where applicable and the investigator/institution should promptly notify the sponsor and provide the sponsor with a detailed written explanation of the termination or suspension.

4.13   Final Report(s) by Investigator

Upon completion of the trial, the investigator, where applicable, should inform the institution; the investigator/institution should provide the IRB/IEC with a summary of the trial's outcome, and the regulatory authority(ies) with any reports required.

5.   SPONSOR

5.1   Quality Assurance and Quality Control

5.1.1   The sponsor is responsible for implementing and maintaining quality assurance and quality control systems with written SOPs to ensure that trials are conducted and data are generated, documented (recorded), and reported in compliance with the protocol, GCP, and the applicable regulatory requirement(s).

(Continued on next page)

Appendix 6. International Conference on Harmonisation Guideline for Good Clinical Practice *(Continued)*

5.1.2	The sponsor is responsible for securing agreement from all involved parties to ensure direct access (see 1.21) to all trial related sites, source data/documents, and reports for the purpose of monitoring and auditing by the sponsor, and inspection by domestic and foreign regulatory authorities.
5.1.3	Quality control should be applied to each stage of data handling to ensure that all data are reliable and have been processed correctly.
5.1.4	Agreements, made by the sponsor with the investigator/institution and any other parties involved with the clinical trial, should be in writing, as part of the protocol or in a separate agreement.
5.2	Contract Research Organization (CRO)
5.2.1	A sponsor may transfer any or all of the sponsor's trial-related duties and functions to a CRO, but the ultimate responsibility for the quality and integrity of the trial data always resides with the sponsor. The CRO should implement quality assurance and quality control.
5.2.2	Any trial-related duty and function that is transferred to and assumed by a CRO should be specified in writing.
5.2.3	Any trial-related duties and functions not specifically transferred to and assumed by a CRO are retained by the sponsor.
5.2.4	All references to a sponsor in this guideline also apply to a CRO to the extent that a CRO has assumed the trial related duties and functions of a sponsor.
5.3	Medical Expertise
	The sponsor should designate appropriately qualified medical personnel who will be readily available to advise on trial related medical questions or problems. If necessary, outside consultant(s) may be appointed for this purpose.
5.4	Trial Design
5.4.1	The sponsor should utilize qualified individuals (e.g. biostatisticians, clinical pharmacologists, and physicians) as appropriate, throughout all stages of the trial process, from designing the protocol and CRFs and planning the analyses to analyzing and preparing interim and final clinical trial reports.
5.4.2	For further guidance: Clinical Trial Protocol and Protocol Amendment(s) (see 6.), the ICH Guideline for Structure and Content of Clinical Study Reports, and other appropriate ICH guidance on trial design, protocol and conduct.
5.5	Trial Management, Data Handling, and Record Keeping
5.5.1	The sponsor should utilize appropriately qualified individuals to supervise the overall conduct of the trial, to handle the data, to verify the data, to conduct the statistical analyses, and to prepare the trial reports.
5.5.2	The sponsor may consider establishing an independent data-monitoring committee (IDMC) to assess the progress of a clinical trial, including the safety data and the critical efficacy endpoints at intervals, and to recommend to the sponsor whether to continue, modify, or stop a trial. The IDMC should have written operating procedures and maintain written records of all its meetings.
5.5.3	When using electronic trial data handling and/or remote electronic trial data systems, the sponsor should:
	(a) Ensure and document that the electronic data processing system(s) conforms to the sponsor's established requirements for completeness, accuracy, reliability, and consistent intended performance (i.e., validation).
	(b) Maintain SOPs for using these systems.
	(c) Ensure that the systems are designed to permit data changes in such a way that the data changes are documented and that there is no deletion of entered data (i.e., maintain an audit trail, data trail, edit trail).
	(d) Maintain a security system that prevents unauthorized access to the data.
	(e) Maintain a list of the individuals who are authorized to make data changes (see 4.1.5 and 4.9.3).
	(f) Maintain adequate backup of the data.
	(g) Safeguard the blinding, if any (e.g. maintain the blinding during data entry and processing).
5.5.4	If data are transformed during processing, it should always be possible to compare the original data and observations with the processed data.
5.5.5	The sponsor should use an unambiguous subject identification code (see 1.58) that allows identification of all the data reported for each subject.
5.5.6	The sponsor, or other owners of the data, should retain all of the sponsor-specific essential documents pertaining to the trial (see 8. Essential Documents for the Conduct of a Clinical Trial).
5.5.7	The sponsor should retain all sponsor-specific essential documents in conformance with the applicable regulatory requirement(s) of the country(ies) where the product is approved, and/or where the sponsor intends to apply for approval(s).
5.5.8	If the sponsor discontinues the clinical development of an investigational product (i.e., for any or all indications, routes of administration, or dosage forms), the sponsor should maintain all sponsor-specific essential documents for at least 2 years after formal discontinuation or in conformance with the applicable regulatory requirement(s).
5.5.9	If the sponsor discontinues the clinical development of an investigational product, the sponsor should notify all the trial investigators/institutions and all the regulatory authorities.
5.5.10	Any transfer of ownership of the data should be reported to the appropriate authority(ies), as required by the applicable regulatory requirement(s).
5.5.11	The sponsor's specific essential documents should be retained until at least 2 years after the last approval of a marketing application in an ICH region and until there are no pending or contemplated marketing applications in an ICH region or at least 2 years have elapsed since the formal discontinuation of clinical development of the investigational product. These documents should be retained for a longer period, however if required by the applicable regulatory requirement(s) or if needed by the sponsor.
5.5.12	The sponsor should inform the investigator(s)/institution(s) in writing of the need for record retention and should notify the investigator(s)/institution(s) in writing when the trial related records are no longer needed.
5.6	Investigator Selection
5.6.1	The sponsor is responsible for selecting the investigator(s)/institution(s). Each investigator should be qualified by training and experience and should have adequate resources (see 4.1, 4.2) to properly conduct the trial for which the investigator is selected. If organization of a coordinating committee and/or selection of coordinating investigator(s) are to be utilized in multicentre trials, their organization and/or selection are the sponsor's responsibility.

(Continued on next page)

Appendix 6. International Conference on Harmonisation Guideline for Good Clinical Practice *(Continued)*

5.6.2   Before entering an agreement with an investigator/institution to conduct a trial, the sponsor should provide the investigator(s)/institution(s) with the protocol and an up-to-date Investigator's Brochure, and should provide sufficient time for the investigator/institution to review the protocol and the information provided.

5.6.3   The sponsor should obtain the investigator's/institution's agreement:

(a)   to conduct the trial in compliance with GCP, with the applicable regulatory requirement(s) (see 4.1.3), and with the protocol agreed to by the sponsor and given approval/favourable opinion by the IRB/IEC (see 4.5.1);

(b)   to comply with procedures for data recording/reporting;

(c)   to permit monitoring, auditing and inspection (see 4.1.4) and

(d)   to retain the trial related essential documents until the sponsor informs the investigator/institution these documents are no longer needed (see 4.9.4 and 5.5.12).

The sponsor and the investigator/institution should sign the protocol, or an alternative document, to confirm this agreement.

5.7   Allocation of Responsibilities

Prior to initiating a trial, the sponsor should define, establish, and allocate all trial-related duties and functions.

5.8   Compensation to Subjects and Investigators

5.8.1   If required by the applicable regulatory requirement(s), the sponsor should provide insurance or should indemnify (legal and financial coverage) the investigator/the institution against claims arising from the trial, except for claims that arise from malpractice and/or negligence.

5.8.2   The sponsor's policies and procedures should address the costs of treatment of trial subjects in the event of trial-related injuries in accordance with the applicable regulatory requirement(s).

5.8.3   When trial subjects receive compensation, the method and manner of compensation should comply with applicable regulatory requirement(s).

5.9   Financing

The financial aspects of the trial should be documented in an agreement between the sponsor and the investigator/institution.

5.10   Notification/Submission to Regulatory Authority(ies)

Before initiating the clinical trial(s), the sponsor (or the sponsor and the investigator, if required by the applicable regulatory requirement(s)) should submit any required application(s) to the appropriate authority(ies) for review, acceptance, and/or permission (as required by the applicable regulatory requirement(s)) to begin the trial(s). Any notification/submission should be dated and contain sufficient information to identify the protocol.

5.11   Confirmation of Review by IRB/IEC

5.11.1   The sponsor should obtain from the investigator/institution:

(a)   The name and address of the investigator's/institution's IRB/IEC.

(b)   A statement obtained from the IRB/IEC that it is organized and operates according to GCP and the applicable laws and regulations.

(c)   Documented IRB/IEC approval/favourable opinion and, if requested by the sponsor, a current copy of protocol, written informed consent form(s) and any other written information to be provided to subjects, subject recruiting procedures, and documents related to payments and compensation available to the subjects, and any other documents that the IRB/IEC may have requested.

5.11.2   If the IRB/IEC conditions its approval/favourable opinion upon change(s) in any aspect of the trial, such as modification(s) of the protocol, written informed consent form and any other written information to be provided to subjects, and/or other procedures, the sponsor should obtain from the investigator/institution a copy of the modification(s) made and the date approval/favourable opinion was given by the IRB/IEC.

5.11.3   The sponsor should obtain from the investigator/institution documentation and dates of any IRB/IEC reapprovals/re-evaluations with favourable opinion, and of any withdrawals or suspensions of approval/favourable opinion.

5.12   Information on Investigational Product(s)

5.12.1   When planning trials, the sponsor should ensure that sufficient safety and efficacy data from nonclinical studies and/or clinical trials are available to support human exposure by the route, at the dosages, for the duration, and in the trial population to be studied.

5.12.2   The sponsor should update the Investigator's Brochure as significant new information becomes available (see 7. Investigator's Brochure).

5.13   Manufacturing, Packaging, Labelling, and Coding Investigational Product(s)

5.13.1   The sponsor should ensure that the investigational product(s) (including active comparator(s) and placebo, if applicable) is characterized as appropriate to the stage of development of the product(s), is manufactured in accordance with any applicable GMP, and is coded and labelled in a manner that protects the blinding, if applicable. In addition, the labelling should comply with applicable regulatory requirement(s).

5.13.2   The sponsor should determine, for the investigational product(s), acceptable storage temperatures, storage conditions (e.g. protection from light), storage times, reconstitution fluids and procedures, and devices for product infusion, if any. The sponsor should inform all involved parties (e.g. monitors, investigators, pharmacists, storage managers) of these determinations.

5.13.3   The investigational product(s) should be packaged to prevent contamination and unacceptable deterioration during transport and storage.

5.13.4   In blinded trials, the coding system for the investigational product(s) should include a mechanism that permits rapid identification of the product(s) in case of a medical emergency, but does not permit undetectable breaks of the blinding.

5.13.5   If significant formulation changes are made in the investigational or comparator product(s) during the course of clinical development, the results of any additional studies of the formulated product(s) (e.g., stability, dissolution rate, bioavailability) needed to assess whether these changes would significantly alter the pharmacokinetic profile of the product should be available prior to the use of the new formulation in clinical trials.

5.14   Supplying and Handling Investigational Product(s)

5.14.1   The sponsor is responsible for supplying the investigator(s)/institution(s) with the investigational product(s).

(Continued on next page)

Appendix 6. International Conference on Harmonisation Guideline for Good Clinical Practice *(Continued)*

5.14.2   The sponsor should not supply an investigator/institution with the investigational product(s) until the sponsor obtains all required documentation (e.g., approval/favourable opinion from IRB/IEC and regulatory authority(ies)).

5.14.3   The sponsor should ensure that written procedures include instructions that the investigator/institution should follow for the handling and storage of investigational product(s) for the trial and documentation thereof. The procedures should address adequate and safe receipt, handling, storage, dispensing, retrieval of unused product from subjects, and return of unused investigational product(s) to the sponsor (or alternative disposition if authorized by the sponsor and in compliance with the applicable regulatory requirement(s)).

5.14.4   The sponsor should:
   (a)   Ensure timely delivery of investigational product(s) to the investigator(s).
   (b)   Maintain records that document shipment, receipt, disposition, return, and destruction of the investigational product(s) (see 8. Essential Documents for the Conduct of a Clinical Trial).
   (c)   Maintain a system for retrieving investigational products and documenting this retrieval (e.g., for deficient product recall, reclaim after trial completion, expired product reclaim).
   (d)   Maintain a system for the disposition of unused investigational product(s) and for the documentation of this disposition.

5.14.5   The sponsor should:
   (a)   Take steps to ensure that the investigational product(s) are stable over the period of use.
   (b)   Maintain sufficient quantities of the investigational product(s) used in the trials to reconfirm specifications, should this become necessary, and maintain records of batch sample analyses and characteristics. To the extent stability permits, samples should be retained either until the analyses of the trial data are complete or as required by the applicable regulatory requirement(s), whichever represents the longer retention period.

5.15   Record Access

5.15.1   The sponsor should ensure that it is specified in the protocol or other written agreement that the investigator(s)/institution(s) provide direct access to source data/documents for trial-related monitoring, audits, IRB/IEC review, and regulatory inspection.

5.15.2   The sponsor should verify that each subject has consented, in writing, to direct access to his/her original medical records for trial-related monitoring, audit, IRB/IEC review, and regulatory inspection.

5.16   Safety Information

5.16.1   The sponsor is responsible for the ongoing safety evaluation of the investigational product(s).

5.16.2   The sponsor should promptly notify all concerned investigator(s)/institution(s) and the regulatory authority(ies) of findings that could affect adversely the safety of subjects, impact the conduct of the trial, or alter the IRB/IEC's approval/favourable opinion to continue the trial.

5.17   Adverse Drug Reaction Reporting

5.17.1   The sponsor should expedite the reporting to all concerned investigator(s)/institutions(s), to the IRB(s)/IEC(s), where required, and to the regulatory authority(ies) of all adverse drug reactions (ADRs) that are both serious and unexpected.

5.17.2   Such expedited reports should comply with the applicable regulatory requirement(s) and with the ICH Guideline for Clinical Safety Data Management: Definitions and Standards for Expedited Reporting.

5.17.3   The sponsor should submit to the regulatory authority(ies) all safety updates and periodic reports, as required by applicable regulatory requirement(s).

5.18   Monitoring

5.18.1   Purpose
   The purposes of trial monitoring are to verify that:
   (a)   The rights and well-being of human subjects are protected.
   (b)   The reported trial data are accurate, complete, and verifiable from source documents.
   (c)   The conduct of the trial is in compliance with the currently approved protocol/amendment(s), with GCP, and with the applicable regulatory requirement(s).

5.18.2   Selection and Qualifications of Monitors
   (a)   Monitors should be appointed by the sponsor.
   (b)   Monitors should be appropriately trained, and should have the scientific and/or clinical knowledge needed to monitor the trial adequately. A monitor's qualifications should be documented.
   (c)   Monitors should be thoroughly familiar with the investigational product(s), the protocol, written informed consent form and any other written information to be provided to subjects, the sponsor's SOPs, GCP, and the applicable regulatory requirement(s).

5.18.3   Extent and Nature of Monitoring
   The sponsor should ensure that the trials are adequately monitored. The sponsor should determine the appropriate extent and nature of monitoring. The determination of the extent and nature of monitoring should be based on considerations such as the objective, purpose, design, complexity, blinding, size, and endpoints of the trial. In general there is a need for on-site monitoring, before, during, and after the trial; however in exceptional circumstances the sponsor may determine that central monitoring in conjunction with procedures such as investigators' training and meetings, and extensive written guidance can assure appropriate conduct of the trial in accordance with GCP. Statistically controlled sampling may be an acceptable method for selecting the data to be verified.

5.18.4   Monitor's Responsibilities
   The monitor(s) in accordance with the sponsor's requirements should ensure that the trial is conducted and documented properly by carrying out the following activities when relevant and necessary to the trial and the trial site:
   (a)   Acting as the main line of communication between the sponsor and the investigator.
   (b)   Verifying that the investigator has adequate qualifications and resources (see 4.1, 4.2, 5.6) and remain adequate throughout the trial period, that facilities, including laboratories, equipment, and staff, are adequate to safely and properly conduct the trial and remain adequate throughout the trial period.
   (c)   Verifying, for the investigational product(s):
     (i)   That storage times and conditions are acceptable, and that supplies are sufficient throughout the trial.

(Continued on next page)

Appendix 6. International Conference on Harmonisation Guideline for Good Clinical Practice *(Continued)*

    (ii)   That the investigational product(s) are supplied only to subjects who are eligible to receive it and at the protocol specified dose(s).

    (iii) That subjects are provided with necessary instruction on properly using, handling, storing, and returning the investigational product(s).

    (iv) That the receipt, use, and return of the investigational product(s) at the trial sites are controlled and documented adequately.

    (v)   That the disposition of unused investigational product(s) at the trial sites complies with applicable regulatory requirement(s) and is in accordance with the sponsor.

(d)   Verifying that the investigator follows the approved protocol and all approved amendment(s), if any.

(e)   Verifying that written informed consent was obtained before each subject's participation in the trial.

(f)   Ensuring that the investigator receives the current Investigator's Brochure, all documents, and all trial supplies needed to conduct the trial properly and to comply with the applicable regulatory requirement(s).

(g)   Ensuring that the investigator and the investigator's trial staff are adequately informed about the trial.

(h)   Verifying that the investigator and the investigator's trial staff are performing the specified trial functions, in accordance with the protocol and any other written agreement between the sponsor and the investigator/institution, and have not delegated these functions to unauthorized individuals.

(i)   Verifying that the investigator is enroling only eligible subjects.

(j)   Reporting the subject recruitment rate.

(k)   Verifying that source documents and other trial records are accurate, complete, kept up-to-date and maintained.

(l)   Verifying that the investigator provides all the required reports, notifications, applications, and submissions, and that these documents are accurate, complete, timely, legible, dated, and identify the trial.

(m) Checking the accuracy and completeness of the CRF entries, source documents and other trial-related records against each other. The monitor specifically should verify that:

    (i)   The data required by the protocol are reported accurately on the CRFs and are consistent with the source documents.

    (ii)   Any dose and/or therapy modifications are well documented for each of the trial subjects.

    (iii) Adverse events, concomitant medications and intercurrent illnesses are reported in accordance with the protocol on the CRFs.

    (iv) Visits that the subjects fail to make, tests that are not conducted, and examinations that are not performed are clearly reported as such on the CRFs.

    (v)   All withdrawals and dropouts of enrolled subjects from the trial are reported and explained on the CRFs.

(n)   Informing the investigator of any CRF entry error, omission, or illegibility. The monitor should ensure that appropriate corrections, additions, or deletions are made, dated, explained (if necessary), and initialled by the investigator or by a member of the investigator's trial staff who is authorized to initial CRF changes for the investigator. This authorization should be documented.

(o)   Determining whether all adverse events (AEs) are appropriately reported within the time periods required by GCP, the protocol, the IRB/IEC, the sponsor, and the applicable regulatory requirement(s).

(p)   Determining whether the investigator is maintaining the essential documents (see 8. Essential Documents for the Conduct of a Clinical Trial).

(q)   Communicating deviations from the protocol, SOPs, GCP, and the applicable regulatory requirements to the investigator and taking appropriate action designed to prevent recurrence of the detected deviations.

5.18.5   Monitoring Procedures

The monitor(s) should follow the sponsor's established written SOPs as well as those procedures that are specified by the sponsor for monitoring a specific trial.

5.18.6   Monitoring Report

(a)   The monitor should submit a written report to the sponsor after each trial-site visit or trial-related communication.

(b)   Reports should include the date, site, name of the monitor, and name of the investigator or other individual(s) contacted.

(c)   Reports should include a summary of what the monitor reviewed and the monitor's statements concerning the significant findings/facts, deviations and deficiencies, conclusions, actions taken or to be taken and/or actions recommended to secure compliance.

(d)   The review and follow-up of the monitoring report with the sponsor should be documented by the sponsor's designated representative.

5.19   Audit

If or when sponsors perform audits, as part of implementing quality assurance, they should consider:

5.19.1   Purpose

The purpose of a sponsor's audit, which is independent of and separate from routine monitoring or quality control functions, should be to evaluate trial conduct and compliance with the protocol, SOPs, GCP, and the applicable regulatory requirements.

5.19.2   Selection and Qualification of Auditors

(a)   The sponsor should appoint individuals, who are independent of the clinical trials/systems, to conduct audits.

(b)   The sponsor should ensure that the auditors are qualified by training and experience to conduct audits properly. An auditor's qualifications should be documented.

5.19.3   Auditing Procedures

(a)   The sponsor should ensure that the auditing of clinical trials/systems is conducted in accordance with the sponsor's written procedures on what to audit, how to audit, the frequency of audits, and the form and content of audit reports.

(b)   The sponsor's audit plan and procedures for a trial audit should be guided by the importance of the trial to submissions to regulatory authorities, the number of subjects in the trial, the type and complexity of the trial, the level of risks to the trial subjects, and any identified problem(s).

(c)   The observations and findings of the auditor(s) should be documented.

(Continued on next page)

Appendix 6. International Conference on Harmonisation Guideline for Good Clinical Practice *(Continued)*

    (d)   To preserve the independence and value of the audit function, the regulatory authority(ies) should not routinely request the audit reports. Regulatory authority(ies) may seek access to an audit report on a case by case basis when evidence of serious GCP non-compliance exists, or in the course of legal proceedings.

    (e)   When required by applicable law or regulation, the sponsor should provide an audit certificate.

5.20   Noncompliance

5.20.1   Noncompliance with the protocol, SOPs, GCP, and/or applicable regulatory requirement(s) by an investigator/institution, or by member(s) of the sponsor's staff should lead to prompt action by the sponsor to secure compliance.

5.20.2   If the monitoring and/or auditing identifies serious and/or persistent noncompliance on the part of an investigator/institution, the sponsor should terminate the investigator's/institution's participation in the trial. When an investigator's/institution's participation is terminated because of noncompliance, the sponsor should notify promptly the regulatory authority(ies).

5.21   Premature Termination or Suspension of a Trial

    If a trial is prematurely terminated or suspended, the sponsor should promptly inform the investigators/institutions, and the regulatory authority(ies) of the termination or suspension and the reason(s) for the termination or suspension. The IRB/IEC should also be informed promptly and provided the reason(s) for the termination or suspension by the sponsor or by the investigator/institution, as specified by the applicable regulatory requirement(s).

5.22   Clinical Trial/Study Reports

    Whether the trial is completed or prematurely terminated, the sponsor should ensure that the clinical trial reports are prepared and provided to the regulatory agency(ies) as required by the applicable regulatory requirement(s). The sponsor should also ensure that the clinical trial reports in marketing applications meet the standards of the ICH Guideline for Structure and Content of Clinical Study Reports. (NOTE: The ICH Guideline for Structure and Content of Clinical Study Reports specifies that abbreviated study reports may be acceptable in certain cases.)

5.23   Multicentre Trials

    For multicentre trials, the sponsor should ensure that:

5.23.1   All investigators conduct the trial in strict compliance with the protocol agreed to by the sponsor and, if required, by the regulatory authority(ies), and given approval/favourable opinion by the IRB/IEC.

5.23.2   The CRFs are designed to capture the required data at all multicentre trial sites. For those investigators who are collecting additional data, supplemental CRFs should also be provided that are designed to capture the additional data.

5.23.3   The responsibilities of coordinating investigator(s) and the other participating investigators are documented prior to the start of the trial.

5.23.4   All investigators are given instructions on following the protocol, on complying with a uniform set of standards for the assessment of clinical and laboratory findings, and on completing the CRFs.

5.23.5   Communication between investigators is facilitated.

6.   CLINICAL TRIAL PROTOCOL AND PROTOCOL AMENDMENT(S)

    The contents of a trial protocol should generally include the following topics. However, site specific information may be provided on separate protocol page(s), or addressed in a separate agreement, and some of the information listed below may be contained in other protocol referenced documents, such as an Investigator's Brochure.

6.1   General Information

6.1.1   Protocol title, protocol identifying number, and date. Any amendment(s) should also bear the amendment number(s) and date(s).

6.1.2   Name and address of the sponsor and monitor (if other than the sponsor).

6.1.3   Name and title of the person(s) authorized to sign the protocol and the protocol amendment(s) for the sponsor.

6.1.4   Name, title, address, and telephone number(s) of the sponsor's medical expert (or dentist when appropriate) for the trial.

6.1.5   Name and title of the investigator(s) who is (are) responsible for conducting the trial, and the address and telephone number(s) of the trial site(s).

6.1.6   Name, title, address, and telephone number(s) of the qualified physician (or dentist, if applicable), who is responsible for all trial-site related medical (or dental) decisions (if other than investigator).

6.1.7   Name(s) and address(es) of the clinical laboratory(ies) and other medical and/or technical department(s) and/or institutions involved in the trial.

6.2   Background Information

6.2.1   Name and description of the investigational product(s).

6.2.2   A summary of findings from nonclinical studies that potentially have clinical significance and from clinical trials that are relevant to the trial.

6.2.3   Summary of the known and potential risks and benefits, if any, to human subjects.

6.2.4   Description of and justification for the route of administration, dosage, dosage regimen, and treatment period(s).

6.2.5   A statement that the trial will be conducted in compliance with the protocol, GCP and the applicable regulatory requirement(s).

6.2.6   Description of the population to be studied.

6.2.7   References to literature and data that are relevant to the trial, and that provide background for the trial.

6.3   Trial Objectives and Purpose

    A detailed description of the objectives and the purpose of the trial.

6.4   Trial Design

    The scientific integrity of the trial and the credibility of the data from the trial depend substantially on the trial design. A description of the trial design, should include:

6.4.1   A specific statement of the primary endpoints and the secondary endpoints, if any, to be measured during the trial.

6.4.2   A description of the type/design of trial to be conducted (e.g. double-blind, placebo-controlled, parallel design) and a schematic diagram of trial design, procedures and stages.

(Continued on next page)

Appendix 6. International Conference on Harmonisation Guideline for Good Clinical Practice *(Continued)*

6.4.3   A description of the measures taken to minimize/avoid bias, including:
 (a)   Randomization.
 (b)   Blinding.

6.4.4   A description of the trial treatment(s) and the dosage and dosage regimen of the investigational product(s). Also include a description of the dosage form, packaging, and labelling of the investigational product(s).

6.4.5   The expected duration of subject participation, and a description of the sequence and duration of all trial periods, including follow-up, if any.

6.4.6   A description of the "stopping rules" or "discontinuation criteria" for individual subjects, parts of trial and entire trial.

6.4.7   Accountability procedures for the investigational product(s), including the placebo(s) and comparator(s), if any.

6.4.8   Maintenance of trial treatment randomization codes and procedures for breaking codes.

6.4.9   The identification of any data to be recorded directly on the CRFs (i.e., no prior written or electronic record of data), and to be considered to be source data.

6.5   Selection and Withdrawal of Subjects

6.5.1   Subject inclusion criteria.

6.5.2   Subject exclusion criteria.

6.5.3   Subject withdrawal criteria (i.e., terminating investigational product treatment/trial treatment) and procedures specifying:
 (a)   When and how to withdraw subjects from the trial/investigational product treatment.
 (b)   The type and timing of the data to be collected for withdrawn subjects.
 (c)   Whether and how subjects are to be replaced.
 (d)   The follow-up for subjects withdrawn from investigational product treatment/trial treatment.

6.6   Treatment of Subjects

6.6.1   The treatment(s) to be administered, including the name(s) of all the product(s), the dose(s), the dosing schedule(s), the route/mode(s) of administration, and the treatment period(s), including the follow-up period(s) for subjects for each investigational product treatment/trial treatment group/arm of the trial.

6.6.2   Medication(s)/treatment(s) permitted (including rescue medication) and not permitted before and/or during the trial.

6.6.3   Procedures for monitoring subject compliance.

6.7   Assessment of Efficacy

6.7.1   Specification of the efficacy parameters.

6.7.2   Methods and timing for assessing, recording, and analysing of efficacy parameters.

6.8   Assessment of Safety

6.8.1   Specification of safety parameters.

6.8.2   The methods and timing for assessing, recording, and analysing safety parameters.

6.8.3   Procedures for eliciting reports of and for recording and reporting adverse event and intercurrent illnesses.

6.8.4   The type and duration of the follow-up of subjects after adverse events.

6.9   Statistics

6.9.1   A description of the statistical methods to be employed, including timing of any planned interim analysis(ses).

6.9.2   The number of subjects planned to be enrolled. In multicentre trials, the numbers of enrolled subjects projected for each trial site should be specified. Reason for choice of sample size, including reflections on (or calculations of) the power of the trial and clinical justification.

6.9.3   The level of significance to be used.

6.9.4   Criteria for the termination of the trial.

6.9.5   Procedure for accounting for missing, unused, and spurious data.

6.9.6   Procedures for reporting any deviation(s) from the original statistical plan (any deviation(s) from the original statistical plan should be described and justified in protocol and/or in the final report, as appropriate).

6.9.7   The selection of subjects to be included in the analyses (e.g., all randomized subjects, all dosed subjects, all eligible subjects, evaluable subjects).

6.10   Direct Access to Source Data/Documents
The sponsor should ensure that it is specified in the protocol or other written agreement that the investigator(s)/institution(s) will permit trial-related monitoring, audits, IRB/IEC review, and regulatory inspection(s), providing direct access to source data/documents.

6.11   Quality Control and Quality Assurance

6.12   Ethics
Description of ethical considerations relating to the trial.

6.13   Data Handling and Record Keeping

6.14   Financing and Insurance
Financing and insurance if not addressed in a separate agreement.

6.15   Publication Policy
Publication policy, if not addressed in a separate agreement.

6.16   Supplements
(NOTE: Since the protocol and the clinical trial/study report are closely related, further relevant information can be found in the ICH Guideline for Structure and Content of Clinical Study Reports.)

(Continued on next page)

Appendix 6. International Conference on Harmonisation Guideline for Good Clinical Practice *(Continued)*

7.   INVESTIGATOR'S BROCHURE

7.1   Introduction

The Investigator's Brochure (IB) is a compilation of the clinical and nonclinical data on the investigational product(s) that are relevant to the study of the product(s) in human subjects. Its purpose is to provide the investigators and others involved in the trial with the information to facilitate their understanding of the rationale for, and their compliance with, many key features of the protocol, such as the dose, dose frequency/interval, methods of administration: and safety monitoring procedures. The IB also provides insight to support the clinical management of the study subjects during the course of the clinical trial. The information should be presented in a concise, simple, objective, balanced, and non-promotional form that enables a clinician, or potential investigator, to understand it and make his/her own unbiased risk-benefit assessment of the appropriateness of the proposed trial. For this reason, a medically qualified person should generally participate in the editing of an IB, but the contents of the IB should be approved by the disciplines that generated the described data.

This guideline delineates the minimum information that should be included in an IB and provides suggestions for its layout. It is expected that the type and extent of information available will vary with the stage of development of the investigational product. If the investigational product is marketed and its pharmacology is widely understood by medical practitioners, an extensive IB may not be necessary. Where permitted by regulatory authorities, a basic product information brochure, package leaflet, or labelling may be an appropriate alternative, provided that it includes current, comprehensive, and detailed information on all aspects of the investigational product that might be of importance to the investigator. If a marketed product is being studied for a new use (i.e., a new indication), an IB specific to that new use should be prepared. The IB should be reviewed at least annually and revised as necessary in compliance with a sponsor's written procedures. More frequent revision may be appropriate depending on the stage of development and the generation of relevant new information. However, in accordance with Good Clinical Practice, relevant new information may be so important that it should be communicated to the investigators, and possibly to the Institutional Review Boards (IRBs)/Independent Ethics Committees (IECs) and/or regulatory authorities before it is included in a revised IB.

Generally, the sponsor is responsible for ensuring that an up-to-date IB is made available to the investigator(s) and the investigators are responsible for providing the up-to-date IB to the responsible IRBs/IECs. In the case of an investigator sponsored trial, the sponsor-investigator should determine whether a brochure is available from the commercial manufacturer. If the investigational product is provided by the sponsor-investigator, then he or she should provide the necessary information to the trial personnel. In cases where preparation of a formal IB is impractical, the sponsor-investigator should provide, as a substitute, an expanded background information section in the trial protocol that contains the minimum current information described in this guideline.

7.2   General Considerations

The IB should include:

7.2.1   Title Page

This should provide the sponsor's name, the identity of each investigational product (i.e., research number, chemical or approved generic name, and trade name(s) where legally permissible and desired by the sponsor), and the release date. It is also suggested that an edition number, and a reference to the number and date of the edition it supersedes, be provided. An example is given in Appendix 1.

7.2.2   Confidentiality Statement

The sponsor may wish to include a statement instructing the investigator/recipients to treat the IB as a confidential document for the sole information and use of the investigator's team and the IRB/IEC.

7.3   Contents of the Investigator's Brochure

The IB should contain the following sections, each with literature references where appropriate:

7.3.1   Table of Contents

An example of the Table of Contents is given in Appendix 2

7.3.2   Summary

A brief summary (preferably not exceeding two pages) should be given, highlighting the significant physical, chemical, pharmaceutical, pharmacological, toxicological, pharmacokinetic, metabolic, and clinical information available that is relevant to the stage of clinical development of the investigational product.

7.3.3   Introduction

A brief introductory statement should be provided that contains the chemical name (and generic and trade name(s) when approved) of the investigational product(s), all active ingredients, the investigational product (s) pharmacological class and its expected position within this class (e.g., advantages), the rationale for performing research with the investigational product(s), and the anticipated prophylactic, therapeutic, or diagnostic indication(s). Finally, the introductory statement should provide the general approach to be followed in evaluating the investigational product.

7.3.4   Physical, Chemical, and Pharmaceutical Properties and Formulation

A description should be provided of the investigational product substance(s) (including the chemical and/or structural formula(e)), and a brief summary should be given of the relevant physical, chemical, and pharmaceutical properties.

To permit appropriate safety measures to be taken in the course of the trial, a description of the formulation(s) to be used, including excipients, should be provided and justified if clinically relevant. Instructions for the storage and handling of the dosage form(s) should also be given.

Any structural similarities to other known compounds should be mentioned.

7.3.5   Nonclinical Studies

Introduction:

The results of all relevant nonclinical pharmacology, toxicology, pharmacokinetic, and investigational product metabolism studies should be provided in summary form. This summary should address the methodology used, the results, and a discussion of the relevance of the findings to the investigated therapeutic and the possible unfavourable and unintended effects in humans.

(Continued on next page)

Appendix 6. International Conference on Harmonisation Guideline for Good Clinical Practice *(Continued)*

The information provided may include the following, as appropriate, if known/available:

- Species tested
- Number and sex of animals in each group
- Unit dose (e.g., milligram/kilogram (mg/kg))
- Dose interval
- Route of administration
- Duration of dosing
- Information on systemic distribution
- Duration of post-exposure follow-up
- Results, including the following aspects:
  - Nature and frequency of pharmacological or toxic effects
  - Severity or intensity of pharmacological or toxic effects
  - Time to onset of effects
  - Reversibility of effects
  - Duration of effects
  - Dose response

Tabular format/listings should be used whenever possible to enhance the clarity of the presentation.

The following sections should discuss the most important findings from the studies, including the dose response of observed effects, the relevance to humans, and any aspects to be studied in humans. If applicable, the effective and nontoxic dose findings in the same animal species should be compared (i.e., the therapeutic index should be discussed). The relevance of this information to the proposed human dosing should be addressed. Whenever possible, comparisons should be made in terms of blood/tissue levels rather than on a mg/kg basis.

(a) Nonclinical Pharmacology

A summary of the pharmacological aspects of the investigational product and, where appropriate, its significant metabolites studied in animals, should be included. Such a summary should incorporate studies that assess potential therapeutic activity (e.g. efficacy models, receptor binding, and specificity) as well as those that assess safety (e.g., special studies to assess pharmacological actions other than the intended therapeutic effect(s)).

(b) Pharmacokinetics and Product Metabolism in Animals

A summary of the pharmacokinetics and biological transformation and disposition of the investigational product in all species studied should be given. The discussion of the findings should address the absorption and the local and systemic bioavailability of the investigational product and its metabolites, and their relationship to the pharmacological and toxicological findings in animal species.

(c) Toxicology

A summary of the toxicological effects found in relevant studies conducted in different animal species should be described under the following headings where appropriate:

- Single dose
- Repeated dose
- Carcinogenicity
- Special studies (e.g., irritancy and sensitisation)
- Reproductive toxicity
- Genotoxicity (mutagenicity)

7.3.6 Effects in Humans

Introduction:

A thorough discussion of the known effects of the investigational product(s) in humans should be provided, including information on pharmacokinetics, metabolism, pharmacodynamics, dose response, safety, efficacy, and other pharmacological activities. Where possible, a summary of each completed clinical trial should be provided. Information should also be provided regarding results of any use of the investigational product(s) other than from in clinical trials, such as from experience during marketing.

(a) Pharmacokinetics and Product Metabolism in Humans

- A summary of information on the pharmacokinetics of the investigational product(s) should be presented, including the following, if available:
- Pharmacokinetics (including metabolism, as appropriate, and absorption, plasma protein binding, distribution, and elimination).
- Bioavailability of the investigational product (absolute, where possible, and/or relative) using a reference dosage form.
- Population subgroups (e.g., gender, age, and impaired organ function).
- Interactions (e.g., product-product interactions and effects of food).
- Other pharmacokinetic data (e.g., results of population studies performed within clinical trial(s).

(b) Safety and Efficacy

A summary of information should be provided about the investigational product's/products' (including metabolites, where appropriate) safety, pharmacodynamics, efficacy, and dose response that were obtained from preceding trials in humans (healthy volunteers and/or patients). The implications of this information should be discussed. In cases where a number of clinical trials have been completed, the use of summaries of safety and efficacy across multiple trials by indications in subgroups may provide a clear presentation of the data. Tabular summaries of adverse drug reactions for all the clinical trials (including those for all the studied indications) would be useful. Important differences in adverse drug reaction patterns/incidences across indications or subgroups should be discussed.

The IB should provide a description of the possible risks and adverse drug reactions to be anticipated on the basis of prior experiences with the product under investigation and with related products. A description should also be provided of the precautions or special monitoring to be done as part of the investigational use of the product(s).

(Continued on next page)

Appendix 6. International Conference on Harmonisation Guideline for Good Clinical Practice *(Continued)*

(c) Marketing Experience

The IB should identify countries where the investigational product has been marketed or approved. Any significant information arising from the marketed use should be summarised (e.g., formulations, dosages, routes of administration, and adverse product reactions). The IB should also identify all the countries where the investigational product did not receive approval/registration for marketing or was withdrawn from marketing/registration.

7.3.7 Summary of Data and Guidance for the Investigator

This section should provide an overall discussion of the nonclinical and clinical data, and should summarise the information from various sources on different aspects of the investigational product(s), wherever possible. In this way, the investigator can be provided with the most informative interpretation of the available data and with an assessment of the implications of the information for future clinical trials.

Where appropriate, the published reports on related products should be discussed. This could help the investigator to anticipate adverse drug reactions or other problems in clinical trials.

The overall aim of this section is to provide the investigator with a clear understanding of the possible risks and adverse reactions, and of the specific tests, observations, and precautions that may be needed for a clinical trial. This understanding should be based on the available physical, chemical, pharmaceutical, pharmacological, toxicological, and clinical information on the investigational product(s). Guidance should also be provided to the clinical investigator on the recognition and treatment of possible overdose and adverse drug reactions that is based on previous human experience and on the pharmacology of the investigational product.

7.4 Appendix 1:

TITLE PAGE *(Example)*

SPONSOR'S NAME

Product:
Research Number:
Name(s): Chemical, Generic (if approved)
Trade Name(s) (if legally permissible and desired by the sponsor)

INVESTIGATOR'S BROCHURE

Edition Number:
Release Date:

Replaces Previous Edition Number:
Date:

7.5 Appendix 2:

TABLE OF CONTENTS OF INVESTIGATOR'S BROCHURE *(Example)*

-       Confidentiality Statement (optional)
-       Signature Page (optional)
1   Table of Contents
2   Summary
3   Introduction
4   Physical, Chemical, and Pharmaceutical Properties and Formulation
5   Nonclinical Studies
5.1   Nonclinical Pharmacology
5.2   Pharmacokinetics and Product Metabolism in Animals
5.3   Toxicology
6   Effects in Humans
6.1   Pharmacokinetics and Product Metabolism in Humans
6.2   Safety and Efficacy
6.3   Marketing Experience
7   Summary of Data and Guidance for the Investigator

NB: References on
1.   Publications
2.   Reports
These references should be found at the end of each chapter
Appendices (if any)

(Continued on next page)

Appendix 6. International Conference on Harmonisation Guideline for Good Clinical Practice *(Continued)*

8.   ESSENTIAL DOCUMENTS FOR THE CONDUCT OF A CLINICAL TRIAL

8.1   Introduction

Essential Documents are those documents which individually and collectively permit evaluation of the conduct of a trial and the quality of the data produced. These documents serve to demonstrate the compliance of the investigator, sponsor and monitor with the standards of Good Clinical Practice and with all applicable regulatory requirements.

Essential Documents also serve a number of other important purposes. Filing essential documents at the investigator/institution and sponsor sites in a timely manner can greatly assist in the successful management of a trial by the investigator, sponsor and monitor. These documents are also the ones which are usually audited by the sponsor's independent audit function and inspected by the regulatory authority(ies) as part of the process to confirm the validity of the trial conduct and the integrity of data collected.

The minimum list of essential documents which has been developed follows. The various documents are grouped in three sections according to the stage of the trial during which they will normally be generated: 1) before the clinical phase of the trial commences, 2) during the clinical conduct of the trial, and 3) after completion or termination of the trial. A description is given of the purpose of each document, and whether it should be filed in either the investigator/institution or sponsor files, or both. It is acceptable to combine some of the documents, provided the individual elements are readily identifiable.

Trial master files should be established at the beginning of the trial, both at the investigator/institution's site and at the sponsor's office. A final close-out of a trial can only be done when the monitor has reviewed both investigator/institution and sponsor files and confirmed that all necessary documents are in the appropriate files.

Any or all of the documents addressed in this guideline may be subject to, and should be available for, audit by the sponsor's auditor and inspection by the regulatory authority(ies).

8.2   Before the Clinical Phase of the Trial Commences
During this planning stage the following documents should be generated and should be on file before the trial formally starts

| | | Located in Files of | |
| | | Investigator/ | |
Title of Document	Purpose	Institution	Sponsor
8.2.1 Investigator's Brochure	To document that relevant and current scientific information about the investigational product has been provided to the investigator	X	X
8.2.2 Signed Protocol and Amendments, if any, and sample Case Report Form (CRF)	To document investigator and sponsor agreement to the protocol/amendment(s) and CRF	X	X
8.2.3 Information Given to Trial Subject		X	X
• Informed Consent Form (including all applicable translations)	To document the informed consent		
• Any other written information	To document that subjects will be given appropriate written information (content and wording) to support their ability to give fully informed consent	X	X
• Advertisement for Subject Recruitment (if used)	To document that recruitment measures are appropriate and not coercive	X	
8.2.4 Financial Aspects of the Trial	To document the financial agreement between the investigator/institution and the sponsor for the trial	X	X
8.2.5 Insurance Statement (where required)	To document that compensation to subject(s) for trial-related injury will be available	X	X
8.2.6 Signed Agreement Between Involved Parties, e.g.:	To document agreements		
• Investigator/Institution and Sponsor Investigator/Institution and CRO		X X	X X (where required)
• Sponsor and CRO			X
• Investigator/Institution and Authority(ies) (where required)		X	X

(Continued on next page)

Appendix 6. International Conference on Harmonisation Guideline for Good Clinical Practice *(Continued)*

	Title of Document	Purpose	Located in Files of Investigator/ Institution	Sponsor
8.2.7	Dated, Documented Approval/Favourable Opinion of Institutional Review Board (IRB)/Independent Ethics Committee (IEC) of The Following: • Protocol and any Amendments • CRF (if applicable) • Informed Consent Form(s) • Any Other Written Information to be Provided to the Subject(s) • Advertisement for Subject Recruitment (if used) • Subject Compensation (if any) • Any Other Documents Given Approval/ Favourable Opinion	To document that the trial has been subject to IRB/IEC review and given approval/favourable opinion. To identify the version number and date of the document(s)	X	X
8.2.8	Institutional Review Board/Independent Ethics Committee Composition	To document that the IRB/IEC is constituted in agreement with GCP	X	X (where required)
8.2.9	Regulatory Authority(IES) Authorisation/Approval/ Notification of Protocol (where required)	To document appropriate authorisation/approval/notification by the regulatory authority(ies) has been obtained prior to initiation of the trial in compliance with the applicable regulatory requirement(s)	X (where required)	X (where required)
8.2.10	Curriculum Vitae and/or Other Relevant Documents Evidencing Qualifications of Investigator(s) and Sub-Investigator(s)	To document qualifications and eligibility to conduct trial and/or provide medical supervision of subjects	X	X
8.2.11	Normal Value(s)/Range(s) for Medical/ Laboratory/Technical Procedure(s) and/or Test(s) Included in the Protocol	To document normal values and/or ranges of the tests	X	X
8.2.12	Medical/Laboratory/Technical Procedures/Tests • Certification or • Accreditation or • Established Quality Control and/or External Quality Assessment or • Other Validation (where required)	To document competence of facility to perform required test(s), and support reliability of results	X (where required)	X
8.2.13	Sample of Label(s) Attached to Investigational Product Container(s)	To document compliance with applicable labelling regulations and appropriateness of instructions provided to the subjects		X
8.2.14	Instructions for Handling of Investigational Product(s) And Trial-Related Materials (if not included In Protocol or Investigator's Brochure)	To document instructions needed to ensure proper storage, packaging, dispensing and disposition of investigational products and trial-related materials	X	X
8.2.15	Shipping Records for Investigational Product(s) and Trial-Related Materials	To document shipment dates, batch numbers and method of shipment of investigational product(s) and trial-related materials. Allows tracking of product batch, review of shipping conditions, and accountability	X	X
8.2.16	Certificate(s) of Analysis of Investigational Product(s) Shipped	To document identity, purity, and strength of investigational product(s) to be used in the trial		X
8.2.17	Decoding Procedures for Blinded Trials	To document how, in case of an emergency, identity of blinded investigational product can be revealed without breaking the blind for the remaining subjects' treatment	X	X (third party if applicable)
8.2.18	Master Randomisation List	To document method for randomisation of trial population		X (third party if applicable)
8.2.19	Pre-Trial Monitoring Report	To document that the site is suitable for the trial (may be combined with 8.2.20)		X

(Continued on next page)

Appendix 6. International Conference on Harmonisation Guideline for Good Clinical Practice *(Continued)*

	Title of Document	Purpose	Located in Files of Investigator/ Institution	Sponsor
8.2.20	Trial Initiation Monitoring Report	To document that trial procedures were reviewed with the investigator and the investigator's trial staff (may be combined with 8.2.19)	X	X

8.3   During the Clinical Conduct of the Trial
In addition to having on file the above documents, the following should be added to the files during the trial as evidence that all new relevant information is documented as it becomes available.

	Title of Document	Purpose	Located in Files of Investigator/ Institution	Sponsor
8.3.1	Investigator's Brochure Updates	To document that investigator is informed in a timely manner of relevant information as it becomes available	X	X
8.3.2	Any revision to: • Protocol/Amendment(s) and CRF • Informed Consent Form • Any Other Written Information Provided to Subjects • Advertisement for Subject Recruitment (if used)	To document revisions of these trial related documents that take effect during trial	X	X

8.3.3	Dated, Documented Approval/Favourable Opinion of Institutional Review Board (IRB)/Independent Ethics Committee of the following:
	• Protocol Amendment(s)
	• Revision(s) of:
	  - Informed Consent Form
	  - Any Other Written Information to be Provided to the Subject
	  - Advertisement for Subject Recruitment (if used)
	• Any Other Documents Given Approval/ Favourable Opinion
	• Continuing Review of Trial (where required)
		To document that the amendment(s) and/or revision(s) have been subject to IRB/IEC review and were given approval/favourable opinion. To identify the version number and date of the document(s).	X	X

8.3.4	Regulatory Authority(ies) Authorisations/ approvals/Notifications where required for: • Protocol Amendment(s) and other documents	To document compliance with applicable regulatory requirements	X (where required)	X
8.3.5	Curriculum Vitae for New Investigator(s) and/or Sub-Investigator(s)	(see 8.2.10)	X	X
8.3.6	Updates to Normal Value(s)/Range(s) for Medical/Laboratory/Technical Procedure(s)/Test(s) included in the protocol	To document normal values and ranges that are revised during the trial (see 8.2.11)	X	X
8.3.7	Updates Of Medical/Laboratory/Technical Procedures/Tests • Certification or • Accreditation or • Established Quality Control and/or External Quality Assessment or • Other validation (where required)	To document that tests remain adequate throughout the trial period (see 8.2.12)	X (where required)	X

(Continued on next page)

Appendix 6. International Conference on Harmonisation Guideline for Good Clinical Practice *(Continued)*

	Title of Document	Purpose	Investigator/ Institution	Sponsor
			Located in Files of	
8.3.8	Documentation of Investigational Product(s) and Trial-Related Materials Shipment	(see 8.2.15.)	X	X
8.3.9	Certificate(s) of Analysis for New Batches of Investigational Products	(see 8.2.16)		X
8.3.10	Monitoring Visit Reports	To document site visits by, and findings of, the monitor		X
8.3.11	Relevant Communications Other Than Site Visits • Letters • Meeting notes • Notes of telephone calls	To document any agreements or significant discussions regarding trial administration, protocol violations, trial conduct, adverse event (AE) reporting	X	X
8.3.12	Signed Informed Consent Forms	To document that consent is obtained in accordance with GCP and protocol and dated prior to participation of each subject in trial. Also to document direct access permission (see 8.2.3)	X	
8.3.13	Source Documents	To document the existence of the subject and substantiate integrity of trial data collected. To include original documents related to the trial, to medical treatment, and history of subject	X	
8.3.14	Signed, dated and completed Case Report Forms (CRF)	To document that the investigator or authorised member of the investigator's staff confirms the observations recorded	X (copy)	X (original)
8.3.15	Documentation of CRF Corrections	To document all changes/additions or corrections made to CRF after initial data were recorded	X (copy)	X (original)
8.3.16	Notification By Originating Investigator to Sponsor of Serious Adverse Events and Related Reports	Notification by originating investigator to sponsor of serious adverse events and related reports in accordance with 4.11	X	X
8.3.17	Notification by Sponsor and/or Investigator, where applicable, to regulatory authority(ies) and IRB(s)/IEC(s) of Unexpected Serious Adverse Drug Reactions and of Other Safety Information	Notification by sponsor and/or investigator, where applicable, to regulatory authorities and IRB(s)/IEC(s) of unexpected serious adverse drug reactions in accordance with 5.17 and 4.11.1 and of other safety information in accordance with 5.16.2 and 4.11.2	X (where required)	X
8.3.18	Notification by Sponsor to Investigators of Safety Information	Notification by sponsor to investigators of safety information in accordance with 5.16.2	X	X
8.3.19	Interim or Annual Reports to IRB/IEC and Authority(ies)	Interim or annual reports provided to IRB/IEC in accordance with 4.10 and to authority(ies) in accordance with 5.17.3	X	X (where required)
8.3.20	Subject Screening Log	To document identification of subjects who entered pre-trial screening	X	X (where required)
8.3.21	Subject Identification Code List	To document that investigator/institution keeps a confidential list of names of all subjects allocated to trial numbers on enrolling in the trial. Allows investigator/institution to reveal identity of any subject	X	
8.3.22	Subject Enrollment Log	To document chronological enrollment of subjects by trial number	X	
8.3.23	Investigational Products Accountability at the Site	To document that investigational product(s) have been used according to the protocol	X	X
8.3.24	Signature Sheet	To document signatures and initials of all persons authorised to make entries and/or corrections on CRFs	X	X
8.3.25	Record of Retained Body Fluids/Tissue Samples (if any)	To document location and identification of retained samples if assays need to be repeated	X	X

(Continued on next page)

Appendix 6. International Conference on Harmonisation Guideline for Good Clinical Practice *(Continued)*

8.4   After Completion or Termination of the Trial
After completion or termination of the trial, all of the documents identified in sections 8.2 and 8.3 should be in the file together with the following

	Title of Document	Purpose	Located in Files of Investigator/ Institution	Sponsor
8.4.1	Investigational Product(s) Accountability at Site	To document that the investigational product(s) have been used according to the protocol. To document the final accounting of investigational product(s) received at the site, dispensed to subjects, returned by the subjects, and returned to sponsor	X	X
8.4.2	Documentation of Investigational Product Destruction	To document destruction of unused investigational products by sponsor or at site	X (if destroyed at site)	X
8.4.3	Completed Subject Identification Code List	To permit identification of all subjects enrolled in the trial in case follow-up is required. List should be kept in a confidential manner and for agreed upon time	X	
8.4.4	Audit Certificate (if available)	To document that audit was performed		X
8.4.5	Final Trial Close-out Monitoring Report	To document that all activities required for trial close-out are completed, and copies of essential documents are held in the appropriate files		X
8.4.6	Treatment Allocation and Decoding documentation	Returned to sponsor to document any decoding that may have occurred		X
8.4.7	Final Report by Investigator to IRB/IEC where required, and where applicable, to the regulatory authority(ies)	To document completion of the trial	X	
8.4.8	Clinical Study Report	To document results and interpretation of trial	X (if applicable)	X

Note. From *Guideline for Good Clinical Practice E6(R1),* by ICH Secretariat, International Conference on Harmonisation of Technical Requirements for Registration of Pharmaceuticals for Human Use, 1996. Retrieved December 13, 2007, from http://www.ich.org/cache/compo/475-272-1.html. The complete updated ICH texts are available free of charge from the ICH Web site: http://www.ich.org.

Appendix 7. Federalwide Assurance Terms

Version Date 1/6/2005
FEDERALWIDE ASSURANCE (FWA) FOR THE PROTECTION OF HUMAN SUBJECTS
U. S. Department of Health and Human Services (HHS)
Office for Human Research Protections (OHRP)

A. TERMS OF THE FEDERALWIDE ASSURANCE (FWA) FOR INSTITUTIONS WITHIN THE UNITED STATES

1. Human Subjects Research Must be Guided by Ethical Principles

All of the Institution's human subjects research activities, regardless of whether the research is subject to federal regulations, will be guided by the ethical principles in: (a) The Belmont Report: Ethical Principles and Guidelines for the Protection of Human Subjects of Research of the National Commission for the Protection of Human Subjects of Biomedical and Behavioral Research, or (b) other appropriate ethical standards recognized by federal departments and agencies that have adopted the Federal Policy for the Protection of Human Subjects, known as the Common Rule.

2. Applicability

These terms apply whenever the Institution becomes engaged in human subjects research conducted or supported* by any federal department or agency that has adopted the Common Rule, unless the research is otherwise exempt from the requirements of the Common Rule or a department or agency conducting or supporting the research determines that the research shall be conducted under a separate assurance. In general, the Institution becomes so engaged whenever (a) the Institution's employees or agents intervene or interact with human subjects for purposes of federally-conducted or -supported research; (b) the Institution's employees or agents obtain individually identifiable private information about human subjects for purposes of federally-conducted or -supported research; or (c) the Institution receives a direct federal award to conduct human subjects research, even where all activities involving human subjects are carried out by a subcontractor or collaborator.

[*Federally-supported is defined throughout the FWA and the Terms of Assurance as the U.S. Government providing any funding or other support.]

3. Compliance with the Federal Policy for the Protection of Human Subjects and Other Applicable Federal, State, Local, or Institutional Laws, Regulations, and Policies

When the Institution becomes engaged in federally-conducted or -supported human subjects research to which the FWA applies, the Institution and the institutional review boards (IRBs) designated under the Institution's Assurance will comply with the Federal Policy for the Protection of Human Subjects.

The reference in the Code of Federal Regulations is shown below for each department and agency which has adopted the Common Rule:

7 CFR part 1c	Department of Agriculture
10 CFR part 745	Department of Energy
14 CFR part1230	National Aeronautics and Space Administration
15 CFR part 27	Department of Commerce
16 CFR part 1028	Consumer Product Safety Commission
22 CFR part 225	Agency for International Development
24 CFR part 60	Department of Housing and Urban Development
28 CFR part 46	Department of Justice
32 CFR part 219	Department of Defense
34 CFR part 97	Department of Education
38 CFR part 16	Department of Veterans Affairs
40 CFR part 26	Environmental Protection Agency
45 CFR part 46	Department of Health and Human Services
45 CFR part 46	Central Intelligence Agency
(by Executive Order 12333)	
45 CFR part 690	National Science Foundation
49 CFR part 11	Department of Transportation

For any federally-conducted or -supported human subjects research to which the FWA applies, the Institution also will comply with any additional human subjects regulations and policies of the department or agency which conducts or supports the research and any other applicable federal, state, local, or institutional laws, regulations, and policies. When the Institution is engaged in human subjects research conducted or supported by the Department of Health and Human Services (HHS), the Institution will comply with all subparts of the HHS regulations at Title 45 Code of Federal Regulations part 46 (45 CFR part 46, subparts A, B, C, and D).

Human subjects research conducted or supported by each federal department or agency listed above will be governed by the regulations as implemented by the respective department or agency. The head of the department or agency retains final judgment as to whether a particular activity conducted or supported by the respective department or agency is covered by the Common Rule. If the Institution needs guidance regarding implementation of the Common Rule and other applicable federal regulations, the Institution should contact appropriate officials at the department or agency conducting or supporting the research. For federally-conducted or -supported research covered by the FWA, the department or agency that conducts or supports the research retains final authority for determining whether the Institution complies with the Terms of Assurance. If HHS receives an allegation or indication of noncompliance related to human subjects research that is covered by the FWA and is conducted or supported solely by a Common Rule department or agency other than HHS, HHS will refer the matter to the other department or agency for review and action as appropriate.

(Continued on next page)

Appendix 7. Federalwide Assurance Terms *(Continued)*

Please note that if the Institution voluntarily extends the Common Rule or the Common Rule and subparts B, C, and D of the HHS regulations at 45 CFR part 46 to all research regardless of support, OHRP will have the authority to ensure that the Institution complies with this commitment for all research to which the FWA applies that is not federally-conducted or -supported.

4. Written Procedures*

a) The Institution submitting the FWA has written procedures* for ensuring prompt reporting to the IRB, appropriate institutional officials, the head of any department or agency conducting or supporting the research (or designee), any applicable regulatory body, and OHRP of any:

1. unanticipated problems involving risks to subjects or others;
2. serious or continuing noncompliance with the federal regulations or the requirements or determinations of the IRB(s); and
3. suspension or termination of IRB approval.

Upon request, the Institution will provide a copy of these written procedures to OHRP and any department or agency conducting or supporting research covered by the FWA.

b) The Institution must ensure that the IRB(s) designated under the FWA has established written procedures* for:

1. conducting IRB initial and continuing review (not less than once per year) of research, and reporting IRB findings to the investigator and the Institution;
2. determining which projects require review more often than annually and which projects need verification from sources other than the investigator that no material changes have occurred since the previous IRB review; and
3. ensuring prompt reporting to the IRB of proposed changes in a research activity and for ensuring that such changes in approved research, during the period for which IRB approval has already been given, may not be initiated without IRB review and approval, except when necessary to eliminate apparent immediate hazards to the subjects.

Upon request, the Institution will provide a copy of these written procedures to OHRP and any department or agency conducting or supporting research covered by the FWA.

[*For HHS-conducted or -supported human subjects research, see OHRP guidance on written IRB procedures on the OHRP website at http://www.hhs.gov/ohrp/humansubjects/guidance/irbgd702.htm.]

5. Scope of IRB(s)'s Responsibilities

All human subjects research to which the FWA applies, except for research exempted or waived in accordance with Sections 101(b) or 101(i) of the Common Rule, will be reviewed, prospectively approved, and subject to continuing review at least annually by the designated IRB(s). The IRB(s) will have authority to approve, require modifications in, or disapprove the covered human subjects research. For research approved by the IRB(s), further appropriate review and approval by any department or agency conducting or supporting the research or by officials of the institution holding the FWA may be required.

6. Informed Consent Requirements

Except for research exempted or waived in accordance with Sections 101(b) or 101(i) of the Common Rule, informed consent for research to which the FWA applies will be:

a) sought from each prospective subject or the subject's legally authorized representative, in accordance with, and to the extent required by, Section 116 of the Common Rule; and

b) appropriately documented, in accordance with, and to the extent required by, Section 117 of the Common Rule.

7. Requirement for Assurances for Collaborating Institutions

When the Institution holding the FWA is either a) the primary awardee under a federal grant, contract, or cooperative agreement supporting research to which the FWA applies, or b) the coordinating center for federally-conducted or -supported research to which the FWA applies, the Institution is responsible for ensuring that all collaborating institutions engaged in such research operate under an appropriate OHRP-approved or other federally-approved assurance for the protection of human subjects.

An institution holding an FWA may collaborate with another institution that does not have an FWA. In such circumstances, a collaborating institution may operate under the FWA with the approval of the department or agency conducting or supporting the research and the institution holding the FWA.

For federally-conducted or -supported research covered by the FWA, the department or agency that conducts or supports the research retains final authority for determining which institutions are engaged in the research and need to hold an assurance for the protection of human subjects.

8. Written Agreements with Independent Investigators Who are not Otherwise Affiliated with the Institution

When the Institution holding the FWA is either a) the primary awardee under a federal grant, contract, or cooperative agreement supporting research to which the FWA applies, or b) the coordinating center for federally-conducted or -supported research to which the FWA applies, the Institution is responsible for ensuring that all collaborating independent investigators engaged in such research operate under an appropriate OHRP-approved or other federally-approved assurance for the protection of human subjects.

(Continued on next page)

Appendix 7. Federalwide Assurance Terms *(Continued)*

The engagement in federally-conducted or -supported human subjects research activities to which the FWA applies by each independent investigator who is not otherwise an employee or agent of the Institution may be covered under the FWA only in accordance with a formal, written agreement of commitment to relevant human subject protection policies and IRB review. OHRP's sample Individual Investigator Agreement (see http://www.hhs.gov/ohrp/humansubjects/assurance/unaflsup.rtf) may be used or adapted for this purpose, or the Institution may develop its own commitment agreement in coordination with the department or agency conducting or supporting the research. Institutions must maintain commitment agreements on file and provide copies upon request to OHRP and any department or agency conducting or supporting the research.

For federally-conducted or -supported research covered by the FWA, the department or agency that conducts or supports the research retains final authority for determining which independent investigators are engaged in the research and need to be covered by a written commitment agreement with the institution holding the FWA.

9. **Institutional Support for the IRB(s)**
   The Institution will ensure that each IRB designated under the FWA has meeting space and sufficient staff to support the IRB's review and recordkeeping duties.

10. **Compliance with the Terms of Assurance**
   The Institution accepts and will follow items 1–9 above and is responsible for ensuring that (a) the IRB(s) designated under the FWA agree to comply with these terms; and (b) the IRB(s) possess appropriate knowledge of the local research context for all research to which the FWA applies (please refer to the OHRP Guidance on IRB Knowledge of Local Research Context on the OHRP website at http://www.hhs.gov/ohrp/humansubjects/guidance/local.htm).

   Any designation under the FWA of the IRB of another institution or organization must be documented by a written agreement between the Institution holding the FWA and the IRB organization outlining their relationship and include a commitment that the designated IRB will adhere to the requirements of the FWA. OHRP's sample IRB Authorization Agreement may be used for such purpose, or the parties involved may develop their own agreement. This agreement should be kept on file at both institutions/organizations and made available upon request to OHRP and any department or agency conducting or supporting research covered by the FWA.

11. **Assurance Training**
   The OHRP Assurance Training Modules (see http://137.187.172.153/CBTs/Assurance/login.asp) describe the major responsibilities of the Institutional Signatory Official, the Human Protection Administrator (e.g., Human Subjects Administrator or Human Subjects Contact Person), and the IRB Chair(s) that must be fulfilled under the FWA. OHRP strongly recommends that the Institutional Signatory Official, the Human Protections Administrator, and the IRB Chair(s) personally complete the relevant OHRP Assurance Training Modules, or comparable training that includes the content of these modules, prior to submitting the FWA.

12. **Educational Training**
   OHRP strongly recommends that the Institution and the designated IRB(s) establish educational training and oversight mechanisms (appropriate to the nature and volume of its research) to ensure that research investigators, IRB members and staff, and other appropriate personnel maintain continuing knowledge of, and comply with, the following: relevant ethical principles; relevant federal regulations; written IRB procedures; OHRP guidance; other applicable guidance, state and local laws; and institutional policies for the protection of human subjects. Furthermore, OHRP recommends that a) IRB members and staff complete relevant educational training before reviewing human subjects research; and b) research investigators complete appropriate institutional educational training before conducting human subjects research.

13. **Renewal of Assurance**
   All information provided under the FWA must be renewed or updated at least every 36 months (3 years), even if no changes have occurred, in order to maintain an active FWA. Failure to update this information may result in restriction, suspension, or termination of the Institution's FWA for the protection of human subjects.

DOMESTIC INSTITUTIONS ACCEPTING THESE TERMS MAY PROCEED WITH THE ASSURANCE FILING PROCESS

B. **TERMS OF THE FEDERALWIDE ASSURANCE (FWA) FOR INTERNATIONAL (NON-U.S.) INSTITUTIONS**
   1. **Human Subjects Research Must Be Guided by Ethical Principles**
      All of the Institution's human subjects research activities, regardless of whether the research is subject to U.S. federal regulations, will be guided by one of the following statements of ethical principles: (a) The World Medical Association's Declaration of Helsinki (as adopted in 1996 or 2000); (b) The Belmont Report: Ethical Principles and Guidelines for the Protection of Human Subjects of Research of the U.S. National Commission for the Protection of Human Subjects of Biomedical and Behavioral Research; or (c) other appropriate international ethical standards recognized by U.S. federal departments and agencies that have adopted the U.S. Federal Policy for the Protection of Human Subjects, known as the Common Rule.

(Continued on next page)

Appendix 7. Federalwide Assurance Terms *(Continued)*

2. **Applicability**

   These terms apply whenever the Institution becomes engaged in human subjects research conducted or supported* by any U.S. department or agency that has adopted the Common Rule, unless the research is otherwise exempt from the requirements of the Common Rule or a U.S. federal department or agency conducting or supporting the research determines that the research shall be conducted under a separate assurance. In general, the Institution becomes so engaged whenever (a) the Institution's employees or agents intervene or interact with human subjects for purposes of U.S. federally-conducted or -supported research; (b) the Institution's employees or agents obtain individually identifiable private information about human subjects for purposes of U.S. federally-conducted or -supported research; or (c) the Institution receives a direct award to conduct U.S. federally-supported human subjects research, even where all activities involving human subjects are carried out by a subcontractor or collaborator.

   If a U.S. federal department or agency head determines that the procedures prescribed by the Institution afford protections that are at least equivalent to those provided by the U.S. Federal Policy for the Protection of Human Subjects, the department or agency head may approve the substitution of the foreign procedures in lieu of the procedural requirements provided above, consistent with the requirements of section 101(h) of the U.S. Federal Policy for the Protection of Human Subjects.
   [*Federally-supported is defined throughout the Assurance document and the Terms of Assurance as the U.S. Government providing any funding or other support.]

3. **Compliance with Laws, Regulations, Policies, and Guidelines**

   When the Institution becomes engaged in U.S. federally-conducted or -supported human subjects research to which the FWA applies, the Institution and institutional review boards (IRBs) or independent ethics committees (IECs) designated under the FWA at a minimum will comply with one or more of the following:
   a) The U.S. Federal Policy for the Protection of Human Subjects (see section 3 of the Terms of the FWA for Institutions within the United States for a list of U.S. federal departments and agencies that have adopted the Common Rule);
   b) The Common Rule and subparts B, C, and D of the U.S. Department of Health and Human Services (HHS) regulations at 45 CFR part 46;
   c) The U.S. Food and Drug Administration (FDA) regulations at 21 CFR parts 50 and 56;
   d) The May 1, 1996, International Conference on Harmonization E-6 Guidelines for Good Clinical Practice (ICH-GCP-E6), Sections 1 through 4;
   e) The 1993 Council for International Organizations of Medical Sciences (CIOMS) International Ethical Guidelines for Biomedical Research Involving Human Subjects;
   f) The 1998 Medical Research Council of Canada Tri-Council Policy Statement on Ethical Conduct for Research Involving Humans;
   g) The 2000 Indian Council of Medical Research Ethical Guidelines for Biomedical Research on Human Subjects; or
   h) Other standard(s) for the protection of human subjects recognized by U.S. federal departments and agencies which have adopted the U.S. Federal Policy for the Protection of Human Subjects.

   All U.S. federally-conducted or -supported human subjects research to which the FWA applies will also comply with any additional human subjects regulations and policies of the U.S. federal department or agency which conducts or supports the research and any other applicable U.S. federal, international, state, local, or institutional laws, regulations, and policies.

   The head of the U.S. federal department or agency retains final judgment as to whether a particular activity conducted or supported by the respective department or agency is covered by the Common Rule. If the Institution needs guidance regarding implementation of the Common Rule and/or other applicable U.S. federal regulations, the Institution should contact appropriate officials at the U.S. federal department or agency conducting or supporting the research. For U.S. federally-conducted or -supported research covered by the FWA, the U.S. federal department or agency that conducts or supports the research retains final authority for determining whether the Institution complies with the Terms of Assurance. If HHS receives an allegation or indication of noncompliance related to human subjects research that is covered by the FWA and is conducted or supported solely by a Common Rule department or agency other than HHS, HHS will refer the matter to the other U.S. federal department or agency for review and action as appropriate.

4. **IRB/IEC Written Procedures***
   a) The Institution submitting the FWA has established written procedures* for ensuring prompt reporting to the IRB/IEC, appropriate institutional officials, the head of any U.S. federal department or agency conducting or supporting the research (or designee), any applicable regulatory body, and OHRP of any:
      1. unanticipated problems involving risks to subjects or others;
      2. serious or continuing noncompliance with the applicable U.S. federal regulations or the requirements or determinations of the IRB(s)/IEC(s); and
      3. suspension or termination of IRB/IEC approval.
      Upon request, the Institution will provide a copy of these written procedures to OHRP and any department or agency conducting or supporting research covered by the FWA.
   b) The Institution must ensure that the IRB(s)/IEC(s) designated under the FWA has established written procedures* for:
      1. conducting IRB/IEC initial and continuing review (not less than once per year), of research, and reporting IRB/IEC findings to the investigator and the Institution;
      2. determining which projects require review more often than annually and which projects need verification from sources other than the investigator that no material changes have occurred since the previous IRB/IEC review; and
      3. ensuring prompt reporting to the IRB/IEC of proposed changes in a research activity, and for ensuring that such changes in approved research, during the period for which IRB/IEC approval has already been given, may not be initiated without IRB/IEC review and approval, except when necessary to eliminate apparent immediate hazards to the subjects.

(Continued on next page)

Appendix 7. Federalwide Assurance Terms *(Continued)*

Upon request, the Institution will provide a copy of these written procedures to OHRP and any department or agency conducting or supporting research covered by the FWA.

[*For HHS-conducted or -supported human subjects research, see OHRP guidance on written IRB procedures on the OHRP website at http://www.hhs.gov/ohrp/humansubjects/guidance/irbgd702.htm.]

5. **Scope of IRB(s)/IEC(s)'s Responsibilities**

   All U.S. federally-conducted or -supported research to which the FWA applies, except for research exempted or waived in accordance with sections 101(b) or 101(i) of the U.S. Common Rule, will be reviewed, prospectively approved, and subject to continuing review at least annually by the designated IRB(s)/IEC(s). The IRB(s)/IEC(s) shall have authority to approve, require modifications in, or disapprove the covered human subjects research. For research approved by the IRB(s)/IEC(s), further appropriate review and approval by any U.S. federal department or agency conducting or supporting the research or by officials of the institution holding the FWA may be required.

6. **Informed Consent Requirements**

   Except for research exempted or waived in accordance with Sections 101(b) or 101(i) of the U.S. Common Rule, informed consent for research to which the FWA applies will be:
   a) sought from each prospective subject or the subject's legally authorized representative, in accordance with, and to the extent required by, Section 116 of the U.S. Common Rule; and
   b) appropriately documented, in accordance with, and to the extent required by, Section 117 of the U.S. Common Rule.

7. **Considerations for Special Class of Subjects**

   For HHS-conducted or supported human subjects research, the Institution will comply with the HHS regulations at 45 CFR part 46, subparts B, C, and D, prior to the involvement of pregnant women, fetuses, or neonates; prisoners; or children, respectively. For non-HHS U.S. federally-supported human subjects research, the Institution will comply with any human subject regulations and/or policies of the supporting U.S. federal department or agency for these classes of subjects.

8. **Requirement for Assurances for Collaborating Institutions**

   When the Institution holding the FWA is either a) the primary awardee under a U.S. federal grant, contract, or cooperative agreement supporting research to which the FWA applies, or b) the coordinating center for U.S. federally-conducted or -supported research to which the FWA applies, the Institution is responsible for ensuring that all collaborating institutions engaged in such research operate under an appropriate OHRP-approved or other U.S. federally-approved assurance for the protection of human subjects.

   An institution holding an FWA may collaborate with another institution that does not have an FWA. In such circumstances, a collaborating institution may operate under the FWA with the approval of the U.S. federal department or agency conducting or supporting the research and the institution holding the FWA.

   For U.S. federally-conducted or -supported research covered by the FWA, the U.S. federal department or agency that conducts or supports the research retains final authority for determining which institutions are engaged in the research and need to hold an assurance for the protection of human subjects.

9. **Written Agreements with Independent Investigators Who are not Otherwise Affiliated with the Institution**

   When the Institution holding the FWA is either a) the primary awardee under a U.S. federal grant, contract, or cooperative agreement supporting research to which the FWA applies, or b) the coordinating center for U.S. federally-conducted or -supported research to which the FWA applies, the Institution is responsible for ensuring that all collaborating independent investigators engaged in such research operate under an appropriate OHRP-approved or other U.S. federally-approved assurance for the protection of human subjects.

   The engagement in U.S. federally-conducted or -supported human subjects research activities to which the FWA applies by each independent investigator who is not otherwise an employee or agent of the Institution may be covered under the FWA only in accordance with a formal, written agreement of commitment to relevant human subject protection policies and IRB/IEC review. OHRP's sample Individual Investigator Agreement (see http://www.hhs.gov/ohrp/humansubjects/assurance/unaflsup.rtf) may be used or adapted for this purpose, or the Institution may develop its own commitment agreement in coordination with the U.S. federal department or agency conducting or supporting the research. Institutions should maintain commitment agreements on file and provide copies upon request to OHRP or any U.S. federal department or agency conducting or supporting the research.

   For U.S. federally-conducted or -supported research covered by the FWA, the U.S. federal department or agency that conducts or supports the research retains final authority for determining which independent investigators are engaged in the research and need to be covered by a written commitment agreement with the institution holding the FWA.

10. **Institutional Support for the IRB(s)/IEC(s)**

    The Institution will ensure that each IRB(s)/IEC(s) designated under the FWA has meeting space and sufficient staff to support the IRB's/IEC's review and recordkeeping duties.

(Continued on next page)

Appendix 7. Federalwide Assurance Terms *(Continued)*

11. **Compliance with the Terms of Assurance**

The Institution accepts and will follow items 1–10 above and is responsible for ensuring that (a) the IRB(s)/IEC(s) designated under the FWA agree to comply with these terms, and (b) the IRB(s)/IEC(s) possess appropriate knowledge of the local research context for all research to which the FWA applies (please refer to the OHRP Guidance on IRB Knowledge of Local Research Context on the OHRP website at http://www.hhs.gov/ohrp/humansubjects/guidance/local.htm).

Any designation under the FWA of the IRB/IEC or another institution or organization should be documented by a written agreement between the Institution holding the FWA and the IRB/IEC organization outlining their relationship and include a commitment that the designated IRB/IEC will adhere to the requirements of the FWA. OHRP's sample IRB Authorization Agreement may be used for such purpose, or the parties involved may develop their own agreement. This agreement should be kept on file at both institutions/organizations and made available upon request to OHRP and any U.S. federal department or agency conducting or supporting research covered by the FWA.

12. **Assurance Training**

The OHRP Assurance Training Modules (see http://137.187.172.153/CBTs/Assurance/login.asp) describe the major responsibilities of the Institutional Signatory Official, the Human Protection Administrator (e.g., Human Subjects Administrator or Human Subjects Contact Person), and the IRB/IEC Chair(s) that must be fulfilled under the FWA. OHRP strongly recommends that the Institutional Signatory Official, the Human Protections Administrator, and the IRB/IEC Chair(s) personally complete the relevant OHRP Assurance Training Modules, or comparable training that includes the content of these Modules, prior to submitting the FWA.

13. **Educational Training**

OHRP strongly recommends that the Institution and the designated IRB(s)/IEC(s) establish educational training and oversight mechanisms (appropriate to the nature and volume of its research) to ensure that research investigators, IRB/IEC members and staff, and other appropriate personnel maintain continuing knowledge of, and comply with the following: relevant ethical principles; relevant U.S. regulations; written IRB/IEC procedures; OHRP guidance; other applicable guidance; national, state and local laws; and institutional policies for the protection of human subjects. Furthermore, OHRP recommends that a) IRB/IEC members and staff complete relevant educational training before reviewing human subjects research; and b) research investigators complete appropriate institutional educational training before conducting human subjects research.

14. **Renewal of Assurance**

All information provided under the FWA should be renewed or updated every 36 months (3 years), even if no changes have occurred, in order to maintain an active FWA. Failure to update this information may result in restriction, suspension, or termination of the Institution's FWA for the protection of human subjects.

Appendix 8. Federalwide Assurance Template

OMB No. 0990-0278
Approved for use through 01/31/2008

Federalwide Assurance (FWA) for the Protection of Human Subjects for Institutions Within the United States

[ ] New Filing   [ ] Update or Renewal for FWA Number:_____

1. **Institution Filing Assurance**
   Legal Name:

   City: State:

   HHS Institution Profile File (IPF) code, if known:

   Federal Entity Identification Number (EIN), if known:

   If this Assurance replaces an MPA or CPA, please provide the "M" or "T" number:

2. **Institutional Components**
   List below all components over which the Institution has legal authority <u>that operate under a different name</u>. Also list with an asterisk (*) any <u>alternate names</u> under which the Institution operates. The Institution should have available for review by the Office for Human Research Protections (OHRP) upon request a brief description and line diagram explaining the interrelationships among the Assurance Signatory Official, the Institutional Review Board(s) (IRB), IRB support staff, and investigators in these various components.

   NOTE: The Signatory Official signing this Assurance must be legally authorized to represent the Institution providing this Assurance and all components listed below. Entities that the Signatory Official is not legally authorized to represent may <u>not</u> be listed here without the prior approval of OHRP.

   [ ] Please check here if there are no such components or alternate names.

Name of Component or Alternate Names Used	City	State (or Country if Outside U.S.)

3. **Statement of Principles**
   This Institution assures that all of its activities related to human subjects research, regardless of the source of support, will be guided by the ethical principles in the following document(s): (*indicate below*)

   [ ] *The Belmont Report*

   [ ] *Other:* (*Please submit copy to OHRP with this Assurance*)

4. **Applicability**
   (a) This Institution assures that whenever it engages in human subjects research conducted or supported by any federal department or agency that has adopted the Federal Policy for the Protection of Human Subjects, known as the Common Rule, the Institution will comply with the **Terms of the Federalwide Assurance for Institutions Within the United States (contained in a separate document on the OHRP website)**, unless the research is otherwise exempt from the requirements of the Common Rule or a department or agency conducting or supporting the research has determined that the research shall be covered by a separate assurance.
   (b) *Optional:* This Institution elects to apply the following to all of its human subjects research regardless of the source of support, except for research that is covered by a separate assurance:

   [ ] *The Common Rule (see section 3 of the Terms of the FWA for Institutions Within the United States for a list of departments and agencies that have adopted the Common Rule and the applicable citations to the Code of Federal Regulations)*

   [ ] *The Common Rule and subparts B, C, and D of the HHS regulations at 45 CFR part 46*

5. **Designation of Institutional Review Boards (IRBs)**
   This Institution designates the following IRB(s) for review of research under this Assurance (*if the IRB has not previously registered with HHS or has not provided a membership roster to HHS, please submit to OHRP the appropriate IRB registration materials which are available on the OHRP website*).

(Continued on next page)

Appendix 8. Federalwide Assurance Template *(Continued)*

NOTE: Reliance on the IRB of another institution or organization or an independent IRB must be documented by a written agreement that is available for review by OHRP upon request. OHRP's sample IRB Authorization Agreement may be used for this purpose, or the parties involved may develop their own agreement. Future designation of other IRBs requires an update of the FWA.

HHS IRB Registration Number	Name of IRB as Registered with HHS

6. **Human Protections Administrator (e.g., Human Subjects Administrator or Human Subjects Contact Person)**
    First Name: Middle Initial: Last Name:

    Degrees or Suffix: Institutional Title:

    Institution:

    Telephone: FAX: E-Mail:

    Address:

    City: State: Zip Code:

7. **Signatory Official (i.e., Official Legally Authorized to Represent the Institution -- Cannot be IRB Chairperson or IRB Member)**
    I understand that the Assurance Training Modules on the OHRP website describe the responsibilities of the Signatory Official, the IRB Chair(s), and the Human Protections Administrator under this Assurance. Additionally, I recognize that providing research investigators, IRB members and staff, and other relevant personnel with appropriate initial and continuing education about human subject protections will help ensure that the requirements of this Assurance are satisfied.

    Acting officially in an authorized capacity on behalf of this Institution and with an understanding of the Institution's responsibilities under this Assurance, I assure protections for human subjects as specified above. The IRB(s) designated above are to provide review for all research to which this Assurance applies. The designated IRB(s) will comply with the Terms of the Federalwide Assurance for Institutions Within the United States and possess appropriate knowledge of the local context in which this Institution's research will be conducted.

    All information provided with this Assurance is up-to-date and accurate. *I am aware that false statements could be cause for invalidating this Assurance and may lead to other administrative or legal action.*

    Signature _____ Date: _____
    First Name: Middle Initial: Last Name:
    Degrees or Suffix: Institutional Title:
    Institution:
    Telephone: FAX: E-Mail:
    Address:
    City: State: Zip Code:

    NOTE: Institutions operated by the U.S. Government may need to obtain department or agency clearance prior to submission of the FWA to OHRP. Please contact the relevant department or agency Human Subject Protections Officer before forwarding this Assurance to OHRP.

8. **FWA Approval**
    The Federalwide Assurance for the Protection of Human Subjects for Institutions Within the United States submitted to HHS by the above Institution is hereby approved.

    Assurance Number: Expiration Date:

    Signature of HHS Approving Official: _____ Date: _____

    Public burden for this collection of information is estimated to average two hours for a new FWA filing and less than an hour for an FWA renewal or update. An agency may not conduct or sponsor, and a person is not required to respond to, a collection of information unless it displays a currently valid OMB control number. Send comments regarding this burden estimate or any other aspect of this collection of information, including suggestions for reducing this burden to: OS Reports Clearance Officer, Room 503, 200 Independence Avenue, SW., Washington, DC 20201. *Do not return the completed form to this address.*

Appendix 9. Individual Investigator Agreement

Sample Commitment Statement of an Individual Investigator to Institutional Human Subject Protection Policies and IRB/IEC Oversight (institutions may use this text or develop their own agreement)

Individual Investigator Agreement

Name of Institution with the Federalwide Assurance (FWA): _____

Applicable FWA #: _____

Individual Investigator's Name: _____

Specify Research Covered by this Agreement: _____

(1) The above-named Individual Investigator has reviewed: 1) The Belmont Report: Ethical Principles and Guidelines for the Protection of Human Subjects of Research (or other internationally recognized equivalent; see section B.1. of the Terms of the Federalwide Assurance (FWA) for International (Non-U.S.) Institutions); 2) the U.S. Department of Health and Human Services (HHS) regulations for the protection of human subjects at 45 CFR part 46 (or other procedural standards; see section B.3. of the Terms of the FWA for International (Non-U.S.) Institutions); 3) the FWA and applicable Terms of the FWA for the institution referenced above; and 4) the relevant institutional policies and procedures for the protection of human subjects.

(2) The Investigator understands and hereby accepts the responsibility to comply with the standards and requirements stipulated in the above documents and to protect the rights and welfare of human subjects involved in research conducted under this Agreement.

(3) The Investigator will comply with all other applicable federal, international, state, and local laws, regulations, and policies that may provide additional protection for human subjects participating in research conducted under this agreement.

(4) The Investigator will abide by all determinations of the Institutional Review Board (IRB)/Independent Ethics Committee (IEC) designated under the above FWA and will accept the final authority and decisions of the IRB/IEC, including but not limited to directives to terminate participation in designated research activities.

(5) The Investigator will complete any educational training required by the Institution and/or the IRB/IEC prior to initiating research covered under this Agreement.

(6) The Investigator will report promptly to the IRB/IEC any proposed changes in the research conducted under this Agreement. The investigator will not initiate changes in the research without prior IRB/IEC review and approval, except where necessary to eliminate apparent immediate hazards to subjects.

(7) The Investigator will report immediately to the IRB/IEC any unanticipated problems involving risks to subjects or others in research covered under this Agreement.

(8) The Investigator, when responsible for enrolling subjects, will obtain, document, and maintain records of informed consent for each such subject or each subject's legally authorized representative as required under HHS regulations at 45 CFR part 46 (or any other international or national procedural standards selected on the FWA for the institution referenced above) and stipulated by the IRB/IEC.

(9) The Investigator acknowledges and agrees to cooperate in the IRB/IEC's responsibility for initial and continuing review, record keeping, reporting, and certification for the research referenced above. The Investigator will provide all information requested by the IRB/IEC in a timely fashion.

(10) The Investigator will not enroll subjects in research under this Agreement prior to its review and approval by the IRB/IEC.

(11) Emergency medical care may be delivered without IRB/IEC review and approval to the extent permitted under applicable federal regulations and state law.

(12) This Agreement does not preclude the Investigator from taking part in research not covered by this Agreement.

(13) The Investigator acknowledges that he/she is primarily responsible for safeguarding the rights and welfare of each research subject, and that the subject's rights and welfare must take precedence over the goals and requirements of the research.

Investigator Signature: _____ Date _____

Name: _____ Degree(s): _____
      (Last)   *(First)*   *(Middle Initial)*

Address: _____ Phone #: _____

_____
      (City)   *(State/Province)*   *(Zip/Country)*

FWA Institutional Official (or Designee): _____ Date _____

Name: _____ Institution Title: _____
      (Last)   *(First)*   *(Middle Initial)*

Address: _____ Phone #: _____

_____
      (City)   *(State/Province)*   *(Zip/Country)*

Appendix 10. Informed Consent Document Template

Informed Consent Template for Cancer Treatment Trials
(English Language)

*NOTES FOR INFORMED CONSENT AUTHORS:

- Model text suggested for use in the informed consent form is in **bold**. It is recommended that the **bold** text be retained when adapting the template to a specific protocol.
- Instructions and examples for informed consent authors are in *[italics]*.
- A blank line, _____, indicates that the local investigator should provide the appropriate information before the document is reviewed with the prospective research participant.
- The term 'study doctor' has been used throughout the template because the Principal Investigator of a cancer treatment trial is a physician. If this template is used for a trial where the Principal Investigator is not a physician, another appropriate term should be used instead of 'study doctor'.
- The template date in the header is for reference to this template only and should not be included in the informed consent form given to the prospective research participant.

*NOTES FOR LOCAL INVESTIGATORS:

- The goal of the informed consent process is to provide people with sufficient information for making informed choices. The informed consent form provides a summary of the clinical study and the individual's rights as a research participant. It serves as a starting point for the necessary exchange of information between the investigator and potential research participant. This template for the informed consent form is only one part of the larger process of informed consent. For more information about informed consent, review the "Recommendations for the Development of Informed Consent Documents for Cancer Clinical Trials" prepared by the Comprehensive Working Group on Informed Consent in Cancer Clinical Trials for the National Cancer Institute. The Web site address for this document is http://www.cancer.gov/clinicaltrials/understanding/simplification-of-informed-consent-docs/
- A blank line, _____, indicates that the local investigator should provide the appropriate information before the document is reviewed with the prospective research participant.
- Suggestion for Local Investigators: An NCI pamphlet explaining clinical trials is available for your patients. The pamphlet is entitled: "If You Have Cancer…What You Should Know about Clinical Trials". This pamphlet may be ordered on the NCI Web site at https://cissecure.nci.nih.gov/ncipubs/ or call 1-800-4-CANCER (1-800-422-6237) to request a free copy.
- Optional feature for Local Investigators: Reference and attach drug sheets, pharmaceutical information for the public, or other material on risks. Check with your local IRB regarding review of additional materials.

*These notes for authors and investigators are instructional and should not be included in the informed consent form given to the prospective research participant.

Study Title

This is a clinical trial, a type of research study. Your study doctor will explain the clinical trial to you. Clinical trials include only people who choose to take part. Please take your time to make your decision about taking part. You may discuss your decision with your friends and family. You can also discuss it with your health care team. If you have any questions, you can ask your study doctor for more explanation.

You are being asked to take part in this study because you have *[Type/stage/presentation of cancer being studied is briefly described here. For example: "Colon cancer that has spread and has not responded to one treatment".]*

Why is this study being done?

The purpose of this study is to…. *[Limit explanation to why study is being done. Explain in 1-2 sentences. Some examples are provided.]*

[Example: Phase 1 study]

Test the safety of [drug/intervention] at different dose levels. We want to find out what effects, good and/or bad, it has on you and your [specify type/stage/presentation of] cancer.

[Example: Phase 2 study]

Find out what effects, good and/or bad, [drug/intervention] has on you and your [specify type/stage/presentation of] cancer.

(Continued on next page)

Appendix 10. Informed Consent Document Template *(Continued)*

[Example: Phase 3 study]

Compare the effects, good and/or bad, of [drug/intervention] with [commonly-used drug/intervention] on you and your [specify type/stage/presentation of] cancer to find out which is better. In this study, you will get either the [drug/intervention] or the [commonly-used drug/intervention]. You will not get both.

How many people will take part in the study?

About *[state total accrual goal here]* **people will take part in this study.** *[If appropriate, a short description about cohorts can be given here. For example: "At the beginning of the study, (enter number of first cohort) patients will be treated with a low dose of the drug. If this dose does not cause bad side effects, it will slowly be made higher as new patients take part in the study. A total of (enter maximum number) patients are the most that would be able to enter the study".]*

What will happen if I take part in this research study?

- *[List tests and procedures and their frequency under the categories below. Include whether a patient will be at home, in the hospital, or in an outpatient setting.]*

Before you begin the study ...

You will need to have the following exams, tests or procedures to find out if you can be in the study. These exams, tests or procedures are part of regular cancer care and may be done even if you do not join the study. If you have had some of them recently, they may not need to be repeated. This will be up to your study doctor.

- *[List tests and procedures as appropriate. Use bulleted format.]*

During the study ...

If the exams, tests and procedures show that you can be in the study, and you choose to take part, then you will need the following tests and procedures. They are part of regular cancer care.

- *[List tests and procedures as appropriate. Use bulleted format.]*

You will need these tests and procedures that are part of regular cancer care. They are being done more often because you are in this study.

- *[List tests and procedures as appropriate. Use bulleted format. Omit this section if no tests or procedures are being done more often than usual.]*

You will need these tests and procedures that are either being tested in this study or being done to see how the study is affecting your body.

- *[List tests and procedures as appropriate. Use bulleted format. Omit this section if no tests or procedures are being tested in this study or required for safety monitoring.]*

[For randomized studies:]   **You will be "randomized" into one of the study groups described below. Randomization means that you are put into a group by chance. A computer program will place you in one of the study groups. Neither you nor your doctor can choose the group you will be in. You will have an** *[equal/one in three/etc.]* **chance of being placed in any group.**

> **If you are in group 1 (often called "Arm A") ...** *[Explain what will happen for this group with clear indication of which interventions depart from routine care.]*

> **If you are in group 2 (often called "Arm B")...** *[Explain what will happen for this group with clear indication of which interventions depart from routine care.]*

> *[For studies with more than two groups, an explanatory paragraph containing the same type of information should be included for each group.]*

(Continued on next page)

Appendix 10. Informed Consent Document Template *(Continued)*

When I am finished taking *[drugs or intervention]...[Explain the follow-up tests, procedures, exams, etc. required, including the timing of each and whether they are part of standard cancer care or part of standard care but being performed more often than usual or being tested in this study. Define the length of follow-up.]*

[Optional Feature: In addition to the mandatory narrative explanation found in the preceding text, a simplified calendar (study chart) or schema (study plan) may be inserted here. The schema from the protocol should not be used as it is too complex, however a simplified version of the schema is encouraged. Instructions for reading the calendar or schema should be included. See examples.]

Study Chart *[Example]*

You will receive *[drug(s) or intervention]* **every** *[insert appropriate number of days or weeks]* **in this study. This** *[insert appropriate number of days or weeks]* **period of time is called a cycle. The cycle will be repeated** *[insert appropriate number]* **times. Each cycle is numbered in order. The chart below shows what will happen to you during Cycle 1 and future treatment cycles as explained previously. The left-hand column shows the day in the cycle and the right-hand column tells you what to do on that day.**

Cycle 1	
Day	**What you do**
Two days before starting study	• Get routine blood tests.
Day before starting study	• Check-in to _____ the evening before starting study.
Day 1	• Begin taking _____ once a day. Keep taking _____ until the end of study, unless told to stop by your health care team.
Day 2	• Leave _____ and go to where you are staying.
Day 8	• Get routine blood tests.
Day 15	• Get routine blood tests.
Day 22	• Get routine blood tests.
Day 28	• Get routine blood tests and exams. • Get 2nd chest x-ray for research purposes.
Day 29	• Return to your doctor's office at _____ *[insert appointment time]* for your next exam and to begin the next cycle.

Future cycles	
Day	**What you do**
Days 1-28	• Keep taking _____ once a day if you have no bad side effects and cancer is not getting worse. Call the doctor at _____ *[insert phone number]* if you do not know what to do. • Get routine blood tests each week (more if your doctor tells you to). • Get routine blood tests and exams every cycle (more if your doctor tells you to). • Get routine X-rays, CT scans, or MRIs every other cycle (more if your doctor tells you to).
Day 29	• Return to your doctor's office at _____ *[insert appointment time]* for your next exam and to begin the next cycle.

(Continued on next page)

Appendix 10. Informed Consent Document Template *(Continued)*

Study Plan *[Example]*

Another way to find out what will happen to you during the study is to read the chart below. Start reading at the top and read down the list, following the lines and arrows.

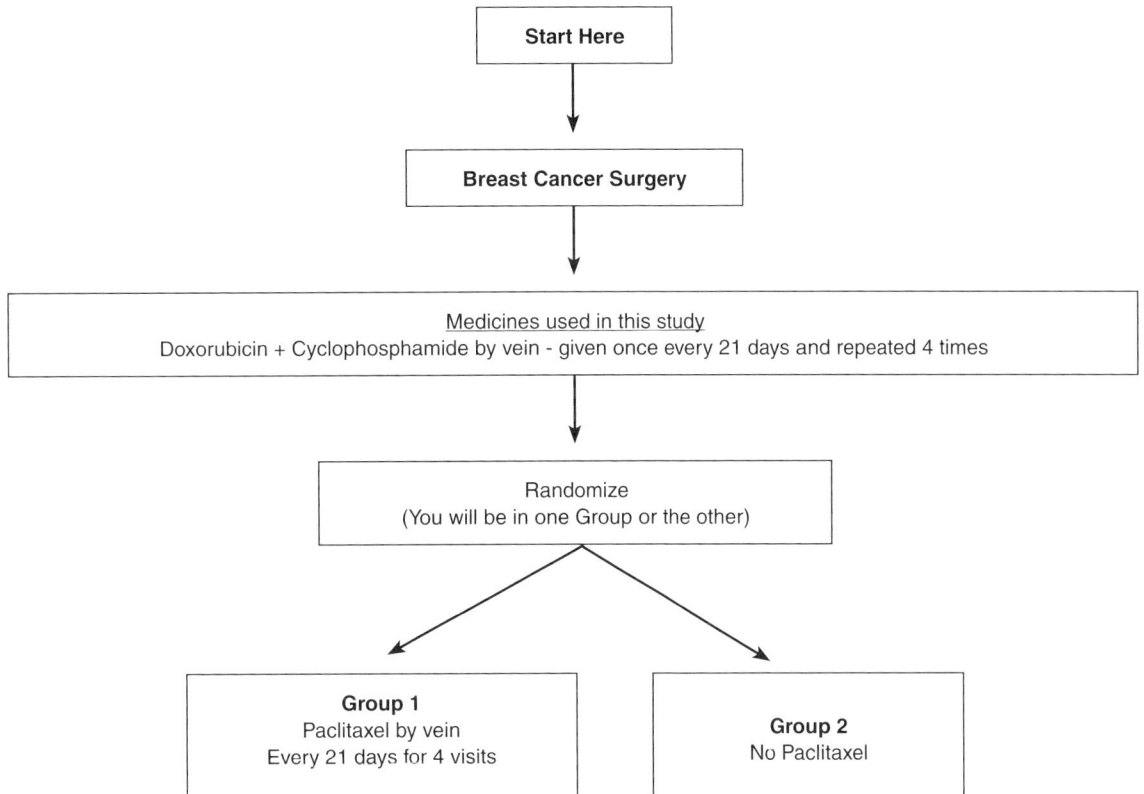

How long will I be in the study?

You will be asked to take *[drugs or intervention]* **for** *(months, weeks/until a certain event).* **After you are finished taking** *[drugs or intervention],* **the study doctor will ask you to visit the office for follow-up exams for at least** *[indicate time frames and requirements of follow-up. When appropriate, state that the study will involve long-term follow-up and specify time frames and requirements of long-term follow-up. For example, "We would like to keep track of your medical condition for the rest of your life. We would like to do this by calling you on the telephone once a year to see how you are doing. Keeping in touch with you and checking on your condition every year helps us look at the long-term effects of the study."]*

Can I stop being in the study?

Yes. You can decide to stop at any time. Tell the study doctor if you are thinking about stopping or decide to stop. He or she will tell you how to stop safely.

It is important to tell the study doctor if you are thinking about stopping so any risks from the *[drugs or intervention]* **can be evaluated by your doctor. Another reason to tell your doctor that you are thinking about stopping is to discuss what followup care and testing could be most helpful for you.**

The study doctor may stop you from taking part in this study at any time if he/she believes it is in your best interest; if you do not follow the study rules; or if the study is stopped.

(Continued on next page)

Appendix 10. Informed Consent Document Template *(Continued)*

What side effects or risks can I expect from being in the study?

You may have side effects while on the study. Everyone taking part in the study will be watched carefully for any side effects. However, doctors don't know all the side effects that may happen. Side effects may be mild or very serious. Your health care team may give you medicines to help lessen side effects. Many side effects go away soon after you stop taking the *[drug(s) or intervention]*. In some cases, side effects can be serious, long lasting, or may never go away. *[The next sentence should be included if appropriate. There also is a risk of death.]*

You should talk to your study doctor about any side effects that you have while taking part in the study.

Risks and side effects related to the *[procedures, drugs, interventions, devices]* include those which are:

<u>Likely</u>

•
•
•
•

<u>Less Likely</u>

•
•
•
•

<u>Rare but serious</u>

•
•
•
•

[Notes for consent form authors regarding the presentation of risks and side effects:

• *Using a bulleted format, list risks and side effects related to the investigational aspects of the trial. Side effects of supportive medications should not be listed unless they are mandated by the study.*

• *List by regimen the physical and nonphysical risks and side effects of participating in the study in three categories: 1. "likely"; 2. "less likely"; 3. "rare but serious".*

• *There is no standard definition of "likely" and "less likely". As a guideline, "likely" can be viewed as occurring in greater than 20% of patients and "less likely" in less than or equal to 20% of patients. However, this categorization should be adapted to specific study agents by the principal investigator.*

• *In the "likely" and "less likely" categories, identify those side effects that may be 'serious'. 'Serious' is defined as side effects that may require hospitalization or may be irreversible, long-term, life threatening or fatal.*

• *Side effects that occur in less than 2-3% of patients do not have to be listed unless they are serious, and should then appear in the "rare but serious" category.*

• *Physical and nonphysical risks and side effects should include such things as the inability to work. Whenever possible, describe side effects by how they make a patient feel, for example, "Loss of red blood cells, also called anemia, can cause tiredness, weakness and shortness of breath."*

• *For some investigational drugs/interventions/devices there may be side effects that have been noted during treatment however not enough data is available to determine if the side effect is related to the drug/intervention/device. Because some local IRBs request to be informed of these possible side effects, this information, when available, is provided to the study chair. Inclusion of this information in the informed consent document is not mandatory. However, if included, these side effects should be listed under a separate category titled "Side effects reported by patients, but not proven to be caused by (drug/intervention/device)". Side effects in this category do not have to be labeled as "likely", "less likely" or "rare but serious" and should not be repeated here if they appear in a previous category. Similar to the other categories, these side effects should be listed in a bulleted format.]*

(Continued on next page)

Appendix 10. Informed Consent Document Template *(Continued)*

Reproductive risks: You should not become pregnant or father a baby while on this study because the drugs in this study can affect an unborn baby. Women should not breastfeed a baby while on this study. It is important you understand that you need to use birth control while on this study. Check with your study doctor about what kind of birth control methods to use and how long to use them. Some methods might not be approved for use in this study. *[Include a statement about possible sterility when appropriate. For example, "Some of the drugs used in the study may make you unable to have children in the future." If appropriate include a statement that pregnancy testing may be required.]*

For more information about risks and side effects, ask your study doctor.

Are there benefits to taking part in the study?

Taking part in this study may or may not make your health better. While doctors hope *[procedures, drugs, interventions, devices]* will be more useful against cancer compared to the usual treatment, there is no proof of this yet. We do know that the information from this study will help doctors learn more about *[procedures, drugs, interventions, devices]* as a treatment for cancer. This information could help future cancer patients.

What other choices do I have if I do not take part in this study?

Your other choices may include:

- Getting treatment or care for your cancer without being in a study
- Taking part in another study
- Getting no treatment

[Additional bullets should include, when appropriate, alternative specific procedures or treatments.]

- *[For studies involving end-stage cancer, add the following paragraph as an additional bullet.]* **Getting comfort care, also called palliative care. This type of care helps reduce pain, tiredness, appetite problems and other problems caused by the cancer. It does not treat the cancer directly, but instead tries to improve how you feel. Comfort care tries to keep you as active and comfortable as possible.**

Talk to your doctor about your choices before you decide if you will take part in this study.

Will my medical information be kept private?

We will do our best to make sure that the personal information in your medical record will be kept private. However, we cannot guarantee total privacy. Your personal information may be given out if required by law. If information from this study is published or presented at scientific meetings, your name and other personal information will not be used.

Organizations that may look at and/or copy your medical records for research, quality assurance, and data analysis include:

- *[List relevant organizations like study sponsor(s), pharmaceutical company collaborators, local IRB, etc.]*
- **The National Cancer Institute (NCI) and other government agencies, like the Food and Drug Administration (FDA), involved in keeping research safe for people**

[Note to Local Investigators: The NCI has recommended that HIPAA regulations be addressed by the local institution. The regulations may or may not be included in the informed consent form depending on local institutional policy.]

What are the costs of taking part in this study?

You and/or your health plan/insurance company will need to pay for some or all of the costs of treating your cancer in this study. Some health plans will not pay these costs for people taking part in studies. Check with your health plan or insurance company to find out what they will pay for. Taking part in this study may or may not cost your insurance company more than the cost of getting regular cancer treatment.

(Continued on next page)

Appendix 10. Informed Consent Document Template *(Continued)*

[If applicable, inform the patient of any tests, procedures or agents for which there is no charge. The explanation, when applicable, should clearly state that there are charges resulting from performance of the test or drug administration that will be billed to the patient and/or health plan. For example, "The NCI (if not the NCI, state other study sponsor here) is supplying (drug) at no cost to you. However, you or your health plan may need to pay for costs of the supplies and personnel who give you the (drug)."]

[Include the following sentence if appropriate:]

The study agent, *[study drug]*, will be provided free of charge while you are participating in this study. However, if you should need to take the study agent much longer than is usual, it is possible that the supply of free study agent that has been supplied to *[the NCI or other study sponsor, as appropriate]* could run out. If this happens, your study doctor will discuss with you how to obtain additional drug from the manufacturer and you may be asked to pay for it.

You will not be paid for taking part in this study.

For more information on clinical trials and insurance coverage, you can visit the National Cancer Institute's Web site at http://www.cancer.gov/clinicaltrials/understanding/insurance-coverage. You can print a copy of the "Clinical Trials and Insurance Coverage" information from this Web site.

Another way to get the information is to call 1-800-4-CANCER (1-800-422-6237) and ask them to send you a free copy.

What happens if I am injured because I took part in this study?

It is important that you tell your study doctor, _____ *[investigator's name(s)]*, if you feel that you have been injured because of taking part in this study. You can tell the doctor in person or call him/her at _____ *[telephone number]*.

You will get medical treatment if you are injured as a result of taking part in this study. You and/or your health plan will be charged for this treatment. The study will not pay for medical treatment.

What are my rights if I take part in this study?

Taking part in this study is your choice. You may choose either to take part or not to take part in the study. If you decide to take part in this study, you may leave the study at any time. No matter what decision you make, there will be no penalty to you and you will not lose any of your regular benefits. Leaving the study will not affect your medical care. You can still get your medical care from our institution.

We will tell you about new information or changes in the study that may affect your health or your willingness to continue in the study.

In the case of injury resulting from this study, you do not lose any of your legal rights to seek payment by signing this form.

Who can answer my questions about the study?

You can talk to your study doctor about any questions or concerns you have about this study. Contact your study doctor _____ _____ *[name(s)]* at _____ *[telephone number]*.

(Continued on next page)

Appendix 10. Informed Consent Document Template *(Continued)*

For questions about your rights while taking part in this study, call the _____ *[name of center]* **Institutional Review Board (a group of people who review the research to protect your rights) at _____** *(telephone number).* *[Note to Local Investigator: Contact information for patient representatives or other individuals in a local institution who are not on the IRB or research team but take calls regarding clinical trial questions can be listed here.]*

*You may also call the Operations Office of the NCI Central Institutional Review Board (CIRB) at 888-657-3711 (from the continental US only). *[*Only applies to sites using the CIRB.]*

Please note: This section of the informed consent form is about additional research studies that are being done with people who are taking part in the main study. You may take part in these additional studies if you want to. You can still be a part of the main study even if you say 'no' to taking part in any of these additional studies.

You can say "yes" or "no" to each of the following studies. Please mark your choice for each study.

[Insert information about companion studies here. Provide yes/no options at each decision point. The following studies are included as examples therefore are written with italicized font. Any text provided for patients should use the same non-italicized font as used for the rest of the informed consent document.]

[Example: Quality of Life study]

Quality of Life Study

We want to know your view of how your life has been affected by cancer and its treatment. This "Quality of life" study looks at how you are feeling physically and emotionally during your cancer treatment. It also looks at how you are able to carry out your day-to-day activities.

This information will help doctors better understand how patients feel during treatments and what effects the medicines are having. In the future, this information may help patients and doctors as they decide which medicines to use to treat cancer.

You will be asked to complete 3 questionnaires: one on your first visit, one 6 months later, and the last one 12 months after your first visit. It takes about 15 minutes to fill out each questionnaire.

If any questions make you feel uncomfortable, you may skip those questions and not give an answer.

If you decide to take part in this study, the only thing you will be asked to do is fill out the three questionnaires. You may change your mind about completing the questionnaires at any time.

Just like in the main study, we will do our best to make sure that your personal information will be kept private.

Please circle your answer.

I choose to take part in the Quality of Life Study. I agree to fill out the three Quality of Life Questionnaires.

YES   NO

(Continued on next page)

Appendix 10. Informed Consent Document Template *(Continued)*

[Example: Use of Tissue for Research]

[The following example of tissue consent has been taken from the NCI Cancer Diagnosis Program's model tissue consent form found at the following URL http://www.cancerdiagnosis.nci.nih.gov/specimens/model.pdf]

Consent Form for Use of Tissue for Research

About Using Tissue for Research

You are going to have a biopsy (or surgery) to see if you have cancer. Your doctor will remove some body tissue to do some tests. The results of these tests will be given to you by your doctor and will be used to plan your care.

We would like to keep some of the tissue that is left over for future research. If you agree, this tissue will be kept and may be used in research to learn more about cancer and other diseases. Please read the information sheet called "How is Tissue Used for Research" to learn more about tissue research.

Your tissue may be helpful for research whether you do or do not have cancer. The research that may be done with your tissue is not designed specifically to help you. It might help people who have cancer and other diseases in the future.

Reports about research done with your tissue will not be given to you or your doctor. These reports will not be put in your health record. The research will not have an effect on your care.

Things to Think About

The choice to let us keep the left over tissue for future research is up to you. No matter what you decide to do, it will not affect your care.

If you decide now that your tissue can be kept for research, you can change your mind at any time. Just contact us and let us know that you do not want us to use your tissue. Then any tissue that remains will no longer be used for research.

In the future, people who do research may need to know more about your health. While the xyz may give them reports about your health, it will not give them your name, address, phone number, or any other information that will let the researchers know who you are.

Sometimes tissue is used for genetic research (about diseases that are passed on in families). Even if your tissue is used for this kind of research, the results will not be put in your health records.

Your tissue will be used only for research and will not be sold. The research done with your tissue may help to develop new products in the future.

Benefits

The benefits of research using tissue include learning more about what causes cancer and other diseases, how to prevent them, and how to treat them.

Risks

The greatest risk to you is the release of information from your health records. We will do our best to make sure that your personal information will be kept private. The chance that this information will be given to someone else is very small.

Making Your Choice

Please read each sentence below and think about your choice. After reading each sentence, circle "Yes" or "No". If you have any questions, please talk to your doctor or nurse, or call our research review board at IRB's phone number.

No matter what you decide to do, it will not affect your care.

1. My tissue may be kept for use in research to learn about, prevent, or treat cancer.

☐ *YES*   ☐ *NO*

2. My tissue may be kept for use in research to learn about, prevent or treat other health problems (for example: diabetes, Alzheimer's disease, or heart disease).

☐ *YES*   ☐ *NO*

3. Someone may contact me in the future to ask me to take part in more research.

☐ *YES*   ☐ *NO*

(Continued on next page)

Appendix 10. Informed Consent Document Template *(Continued)*

Where can I get more information?

You may call the National Cancer Institute's Cancer Information Service at:

1-800-4-CANCER (1-800-422-6237) or TTY: 1-800-332-8615

You may also visit the NCI Web site at http://www.cancer.gov/

- For NCI's clinical trials information, go to: http://www.cancer.gov/clinicaltrials/
- For NCI's general information about cancer, go to http://www.cancer.gov/cancertopics/

You will get a copy of this form.   If you want more information about this study, ask your study doctor.

Signature_____

I have been given a copy of all _____ *[insert total of number of pages]* **pages of this form. I have read it or it has been read to me. I understand the information and have had my questions answered. I agree to take part in this study.**

Participant _____

Date _____

Appendix 11. National Cancer Institute Return Agent Form

NIH-986 (REV. 2/97)

National Institutes of Health
National Cancer Institute

Division of Cancer Treatment and Diagnosis
Cancer Therapy Evaluation Program

Return Drug List

Return only agents supplied by the
National Cancer Institute

The agents listed below were ordered by (one investigator per form only):

Dr.

Address: (Including Institution)

NCI Investigator No.:

☐ Check here if returned receipt should be mailed to the above address, OR fill in a fax number below

	NSC Number	Agent Name	NCI Protocol Number	Strength, Unit, & Dose (Specify vials, capsules, or tablets)	Lot Number (or Patient ID for Blinded Trial)	Manufacturer	Quantity (Specify whole or partial containers)	Container Number	Action
1									
	Reason for return:	☐ Agent expired	☐ All patient(s) off treatment.	☐ Protocol complete	☐ Other:				
2									
	Reason for return:	☐ Agent expired	☐ All patient(s) off treatment.	☐ Protocol complete	☐ Other:				
3									
	Reason for return:	☐ Agent expired	☐ All patient(s) off treatment.	☐ Protocol complete	☐ Other:				
4									
	Reason for return:	☐ Agent expired	☐ All patient(s) off treatment.	☐ Protocol complete	☐ Other:				
5									
	Reason for return:	☐ Agent expired	☐ All patient(s) off treatment.	☐ Protocol complete	☐ Other:				
6									
	Reason for return:	☐ Agent expired	☐ All patient(s) off treatment.	☐ Protocol complete	☐ Other:				

FOR NCI USE ONLY

Return. No.:

Signature of Authorizing Official:

Date of Authorization:

Date Received:

RETURN RECEIPT: To obtain a return receipt by fax, provide your number in the space below.

INSTRUCTIONS:

1. Properly complete all sections to receive credit for the return.
2. Type all information–one item, lot, or protocol per line.
3. DO NOT mark in shaded areas.
4. Investigator signature or signature of individual preparing this form:
5. Pack the agent(s) well to minimize breakage and leakage.
6. All agents may be returned via room temperature
7. Enclose the completed list with the agent(s) and return to:

✂

NCI Clinical Repository
627 Lofstrand Lane
Rockville, MD 20850
Attn: Returns

Signature / Printed Name _____ Date _____

Title _____

Phone No. _____

06/06

Appendix 12. National Cancer Institute Transfer Investigational Agent Form

06/06

Cancer Therapy Evaluation Program
Division of Cancer Treatment and Diagnosis
National Cancer Institute
National Institutes of Health

Transfer Investigational Agent Form

This form is to be used for an intra-institutional transfer, one transfer/form.

TRANSFER FROM:

Investigator transferring agent:
Dr.

NCI Investigator Number:

Date of transfer:

Name of Institution:

Street Address:

City:

State:

Zip Code:

Reason for transfer request: ☐ Protocol closed/complete ☐ Unused agent obtained for Special Exception ☐ Agent has short dating ☐ Other**

(**Requires verbal clarification with PMB before approval)

TRANSFER TO:

Investigator receiving agent:
Dr.

NCI Investigator Number:

The following PMB-supplied agent for NCI-approved protocol is being transferred to NCI-approved protocol:

Received on NCI Protocol Number	Transferred to NCI Protocol Number	NSC Number	Agent Name	Strength and Formulation	Quantity	Manufacturer and Lot Number

Authorized Signature (Investigator or Designee)

Printed Name

Telephone Number   _Fax Number_

Email Address

See http://ctep.cancer.gov/requisition/agents.html for further information.

All requested information MUST be supplied for form to be valid.

Return form to:
Pharmaceutical Management Branch
Cancer Therapy Evaluation Program
Division of Cancer Treatment and Diagnosis, NCI, NIH
Executive Plaza North, Room 7149
Bethesda, MD 20892

FAX: 301-402-0429

Appendix 13. Internet Resource List

Introduction

Many of the resources listed in this appendix are identified in previous chapters of this manual. These Web-based resources, as well as many others, have been compiled to facilitate their use (the addresses are current as of the time of this printing). Because the Internet is a dynamic entity, new resources frequently are being added, while others are being deleted or moved to different Internet addresses. Additionally, many of these Web sites are accessible through the Oncology Nursing Society's (ONS's) Web site, www.ons.org, where the links continually are verified and updated as needed.

U.S. GOVERNMENT RESOURCES

Providing a search function is one of the requirements for a federal Web site, as outlined in *OMB Policy 3: Establish and Enforce Agency-Wide Linking Policies* by the Web Content Managers Advisory Council (www.usa.gov/webcontent/reqs_bestpractices/omb_policies/linking.shtml). A search engine helps the public to find government information and services available at a Web site.

U.S. Department of Health and Human Services (DHHS) Reference Collections www.hhs.gov/reference/index.html	DHHS is the U.S. government's principal agency for protecting the health of all Americans and providing essential human services, especially for those who are least able to help themselves. The department includes more than 300 programs, covering a broad range of activities. The Reference Collections Web page provides links to dictionaries, glossaries, electronic databases, encyclopedias, publications, reports, statistical data, and more.
MedlinePlus www.nlm.nih.gov/medlineplus	MedlinePlus directs visitors to information to help answer health questions. MedlinePlus brings together, by health topic, authoritative information from the National Library of Medicine, the National Institutes of Health (NIH), and other government, nonprofit, and other health-related organizations. Preformulated MEDLINE® searches are included in MedlinePlus which provides easy access to the medical research literature, along with a database of full-text drug information and an illustrated medical encyclopedia.
National Institutes of Health (NIH) www.nih.gov NIH and Clinical Research http://clinicalresearch.nih.gov	NIH, which is part of DHHS, is the primary federal agency for conducting and supporting medical research. Composed of 27 institutes and centers, NIH provides leadership and financial support to researchers in every state and throughout the world.
National Cancer Institute (NCI) www.cancer.gov	NCI is a component of the NIH. NCI coordinates the National Cancer Program, which conducts and supports research, training, health information dissemination, and other programs with respect to the cause, diagnosis, prevention, and treatment of cancer. NCI provides a vast amount of cancer-related information online. An index of Web sites for major NCI units, programs, and projects is available at www.cancer.gov/aboutnci/ncisites.
• NCI Dictionary of Cancer Terms www.cancer.gov/dictionary	This NCI site contains definitions for more than 4,000 terms related to cancer and medicine.
• NCI Drug Dictionary www.cancer.gov/drugdictionary	The NCI Drug Dictionary contains technical definitions and synonyms for drugs and agents used to treat patients with cancer or conditions related to cancer.
U.S. Food and Drug Administration (FDA) www.fda.gov	The FDA is a federal agency within the DHHS that regulates and evaluates products for human and animal use that are applied to or taken into the body.
• FDA Database Search www.fda.gov/search/databases.html	The FDA provides a directory of its databases, which can be accessed separately using the links on this page. Following each link is a brief description of the database.
Office for Human Research Protections (OHRP) www.hhs.gov/ohrp	OHRP provides leadership to the nation's system for protecting volunteers in research that is conducted or supported by the DHHS. OHRP provides clarification and guidance to research institutions and develops educational programs and materials. Nearly 10,000 universities, hospitals, and other research institutions in the United States and abroad have formal agreements (assurances) with OHRP to comply with the regulations pertaining to human subject protections.

CLINICAL TRIAL DATABASES

ClinicalTrials.gov www.clinicaltrials.gov	ClinicalTrials.gov provides regularly updated information about federally and privately supported clinical research in human volunteers. NIH, through the NLM, developed this site in collaboration with the FDA. ClinicalTrials.gov contains more than 41,000 clinical studies sponsored by the NIH, other federal agencies, and private industry.
MetaRegister of Controlled Trials (*m*RCT) www.controlled-trials.com/mrct	The *m*RCT is an international searchable database of ongoing randomized controlled trials in all areas of health care, built by combining registers held by public, nonprofit, and commercial sponsors of trials.

(Continued on next page)

Appendix 13. Internet Resource List *(Continued)*	
Pharmaceutical Research and Manufacturers of America (PhRMA) Clinical Study Results Database www.clinicalstudyresults.org	The PhRMA sponsors this online database for clinical study results in a reader-friendly, standardized format. The site was created to improve accessibility to and transparency of the results of clinical studies.
Thomson CenterWatch Clinical Trials Listing Service™ www.centerwatch.com	Thomson CenterWatch's service provides in-depth information about clinical research, including listings of active industry- and government-sponsored clinical trials.
World Health Organization International Clinical Trials Registry Platform (ICTRP) www.who.int/ictrp	ICTRP enables users to search a central database that contains the trial registration data sets provided by primary registers.
MAILING LISTS	
CataList www.lsoft.com/lists/listref.html	*CataList* is the catalog of Listserv® lists. From this page, visitors can browse more than 53,000 public Listserv lists on the Internet, search for mailing lists of interest, and get information about Listserv host sites.
FDA E-Mail Lists www.fda.gov/emaillist.html	Users can subscribe to any number of the FDA's free e-mail lists on myriad topics, such as consumer health information, drugs, diseases and conditions, guidance documents, regulations, and research.
NIH Listserv https://list.nih.gov	From the NIH Listserv home page, visitors can browse through all of the available NIH mailings lists.
JOURNALS	
BioMed Central www.biomedcentral.com	BioMed Central is an independent publisher that provides 184 open-access, peer-reviewed journals online.
Applied Clinical Trials www.actmagazine.com	*Applied Clinical Trials* is a global, peer-reviewed journal about clinical trial management. The journal annually compiles a directory of education and training opportunities for clinical research professionals.
Journal of Clinical Research Best Practices www.firstclinical.whsites.net/journal	The *Journal of Clinical Research Best Practices* is a forum for sharing material of practical use in clinical research. This journal is a refuge for material that is too controversial, time sensitive, or nontraditional for other publications.
PROFESSIONAL MEMBERSHIP ORGANIZATIONS	
The number of professional organizations solely or partially dedicated to clinical research continues to increase. Several organizations are listed and described here to reflect the variety of membership opportunities. In addition, an online directory of more than 150 clinical research associations is available at www.firstclinical.whsites.net/directories.	
American Society of Clinical Oncology (ASCO) www.asco.org	ASCO, founded in 1964, is a nonprofit organization with goals of improving cancer care and prevention and ensuring that all patients with cancer receive the highest quality care. The organization has more than 25,000 members representing all oncology disciplines and sub-specialties. ASCO is committed to advancing oncology education for healthcare professionals, advocating for policies to provide access to high-quality cancer care, and supporting clinical trials and the need for increased clinical and translational research.
Association of Clinical Research Professionals (ACRP) www.acrpnet.org	ACRP is an international association of more than 20,000 individuals dedicated to clinical research and development. ACRP is a resource for clinical research professionals in the pharmaceutical, biotechnology, and medical device industries, as well as those in hospitals, academic medical centers, and physician office settings.
Drug Information Association (DIA) www.diahome.org	DIA is a nonprofit scientific association with a membership of more than 20,000. These members primarily are from the international pharmaceutical industry, regulatory agencies, and academia. DIA provides educational programs and publications to its members on issues regarding pharmaceuticals and related products.

(Continued on next page)

Appendix 13. Internet Resource List *(Continued)*	
Oncology Nursing Society (ONS) www.ons.org	ONS is a national organization of more than 35,000 RNs and other healthcare professionals dedicated to excellence in patient care, teaching, research, administration, and education in the field of oncology. ONS recognizes the value of subspecialty practice and the unique needs of nurses who provide specialized care. The Society offers members the opportunity to join any of 30 special interest groups (SIGs), including the Clinical Trial Nurses SIG.
Regulatory Affairs Professionals Society (RAPS) www.raps.org	RAPS is a worldwide member organization devoted to the health product regulatory profession and has more than 11,000 individual members from industry, government, research, clinical, and academic organizations in more than 50 countries. RAPS develops professional standards for knowledge, competency, and ethics.
Society for Clinical Data Management (SCDM) www.scdm.org	SCDM is a nonprofit professional society founded to advance the discipline of clinical data management. The interest of all SCDM members is quality clinical data management practices. The society offers certification and publishes a quarterly newsletter.
Society for Clinical Trials (SCT) www.sctweb.org	SCT is an international professional organization dedicated to the development and dissemination of knowledge about the design and conduct of clinical trials and related healthcare research methodologies.
Society of Clinical Research Associates (SoCRA) www.socra.org	SoCRA is a nonprofit professional organization dedicated to the advancement and continuing education of clinical research professionals. The society offers certification and publishes a journal, *SoCRA Source*.
Society of Quality Assurance (SQA) www.sqa.org	SQA is a professional membership organization dedicated to providing a forum for information exchange and utilization of knowledge in research and regulatory quality assurance, enhancing knowledge of regulatory and quality assurance concerns that affect research, and fostering the recognition of the quality assurance profession worldwide.
OTHER ORGANIZATIONS	
Association of Clinical Research Organizations (ACRO) www.acrohealth.org	ACRO represents clinical research organizations worldwide. ACRO's members provide specialized services that are integral to the development of drugs, biologics, and medical devices. ACRO advances clinical outsourcing to improve the quality, efficiency, and safety of biomedical research.
International Federation of Pharmaceutical Manufacturers and Associations (IFPMA) www.ifpma.org	IFPMA is a nonprofit, nongovernmental organization representing national industry associations and companies from both developed and developing countries. Member companies of the IFPMA are research-based pharmaceutical, biotech, and vaccine companies.
Pharmaceutical Research and Manufacturers of America (PhRMA) www.phrma.org	PhRMA represents pharmaceutical research and biotechnology companies. The organization conducts effective advocacy for public policies that encourage discovery of important new medicines for patients by pharmaceutical and biotechnology research companies.
International Conference on Harmonisation of Technical Requirements for Registration of Pharmaceuticals for Human Use www.ich.org	The ICH brings together the regulatory authorities of Europe, Japan, and the United States and experts from the pharmaceutical industry in the three regions to discuss scientific and technical aspects of product registration.
Summary New Web-based resources will continue to become available. These resources provide clinical trial nurses with easily accessible information. Today, nurses' abilities to access and skillfully use digital information are critical to the integrity of clinical trials and the safety and well-being of their patients.	
Note. Created by Heidi E. Deininger, PhD, RN, AOCN®.	

Index

Index

The letter f after a page number indicates that relevant content appears in a figure; the letter t, in a table.

B

C

D

O

P

T

U

V

W